Hydrogel for Sustained Delivery of Therapeutic Agents (2nd Edition)

Hydrogel for Sustained Delivery of Therapeutic Agents (2nd Edition)

Guest Editors

Adina Magdalena Musuc
Magdalena Mititelu
Mariana Chelu

MDPI

Basel • Beijing • Wuhan • Barcelona • Belgrade • Novi Sad • Cluj • Manchester

Guest Editors

Adina Magdalena Musuc
Chemical Kinetics
"Ilie Murgulescu" Institute of Physical Chemistry of Romanian Academy
Bucharest
Romania

Magdalena Mititelu
Clinical Laboratory and Food Safety of Faculty of Pharmacy
"Carol Davila" University of Medicine and Pharmacy
Bucharest
Romania

Mariana Chelu
Surface Chemistry and Catalysis
"Ilie Murgulescu" Institute of Physical Chemistry of Romanian Academy
Bucharest
Romania

Editorial Office

MDPI AG
Grosspeteranlage 5
4052 Basel, Switzerland

This is a reprint of the Special Issue, published open access by the journal *Gels* (ISSN 2310-2861), freely accessible at: https://www.mdpi.com/journal/gels/special_issues/81EVVPVPDH.

For citation purposes, cite each article independently as indicated on the article page online and as indicated below:

Lastname, A.A.; Lastname, B.B. Article Title. *Journal Name* **Year**, *Volume Number*, Page Range.

ISBN 978-3-7258-7607-5 (Hbk)
ISBN 978-3-7258-7608-2 (PDF)
https://doi.org/10.3390/books978-3-7258-7608-2

Contents

About the Editors

Adina Magdalena Musuc

Adina Magdalena Musuc is a Senior Researcher and Head of the Chemical Kinetics Department at the Institute of Physical Chemistry "Ilie Murgulescu" of the Romanian Academy, Bucharest, with over 25 years of experience. She holds a B.Sc., M.Sc., Ph.D., and habilitation in chemistry from the University of Bucharest. She has received the "Gheorghe Spacu" Medal (2018 and 2024) and the "Nicolae Teclu" Award (2014). She has published more than 100 ISI papers, holds three patents, and is Vice President of the Romanian Society of Chemistry. Her research interests include physical chemistry, green chemistry, biopolymers, nanomaterials, drug delivery, and environmental applications.

Magdalena Mititelu

Magdalena Mititelu is affiliated with the Faculty of Pharmacy, University of Medicine and Pharmacy Carol Davila, Bucharest. She holds degrees in pharmacy, economics, and physical chemistry and is a senior pharmacist, nutrition consultant, and dietitian. She has published more than 250 articles, holds 11 patents, and has won four medals at international invention exhibitions. She is the author of 13 specialized books. Her expertise includes innovative therapeutic formulas, marine biotechnology, toxicological analysis, and clinical nutrition.

Mariana Chelu

Mariana Chelu is a Scientific Researcher at the Institute of Physical Chemistry "Ilie Murgulescu" of the Romanian Academy, where she earned her Ph.D. in 2021. Her research focuses on green chemistry, sol–gel processes, nanostructured materials, hydrogels, drug delivery systems, and advanced polymer composites for biomedical and environmental applications.

gels

MDPI

Review

Development and Applications of PLGA Hydrogels for Sustained Delivery of Therapeutic Agents

Anita Ioana Visan and Irina Negut *

National Institute for Lasers, Plasma and Radiation Physics, 409 Atomistilor Street, 077125 Magurele, Romania; anita.visan@inflpr.ro
* Correspondence: negut.irina@inflpr.ro

Abstract: Poly(lactic-co-glycolic acid) (PLGA) hydrogels are highly utilized in biomedical research due to their biocompatibility, biodegradability, and other versatile properties. This review comprehensively explores their synthesis, properties, sustained release mechanisms, and applications in drug delivery. The introduction underscores the significance of PLGA hydrogels in addressing challenges like short half-lives and systemic toxicity in conventional drug formulations. Synthesis methods, including emulsion solvent evaporation, solvent casting, electrospinning, thermal gelation, and photopolymerization, are described in detail and their role in tailoring hydrogel properties for specific applications is highlighted. Sustained release mechanisms—such as diffusion-controlled, degradation-controlled, swelling-controlled, and combined systems—are analyzed alongside key kinetic models (zero-order, first-order, Higuchi, and Peppas models) for designing controlled drug delivery systems. Applications of PLGA hydrogels in drug delivery are discussed, highlighting their effectiveness in localized and sustained chemotherapy for cancer, as well as in the delivery of antibiotics and antimicrobials to combat infections. Challenges and future prospects in PLGA hydrogel research are discussed, with a focus on improving drug loading efficiency, improving release control mechanisms, and promoting clinical translation. In summary, PLGA hydrogels provide a promising platform for the sustained delivery of therapeutic agents and meet diverse biomedical requirements. Future advancements in materials science and biomedical engineering are anticipated to further optimize their efficacy and applicability in clinical settings. This review consolidates the current understanding and outlines future research directions for PLGA hydrogels, emphasizing their potential to revolutionize therapeutic delivery and improve patient outcomes.

Keywords: poly(lactic-co-glycolic acid) (PLGA); hydrogels; sustained delivery; therapeutic agents

1. Introduction

With the exponential growth of scientific knowledge, the field of poly(l-lactide-co-glycolide) (PLGA) hydrogels has witnessed remarkable progress. This study aims to explore details of the synthesis techniques employed in creating PLGA hydrogels, highlighting factors that govern the formation process. Furthermore, it meticulously examines the special properties exhibited by these hydrogels, considering their biodegradability, biocompatibility, and tunable mechanical characteristics. The applications of PLGA hydrogels in the biomedical domain are truly remarkable. Their versatility and ability to encapsulate and deliver therapeutic agents have garnered significant attention. By expanding the horizons of drug delivery systems, tissue engineering, regenerative medicine, and wound healing, PLGA hydrogels exhibit immense promise. Continuous research in this field furthers our understanding and fosters the development of innovative strategies, pushing the boundaries of medical technology. Therefore, this detailed extended review serves as an invaluable resource for researchers, scientists, and medical practitioners, providing comprehensive insights into the advancements, potential challenges, and exciting prospects of PLGA hydrogels in the field of biomedical applications [1]. Over the years, hydrogels have continued to evolve, as no single material can meet the growing technological demand. Various synthesis techniques have been developed to design smart hydrogels suitable for diverse applications, enabling the fabrication and modification of the structural, mechanical, and sensitive properties of these outstanding materials. Smart hydrogels are fascinating materials between elastomers and gels that are characterized by their ability to swell and shrink in response to environmental stimuli such as pH, temperature, light, ions, enzymes, electric or magnetic fields, and biomolecules. This property has led to a growing interest in using hydrogels for various applications in the fields of drug delivery release, wound healing, tissue engineering, and regenerative medicine. At the same time, synthetic advances have created a new generation of hydrogels, ensuring the applicability of smart, responsive materials in the most complex physiological environments, inspired by nature's small building units [2–5].

Figure 1 illustrates the various external stimuli—such as pH, temperature, electricity, magnetics, light, and biomolecules (including glucose and enzymes)—that can control drug release from a smart hydrogel, highlighting their potential biomedical applications.

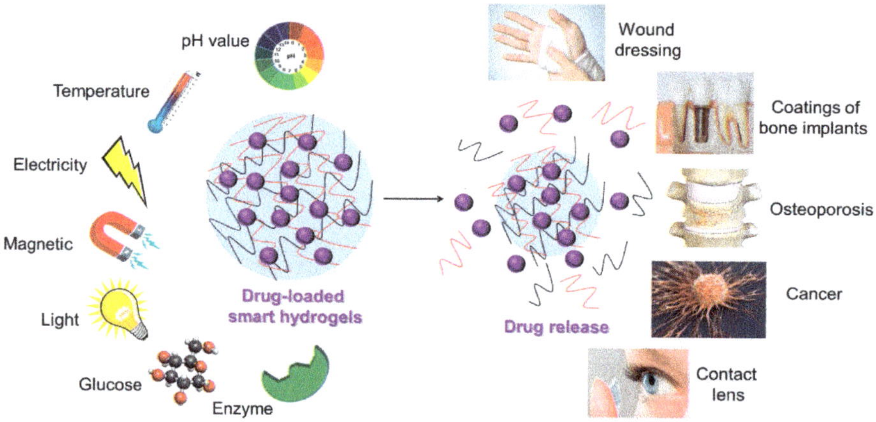

Figure 1. Illustration of various external stimuli, including pH, temperature, electricity, magnetics, light, and biomolecules (including glucose and enzymes), which are controlling the drug release from a smart hydrogel, and their biomedical applications [6].

The topic of composite hydrogels for sustained release of therapeutic agents has been extensively reviewed in the literature. For instance, Liu, Nakamura, and Lowman (2003) conducted a comprehensive review identifying the potential of composite hydrogels in providing controlled and sustained release of therapeutic agents, highlighting their ability to enhance drug stability and bioavailability [7]. Similarly, Liu et al. (2023) explored the application and development of hydrogel biomaterials for the treatment of intervertebral disc degeneration, concluding that hydrogels can effectively mimic the natural extracellular matrix, providing mechanical support and promoting tissue regeneration [8].

Despite these valuable contributions, there remain significant gaps, particularly in the areas of long-term controlled release and the development of hydrogels with enhanced mechanical properties. For instance, Cisneros et al. (2021) discussed the long-term controlled release of simvastatin from photoprinted triple-networked hydrogels, composed of modified chitosan and PLA–PEG micelles, yet there is still a need for further research into the scalability and clinical applicability of these systems [9]. Additionally, Alsaab et al. (2022) reviewed the advancements in PLGA-based nanomedicine, underscoring the importance of developing nanocomposite hydrogels for improved therapeutic efficacy and targeting [10].

These gaps are crucial because they highlight the need for more robust and versatile hydrogel systems that can be tailored to specific therapeutic needs. Therefore, by building on the foundational work of previous reviews, this review seeks to advance the application of hydrogel biomaterials in drug delivery, ultimately contributing to the identification of more effective therapeutic strategies.

The need to review the development and application of PLGA hydrogels for the sustained delivery of therapeutic agents arises from the growing importance of this biodegradable polymer in the field of drug delivery systems. PLGA hydrogels provide a versatile and efficient platform for the controlled release of a variety of therapeutic agents, including small molecules, proteins, and nucleic acids. Their biocompatibility, adjustable degradation rates, and ability to encapsulate different types of drugs make them ideal for various medical applications. This review not only summarizes the latest advances and innovations in PLGA hydrogel formulations but also highlights their clinical implications and addresses the current challenges and future directions. This provides researchers and healthcare professionals with a valuable resource to advance further research and development and ultimately improve patient outcomes through more effective and targeted therapies.

Definition and Composition of PLGA Hydrogels

PLGA is a biodegradable and biocompatible polymer widely used in biomedical applications, particularly in drug delivery systems, tissue engineering, and regenerative medicine. The hydrogel form of PLGA combines the advantageous properties of hydrogels—such as its high water content and tunable mechanical properties—with the favorable characteristics of PLGA, including its degradability and versatility in drug release profiles [11].

PLGA is a copolymer of lactic acid and glycolic acid. When combined, they form a hydrogel that can absorb and retain water. The ratio of lactic acid to glycolic acid affects the hydrogel's properties and degradation rate. Common ratios are 50:50, 75:25, or 25:75, each suitable for different applications [12].

PLGA's structural formula comprises repeating units of lactic acid and glycolic acid, which degrade into biocompatible and metabolizable by-products.

The general structural formula of PLGA (Figure 2) can be written as follows:

$$\text{-[O-CH(CH}_3\text{)-CO]}_m\text{-[O-CH}_2\text{-CO]}_n\text{–} \quad (1)$$

where

- m represents the number of lactic acid units.
- n represents the number of glycolic acid units.

The ratio of m to n can vary depending on the specific type of PLGA used. For example, PLGA with a 50:50 ratio of lactic acid to glycolic acid would have equal numbers of m and n. The structure can be visualized as alternating chains of the lactic acid and glycolic acid units. The ratio of these units determines the polymer's physical and chemical properties, such as its degradation rate and mechanical strength [13].

To form a hydrogel, PLGA polymers are crosslinked, which can be achieved through various chemical or physical methods.

Chemical crosslinking involves covalent bonding, often using agents such as glutaraldehyde, carbodiimides, or photoinitiators that activate under UV light [14].

Physical crosslinking can involve processes such as ionic interactions or crystallization. As a hydrogel, PLGA networks incorporate water into their structure, significantly influencing their mechanical properties and biological interactions [15]. The water content allows the hydrogel to swell, providing a moist environment conducive to cellular activities and facilitating the controlled release of therapeutic agents. To enhance the functionality of PLGA hydrogels, various additives can be included. These may include bioactive molecules like growth factors or drugs, nanoparticles for targeted delivery, or other polymers to modify mechanical properties or degradation rates [16]. Fillers such as hydroxyapatite or bioactive glass can be added to improve bioactivity, especially for bone tissue engineering applications [17].

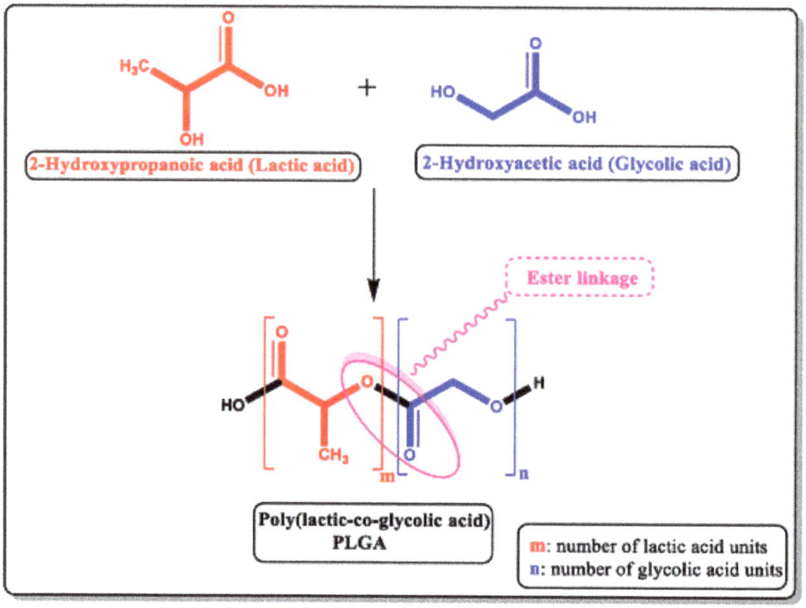

Figure 2. The structural formula of PLGA [10].

SEM micrographs play a pivotal role in the development and characterization of PLGA-based biomedical applications. They provide critical insights into the morphology, size, and surface properties of PLGA particles which are essential for optimizing their performance in drug delivery systems and tissue engineering scaffolds. The detailed visualization afforded by SEM ensures that PLGA-based systems are designed with the precision necessary for effective clinical outcomes. A study by Silvestri et al. [18] explored the effects of surface hydrophilicity on PLGA–poloxamer nanoparticles in an in vivo animal model. SEM micrographs revealed significant details about the surface texture and porosity of the PLGA hydrogels. Hydrogels with varying degrees of hydrophilicity were synthesized, and SEM imaging demonstrated how these variations impacted the surface morphology. Hydrogels with higher hydrophilicity showed more porous structures, which can facilitate better cell infiltration and nutrient diffusion, enhancing their suitability for biomedical applications (Figure 3).

In another study [19], the synthesis and characterization of PLGA nanoparticle/4-arm-PEG hybrid hydrogels with controlled porous structures were reported. SEM micrographs from this study provided a comprehensive view of the internal and external morphology of the hydrogels. The hybrid hydrogels displayed a well-defined porous network, which is essential for drug delivery systems as it influences the release rate of encapsulated drugs. The controlled porosity observed in the SEM images indicates the effectiveness of the synthesis method in producing hydrogels with specific structural characteristics can be found in Ref. [19].

These micrographs are essential in understanding the physical attributes of PLGA-based delivery systems which directly influence their performance in biomedical applications.

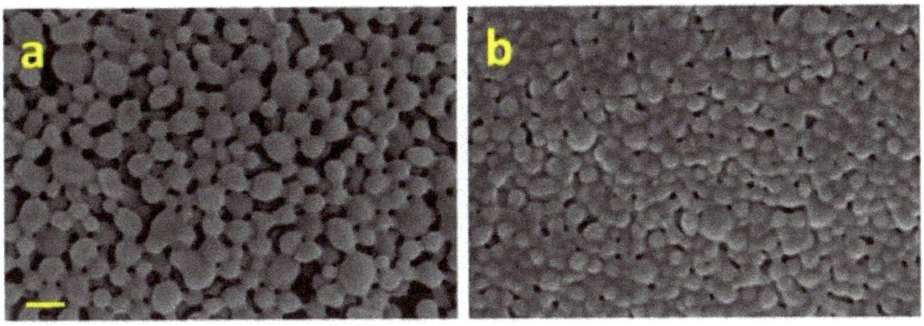

Figure 3. Scanning electron microscopy (SEM) images of (**a**) poly(lactic-co-glycolic) acid (PLGA) nanoparticles (P NPs) and PLGA–poloxamer nanoparticles (PP NPs); (**b**) PLGA–poloxamer nanoparticles (PP NPs). The scale bar is 200 nm [18].

SEM images typically show that PLGA particles exhibit a spherical shape with a smooth surface. The size of these particles can vary significantly based on the preparation method. For instance, Wang et al. demonstrated that the particle size distribution of PLGA nanoparticles could be controlled to enhance the efficacy of localized chemotherapy for tumors [20]. Similarly, Hsu et al. highlighted the importance of particle size in the development of nanoparticle–hydrogel composites for ocular drug delivery, showing that SEM micrographs helped confirm the uniformity and desirable size of the PLGA nanoparticles used [21].

The surface texture observed in SEM micrographs can provide insights into the encapsulation efficiency and drug release profiles. For example, a study by Wang et al. showed that the surface of PLGA nanoparticles loaded with sorafenib was smooth, indicating efficient drug encapsulation within the particles [22]. Similarly, Kong et al. utilized SEM to confirm the smooth texture of PLGA-based hydrogels, which is crucial for controlled drug release during in situ therapies [23].

PLGA's versatility in drug delivery is well-documented across various studies. The incorporation of PLGA nanoparticles into hydrogels can create composite systems with enhanced drug release properties. For instance, Folle et al. used SEM to analyze the integration of thyme-oil-loaded PLGA nanoparticles into a hydrogel matrix, designed for treating skin inflammation. The micrographs confirmed the successful embedding of nanoparticles within the hydrogel, crucial for ensuring the sustained release of the active ingredient [24].

The unique combination of properties makes PLGA hydrogel an excellent candidate for a wide range of biomedical applications. In drug delivery, its degradability allows for the controlled release of drugs over a sustained period. In tissue engineering, its biocompatibility and ability to mimic the extracellular matrix environment support cell proliferation and differentiation [16]. Furthermore, the flexibility in its composition enables customization to fulfill particular medical requirements. While PLGA is generally considered safe and biocompatible, understanding its degradation behavior and potential for localized toxicity is important for its application in biomedical devices. Proper design and formulation can mitigate adverse effects, ensuring PLGA remains a valuable material in the medical and pharmaceutical fields [10].

PLGA is generally considered biocompatible. When implanted in the body, it degrades into its monomers, lactic acid and glycolic acid, which are naturally metabolized and eliminated by the body. Lactic acid enters the tricarboxylic acid (TCA) cycle and is metabolized to carbon dioxide and water, while glycolic acid is either excreted through the kidneys or metabolized into glycine, which enters the TCA cycle. The degradation of PLGA results in the production of lactic acid and glycolic acid. While both are naturally occurring substances in the body, an excessive accumulation can lead to localized pH changes and inflammation. This can be particularly problematic if large amounts of PLGA are used, leading to acidic microenvironments which can affect cell viability and function [25]. Excessive acidity from PLGA degradation can cause a range of cellular responses. These may include apoptosis or necrosis if the local environment becomes too acidic, affecting the surrounding tissues. Additionally, an increase in the concentration of glycolic acid can cause metabolic acidosis if the body's buffering capacity is overwhelmed, although this is rare and typically only occurs with very high doses [26].

The immune response to PLGA is typically minimal, but it can vary depending on the specific formulation, molecular weight, and degradation rate of the polymer. In some cases, the body may recognize PLGA as a foreign material, leading to a mild inflammatory response. This is usually transient and resolves as the polymer degrades and is cleared from the body [25]. Macrophages and other immune cells may infiltrate the area where PLGA is degrading, which can sometimes lead to fibrous encapsulation, a common response to foreign materials. However, this reaction is generally mild and can be managed through the careful design and placement of PLGA-based devices [27].

Long-term studies on the use of PLGA in humans have generally shown it to be safe. However, prolonged exposure to the degradation products can potentially cause issues in sensitive tissues or organs. Therefore, the design of PLGA-based devices often includes considerations to control the degradation rate and ensure the safe elimination of by-products [13].

For instance, devices that slowly degrade over time are less likely to cause a sudden spike in lactic and glycolic acid concentrations, reducing the risk of localized toxicity. Additionally, the molecular weight and copolymer ratio can be adjusted to tailor the degradation rate to match the intended use [25].

To conclude, PLGA hydrogel represents a sophisticated material combining the advantageous properties of both PLGA polymers and hydrogels. Its tunable composition and favorable characteristics make it a powerful tool in advancing medical science and improving patient care through innovative drug delivery systems and tissue engineering solutions [28].

2. Synthesis Methods of PLGA Hydrogels

In the following section, we will summarize several common syntheses approaches for drug-loaded PLGA hydrogels. The state-of-the-art synthesis strategies and the corresponding properties of the PLGA hydrogel are also presented. In recently published studies, great effort has been devoted to optimizing the properties to fit the specific requirements in different applications, and the related knowledge is summarized.

To predominate therapeutic applications, PLGA hydrogels, as well as many other hydrogels, should have a uniform shape for further research and subsequent transition injectable properties to be used for minimally invasive local therapy, especially those administered via minimally invasive techniques, e.g., syringe injection. Therefore, the following synthesis methods are good enough in the two stated perspectives and are generally considered easily controllable and reproducible methods for PLGA hydrogel and need no or fewer harmful chemical reagents [29].

The properties, notably the temperature, pH, and solvent, associated with biomedical applications can be easily controlled to fit the various clinical applications using traditional synthesis methods; for example, a PLGA solution in an acid organic solvent can be easily prepared by adjusting the solvent component before injection. After the hydrogel is formed, the temperature of the body plays the most important role in the sol-gel transition process [30].

Figure 4 provides an overview of the different fabrication techniques for PLGA for drug-loaded PLGA hydrogels, highlighting factors related to its degradation, characteristics, responsiveness, and advantages and disadvantages. Given its biodegradability and biocompatibility, PLGA is extensively utilized as a hydrophobic polymer to create various carriers, such as polymersomes, emulsions, polymeric micelles, and more, making it a versatile choice in drug delivery systems.

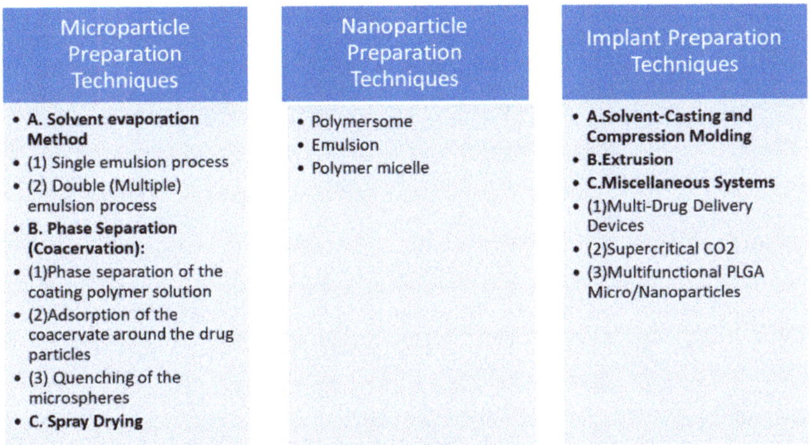

Figure 4. The figure shows the different and main fabrication techniques for drug-loaded PLGA hydrogels and the factors related to their degradation besides their characteristics, responsiveness, advantages, and disadvantages [10].

PLGA exhibits both hydrophilic and hydrophobic characteristics, which depend on its copolymer composition and the ratio of lactic acid to glycolic acid. Generally, the glycolic acid units are more hydrophilic, while the lactic acid units are more hydrophobic due to the presence of the methyl group. Consequently, the overall hydrophilicity or hydrophobicity of PLGA can be tailored by adjusting the lactic to glycolic acid ratio. For instance, a higher content of glycolic acid increases the hydrophilicity, whereas a higher content of lactic acid enhances the hydrophobicity. When PLGA has a higher ratio of lactic acid, it tends to be more hydrophobic. The methyl groups in the lactic acid units repel water, reducing the polymer's affinity for water. Increasing the glycolic acid content makes the polymer slightly less hydrophobic. Glycolic acid lacks the hydrophobic methyl group, making it more polar than lactic acid. Consequently, PLGA with a higher glycolic acid content has better water affinity, although it remains predominantly hydrophobic [31].

PLGA hydrogel synthesis is mainly done through physical or chemical crosslinking methods. The physical crosslinking method relies on the chemical modification of a PLGA polymer, e.g., thiol modification of the PLGA end group, to reduce the critical association concentration. The chemical crosslinking method relies on the introduction of a third component to react with the PLGA polymer more or less. In general, the chemical crosslinking method achieves a tighter network structure and higher modulus than the physical one, due to the generation of additional crosslink sites by introducing a third component [32].

2.1. Chemical Crosslinking

The role of crosslinking in the preparation of PLGA hydrogels is to hold the polymer in a 3D structure. When prepared as hydrogels, hydrophilic polymer chains are propagated in the preparation system. Without crosslinking, these chains would dissolve when heated or stirred. Permanent polymer crosslinking holds the network in place and prevents dissolution. Crosslinking within the polymer network can occur with or without external crosslinking agents. External crosslinking often involves covalent bonds between the polymer chains, requiring the presence of functional groups on the polymer chain. However, monomer or oligomer compounds without external crosslinking effects cannot form covalent bonds [33].

For the external charging method, the presence of functional groups is essential as they can serve as binding sites between the polymer chains. If the appropriate concentration of functional groups is present in the polymer, crosslinking can be achieved by adjusting the concentration of monomers or oligomers. The addition of external energy facilitates the formation of covalent bonds, resulting in the final curing of the polymer network structure. On the other hand, due to the dual-phase nature of PLGA hydrogels, with hydrophobicity in the central region and hydrophilicity in the head and tail, ammonolysis or aminolysis reactions are typically used to achieve crosslinking. In this article, we summarize the preparation method, properties, and biomedical applications of chemically crosslinked PLGA hydrogels. Additionally, we provide future trends for PLGA hydrogels in the concluding section [34].

2.2. Physical Crosslinking

Techniques based on the physical interaction of polymer chains do not destroy the polymer microstructure and maintain the sol-gel transition properties. Many of the desirable features of chemical hydrogel crosslinking can also be approached through proper physical hydrogel formation. The major advantage of this class of hydrogels is the lack of potential for cytotoxic residue or the need to use cytotoxically controlled chemicals or irradiation sources. Thus, these hydrogels are very useful when interacting with living systems [35].

H-bond crosslink hydrogels are derived from polymers possessing H-bonding sites. These sites form intermolecular or intramolecular H-bonded secondary structures. Although H-bonding-based hydrogels are mostly derived from self-associative polymers, H-bonding sites can also be incorporated into synthetic polymers in a bioinspired manner. In these cases, the H-bonded sites are built into the hydrogel by conjugating natural, amino acid-derived, and/or peptidic moieties into the polymer chain. Such mutations create nanostructures that can form H-bonds amongst each other. In the case of self-associative polymers, no external driving force is needed for gelation [2].

2.3. Fabrication Techniques for PLGA Hydrogels

The development of hydrogels as delivery platforms for therapeutic agents, for example, drugs, peptides, proteins, and growth factors, has received more attention due to their unique hydration and physical properties. Conventional hydrogels are prepared with physical or chemical crosslinking and, in most cases, lack loading capacity for hydrophobic molecules. These hydrogels, derived from compressed PLGA, exhibit fascinating phase behavior near the glass transition temperature (Tg). They are fabricated through casting/quenching processing and applied for the sustained delivery of various drugs at the same time, feasible for model drugs with different hydrophilicities [36]. Different drugs can achieve different sustained release profiles through these PLGA hydrogels, suggesting they are versatile for the delivery of many therapeutic agents. The phase transition temperature of the hydrogel is potentially used as a guideline for sustained release (burst or slow release) of the drugs [37]. The ability to control the release rate of drugs is a critical aspect in modern pharmaceutics. Hydrogel-based delivery systems have garnered considerable attention due to their unique properties, including their biocompatibility, excellent mechanical strength, and tunable release profiles. Notably, hydrogels have emerged as promising carriers for a diverse range of therapeutic agents, including small drug molecules, peptides, proteins, and growth factors [38]. One key advantage of PLGA hydrogels is their ability to facilitate sustained drug delivery. Regardless of the hydrophilicity of the model drug, these hydrogels have demonstrated immense versatility in accommodating a wide variety of therapeutic agents. Consequently, different drugs have exhibited distinct sustained release profiles within the PLGA hydrogel matrix. This observation underscores the potential of PLGA hydrogels as a promising platform for efficient drug delivery [39]. An interesting perspective is to use the Tg of the PLGA hydrogel as a crucial guideline for regulating sustained release mechanisms. By carefully manipulating temperature, the desired drug release kinetics can be achieved, be it burst release or slower, controlled release over a longer period of time. This temperature-dependent control of drug release holds promise for tailoring hydrogel-based delivery systems to specific therapeutic needs [40].

The synthesis of PLGA hydrogels specifically for sustained drug delivery involves several methods designed to optimize the encapsulation, release profiles, and biocompatibility of therapeutic agents [41]. Emulsion solvent evaporation involves dissolving PLGA and the drug in an organic solvent, followed by emulsification in an aqueous phase. The organic solvent is then evaporated, leading to the formation of drug-loaded PLGA nanoparticles or microspheres that can be crosslinked to form hydrogels, ensuring sustained release of the drug [31].

Solvent casting/particulate leaching implies that the PLGA is dissolved in a solvent along with the drug, cast into a mold containing a leachable particulate (e.g., salt or sugar), and then the solvent is evaporated. The particles are then released to create a porous hydrogel structure that enables sustained drug release [42].

In the case of the electrospinning technique, PLGA and the drug are dissolved in a solvent, and the solution is electrospun to create fine fibers. These fibers are then collected and crosslinked to form a hydrogel matrix. The porous structure of the electrospun fibers facilitates controlled and sustained drug release. Solvent casting employs water-soluble particulates like salt or sugar, which are leached out to create porous structures, reducing environmental impact [43].

Another synthesis technique is thermal gelation. PLGA copolymers are designed to undergo gelation at specific temperatures. The drug is mixed with the PLGA solution, which then forms a hydrogel upon a temperature change. This method allows the hydrogel to encapsulate the drug efficiently and release it in a controlled manner. Thermal gelation does not require organic solvents, thus reducing the potential toxicological impacts [44].

In the photopolymerization method, PLGA can be functionalized with photoreactive groups, and the active ingredient can be mixed into this solution. When exposed to light, crosslinking occurs, forming a hydrogel. Photopolymerization provides precise control over the gelation process and drug distribution within the hydrogel. Moreover, this method eliminates the need for chemical crosslinkers and reduces the generation of hazardous waste [45].

Table 1 provides an overview of different synthesis methods for PLGA hydrogels, highlighting their advantages and disadvantages and providing case examples.

Table 1. Overview of Different Synthesis Methods for PLGA Hydrogels.

Synthesis Method	Advantages	Disadvantages	Case Example (Drug Released)	Ref.
Emulsion Solvent Evaporation	Good control over particle size; high drug loading	Requires use of organic solvents	Dexamethasone	[41]
Solvent Casting/Particulate Leaching	Creates porous structure; simple method	Potential residual solvents; limited to small-scale production	Vancomycin	[46]
Electrospinning	High surface area; controlled release profile	Complex setup; requires high voltage	Ciprofloxacin	[47]
Thermal Gelation	No need for organic solvents; temperature-controlled gelation	Limited to thermosensitive drugs; potential thermal degradation	BSA (Bovine Serum Albumin)	[48]
Photopolymerization	Precise control over gelation; spatial control	Requires photoinitiators; potential UV damage to drugs	Methotrexate	[49]

2.4. Emulsion Solvent Evaporation Technique

The emulsion technique for PLGA hydrogel fabrication involves the careful selection of solvents, emulsification of PLGA, hardening of emulsion droplets, and formation of porous structures [31]. Typically, to prepare PLGA hydrogels using the emulsion technique, a porogen or polymer blend is prepared with a hydrogel solvent, followed by PLGA dissolution in the polymer. Solvents are carefully chosen such that they can effectively dissolve PLGA and porogens, ensuring a thorough mixture. In addition, these solvents must be partially miscible with each other to enable controlled phase separation of these two polymers. This controlled phase separation is crucial in achieving the desired structure and properties of the hydrogel [50]. Moreover, it is essential for the chosen solvents to be non-toxic and low-boiling. This enables easy removal of the solvents at biological temperatures, preventing any potential harm to the surrounding environment or biological systems. Therefore, the selection of suitable solvents is a critical step in the fabrication process [50].

To promote emulsion formation, an emulsifying agent is then dissolved in the solvent or polymer mixture. This emulsifying agent aids in achieving a stable and uniform dispersion of PLGA within the solvent or polymer solution. By ensuring the successful emulsification of the components, the subsequent steps of the fabrication process can proceed smoothly [51]. Following emulsification, the emulsified ethyl acetate (or other organic solution) droplets are then hardened. These hardened droplets serve as pores or void spaces in the co-solvent/extraction polymer. The formation of these porous structures is significant as it impacts the overall characteristics of the resulting hydrogel. The porosity and void space allow for the effective loading and release of drugs or other bioactive agents within the hydrogel matrix. Importantly, the one-step particle-leaching process employed in this technique is suitable for a broad range of polymers [52].

This versatility makes it highly applicable in various biomedical and tissue engineering applications. Additionally, the particle-leaching process is scalable, allowing for the fabrication of hydrogels with a general microsphere size. This scalability is advantageous as it permits the production of hydrogels in different sizes, catering to specific requirements and applications. The emulsion method is the most widely used method for preparing PLGA hydrogels and provides a versatile platform for biomedical applications [53]. By immersing a crosslinked porous polymer into PLGA dissolved in a suitable non-toxic solvent, and subsequently evaporating the solvent while initiating the crosslinking process, a single-phase hydrogel with open channels can be obtained. Researchers have reported various strategies to produce desirable PLGA hydrogels using the emulsion method, often involving the incorporation of surfactant dispersion. This allows the formation of stable emulsion droplets which eventually harden into the desired heterogeneous solid matrix, offering enhanced mechanical properties and controlled release capabilities [54].

2.5. Solvent Casting

Generally, a PLGA matrix is formed by solvent evaporation or diffusion. The most commonly used method, solvent casting, has been widely employed to mold various forms of PLGA matrices, including films, foils, fibers, and microparticles. In the solvent casting process, the polymer, along with other dissolved bioactive agents, is dissolved in commonly used solvents, such as chloroform and acetone, to obtain a homogeneous solution. This solution is then cast into a suitable mold or spread onto a substrate. As the solvent gradually migrates from the polymer/solvent solution to the surrounding air, a solid film is formed. During the solvent evaporation process, the solvent present in the polymer solution diffuses towards the air/polymer interface, resulting in the formation of a flat film [41]. It is worth noting that by manipulating the surface properties, the cross-section of the films can be significantly altered. This can lead to the formation of distinct features, such as finger-like layers or porous microsponges within the PLGA matrix [52]. Through careful optimization, an ideal release profile for hydrophobic drugs encapsulated within the solvent casting systems has been achieved. However, it is important to address the challenges associated with organic dissolution or phase separation, as they can hinder the sustained release of bioactive agents from the PLGA matrix. The major drawback is that the hydration and degradation of solvent casting systems are often insufficient to provide effective release characteristics [55]. This limitation significantly hinders the potential applications of these systems. Consequently, many researchers around the world have tirelessly explored and experimented with various approaches to overcome this deficiency. Unfortunately, despite their efforts, the release characteristics of the resulting systems has still turned out to be flawed in several respects. In response to this challenge, there have been promising advancements in the field of medicated polymer matrices and other modified systems. These advances aim to improve the delivery characteristics of therapeutic administrations by incorporating innovative concepts and technologies. However, it is important to note that these potential strategies are currently limited by an incomplete understanding of the fundamental mass transport and mechanistic interactions of the polymer matrix [56]. To address these limitations and "unlock" the full potential of therapeutic administrations, various strategies have been explored. For instance, after the films are dried, the hydrophobic polymer and any residual virtual solvent are allowed to evaporate, resulting in the formation of a PLGA nano-fiber matrix. This nano-fiber matrix has shown promising results in effectively encapsulating small water-insoluble drugs within its rough surface morphology. However, it should be noted that the sustained release of drugs from this matrix is still an area that requires further investigation. In order to achieve sustained or semi-sustained release, as well as zero-order release kinetics, additional hydrophobic additives can be blended with the polymer/solution and encapsulated drugs [31]. The incorporation of these additives allows for variations in the polymer chains or the crystallinity of the polymer matrix, thereby enabling control over the drug release. This approach has shown potential in expanding the capabilities of PLGA matrices and tailoring their release profiles for different therapeutic applications [56].

2.6. Electrospinning

Using electrospinning to obtain PLGA hydrogels has emerged as a versatile and promising technique for achieving sustained drug delivery in biomedical applications. This method combines the inherent properties of PLGA polymers with the unique advantages of electrospinning, enabling the production of nano- to micro-scale fibers with controlled drug release profiles. Electrospinning uses an electric field to draw or melt a polymer solution into ultrafine fibers. The process typically involves a syringe or pump to deliver the polymer solution through a needle or spinneret, which is connected to a high-voltage power supply. When the electric field is applied, electrostatic forces overcome the surface tension of the polymer solution, forming a jet that expands and solidifies into fibers as the solvent evaporates or coagulates in a collection medium. The resulting fibers can range in diameter from nanometers to micrometers and offer a high surface area-to-volume ratio and a porous structure that promotes drug loading and release [57].

The advantages of electrospinning include controlled release profiles, high drug loading capacity, biocompatibility, biodegradability, ease of scalability, and versatility [58]. Electrospun PLGA fibers allow for precise control over the release kinetics of encapsulated drugs. Factors such as polymer composition, fiber morphology, and drug loading can be tailored to achieve sustained release over extended periods. The high surface area and porous structure of electrospun fibers facilitate the efficient encapsulation of a wide range of drugs, including hydrophobic and hydrophilic compounds, proteins, and growth factors [59]. Electrospinning can incorporate multiple drugs or bioactive agents within the same scaffold, enabling combination therapies or the sequential release of different agents. Moreover, it is a scalable technique that can be adapted for the industrial production of drug delivery systems, ensuring reproducibility and uniformity in fiber morphology and drug release characteristics [60].

Despite its advantages, electrospinning presents some challenges, such as process optimization, potential drug degradation, or poor mechanical properties. Parameters such as polymer concentration, solvent selection, voltage, and the distance between spinneret and collector must be carefully optimized to achieve the desired fiber morphology and drug release kinetics [61]. Some drugs may degrade or lose activity during the electrospinning process due to exposure to solvents, electric fields, or prolonged processing times. Electrospun fibers may exhibit lower mechanical strength compared to bulk materials, requiring strategies to enhance scaffold stability and durability [60].

Electrospun PLGA hydrogels have been utilized in various biomedical applications, including wound healing [62], for the delivery of growth factors and antimicrobial agents to promote tissue regeneration and prevent infection [58]. In orthopedics, electrospun PLGA hydrogels have been utilized to control the release of analgesics and anti-inflammatory drugs for the management of musculoskeletal disorders such as osteoarthritis [43]. In neuroscience, electrospun PLGA hydrogels have been applied for the localized delivery of neuroprotective agents or growth factors for the treatment of neurodegenerative diseases or spinal cord injuries [63]. The electrospinning of PLGA hydrogels represents a promising strategy for achieving sustained drug delivery in biomedical applications. By harnessing the advantages of PLGA polymers and electrospinning technology, researchers can tailor drug release profiles to meet specific therapeutic needs while ensuring biocompatibility and biodegradability. Continuous advances in materials science and process optimization are expected to further improve the efficacy and clinical implementation of electrospun PLGA hydrogel-based drug delivery systems.

2.7. Thermal Gelation

Thermal gelation of PLGA hydrogels is a versatile technique that leverages the thermoresponsive properties of PLGA to form hydrogels under controlled temperature conditions. PLGA hydrogels are typically prepared using block copolymers or blends where PLGA serves as the hydrophobic segment. Below a critical gelation temperature, these polymers remain in solution due to their solvency in aqueous environments. However, upon reaching the gelation temperature, which is often slightly above physiological temperatures (~37 °C), the polymer undergoes a phase transition from a liquid solution to a gel state. This transition occurs due to the dehydration of the polymer chains and subsequent physical entanglement or aggregation, resulting in the formation of a three-dimensional structure [48].

One of the significant advantages of thermal gelation is its injectability. The polymer solution can be injected as a liquid precursor into the target site within the body, where it undergoes gelation upon exposure to body heat. This property makes it suitable for minimally invasive procedures [64]. The gelation process itself is non-toxic and does not require harsh chemicals or crosslinking agents that could potentially harm biological tissues [65]. The gel structure formed by thermal gelation can encapsulate drugs or bioactive molecules. The sustained release of these substances can be achieved by modulating the polymer composition and gelation parameters, ensuring controlled drug delivery over a prolonged period of time [65].

The thermal gelation of PLGA hydrogels has been employed in various biomedical fields, including controlled drug delivery systems, tissue engineering scaffolds, and wound healing applications. Its adaptability allows for the incorporation of different therapeutic agents tailored to specific medical needs [66].

However, there are some challenges that should be taken into account. In recent years, researchers have focused on improving the delivery systems for these materials, particularly in bone regenerative medicine. Although hydrogels have shown promise in this regard, their application has been limited to areas with small cavities and irregular shapes [67]. This is mainly due to the challenges associated with their administration and distribution within the targeted region. Interstitial injections of hydrogels have proven to be a complex and intricate procedure. Precise delivery of these materials to the intended location requires surgical expertise and meticulous care. Furthermore, both therapeutic agents and PLGA materials require high drug loads, zero-order release, easier handling during treatment, and careful design and physical forms for efficient drug delivery. To meet these needs, scientists have developed thermoresponsive hydrogel PLGA for cellular or therapeutic drug delivery which belongs to a novel class of biological gels with broad applications in tissue regeneration, drug delivery, and numerous other areas of biomedicine. In general, thermoresponsive PLGA gels exhibit liquid properties at both low and high temperatures. However, when exposed to human body temperature, the solution quickly turns into a non-finishing semi-liquid gel, improving its performance as a drug delivery system [68].

Furthermore, when compared to the use of simple PLA/PLGA microspheres, hydrogels have shown certain drawbacks. These include a lower drug load capacity, a peak release rate, and potential irradiation of the therapeutic agent. Such shortcomings can significantly impact the chemical and physical properties of the drug, jeopardizing its efficacy and overall therapeutic outcome. Considering these observations, ongoing research aims to overcome these limitations and optimize the use of PLA and PLGA for biomedical applications. Scientists are exploring new approaches to maximize drug loading, regulate release rates, and minimize adverse effects on the therapeutic agent. By overcoming these challenges and refining the chemical and physical properties of PLA and PLGA, researchers hope to unlock their full potential in various therapeutic applications [68].

The gelation temperature must be precisely controlled to ensure gel formation occurs at the intended physiological conditions. Variations in temperature or polymer concentration can affect the gelation kinetics and mechanical properties of the hydrogel. While PLGA hydrogels formed by thermal gelation are injectable, they may have lower mechanical strength compared to crosslinked hydrogels. Strategies to improve mechanical properties without compromising injectability are being actively researched. The degradation rate of PLGA hydrogels must be compatible with the intended application. The balance between degradation kinetics and drug release profiles is crucial for maintaining therapeutic efficacy over the desired timeframe [67].

The thermal gelation of PLGA hydrogels is used to encapsulate and deliver drugs for localized therapies, such as cancer treatment [69] or chronic wounds [70]. These hydrogels serve as scaffolds to support cell growth and tissue regeneration, particularly in musculoskeletal and cardiovascular applications [71]. In ocular applications, thermal gelling PLGA hydrogels have been investigated for sustained drug release to treat diseases such as glaucoma or macular degeneration [72]. Continued advances in materials science and gelation techniques are expected to further increase the utility and effectiveness of these hydrogels in diverse therapeutic applications [67].

2.8. Photopolymerization

Photopolymerization of PLGA hydrogels has emerged as a sophisticated approach to precisely control drug release kinetics and spatial distribution in biomedical applications. Photopolymerization involves the use of light-sensitive molecules (photoinitiators) to initiate/trigger polymerization reactions in the presence of monomers or pre-polymers. For PLGA hydrogels, photopolymerization typically involves the functionalization of PLGA with photoreactive groups, such as methacrylate or acrylate moieties, that can crosslink upon exposure to light of specific wavelengths (typically ultraviolet or visible light). The photoinitiator absorbs photons from light and generates reactive species (free radicals or ions) that trigger polymerization and crosslinking reactions, forming a three-dimensional hydrogel network. This process occurs quickly and can be spatially and temporally controlled, enabling the precise encapsulation and release of drugs [73].

The advantages of photopolymerization for PLGA hydrogels involve spatial and temporal control, high efficiency and versatility, tunable properties, and integration with biomolecules for biocompatibility and biodegradability [74].

Photopolymerization enables the localized crosslinking of PLGA hydrogels within seconds to minutes upon exposure to light, allowing for precise control over the spatial distribution of drug-loaded hydrogel matrices. The reaction occurs quickly and efficiently under mild conditions, preserving the bioactivity of sensitive drugs or biological molecules encapsulated within the hydrogel matrix. The mechanical and degradation properties of photopolymerized PLGA hydrogels can be tailored by adjusting parameters such as polymer concentration, photoinitiator type and concentration, light exposure intensity, and duration. PLGA is biocompatible and biodegradable, making photopolymerized PLGA hydrogels suitable for sustained drug delivery applications without inducing significant inflammatory responses [75].

Photopolymerization allows for the incorporation of bioactive molecules, such as growth factors or peptides, into the hydrogel matrix, facilitating synergistic therapeutic effects or tissue regeneration. Despite its advantages, the photopolymerization of PLGA hydrogels presents several challenges: depth of light penetration, photoinitiator toxicity, and shelf stability. Limited light penetration depth restricts the thickness of photopolymerized hydrogels, necessitating strategies for creating thicker constructs for certain applications. Some photoinitiators can be cytotoxic or cause photodamage to encapsulated drugs or biomolecules, requiring careful selection and optimization. Photopolymerizable formulations may require careful handling and storage to maintain photoinitiator stability and prevent premature polymerization [73].

Photopolymerized PLGA hydrogels have been applied in various biomedical fields, including regenerative medicine, for the controlled release of growth factors or stem cell therapies for tissue engineering [76,77] and wound healing applications [78]. In drug delivery systems, photopolymerized PLGA hydrogels have been used for the sustained release of antibiotics, anti-inflammatory drugs, or chemotherapeutic agents for localized treatment of infections, inflammation, or cancers [79,80].

The photopolymerization of PLGA hydrogels represents a powerful tool for developing advanced drug delivery systems with precise spatial and temporal control of drug release. By leveraging the unique properties of PLGA polymers and photopolymerization technology, researchers can develop innovative therapies that have greater efficacy, reduced side effects, and improved patient outcomes in various clinical settings [75].

3. Properties of PLGA Hydrogels

PLGA hydrogels (Scheme 1) exhibit several beneficial properties that make them suitable for various biomedical applications, particularly in drug delivery and tissue engineering. Below are the key properties of PLGA hydrogels, each accompanied by example cases where PLGA hydrogels have been used for sustained drug release.

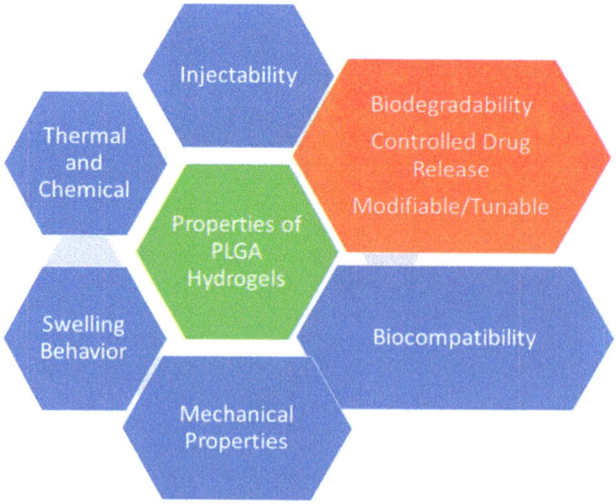

Scheme 1. Properties of PLGA hydrogels.

3.1. Biodegradability

PLGA hydrogels break down into lactic acid and glycolic acid, which are naturally metabolized by the body. The rate of degradation can be controlled by adjusting the ratio of lactic acid to glycolic acid in the copolymer [81]. PLGA hydrogels have been used to create an injectable depot system for the sustained release of insulin. This system provides a steady release of insulin over an extended period, reducing the frequency of injections that diabetics need [31].

In another example, PLGA hydrogels loaded with bone morphogenetic proteins (BMPs) have been applied to sustain the release of these proteins, promoting bone regeneration in orthopedic applications [82].

3.2. Biocompatibility

PLGA hydrogels are highly biocompatible, meaning they do not induce significant inflammatory or immune responses when implanted in the body [83].

PLGA hydrogels have been used to deliver chemotherapeutic drugs like paclitaxel in a sustained manner directly to the tumor site, reducing systemic toxicity and improving therapeutic outcomes [53,84].

For the treatment of ocular diseases, PLGA hydrogels have been used to ensure the sustained release of anti-inflammatory drugs and improve patient compliance by reducing the need for frequent eye drops [85,86].

3.3. Mechanical Properties

Variating the polymer composition, crosslinking density, and the addition of other materials can tailor the mechanical properties of PLGA hydrogels.

PLGA hydrogels designed with appropriate mechanical properties have been used to deliver growth factors for cartilage repair, providing a scaffold that supports the mechanical loads while promoting tissue regeneration [87].

In wound healing, PLGA hydrogels with adjustable mechanical properties have been used to sustain the release of antimicrobial agents, forming a protective barrier while promoting healing [88].

3.4. Controlled Drug Release

PLGA hydrogels provide controlled and sustained drug release which can be fine-tuned by manipulating the degradation rate of the PLGA, the hydrogel's porosity, and the swelling behavior [89].

PLGA hydrogels loaded with antibiotics such as vancomycin have been used to treat bone infections, to ensure sustained release of the drug at the infection site, and to improve the effectiveness of the treatment [90].

For postoperative pain management, PLGA hydrogels have been employed to deliver analgesics like bupivacaine over a prolonged period, reducing the need for frequent dosing [91].

3.5. Swelling Behavior

PLGA hydrogels swell upon contact with aqueous environments, which is important for drug loading and release, as well as providing a hydrated environment for cell growth in tissue engineering applications [92].

PLGA hydrogels with tailored swelling properties have been used for the sustained release of hydration-sensitive drugs, ensuring that the drug release profile is controlled by the swelling behavior of the hydrogel [93].

In tissue engineering, PLGA hydrogels have been utilized to encapsulate cells and provide a sustained release of growth factors, thereby improving cell viability and proliferation [94].

3.6. Thermal and Chemical Stability

PLGA hydrogels are generally stable under physiological conditions, maintaining their structure and function at body temperature and allowing for sterilization using standard methods without significant degradation [95].

PLGA hydrogels stable at body temperature have been used to deliver osteogenic factors for bone tissue engineering, maintaining the release kinetics over several weeks [96,97].

PLGA hydrogels that can be sterilized without degradation have been developed for the sustained delivery of anti-inflammatory drugs in arthritic joints [98].

3.7. Modifiable/Tunable Surface Properties

The surface properties of PLGA hydrogels can be modified to enhance cell attachment, proliferation, and differentiation, making them ideal for creating scaffolds in tissue engineering [99].

PLGA hydrogels functionalized with RGD peptides have been used to improve cell adhesion and promote sustained release of growth factors in wound healing applications [100,101].

PLGA hydrogels coated with nanoparticles have been employed for the sustained release of anti-cancer drugs, improving the targeting and efficacy of the treatment [102].

3.8. Tunable Degradation Kinetics

Adjusting the copolymer composition and molecular weight can fine-tune the degradation kinetics of PLGA hydrogels, allowing for the design of hydrogels that degrade over a specific period [103].

PLGA hydrogels with tailored degradation rates are used for the sustained release of hormones such as leuprolide acetate in hormone replacement therapy, ensuring consistent hormone levels for months [104,105].

In vaccine delivery, PLGA hydrogels have been designed to degrade slowly, providing a sustained release of antigens and enhancing the immune response [106,107].

3.9. Injectability

PLGA hydrogels can be formulated as injectable systems, providing a minimally invasive method for delivering drugs or cells to specific sites in the body [108].

Injectable PLGA hydrogels have been developed for the sustained release of local anesthetics, providing long-lasting pain relief after surgery [25,109].

PLGA hydrogels formulated for injection have been used to deliver stem cells to damaged tissues, where the hydrogel provides a sustained release of growth factors to support cell survival and differentiation [110,111].

4. Sustained Release Mechanisms of PLGA Hydrogels

PLGA hydrogels enable controlled drug release through various kinetic mechanisms influenced by factors such as pH, monomer ratio, and intrinsic viscosity of PLGA. Understanding these factors is crucial for optimizing drug delivery systems to achieve the desired therapeutic outcomes.

The degradation rate of PLGA is significantly influenced by the pH of the environment (Figure 5). As demonstrated by Lu et al. [112], PLGA degrades faster under acidic conditions compared to neutral or basic conditions. This accelerated degradation is due to the hydrolysis of ester bonds in PLGA, which occurs more rapidly in acidic environments. Thus, the pH of the medium is a critical factor in designing PLGA-based drug delivery systems for specific applications [113].

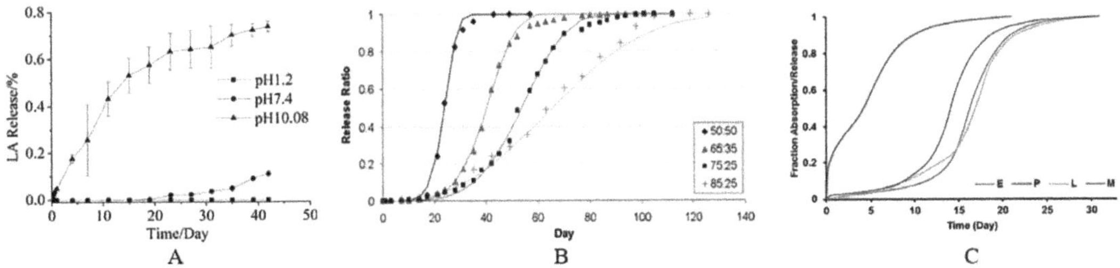

Figure 5. (**A**) Comparison of PLGA degradation rates under different pH conditions. (**B**) Comparison of PLGA degradation rates for different monomer ratios. (**C**) Comparison of the degradation rates of PLGAs with different intrinsic viscosities; the magnitude of the intrinsic viscosities of the four PLGAs is P < L < E < M [112].

The ratio of lactic acid to glycolic acid in PLGA also impacts its degradation rate. Lu et al. [112] illustrate that PLGA with a higher glycolic acid content degrades more quickly than those with higher lactic acid content. This is because glycolic acid contributes to increased hydrophilicity and amorphous characteristics, enhancing water uptake and hydrolysis rates. Adjusting the monomer ratio allows for the customization of degradation and drug release rates according to therapeutic needs [114].

Intrinsic viscosity, indicative of the molecular weight of PLGA, affects its degradation behavior. It was demonstrated that PLGAs with different intrinsic viscosities degrade at varying rates, with the order being P < L < E < M. Higher intrinsic viscosity correlates with a slower degradation rate due to the increased molecular weight, resulting in more extended drug release profiles [115].

The drug release kinetics from PLGA hydrogels can be modulated by manipulating the factors mentioned above. The release mechanisms typically include diffusion, degradation, or a combination of both.

Initially, drug release is often governed by diffusion through the PLGA matrix. This phase may exhibit a burst release, where a significant portion of the drug is rapidly released from the hydrogel's surface.

As the PLGA matrix degrades, the release mechanism transitions to being degradation-controlled. Here, the drug release rate aligns with the degradation rate of the PLGA, which can be fine-tuned by altering the pH, monomer ratio, or intrinsic viscosity.

In many practical applications, the drug release profile is a combination of diffusion and degradation mechanisms. Early stages might be diffusion-dominated, with degradation playing a more significant role as the matrix breaks down over time.

The practical application of these concepts can be seen in the release profile of oxaliplatin from PLGA microparticles. As shown in Figure 6, oxaliplatin release from PLGA microparticles exhibits a sustained release over time compared to oxaliplatin powder. When these microparticles are loaded into different hydrogels, such as HC12, Guardix-Sol®, and HC21, the release profiles differ significantly (A, B, and C, respectively), highlighting the impact of the hydrogel matrix on drug release kinetics. These findings underscore the potential of PLGA-based systems in achieving controlled and sustained drug delivery [116].

Understanding the mechanisms governing the release of therapeutic agents from PLGA hydrogels is crucial for optimizing their performance in biomedical applications. The release mechanisms, including diffusion, degradation, and swelling, can be manipulated through the careful selection of polymer properties and hydrogel formulation. Advances in understanding these mechanisms continue to drive innovations in drug delivery systems, paving the way for more effective and personalized therapies.

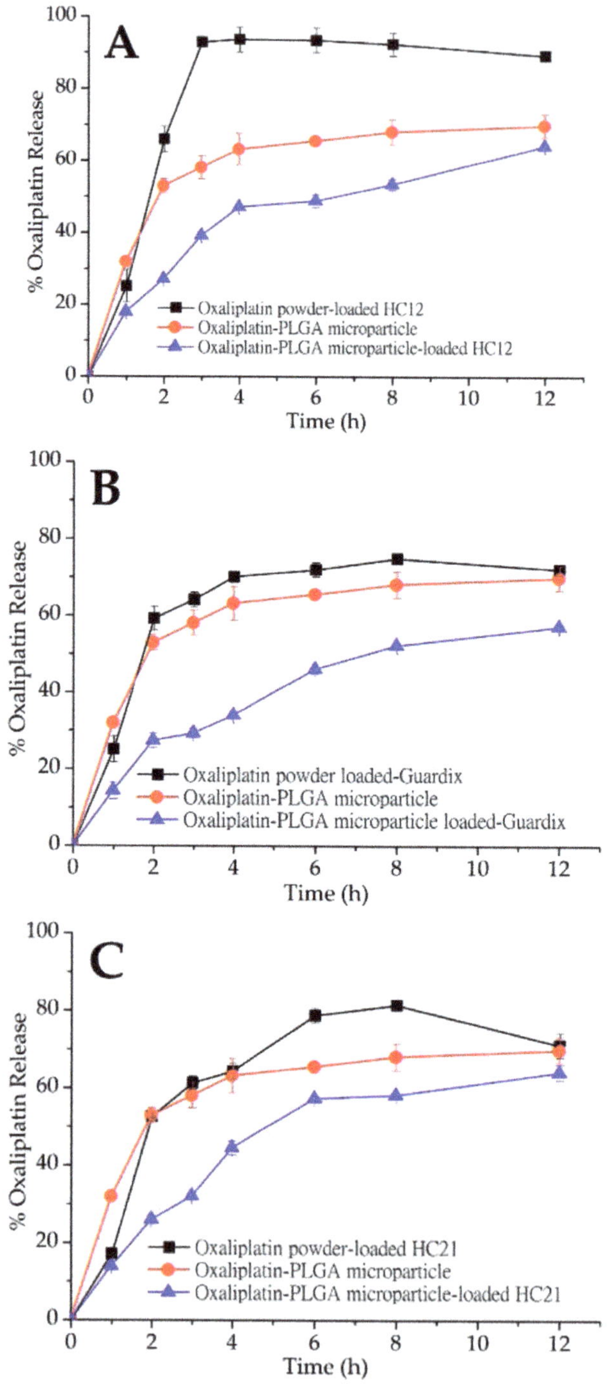

Figure 6. In vitro oxaliplatin release from PLGA microparticles (red, •). Oxaliplatin release profile from oxaliplatin powder and oxaliplatin–PLGA microparticles-loaded in (**A**) HC12; (**B**) Guardix-Sol®; and (**C**) HC21 hydrogel. Mean ± S.D. (n = 3) [116].

4.1. Diffusion-Controlled Drug Release System

One of the main mechanisms of drug release from PLGA hydrogels is diffusion. In this process, molecules are released as a result of their movement through the aqueous pores of the hydrogel matrix. In the initial phase, a burst release takes place. When a drug-loaded PLGA hydrogel is exposed to the physiological environment, an initial burst release occurs. This phase is characterized by a rapid release of a significant amount of drug molecules that are loosely bound or located near the surface of the hydrogel. The mechanism implies that drug molecules diffuse through the aqueous channels and pores within the hydrogel matrix. The release rate is initially high due to the steep concentration gradient between the drug-loaded hydrogel and the surrounding medium.

In a later phase, a sustained release occurs. As diffusion continues, the release rate gradually decreases. This sustained release phase is governed by Fick's law of diffusion, where the rate of release depends on the concentration gradient, the drug's diffusion coefficient, and the thickness of the hydrogel matrix [117].

The diffusion rate can be influenced by the polymer composition (e.g., the ratio of lactic acid to glycolic acid in the PLGA), the molecular weight of the polymer, and the physicochemical properties of the drug (e.g., size and hydrophilicity). The diffusion rate depends on factors such as the molecular size, hydrophilicity, and mesh size of the hydrogel network. Smaller molecules typically diffuse faster than compared to larger ones, resulting in faster release rates over time [31]. The natural or artificial barriers, such as polymer matrices encapsulating drugs or transplanted devices, interact with the drug release scaffold from both the interior and exterior directions. For the drug delivery system of interest, the two flow directions can result in two different control mechanisms: inside-out could induce diffusion-controlled drug release, while the reverse flow from outside-in would cause hydration-controlled or erosion-controlled drug release. When the diffusional release of the drug is controlled, the drug molecules are transported through the polymer matrix, which serves as a rate-limiting barrier, thus forming a diffusion barrier with different properties and configurations [1].

Among various possible mechanisms affecting the release of drugs incorporated into controlled delivery systems, the diffusion-controlled release is one of the most important and effective. The diffusion of drug molecules from the polymer matrix into the surrounding aqueous environment and into the receiving phase or tissues that act as drug sinks could sustain needed release profiles, particularly in the context of pulsatile, continuous, or on-demand delivery [118].

4.1.1. Degradation-Controlled Release System

Degradation-controlled release is another mechanism that often contributes to a prolonged and sustained release of drugs as the hydrogel continues to degrade and erode. PLGA hydrogels degrade through the hydrolysis of ester bonds in the polymer backbone, leading to a gradual breakdown of the matrix [117]. When the polymer degrades, it releases encapsulated drugs, proteins, or small molecules. This degradation-controlled release mechanism can be tuned by adjusting the composition of the PLGA (e.g., the lactide to glycolide ratio), molecular weight, and the degree of crosslinking. A higher crosslinking density generally slows down the degradation and release rate, offering sustained release profiles. By the completion of the delivery through surface erosion that enables the newly formed surface at the interface with the body fluid to disestablish as a potential barrier to mass transfer, the erosion mechanism can be used to foretell when the delivery system transfers to a zero-order drug release regime. Additionally, in certain cases of passive diffusion of biomolecules, erosion specifically occurs in the tumor due to localized factors such as increased enzyme activity, acidic pH, and elevated metabolic rates. These conditions accelerate the degradation of the hydrogel matrix in the tumor environment, thereby promoting localized erosion and targeted drug release. Therefore, degradation-controlled release is a potential mechanism to contribute to anti-cancer activity [119].

One of the most popular mechanisms for rate control is to prevent drug leakage through physical or chemical encapsulation, such as covalent bonding between drugs and PLGA hydrogels. This modulation of the drug release kinetics can be based mainly on drug release during the biodegradation of the hydrogels and is referred to as "degradation-controlled release". The degradation rate of the hydrogel mainly depends on the species and structure of the material. The PLGA provides -(CH_2-CO-O)- units within the framework for the rapid degradation into CO_2 and H_2O molecules, finally leading to a decrease of the delivery system by "bulk erosion" [31].

4.1.2. Swelling-Controlled Release System

Swelling-controlled release of PLGA hydrogels in aqueous environments can also influence the kinetics of drug release. Upon contact with physiological fluids, hydrogels absorb water and swell, increasing the mesh size and facilitating the diffusion of encapsulated molecules. The swelling behavior of PLGA hydrogels depends on parameters such as polymer concentration, pH, and temperature, all of which can be individually adjusted to achieve specific release profiles [31].

4.1.3. Combined Release Mechanisms

Combined mechanisms can occur. In many cases, drug release from PLGA hydrogels involves a combination of diffusion and degradation mechanisms. During the burst release phase, diffusion initially dominates. As degradation progresses, the erosion of the hydrogel matrix becomes more significant and affects the release kinetics over time [41]. Often, drug release from PLGA hydrogels also involves a combination of diffusion, degradation, and swelling mechanisms. For instance, initial burst release may occur due to rapid diffusion of molecules near the surface, followed by sustained release as degradation progresses and the hydrogel swells. Understanding and optimizing these mechanisms are crucial for the development of PLGA hydrogels that meet the desired therapeutic needs, such as controlled release over extended periods or targeted delivery to specific tissues.

4.2. Types of Kinetics of Drug Release Mechanisms

The kinetics of drug release from PLGA hydrogels are pivotal in development of controlled drug delivery systems. In general, hydrogels are porous and possess interconnected pore networks, and drug release occurs through a mixture of molecular diffusion, convective flow, polymer swelling, and relaxation behavior. Therefore, the main drug transport mechanism in most practical hydrogel drug delivery systems is either Fickian diffusion, non-Fickian diffusion, case-II transports, or a combination of two in the same hydrogel system. In this context, clarifying the kinetic types is important for a better understanding and efficient application of PLGA hydrogels in drug delivery. Understanding these mechanisms allows for the design of hydrogels that can provide sustained and targeted release of therapeutic agents. Next, we shortly examine four key models: zero-order kinetics, first-order kinetics, the Higuchi model, and the Peppas model.

4.2.1. Zero-Order Kinetics

Zero-order kinetics is characterized by a drug release rate that remains constant over time, regardless of the drug concentration in the hydrogel. This type of release mechanism is highly sought after in therapeutic applications because it can maintain constant drug levels in the bloodstream and minimize the peaks and troughs that can occur with other release mechanisms [120]. Zero-order drug release is independent of the initial drug concentration or the dimensions of the hydrogel configuration, such as the disc or wafer tested. It is the optimal release kinetics because the kinetics model and parameters for drug release are predictable, attainable, and applicable to controlled drug delivery. Dose-independent, and decoupled from any initial burst release of the drug. The release criteria for zero-order are that $n < 0.43$ for erosion and $r^2 > 0.98$ for drug release. When the release profile is zero-order, the release criteria of zero-order kinetic release can only be obtained with PLGA containing 50% carbopol which is 20% esterified. With the zero-order release kinetic profile, the required mass transport of the drug is uniform, reaching the release area. The drug release is decoupled from the hydrogel matrix gel erosion [121].

Since the release rate is independent of the rate of degradation of the non-drug-filled matrix degradation, zero-order kinetics is generally considered to be the preferred kinetic release profile for a sustained release system. The drug release from the hydrogel is controlled by Fickian diffusion. When the polymer degradation and drug release are decoupled, the in vitro drug release can be rapid, reaching that of the erosion by area. The release criterion is $r^2 > 0.98$ with n approaching 1. The release units for zero-order kinetics are $\mu g/(mm^2 day)$. The zero-order release rate and period are independent of the initial amount of drug in the hydrogel system or the conditions of the experiment, making it the most predictable release kinetics [122].

The selection of the polymer composition is crucial. Variations in the ratio of lactic acid to glycolic acid in PLGA can influence the degradation rate, which is critical for achieving a zero-order release profile [123]. The geometric shape and size of the hydrogel matrix can influence the surface area available for drug release. For instance, cylindrical or disk-shaped matrices could provide more uniform, consistent release rates [124].

A higher initial drug loading can support a zero-order sustained release because the larger drug reservoir helps maintain the concentration gradient necessary for constant release. The extent of crosslinking within the hydrogel affects its degradation rate and mechanical properties, thereby influencing the release rate. Higher crosslinking can slow down degradation, supporting a more consistent release rate [125].

The excipients added, such as polyvinyl pyrrolidone (PVP), hydroxypropyl-β-cyclodextrin (HP-β-CD), polyethylene glycol (PEG), and Span 80, have a noticeable effect on the drug release kinetics [1].

4.2.2. First-Order Kinetics

First-order kinetics describes a drug release mechanism in which the release rate is directly proportional to the drug concentration remaining in the hydrogel. This results in an exponential decrease in the release rate over time, which is typical of many conventional drug delivery systems [126].

Drugs with higher solubility within the hydrogel matrix are more likely to follow first-order kinetics because they can easily diffuse out of the matrix [127].

The degradation rate of the PLGA polymer influences the rate at which the drug is released. Faster degradation can lead to a quicker release [128].

According to the principles of first-order kinetics, higher initial drug concentrations will result in higher initial release rates. The drug's diffusion coefficient within the hydrogel matrix is a critical factor that affects the release kinetics. Higher diffusion coefficients generally result in faster release rates [129].

As long as the kinetic of the phenomenon is slow or only the release of the drug through the external environment is not a thermodynamic process, the equilibrium is never reached, and the spontaneous mixing process cannot take place through the hydrogel network. From the kinetics of drug release, much information is derived on both native hydrogel and the complex drug/hydrogel. The methods of studying the release kinetics from hydrogel depend on many factors, including the nature of the hydrogel, the hydrogel network size, the diffusion of the released molecules, hydrophobic/hydrophilic interactions, electrostatics, steric spheres, and a chain relaxation of hydrogel. The release time depends greatly on the degree of drug loading, the approach to drug equilibrium, and the ability loading to the drug. An understanding of the release mechanism is necessary in the choice of polymers that minimize the initial burst release of a loaded pharmacological agent [130].

Kinetics describes the speed, the order, and the reaction mechanisms with time of the reaction. Kinetic studies allow not only the understanding of the nature of the drug–hydrogel interactions but also the prediction of the hydrogel model needed for different pharmaceutical applications [131]. The evaluation of the kinetics of drug release from the hydrogel is useful to understand the physical–chemical mechanisms involved in the transport of drugs (and other substances) from the environmental bulk, through the hydrogel network, and its further release to the external environment [132].

The diffusion and degradation processes both follow first-order kinetics, and PLGA hydrogels display zero-order kinetics if there is no erosion. The hydrogel displays a prolonged release effect. Its release curve can be divided into the first-order and zero-order release segments, which are influenced by multiple factors [133].

4.3. Higuchi Model

The Higuchi model is the most widely used mass transport equation for drug release in polymer-based drug delivery matrix systems. The Higuchi model for drug release from polymeric solid devices is actually a special case of the diffusion equation and assumes only one-dimensional regular drug distribution in the polymer matrix. It is actually a limiting case of a form of the diffusion equation with fixed concentration boundary conditions at the two infinite parallel surfaces of the slab. Considering this, the Higuchi model is often considered as a square root of time-driven diffusion. Assuming no polymer relaxation, trans-polymer drug release, dose metrics, and cylindrical geometry (radius < thickness), Higuchi's first-dimensional application of Fick's second law of diffusion [134]. Specifically, the Higuchi model describes the release of active ingredients from a matrix system, where the release rate is proportional to the square root of time. This model assumes a homogeneous matrix and is often used for systems where diffusion is the primary release mechanism [128].

The model is applicable to drugs with limited solubility within the matrix. Highly soluble drugs might deviate from the model due to too rapid a release [135]. The initial porosity and the changes in porosity due to matrix erosion can influence drug release rates. A more porous matrix facilitates quicker drug diffusion [136].

The Higuchi model assumes a uniform drug distribution within the matrix. A non-uniform distribution can lead to deviations from the expected release profile.

The drug's diffusion coefficient within the polymer matrix is a critical parameter. The polymer's physical and chemical properties can influence this [137].

4.4. Peppas Model

The Peppas model, also known as the Korsmeyer–Peppas model, is an empirical model used to describe drug release from polymeric systems when the mechanism of release is not well-known or involves multiple processes [137].

The model is described by Equation (1):

$$M_t/M_\infty = kt^n, \tag{2}$$

where M_t/M_∞ is the fraction of drug released at the time, t, k is a release rate constant, and n is the release exponent indicative of the mechanism of release [127].

The degree of swelling can significantly influence the release mechanism, particularly in the transition from diffusive to swelling-controlled release [127].

Non-uniform distribution of the drug within the matrix can cause deviations from the expected release profile [127].

The rate at which the polymer degrades impacts the release exponent, n. Faster degradation can lead to a higher release rate [127].

The density of crosslinks within the hydrogel matrix affects the drug diffusion rate and polymer erosion, which are critical for the Peppas model [137]. The dissolution and release mechanism of the drug from the polymer matrix always involves the mass transfer process of the solvent into the polymer and the redistribution of the drug in the matrix, forming a two-phase system containing drug-rich and polymer-rich phases. Generally, the Peppas model is used to analyze solute mobility, an empirical model that is very efficient for investigating and predicting the efficiency of polymers as drug carriers, studying the underlying mass transfer mechanisms, and deconvolving a set of relaxation times from the drug release curves. Complicated kinetics of the phase transport restraint at the molecular level can be explained within a simple framework, and the results are indicative for solving practical problems in the design of drug carriers at the engineering level [138,139].

Several factors influence the kinetics of drug release from a delivery system, such as the dose, the dosage form (regardless of the polymer or matrix used), the solubility of the drug, the drug loading capacity, and its release profile. These parameters greatly influence how a drug behaves in the body over time. First-order models are often used to describe the dissolution properties of a drug from a solid dosage form and, to a lesser extent, the dissolution of a drug encapsulated in a polymer matrix. However, if one wishes to use a drug delivery system to modulate the original pharmacokinetic profile, other release kinetics such as zero-order, first-order, or Korsmeyer–Peppas should be considered. Recently, extensive research focus has been placed on the development of analytical methods that incorporate in vitro data that can connect to in vivo projections from polymer devices. Depending on the kinetic model used, different results are observed regarding polymer concentrations at the delivery site [140].

5. Applications of PLGA Hydrogels in Drug Delivery

In vivo, drug delivery via hydrogel-based systems encompasses a diverse array of administration routes tailored to specific pathological conditions and anatomical sites [141]. Subcutaneous injection is notable for its pivotal role in evaluating toxicological effects, offering direct access to underlying tissues while facilitating controlled release of therapeutic agents. For skin-related issues, topical or transdermal application proves advantageous, providing localized treatment and bypassing systemic metabolism [142]. Orthotopic and intraperitoneal injections represent non-invasive alternatives that ensure effective therapeutic results depending on the target organ or cavity [31]. However, problems remain with oral administration due to enzymatic degradation in the gastrointestinal tract, limiting its efficacy in delivering hydrogel-based formulations for systemic treatments [143]. Each route of administration offers unique advantages, crucial for optimizing the efficacy and safety of hydrogel-mediated drug delivery systems in clinical applications (Figure 7).

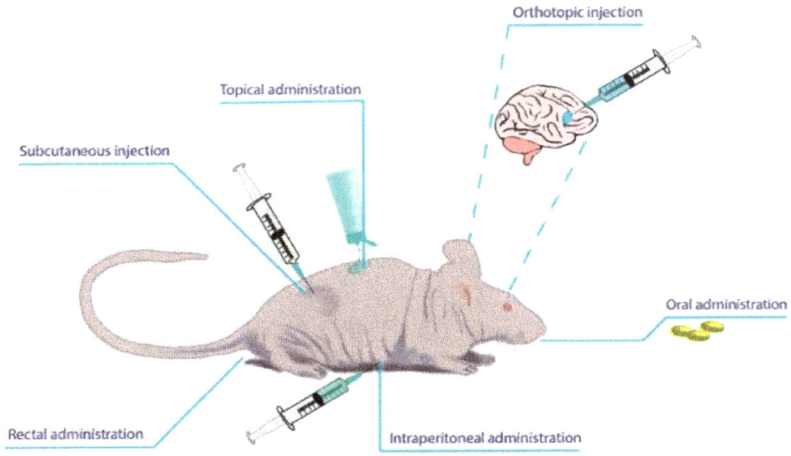

Figure 7. In vivo drug delivery routes of hydrogel administration. There are various methods for in vivo administration of hydrogel-based products depending on the pathological conditions and their localization. Subcutaneous injection plays a crucial role in toxicological effects' evaluation. Topical or transdermal application is preferred for skin-associated problems. Orthotopic and intraperitoneal injections are non-invasive techniques that ensure good therapy results. On the other hand, oral administration has some limitations because of digestive enzymes [144].

5.1. Cancer Therapeutics

Sustained release of PLGA hydrogel formulations is designed to achieve the desired pharmacokinetic profile suitable for localized drug delivery. PLGA, being the most widely used biodegradable polymer in the field of drug delivery, offers the advantage of modulating the release kinetics by tweaking the physicochemical properties, molecular weight, and blend ratio with other biodegradable polymers. Rationally designed PLGA nanoparticles and microspheres integrated within the PLGA hydrogel achieve the sustained release profile. Furthermore, it is shown that the gel matrix can afford synergistic release kinetics. The presence of nanoparticles and microspheres that can hold significant amounts of a drug allows the hydrogel to maintain the initial drug release rates, even for loaded amounts that are potentially higher than what can be offered within the hydrogel itself [145].

Sustained release of chemotherapeutic drugs is an attractive concept in cancer treatment. Certain FDA-approved drugs commonly used in chemotherapy have narrow therapeutic windows where small doses can be therapeutically effective, but higher doses may result in serious side effects. A popular route for localized drug delivery for cancer treatment is through intratumoral injection, where the drug directly enters the tumor. However, intratumoral injection of drugs does away with the dose-sparing effect obtained by using other routes, since a significant amount of the drug is locally or regionally injected. Therefore, a controlled release formulation for local injection can minimize the frequency of drug injections, avoiding declines between repeated injections while maintaining the therapeutic level at the target site for an extended period of time. In the case of localized drug delivery, the requirement of indefinite or chronic expression of the drug to maintain a pharmacological effect essentially translates to the sustained release of the drug [146].

There have been innovations from chemical medicines to immunosuppressive agents and pro-drugs. Use of sustained release is the most significant strategy to extend the block time at the tumor and ensure the least side effects from chemotherapy. Therefore, the innovation should focus on developing various PLGA hydrogels in order to reach comprehensive effects in chemical gene combination chemotherapy based on self-assembly. The hydrogel shell disappears at the moment of contact with apoptosis bodies and exerts excellent properties. Moreover, controllable side-drug release can avoid damage to normal cells. Additionally, controlled release protects the drug in the body by reducing repairs in patients. However, the PLGA hydrogel limits the clinical efficacy because of unsatisfied drug release kinetics for different diseases. Therefore, clinical and global academic innovations are required for various autoimmune diseases [147,148].

Cancer therapeutics are the most developed application of PLGA hydrogels in clinical trials and commercial products. Doxil (Doerr®), which is a rapid slow release of doxorubicin, has been commercially available since 1995. A self-assembled PLGA hydrogel is another delivery platform for the rapid and sustained release of doxorubicin [149]. PLGA-based formulations have shown significant cancer therapeutics potential. In many clinical trials for camptothecin, doxorubicin, paclitaxel, and hydroxycamptothecin intravenous injections, most patients achieved CR (complete remission) or PR (partial remission) among the patients in the effective evaluation group, and the symptoms in the control of the distant tumor were obviously inhibited by the sustained release effect of the drug. The 5-Fu hydrogel implant can prolong the release of the drug, and the blood concentration of the drug reaches a high concentration under continuous action, inhibiting the DNA and RNA metabolism of tumor cells. At the same time, GHCR has achieved great success in the prevention of liver cancer and breast cancer using liquid embolization of polymerized drugs (LEPD) and gel micelles [150].

5.2. Antibiotics and Antimicrobials

Meanwhile, the increasing growth of antibiotic resistance has become an urgent issue and weakens the therapeutic efficacy of antibiotics, leading to a high financial burden and increased mortality, competing with cancer. The question arises of what to do to combat drug resistance and launch the continuous production of new antibiotics with novel mechanisms [151]. In response, 3D printing, known for its high versatility in producing 3D structures with designed architectures, has been widely used to produce 3D scaffolds for bacterial purification and drug release of various antibiotics. In addition, it can be directly integrated with filament formulations of drugs as well as metal oxide nanoparticles to fabricate antibacterial materials by hybrid methods. This technology can not only provide high flexibility for fabricating complex and customized structures but also enable region-controlled drug release and site-specific treatment [152].

PLGA hydrogels are promising for localized drug release, and their development has been moving toward an advanced stage. Over the past decade, hydrogels made with PLGA and polyethylene glycol (PEG) have been extensively developed for the sustained delivery of antibiotics and antimicrobials. These hydrogels have demonstrated excellent performance for anti-infection in vivo. A number of antibiotics, ranging from small molecules like ofloxacin, ciprofloxacin, and gentamicin to large proteins like LL-37, have been successfully encapsulated in PLGA hydrogel and released for an extended period without any loss of original activity. More importantly, through optimized formulations or post-synthesis treatment, the hydrogels do not cause any harm or side effects to the local cells during drug release, both in vitro and in vivo [153].

In skeletal tissue engineering and spinal fusion, PLGA hydrogel has been extensively studied, primarily due to its bone tissue compatibility. A study used PLGA hydrogel to encapsulate gentamicin and reported that PLGA hydrogels exhibited an ability to control gentamicin release and exhibited sustained release over a 56-day study at concentrations remaining above the bacteria sensitivity level. Another study investigated a PLGA hydrogel containing vancomycin and studied the effects of antimicrobial activity and degradation-related cytotoxicity. These results suggest a potential use for PLGA hydrogel in clinical applications requiring localized release of antibiotics at a minimal repeated dose for the prevention of surgical site infections [154,155].

As a class of persistent clinical problems, hardware-associated infection (HAI) is caused by bacterial colonization and biofilm formation on the surface of surgical implants, such as plates, screws, and balance nails, which are often used directly or temporarily in the clinic [156]. For the prevention and treatment of HAI, the local administration of high-concentration antibiotics plays an important role because the systemic administration of antibiotics not only cannot achieve an efficient therapeutic concentration but also results in inevitable side effects. Therefore, a variety of polymers, metal nanoparticles, and fibers have been used to load antibiotics to prepare local antibiotic delivery systems. The high-density pores in hydrogels can provide a reserve for loading growth factors and antibiotics, while the water content satisfies the water environment that is favorable for the activities of transplanted cells [157].

6. Challenges and Future Perspectives in PLGA Hydrogel Research

This section presents the utilization of PLGA hydrogel-based products in clinical trials aimed at achieving sustained drug release. Table 2 provides a comprehensive summary of various completed clinical trials investigating the efficacy and safety of PLGA hydrogels across different medical applications. By examining these studies, we can gain valuable insights into the potential of PLGA hydrogels to improve treatment outcomes and improve patient compliance.

Table 2. Summary of Commercial PLGA-Based Products.

Commercial Product	Drug Release in PLGA Matrix	Benefit	Reference
Lupron Depot	Leuprolide acetate released over 1–6 months	Treats prostate cancer, endometriosis, and uterine fibroids with sustained release	[158]
Zoladex	Goserelin acetate released over 1–3 months	Provides hormone therapy for prostate and breast cancer with controlled release	[159]
Sandostatin LAR	Octreotide acetate released over 1 month	Treats acromegaly and severe diarrhea by sustained drug levels	[160]
Risperdal Consta	Risperidone released over 2 weeks	Treats schizophrenia with prolonged therapeutic effect	[161]

PLGA has low cost and excellent biocompatibility. Moreover, it has been approved by the Food and Drug Administration (US FDA) for therapeutic medicine application. However, it has a hydrophobic nature and the experimental procedures have required toxic reagents. The adding processes only require mechanical force without damage to cell viability at the mixing or injected points. The synthesized PLGA hydrogel has good biocompatibility [162].

Over the last decade, the use of the copolymer poly(l-lactide-co-glycolide) (PLGA) has become widespread, in part due to its versatility and the physical forms that it can be induced to take, such as sutures, pins, screws, films, and microparticles. The desired characteristics of PLGA have been exploited to realize a range of applications that take advantage of its biocompatibility and biodegradability. In addition, hydrogels based on PLGA copolymers have been developed. One of the most versatile polymers currently available in the biomedical field is PLGA, successfully developed for drug therapy, wound healing therapy in the form of adsorbed sheets, and devices in the form of injectable microparticle-based formulations that possess desirable properties [37]. The incorporation of PLGA microparticles into polymeric hydrogels further extends their utility in a broad range of clinical applications and shows this combination to hold the potential to create the ultimate sustained release system. An overview of the development and applications of the PLGA employed as microparticles and the newly developed PLGA hydrogel is given [163]. Biodegradable PLGA hydrogels, in vitro or in vivo, have been applied to collagen, chitosan, gelatin, hyaluronic acid, etc. Usually, based on their own combined self-crosslinking and other crosslinking methods, they are often involved in several analytical methods, including tensile strength, brittleness, biodegradability, adult stem cells, growth factors, enzymes, antibacterial agents, factors with slow release effects, and gene factors. These can be combined to focus on the development of regenerative medicine, cancer treatment, and many other needs [164].

Enhanced Drug Loading and Release Control

PLGA-based nanoparticles have been used to control the drug release through an inactive bake-cast method. Methoxy poly(ethylene glycol)-b-poly(L-lactide-co-N-2-(N′3-aminopropyl)guanidine-L-aspartamide) (mPEG-b-PLA-co-PLGA) or PE, both linked with the luteinizing hormone releasing hormone peptide (LHRH), were incorporated into nanoparticles. Liver tissue differences influenced the safety and anti-tumor efficiency of PLGA–Doxin–LHRH nanoparticles [165].

The ophthalmic drug release and biocompatibility of secnidazole PLGA nanoparticles were tested. Other authors observed that an addition of cyclodextrins can release the in vivo model drug encapsulated by PLGA nanoparticles. The developments should improve the effectiveness and therapeutic index [166].

PLGA hydrogels made by dialysis and low temperature can increase encapsulation rates (or loading rates) to a certain extent. Their sol-gel phase transition occurs at low temperature, which does not damage the encapsulated proteins. A PLGA hydrogel prepared at the controlled release stage showed more sustained delivery profiles, even after the introduction of the fresh active ingredient. The increased therapeutic agent release module was physically trapped in the PLGA hydrogel. H. Chen et al. indicated that the PLGA–Porex hydrogel is also effective in maintaining drug release during multiple dosing systems [167]. The porosity control of hydrogel can effectively inhibit drug burst release and greatly control the uptake capacity [168].

7. Conclusions

PLGA hydrogels have emerged as a highly versatile and effective platform for the sustained delivery of therapeutic agents. Their adjustable biodegradability, biocompatibility, and mechanical properties make them suitable for a wide range of biomedical applications. Through their controlled synthesis and strategic modification, PLGA hydrogels can be engineered to provide precise drug release profiles, addressing the unique requirements of various therapeutic scenarios. The successful application of PLGA hydrogels in drug delivery systems for diseases such as cancer, diabetes, and tissue regeneration highlights their potential to significantly improve treatment efficacy and patient compliance.

Despite these promising advancements, several challenges remain, including optimizing drug loading and release kinetics, scaling up production processes, and ensuring consistent performance in clinical settings. Future research should focus on overcoming these obstacles, exploring novel modifications, and integrating advanced technologies such as nanotechnology and personalized medicine approaches. Overall, PLGA hydrogels represent a robust and adaptable platform with the potential to revolutionize the sustained delivery of therapeutic agents and open new horizons in medical treatments and patient care.

Author Contributions: Conceptualization, A.I.V.; methodology, A.I.V.; software, I.N.; validation, A.I.V.; formal analysis, I.N.; investigation, A.I.V. and I.N.; resources, I.N.; data curation, I.N.; writing—original draft preparation, A.I.V. and I.N.; writing—review and editing, A.I.V.; visualization, I.N.; supervision, A.I.V.; project administration, I.N.; funding acquisition, I.N. All authors have read and agreed to the published version of the manuscript.

Funding: This work was founded by the Romanian Ministry of Education and Research, under Romanian National Nucleu Program LAPLAS VII—contract no. 30N/2023. I.N. acknowledges the support of a grant of the Ministry of Research, Innovation and Digitization, CNCS—UEFISCDI, project no. PN-III-P2-2.1-PED-2021-3178 within PNCDI III.

Institutional Review Board Statement: Not applicable.

Informed Consent Statement: Not applicable.

Data Availability Statement: Not applicable.

Conflicts of Interest: The authors declare no conflicts of interest.

References

1. Rahmani, F.; Atabaki, R.; Behrouzi, S.; Mohamadpour, F.; Kamali, H. The recent advancement in the PLGA-based thermo-sensitive hydrogel for smart drug delivery. *Int. J. Pharm.* **2023**, *631*, 122484. [CrossRef] [PubMed]
2. Jayakumar, A.; Jose, V.K.; Lee, J.M. Hydrogels for medical and environmental applications. *Small Methods* **2020**, *4*, 1900735. [CrossRef]
3. Liu, X.; Gao, M.; Chen, J.; Guo, S.; Zhu, W.; Bai, L.; Zhai, W.; Du, H.; Wu, H.; Yan, C. Recent advances in stimuli-responsive shape-morphing hydrogels. *Adv. Funct. Mater.* **2022**, *32*, 2203323. [CrossRef]
4. Ding, M.; Jing, L.; Yang, H.; Machnicki, C.; Fu, X.; Li, K.; Wong, I.; Chen, P.-Y. Multifunctional soft machines based on stimuli-responsive hydrogels: From freestanding hydrogels to smart integrated systems. *Mater. Today Adv.* **2020**, *8*, 100088. [CrossRef]

5. Gholamali, I. Stimuli-responsive polysaccharide hydrogels for biomedical applications: A review. *Regen. Eng. Transl. Med.* **2021**, *7*, 91–114. [CrossRef]
6. Bordbar-Khiabani, A.; Gasik, M. Smart hydrogels for advanced drug delivery systems. *Int. J. Mol. Sci.* **2022**, *23*, 3665. [CrossRef]
7. Liu, X.; Nakamura, K.; Lowman, A. Composite hydrogels for sustained release of therapeutic agents. *Soft Mater.* **2003**, *1*, 393–408. [CrossRef]
8. Liu, Y.; Zhao, Z.; Guo, C.; Huang, Z.; Zhang, W.; Ma, F.; Wang, Z.; Kong, Q.; Wang, Y. Application and development of hydrogel biomaterials for the treatment of intervertebral disc degeneration: A literature review. *Front. Cell Dev. Biol.* **2023**, *11*, 1286223. [CrossRef]
9. Cisneros, K.; Chowdhury, N.; Coleman, E.; Ferdous, T.; Su, H.; Jennings, J.A.; Bumgardner, J.D.; Fujiwara, T. Long-Term Controlled Release of Simvastatin from Photoprinted Triple-Networked Hydrogels Composed of Modified Chitosan and PLA–PEG Micelles. *Macromol. Biosci.* **2021**, *21*, 2100123. [CrossRef]
10. Alsaab, H.O.; Alharbi, F.D.; Alhibs, A.S.; Alanazi, N.B.; Alshehri, B.Y.; Saleh, M.A.; Alshehri, F.S.; Algarni, M.A.; Almugaiteeb, T.; Uddin, M.N. PLGA-based nanomedicine: History of advancement and development in clinical applications of multiple diseases. *Pharmaceutics* **2022**, *14*, 2728. [CrossRef]
11. Goncalves, A.D.; Balestri, W.; Reinwald, Y. Biomedical implants for regenerative therapies. In *Biomaterials*; IntechOpen: Rijeka, Croatia, 2020; pp. 1–36.
12. Chopra, H.; Singh, I.; Kumar, S.; Bhattacharya, T.; Rahman, M.H.; Akter, R.; Kabir, M.T. A comprehensive review on hydrogels. *Curr. Drug Deliv.* **2022**, *19*, 658–675.
13. Huang, J.; Ali, S. PLGA—A versatile copolymer for design and development of nanoparticles for drug delivery. *J. Anal. Pharm. Res.* **2023**, *12*, 72–78.
14. Ahn, W.; Lee, J.-H.; Kim, S.R.; Lee, J.; Lee, E.J. Designed protein-and peptide-based hydrogels for biomedical sciences. *J. Mater. Chem. B* **2021**, *9*, 1919–1940. [CrossRef]
15. Wall, V.; Nguyen, T.-H.; Nguyen, N.; Tran, P.A. Controlling antibiotic release from polymethylmethacrylate bone cement. *Biomedicines* **2021**, *9*, 26. [CrossRef] [PubMed]
16. Rocha, C.V.; Gonçalves, V.; da Silva, M.C.; Bañobre-López, M.; Gallo, J. PLGA-based composites for various biomedical applications. *Int. J. Mol. Sci.* **2022**, *23*, 2034. [CrossRef]
17. Bhushan, S.; Singh, S.; Maiti, T.K.; Sharma, C.; Dutt, D.; Sharma, S.; Li, C.; Tag Eldin, E.M. Scaffold fabrication techniques of biomaterials for bone tissue engineering: A critical review. *Bioengineering* **2022**, *9*, 728. [CrossRef]
18. Silvestri, T.; Grumetto, L.; Neri, I.; De Falco, M.; Graziano, S.F.; Damiano, S.; Giaquinto, D.; Maruccio, L.; de Girolamo, P.; Villapiano, F. Investigating the effect of surface hydrophilicity on the destiny of PLGA-poloxamer nanoparticles in an in vivo animal model. *Int. J. Mol. Sci.* **2023**, *24*, 14523. [CrossRef]
19. Zhuang, Y.; Shen, H.; Yang, F.; Wang, X.; Wu, D. Synthesis and characterization of PLGA nanoparticle/4-arm-PEG hybrid hydrogels with controlled porous structures. *RSC Adv.* **2016**, *6*, 53804–53812. [CrossRef]
20. Wang, Y.; Li, Q.; Zhou, J.-E.; Tan, J.; Li, M.; Xu, N.; Qu, F.; Chen, J.; Li, J.; Wang, J. A photopolymerized semi-interpenetrating polymer networks-based hydrogel incorporated with nanoparticle for local chemotherapy of tumors. *Pharm. Res.* **2021**, *38*, 669–680. [CrossRef]
21. Hsu, X.-L.; Wu, L.-C.; Hsieh, J.-Y.; Huang, Y.-Y. Nanoparticle-hydrogel composite drug delivery system for potential ocular applications. *Polymers* **2021**, *13*, 642. [CrossRef]
22. Wang, Z.; Liu, B.; Tu, J.; Xiang, J.; Xiong, H.; Wu, Y.; Ding, S.; Zhu, D.; Zhu, D.; Liu, F. PLGA nanoparticles loaded with sorafenib combined with thermosensitive hydrogel system and microwave hyperthermia for multiple sensitized radiotherapy. *Pharmaceutics* **2023**, *15*, 487. [CrossRef]
23. Kong, X.; Houzong, R.; Fu, J.; Shao, K.; Wang, L.; Ma, Y.; Shi, J. Application of a novel thermo-sensitive injectable hydrogel in therapy in situ for drug accurate controlled release. *J. Biomed. Mater. Res. Part B Appl. Biomater.* **2020**, *108*, 3200–3216. [CrossRef]
24. Folle, C.; Díaz-Garrido, N.; Mallandrich, M.; Suñer-Carbó, J.; Sánchez-López, E.; Halbaut, L.; Marqués, A.M.; Espina, M.; Badia, J.; Baldoma, L. Hydrogel of thyme-Oil-PLGA nanoparticles designed for skin inflammation treatment. *Gels* **2024**, *10*, 149. [CrossRef]
25. Anderson, J.M.; Shive, M.S. Biodegradation and biocompatibility of PLA and PLGA microspheres. *Adv. Drug Deliv. Rev.* **1997**, *28*, 5–24. [CrossRef] [PubMed]
26. Gentile, P.; Chiono, V.; Carmagnola, I.; Hatton, P.V. An overview of poly (lactic-co-glycolic) acid (PLGA)-based biomaterials for bone tissue engineering. *Int. J. Mol. Sci.* **2014**, *15*, 3640–3659. [CrossRef]
27. Danhier, F.; Ansorena, E.; Silva, J.M.; Coco, R.; Le Breton, A.; Préat, V. PLGA-based nanoparticles: An overview of biomedical applications. *J. Control. Release* **2012**, *161*, 505–522. [CrossRef] [PubMed]
28. El-Hammadi, M.M.; Arias, J.L. Recent advances in the surface functionalization of PLGA-based nanomedicines. *Nanomaterials* **2022**, *12*, 354. [CrossRef]
29. Jemison, M.; Olabisi, R. Biomaterials for human space exploration: A review of their untapped potential. *Acta Biomater.* **2021**, *128*, 77–99. [CrossRef]
30. Kheder, N.A.; Mabkhot, Y.N. Synthesis and Antimicrobial Studies of Some Novel Bis-[1,3,4] thiadiazole and Bis-thiazole Pendant to Thieno [2,3-b] thiophene Moiety. *Int. J. Mol. Sci.* **2012**, *13*, 3661–3670. [CrossRef] [PubMed]
31. Makadia, H.K.; Siegel, S.J. Poly lactic-co-glycolic acid (PLGA) as biodegradable controlled drug delivery carrier. *Polymers* **2011**, *3*, 1377–1397. [CrossRef]

32. Zhang, Y.; Chan, H.F.; Leong, K.W. Advanced materials and processing for drug delivery: The past and the future. *Adv. Drug Deliv. Rev.* **2013**, *65*, 104–120. [CrossRef] [PubMed]
33. Veld, M.A.; Palmans, A.R. Hydrolases part I: Enzyme mechanism, selectivity and control in the synthesis of well-defined polymers. *Enzym. Polym.* **2011**, *237*, 55–78.
34. Ngwuluka, N.C.; Choonara, Y.E.; Kumar, P.; Du Toit, L.C.; Khan, R.A.; Pillay, V. A novel pH-responsive interpolyelectrolyte hydrogel complex for the oral delivery of levodopa. Part I. IPEC modeling and synthesis. *J. Biomed. Mater. Res. Part A* **2015**, *103*, 1077–1084. [CrossRef] [PubMed]
35. Feng, Q.; Yu, M.-Z.; Wang, J.-C.; Hou, W.-J.; Gao, L.-Y.; Ma, X.-F.; Pei, X.-W.; Niu, Y.-J.; Liu, X.-Y.; Qiu, C. Synergistic inhibition of breast cancer by co-delivery of VEGF siRNA and paclitaxel via vapreotide-modified core–shell nanoparticles. *Biomaterials* **2014**, *35*, 5028–5038. [CrossRef] [PubMed]
36. Hawthorne, D.; Pannala, A.; Sandeman, S.; Lloyd, A. Sustained and targeted delivery of hydrophilic drug compounds: A review of existing and novel technologies from bench to bedside. *J. Drug Deliv. Sci. Technol.* **2022**, *78*, 103936. [CrossRef]
37. Jin, S.; Xia, X.; Huang, J.; Yuan, C.; Zuo, Y.; Li, Y.; Li, J. Recent advances in PLGA-based biomaterials for bone tissue regeneration. *Acta Biomater.* **2021**, *127*, 56–79. [CrossRef] [PubMed]
38. Gebreel, R.M.; Edris, N.A.; Elmofty, H.M.; Tadros, M.I.; El-Nabarawi, M.A.; Hassan, D.H. Development and characterization of PLGA nanoparticle-laden hydrogels for sustained ocular delivery of norfloxacin in the treatment of pseudomonas keratitis: An experimental study. *Drug Des. Dev. Ther.* **2021**, *15*, 399–418. [CrossRef] [PubMed]
39. Elmowafy, M.; Shalaby, K.; Elkomy, M.H.; Alsaidan, O.A.; Gomaa, H.A.; Abdelgawad, M.A.; Mostafa, E.M. Polymeric nanoparticles for delivery of natural bioactive agents: Recent advances and challenges. *Polymers* **2023**, *15*, 1123. [CrossRef]
40. Cellesi, F. Thermoresponsive hydrogels for cellular delivery. *Ther. Deliv.* **2012**, *3*, 1395–1407. [CrossRef]
41. Jain, R.A. The manufacturing techniques of various drug loaded biodegradable poly (lactide-co-glycolide)(PLGA) devices. *Biomaterials* **2000**, *21*, 2475–2490. [CrossRef]
42. Li, Y.; Wei, R.; Ji, S.; Meng, F.; Zhong, Z. Reversibly crosslinked poly (vinyl alcohol) nanoparticles for triggered release of doxorubicin. *J. Control. Release Off. J. Control. Release Soc.* **2011**, *152*, e54–e55. [CrossRef]
43. Agarwal, S.; Wendorff, J.H.; Greiner, A. Use of electrospinning technique for biomedical applications. *Polymer* **2008**, *49*, 5603–5621. [CrossRef]
44. Lamba, J.K.; Lin, Y.S.; Schuetz, E.G.; Thummel, K.E. Genetic contribution to variable human CYP3A-mediated metabolism. *Adv. Drug Deliv. Rev.* **2002**, *54*, 1271–1294. [CrossRef]
45. Burdick, J.A.; Anseth, K.S. Photoencapsulation of osteoblasts in injectable RGD-modified PEG hydrogels for bone tissue engineering. *Biomaterials* **2002**, *23*, 4315–4323. [CrossRef] [PubMed]
46. Lakshmi, S.; Kumar, S.P.; Jayakrishnan, A. Bacterial adhesion onto azidated poly (vinyl chloride) surfaces. *J. Biomed. Mater. Res.* **2002**, *61*, 26–32. [CrossRef] [PubMed]
47. Chiarantini, L.; Cerasi, A.; Fraternale, A.; Millo, E.; Benatti, U.; Sparnacci, K.; Laus, M.; Ballestri, M.; Tondelli, L. Comparison of novel delivery systems for antisense peptide nucleic acids. *J. Control. Release* **2005**, *109*, 24–36. [CrossRef]
48. Jeong, B.; Bae, Y.H.; Lee, D.S.; Kim, S.W. Biodegradable block copolymers as injectable drug-delivery systems. *Nature* **1997**, *388*, 860–862. [CrossRef] [PubMed]
49. Fouassier, J.P.; Ruhlmann, D.; Erddalane, A. Photoinduced polymerization reactions in the presence of light stabilizers: Reactivity of the photoinitiator in solution and in bulk. *Macromolecules* **1993**, *26*, 721–728. [CrossRef]
50. Akhter, A.; Hayashi, Y.; Sakurai, Y.; Ohga, N.; Hida, K.; Harashima, H. Ligand density at the surface of a nanoparticle and different uptake mechanism: Two important factors for successful siRNA delivery to liver endothelial cells. *Int. J. Pharm.* **2014**, *475*, 227–237. [CrossRef]
51. Pondi, S.B. Controlled-Release of Curcumin from Poly (Lactide-Co-Glycolide) Acid/Albumin/Curcumin and Silica/Albumin/Curcumin Drug-Delivery Systems. Ph.D. Thesis, Universiti Teknologi Malaysia, Johor Bharu, Malaysia, 2017.
52. Astete, C.E.; Sabliov, C.M. Synthesis and characterization of PLGA nanoparticles. *J. Biomater. Sci. Polym. Ed.* **2006**, *17*, 247–289. [CrossRef]
53. Feng, S.-S.; Chien, S. Chemotherapeutic engineering: Application and further development of chemical engineering principles for chemotherapy of cancer and other diseases. *Chem. Eng. Sci.* **2003**, *58*, 4087–4114. [CrossRef]
54. Berkland, C.; King, M.; Cox, A.; Kim, K.K.; Pack, D.W. Precise control of PLG microsphere size provides enhanced control of drug release rate. *J. Control. Release* **2002**, *82*, 137–147. [CrossRef]
55. Freiberg, S.; Zhu, X. Polymer microspheres for controlled drug release. *Int. J. Pharm.* **2004**, *282*, 1–18. [CrossRef]
56. Cleek, R.L.; Ting, K.C.; Eskin, S.G.; Mikos, A.G. Microparticles of poly (DL-lactic-co-glycolic acid)/poly (ethylene glycol) blends for controlled drug delivery. *J. Control. Release* **1997**, *48*, 259–268. [CrossRef]
57. Huang, Z.-M.; Zhang, Y.-Z.; Kotaki, M.; Ramakrishna, S. A review on polymer nanofibers by electrospinning and their applications in nanocomposites. *Compos. Sci. Technol.* **2003**, *63*, 2223–2253. [CrossRef]
58. Li, W.J.; Laurencin, C.T.; Caterson, E.J.; Tuan, R.S.; Ko, F.K. Electrospun nanofibrous structure: A novel scaffold for tissue engineering. *J. Biomed. Mater. Res.* **2002**, *60*, 613–621. [CrossRef] [PubMed]
59. Matthews, J.A.; Wnek, G.E.; Simpson, D.G.; Bowlin, G.L. Electrospinning of collagen nanofibers. *Biomacromolecules* **2002**, *3*, 232–238. [CrossRef]

60. Zhang, Y.; Lim, C.T.; Ramakrishna, S.; Huang, Z.-M. Recent development of polymer nanofibers for biomedical and biotechnological applications. *J. Mater. Sci. Mater. Med.* **2005**, *16*, 933–946. [CrossRef] [PubMed]
61. Kenawy, E.R.; Bowlin, G.L.; Mansfield, K.; Layman, J.; Sanders, E.; Simpson, D.G.; Wnek, G.E. Release of tetracycline hydrochloride from electrospun polymers. *J. Control. Release* **2002**, *81*, 57–64. [CrossRef]
62. Knight, P.T.; Kirk, J.T.; Anderson, J.M.; Mather, P.T. In vivo kinetic degradation analysis and biocompatibility of aliphatic polyester polyurethanes. *J. Biomed. Mater. Res. Part A* **2010**, *94*, 333–343. [CrossRef]
63. Peng, L.; Eltgroth, M.L.; LaTempa, T.J.; Grimes, C.A.; Desai, T.A. The effect of TiO_2 nanotubes on endothelial function and smooth muscle proliferation. *Biomaterials* **2009**, *30*, 1268–1272. [CrossRef]
64. Yang, Y.-Y.; Chung, T.-S.; Bai, X.-L.; Chan, W.-K. Effect of preparation conditions on morphology and release profiles of biodegradable polymeric microspheres containing protein fabricated by double-emulsion method. *Chem. Eng. Sci.* **2000**, *55*, 2223–2236. [CrossRef]
65. Schnieders, J.; Gbureck, U.; Thull, R.; Kissel, T. Controlled release of gentamicin from calcium phosphate—Poly (lactic acid-co-glycolic acid) composite bone cement. *Biomaterials* **2006**, *27*, 4239–4249. [CrossRef] [PubMed]
66. Guan, J.; Sacks, M.S.; Beckman, E.J.; Wagner, W.R. Biodegradable poly (ether ester urethane) urea elastomers based on poly (ether ester) triblock copolymers and putrescine: Synthesis, characterization and cytocompatibility. *Biomaterials* **2004**, *25*, 85–96. [CrossRef]
67. Zhang, K.; Xue, K.; Loh, X.J. Thermo-responsive hydrogels: From recent progress to biomedical applications. *Gels* **2021**, *7*, 77. [CrossRef] [PubMed]
68. Maeda, T. Structures and applications of thermoresponsive hydrogels and nanocomposite-hydrogels based on copolymers with poly (Ethylene glycol) and poly (lactide-co-glycolide) blocks. *Bioengineering* **2019**, *6*, 107. [CrossRef] [PubMed]
69. Xue, B.; Qu, Y.; Shi, K.; Zhou, K.; He, X.; Chu, B.; Qian, Z. Advances in the application of injectable thermosensitive hydrogel systems for cancer therapy. *J. Biomed. Nanotechnol.* **2020**, *16*, 1427–1453. [CrossRef] [PubMed]
70. Zawani, M.; Fauzi, M.B. Injectable hydrogels for chronic skin wound management: A concise review. *Biomedicines* **2021**, *9*, 527. [CrossRef]
71. Mantripragada, V.P.; Jayasuriya, A.C. Injectable chitosan microparticles incorporating bone morphogenetic protein-7 for bone tissue regeneration. *J. Biomed. Mater. Res. Part A* **2014**, *102*, 4276–4289. [CrossRef]
72. Giacca, M.; Zacchigna, S. Virus-mediated gene delivery for human gene therapy. *J. Control. Release* **2012**, *161*, 377–388. [CrossRef]
73. Elisseeff, J.; Anseth, K.; Sims, D.; McIntosh, W.; Randolph, M.; Langer, R. Transdermal photopolymerization for minimally invasive implantation. *Proc. Natl. Acad. Sci. USA* **1999**, *96*, 3104–3107. [CrossRef] [PubMed]
74. Elomaa, L.; Teixeira, S.; Hakala, R.; Korhonen, H.; Grijpma, D.W.; Seppälä, J.V. Preparation of poly (ε-caprolactone)-based tissue engineering scaffolds by stereolithography. *Acta Biomater.* **2011**, *7*, 3850–3856. [CrossRef]
75. Ratzinger, G.; Agrawal, P.; Körner, W.; Lonkai, J.; Sanders, H.M.; Terreno, E.; Wirth, M.; Strijkers, G.J.; Nicolay, K.; Gabor, F. Surface modification of PLGA nanospheres with Gd-DTPA and Gd-DOTA for high-relaxivity MRI contrast agents. *Biomaterials* **2010**, *31*, 8716–8723. [CrossRef] [PubMed]
76. Bai, X.; Gao, M.; Syed, S.; Zhuang, J.; Xu, X.; Zhang, X.-Q. Bioactive hydrogels for bone regeneration. *Bioact. Mater.* **2018**, *3*, 401–417. [CrossRef]
77. Ho-Shui-Ling, A.; Bolander, J.; Rustom, L.E.; Johnson, A.W.; Luyten, F.P.; Picart, C. Bone regeneration strategies: Engineered scaffolds, bioactive molecules and stem cells current stage and future perspectives. *Biomaterials* **2018**, *180*, 143–162. [CrossRef] [PubMed]
78. Qi, R.; Guo, R.; Zheng, F.; Liu, H.; Yu, J.; Shi, X. Controlled release and antibacterial activity of antibiotic-loaded electrospun halloysite/poly (lactic-co-glycolic acid) composite nanofibers. *Colloids Surf. B Biointerfaces* **2013**, *110*, 148–155. [CrossRef] [PubMed]
79. Papathanasiou, K.E.; Demadis, K.D. Polymeric matrices for the controlled release of phosphonate active agents for medicinal applications. In *Handbook of Polymers for Pharmaceutical Technologies: Bioactive and Compatible Synthetic/Hybrid Polymers*; Wiley: Hoboken, NJ, USA, 2015; Volume 4, pp. 89–124.
80. Burke, M.D.; Park, J.O.; Srinivasarao, M.; Khan, S.A. A novel enzymatic technique for limiting drug mobility in a hydrogel matrix. *J. Control. Release* **2005**, *104*, 141–153. [CrossRef] [PubMed]
81. Weigel, T.; Schinkel, G.; Lendlein, A. Design and preparation of polymeric scaffolds for tissue engineering. *Expert Rev. Med. Devices* **2006**, *3*, 835–851. [CrossRef] [PubMed]
82. Aksungur, P.; Demirbilek, M.; Denkbaş, E.B.; Vandervoort, J.; Ludwig, A.; Ünlü, N. Development and characterization of Cyclosporine A loaded nanoparticles for ocular drug delivery: Cellular toxicity, uptake, and kinetic studies. *J. Control. Release* **2011**, *151*, 286–294. [CrossRef] [PubMed]
83. Park, J.H.; Ye, M.; Park, K. Biodegradable polymers for microencapsulation of drugs. *Molecules* **2005**, *10*, 146–161. [CrossRef]
84. Kamaly, N.; Xiao, Z.; Valencia, P.M.; Radovic-Moreno, A.F.; Farokhzad, O.C. Targeted polymeric therapeutic nanoparticles: Design, development and clinical translation. *Chem. Soc. Rev.* **2012**, *41*, 2971–3010. [CrossRef]
85. Almeida, H.; Amaral, M.H.; Lobão, P.; Sousa Lobo, J.M. Applications of poloxamers in ophthalmic pharmaceutical formulations: An overview. *Expert Opin. Drug Deliv.* **2013**, *10*, 1223–1237. [CrossRef]
86. Verma, M.S.; Rogowski, J.L.; Jones, L.; Gu, F.X. Colorimetric biosensing of pathogens using gold nanoparticles. *Biotechnol. Adv.* **2015**, *33*, 666–680. [CrossRef]

87. Wassif, R.K.; Elkayal, M.; Shamma, R.N.; Elkheshen, S.A. Recent advances in the local antibiotics delivery systems for management of osteomyelitis. *Drug Deliv.* **2021**, *28*, 2392–2414. [CrossRef]
88. Shichor, I.; Shomron, N.; Lawlor, M.W.; Bae, S.A.; Zoldan, J.; Langer, R.; Kohane, D.S. Toxicogenomic analysis of a sustained release local anesthetic delivery system. *Biomaterials* **2012**, *33*, 3586–3593. [CrossRef]
89. Zheng, Z.; Yin, W.; Zara, J.N.; Li, W.; Kwak, J.; Mamidi, R.; Lee, M.; Siu, R.K.; Ngo, R.; Wang, J. The use of BMP-2 coupled–Nanosilver-PLGA composite grafts to induce bone repair in grossly infected segmental defects. *Biomaterials* **2010**, *31*, 9293–9300. [CrossRef]
90. Sorkin, R.; Kampf, N.; Dror, Y.; Shimoni, E.; Klein, J. Origins of extreme boundary lubrication by phosphatidylcholine liposomes. *Biomaterials* **2013**, *34*, 5465–5475. [CrossRef]
91. Kohane, D.S.; Smith, S.E.; Louis, D.N.; Colombo, G.; Ghoroghchian, P.; Hunfeld, N.G.; Berde, C.B.; Langer, R. Prolonged duration local anesthesia from tetrodotoxin-enhanced local anesthetic microspheres. *Pain* **2003**, *104*, 415–421. [CrossRef]
92. Gref, R.; Minamitake, Y.; Peracchia, M.T.; Trubetskoy, V.; Torchilin, V.; Langer, R. Biodegradable long-circulating polymeric nanospheres. *Science* **1994**, *263*, 1600–1603. [CrossRef]
93. Subramanian, B.; Das, P.; Biswas, S.; Roy, A.; Basak, P. Polymers for Additive Manufacturing and 4D-Printing for Tissue Regenerative Applications. In *Advances in Biomedical Polymers and Composites*; Elsevier: Amsterdam, The Netherlands, 2023; pp. 159–182.
94. Duvvuri, S.; Janoria, K.G.; Mitra, A.K. Development of a novel formulation containing poly (d,l-lactide-co-glycolide) microspheres dispersed in PLGA–PEG–PLGA gel for sustained delivery of ganciclovir. *J. Control. Release* **2005**, *108*, 282–293. [CrossRef]
95. Lu, Y.; Park, K. Polymeric micelles and alternative nanonized delivery vehicles for poorly soluble drugs. *Int. J. Pharm.* **2013**, *453*, 198–214. [CrossRef]
96. Xu, Q.; Xu, H.; Gu, H.; Li, J.; Wang, Y.; Wei, M. Development of lateral flow immunoassay system based on superparamagnetic nanobeads as labels for rapid quantitative detection of cardiac troponin I. *Mater. Sci. Eng. C* **2009**, *29*, 702–707. [CrossRef]
97. Liu, L.; Zhou, X.; Xu, Y.; Zhang, W.; Liu, C.-H.; Wang, X. Controlled release of growth factors for regenerative medicine. *Curr. Pharm. Des.* **2015**, *21*, 1627–1632. [CrossRef] [PubMed]
98. Seo, B.-B.; Kwon, Y.; Kim, J.; Hong, K.H.; Kim, S.-E.; Song, H.-R.; Kim, Y.-M.; Song, S.-C. Injectable polymeric nanoparticle hydrogel system for long-term anti-inflammatory effect to treat osteoarthritis. *Bioact. Mater.* **2022**, *7*, 14–25. [CrossRef] [PubMed]
99. Ciolino, J.B.; Hoare, T.R.; Iwata, N.G.; Behlau, I.; Dohlman, C.H.; Langer, R.; Kohane, D.S. A drug-eluting contact lens. *Investig. Ophthalmol. Vis. Sci.* **2009**, *50*, 3346–3352. [CrossRef] [PubMed]
100. Nguyen, M.K.; Lee, D.S. Injectable biodegradable hydrogels. *Macromol. Biosci.* **2010**, *10*, 563–579. [CrossRef] [PubMed]
101. Liu, P.; Gu, L.; Ren, L.; Chen, J.; Li, T.; Wang, X.; Yang, J.; Chen, C.; Sun, L. Intra-articular injection of etoricoxib-loaded PLGA-PEG-PLGA triblock copolymeric nanoparticles attenuates osteoarthritis progression. *Am. J. Transl. Res.* **2019**, *11*, 6775. [PubMed]
102. Jaiswal, L.; Limayem, A.; Shankar, S. Polysaccharide-based nanomaterials. In *Food, Medical, and Environmental Applications of Nanomaterials*; Elsevier: Amsterdam, The Netherlands, 2022; pp. 95–111.
103. Gaudana, R.; Jwala, J.; Boddu, S.H.; Mitra, A.K. Recent perspectives in ocular drug delivery. *Pharm. Res.* **2009**, *26*, 1197–1216. [CrossRef] [PubMed]
104. Kang, J.; Schwendeman, S.P. Pore closing and opening in biodegradable polymers and their effect on the controlled release of proteins. *Mol. Pharm.* **2007**, *4*, 104–118. [CrossRef]
105. Park, T.G. Degradation of poly (lactic-co-glycolic acid) microspheres: Effect of copolymer composition. *Biomaterials* **1995**, *16*, 1123–1130. [CrossRef]
106. Singh, M.; O'Hagan, D. Advances in vaccine adjuvants. *Nat. Biotechnol.* **1999**, *17*, 1075–1081. [CrossRef] [PubMed]
107. Saroja, C.; Lakshmi, P.; Bhaskaran, S. Recent trends in vaccine delivery systems: A review. *Int. J. Pharm. Investig.* **2011**, *1*, 64. [PubMed]
108. Matichescu, A.; Ardelean, L.C.; Rusu, L.-C.; Craciun, D.; Bratu, E.A.; Babucea, M.; Leretter, M. Advanced biomaterials and techniques for oral tissue engineering and regeneration—A review. *Materials* **2020**, *13*, 5303. [CrossRef] [PubMed]
109. Yang, C.-Y.; Song, B.; Ao, Y.; Nowak, A.P.; Abelowitz, R.B.; Korsak, R.A.; Havton, L.A.; Deming, T.J.; Sofroniew, M.V. Biocompatibility of amphiphilic diblock copolypeptide hydrogels in the central nervous system. *Biomaterials* **2009**, *30*, 2881–2898. [CrossRef] [PubMed]
110. Burdick, J.A.; Mauck, R.L. *Biomaterials for Tissue Engineering Applications: A Review of the Past and Future Trends*; Springer: Vienna, Austria, 2010.
111. Kanczler, J.; Oreffo, R. Osteogenesis and angiogenesis: The potential for engineering bone. *Eur. Cell Mater* **2008**, *15*, 100–114. [CrossRef]
112. Lu, Y.; Cheng, D.; Niu, B.; Wang, X.; Wu, X.; Wang, A. Properties of poly (lactic-co-glycolic acid) and progress of poly (lactic-co-glycolic acid)-based biodegradable materials in biomedical research. *Pharmaceuticals* **2023**, *16*, 454. [CrossRef] [PubMed]
113. Li, J.; Jiang, G.; Ding, F. The effect of pH on the polymer degradation and drug release from PLGA-mPEG microparticles. *J. Appl. Polym. Sci.* **2008**, *109*, 475–482. [CrossRef]
114. Amann, L.C.; Gandal, M.J.; Lin, R.; Liang, Y.; Siegel, S.J. In vitro–in vivo correlations of scalable PLGA-risperidone implants for the treatment of schizophrenia. *Pharm. Res.* **2010**, *27*, 1730–1737. [CrossRef]

115. Wan, B.; Bao, Q.; Burgess, D.J. In vitro-in vivo correlation of PLGA microspheres: Effect of polymer source variation and temperature. *J. Control. Release* **2022**, *347*, 347–355. [CrossRef]
116. Abuzar, S.M.; Ahn, J.-H.; Park, K.S.; Park, E.J.; Baik, S.H.; Hwang, S.-J. Pharmacokinetic profile and anti-adhesive effect of oxaliplatin-PLGA microparticle-loaded hydrogels in rats for colorectal cancer treatment. *Pharmaceutics* **2019**, *11*, 392. [CrossRef]
117. Göpferich, A. Mechanisms of polymer degradation and erosion. In *The Biomaterials: Silver Jubilee Compendium*; Elsevier Science: Oxford, UK, 1996; pp. 117–128.
118. Bermejo, M.; Sanchez-Dengra, B.; Gonzalez-Alvarez, M.; Gonzalez-Alvarez, I. Oral controlled release dosage forms: Dissolution versus diffusion. *Expert Opin. Drug Deliv.* **2020**, *17*, 791–803. [CrossRef]
119. Dhal, C.; Mishra, R. In vitro and in vivo evaluation of gentamicin sulphate-loaded PLGA nanoparticle-based film for the treatment of surgical site infection. *Drug Deliv. Transl. Res.* **2020**, *10*, 1032–1043. [CrossRef]
120. Siepmann, J.; Siepmann, F. Mathematical modeling of drug delivery. *Int. J. Pharm.* **2008**, *364*, 328–343. [CrossRef] [PubMed]
121. Wang, Y.; Fu, M.; Wang, Z.; Zhu, X.; Guan, Y.; Zhang, Y. A sustained zero-order release carrier for long-acting, peakless basal insulin therapy. *J. Mater. Chem. B* **2020**, *8*, 1952–1959. [CrossRef] [PubMed]
122. Mariz, M.; Murta, J.; Gil, M.; Ferreira, P. An ocular insert with zero-order extended delivery: Release kinetics and mathematical models. *Eur. J. Pharm. Biopharm.* **2022**, *181*, 79–87. [CrossRef]
123. Dash, S.; Murthy, P.N.; Nath, L.; Chowdhury, P. Kinetic modeling on drug release from controlled drug delivery systems. *Acta Pol. Pharm.* **2010**, *67*, 217–223.
124. Siepmann, J.; Göpferich, A. Mathematical modeling of bioerodible, polymeric drug delivery systems. *Adv. Drug Deliv. Rev.* **2001**, *48*, 229–247. [CrossRef] [PubMed]
125. Vasir, J.K.; Tambwekar, K.; Garg, S. Bioadhesive microspheres as a controlled drug delivery system. *Int. J. Pharm.* **2003**, *255*, 13–32. [CrossRef]
126. Costa, P.; Lobo, J.M.S. Modeling and comparison of dissolution profiles. *Eur. J. Pharm. Sci.* **2001**, *13*, 123–133. [CrossRef]
127. Ritger, P.L.; Peppas, N.A. A simple equation for description of solute release I. Fickian and non-fickian release from non-swellable devices in the form of slabs, spheres, cylinders or discs. *J. Control. Release* **1987**, *5*, 23–36. [CrossRef]
128. Higuchi, T. Mechanism of sustained-action medication. Theoretical analysis of rate of release of solid drugs dispersed in solid matrices. *J. Pharm. Sci.* **1963**, *52*, 1145–1149. [CrossRef] [PubMed]
129. Noyes, A.A.; Whitney, W.R. The rate of solution of solid substances in their own solutions. *J. Am. Chem. Soc.* **1897**, *19*, 930–934. [CrossRef]
130. Mehryab, F.; Rabbani, S.; Shahhosseini, S.; Shekari, F.; Fatahi, Y.; Baharvand, H.; Haeri, A. Exosomes as a next-generation drug delivery system: An update on drug loading approaches, characterization, and clinical application challenges. *Acta Biomater.* **2020**, *113*, 42–62. [CrossRef] [PubMed]
131. Lim, P.T.; Irwan, R.M.; Li, Z.; Goh, K. Quantifying how drug-polymer interaction and volume phase transition modulate the drug release kinetics from core-shell microgels. *Int. J. Pharm.* **2022**, *622*, 121838. [CrossRef] [PubMed]
132. Vigata, M.; Meinert, C.; Hutmacher, D.W.; Bock, N. Hydrogels as drug delivery systems: A review of current characterization and evaluation techniques. *Pharmaceutics* **2020**, *12*, 1188. [CrossRef] [PubMed]
133. Heredia, N.S.; Vizuete, K.; Flores-Calero, M.; Pazmiño, V.K.; Pilaquinga, F.; Kumar, B.; Debut, A. Comparative statistical analysis of the release kinetics models for nanoprecipitated drug delivery systems based on poly (lactic-co-glycolic acid). *PLoS ONE* **2022**, *17*, e0264825. [CrossRef] [PubMed]
134. Askarizadeh, M.; Esfandiari, N.; Honarvar, B.; Sajadian, S.A.; Azdarpour, A. Kinetic modeling to explain the release of medicine from drug delivery systems. *ChemBioEng Rev.* **2023**, *10*, 1006–1049. [CrossRef]
135. Peppas, N.A.; Korsmeyer, R.W. Dynamically swelling hydrogels in controlled release applications. *Hydrogels Med. Pharm.* **1987**, *3*, 109–136.
136. Siepmann, J.; Peppas, N.A. Modeling of drug release from delivery systems based on hydroxypropyl methylcellulose (HPMC). *Adv. Drug Deliv. Rev.* **2012**, *64*, 163–174. [CrossRef]
137. Harish, N.; Kiran, A.; Rathnanand, M.; Shirwaikar, A.; Shenoy, K. Sustained-release matrix tablets of terbutaline sulphate: Formulation and in vitro evaluation. *Indian Drugs* **2007**, *44*, 233–235.
138. Jafari, S.; Soleimani, M.; Badinezhad, M. Application of different mathematical models for further investigation of in vitro drug release mechanisms based on magnetic nano-composite. *Polym. Bull.* **2022**, *79*, 1021–1038. [CrossRef]
139. Sulttan, S.; Rohani, S. Controlled drug release of smart magnetic self-assembled micelle, kinetics and transport mechanisms. *J. Pharm. Sci.* **2022**, *111*, 2378–2388. [CrossRef] [PubMed]
140. Damodharan, N. Mathematical modelling of dissolution kinetics in dosage forms. *Res. J. Pharm. Technol.* **2020**, *13*, 1339–1345.
141. Ling, Y.; Chen, L.; Huang, M.; Zhou, C.; Yang, L.; Niu, H.; Su, L.; Yang, Y.; Pirraco, R.P.; Reis, R.L. A novel method for the preparation of poly (acrylamide-co-acrylonitrile) upper critical solution temperature thermosensitive hydrogel by the partial dehydration of acrylamide grafted polypropylene sheets. *Gels* **2022**, *8*, 345. [CrossRef]
142. Zhang, Y.; Huang, Y. Rational design of smart hydrogels for biomedical applications. *Front. Chem.* **2021**, *8*, 615665. [CrossRef]
143. Mantha, S.; Pillai, S.; Khayambashi, P.; Upadhyay, A.; Zhang, Y.; Tao, O.; Pham, H.M.; Tran, S.D. Smart hydrogels in tissue engineering and regenerative medicine. *Materials* **2019**, *12*, 3323. [CrossRef] [PubMed]
144. Onaciu, A.; Munteanu, R.A.; Moldovan, A.I.; Moldovan, C.S.; Berindan-Neagoe, I. Hydrogels based drug delivery synthesis, characterization and administration. *Pharmaceutics* **2019**, *11*, 432. [CrossRef] [PubMed]

145. Alvi, M.; Yaqoob, A.; Rehman, K.; Shoaib, S.M.; Akash, M.S.H. PLGA-based nanoparticles for the treatment of cancer: Current strategies and perspectives. *AAPS Open* **2022**, *8*, 12. [CrossRef]
146. Omidi, Y.; Omidian, H. Transformative dynamism in pharmaceutical and biomedical research: Complexity of integration of innovative R & D hubs. *BioImpacts BI* **2021**, *11*, 227–233.
147. Pandey, M.; Choudhury, H.; Abdul-Aziz, A.; Bhattamisra, S.K.; Gorain, B.; Su, J.S.T.; Tan, C.L.; Chin, W.Y.; Yip, K.Y. Advancement on sustained antiviral ocular drug delivery for herpes simplex virus keratitis: Recent update on potential investigation. *Pharmaceutics* **2020**, *13*, 1. [CrossRef]
148. Zhao, Y.; Alakhova, D.Y.; Zhao, X.; Band, V.; Batrakova, E.V.; Kabanov, A.V. Eradication of cancer stem cells in triple negative breast cancer using doxorubicin/pluronic polymeric micelles. *Nanomed. Nanotechnol. Biol. Med.* **2020**, *24*, 102124. [CrossRef] [PubMed]
149. Aloss, K.; Hamar, P. Recent preclinical and clinical progress in liposomal doxorubicin. *Pharmaceutics* **2023**, *15*, 893. [CrossRef] [PubMed]
150. Hiraiwa, M.; Ozaki, K.; Yamada, T.; Iezaki, T.; Park, G.; Fukasawa, K.; Horie, T.; Kamada, H.; Tokumura, K.; Motono, M. mTORC1 activation in osteoclasts prevents bone loss in a mouse model of osteoporosis. *Front. Pharmacol.* **2019**, *10*, 684. [CrossRef] [PubMed]
151. Yang, Q.; Wang, J.; Yang, Y.; Li, S.; Dong, Y.; Sun, Y. In vitro antibacterial effect of vancomycin hydrogel on methicillin-resistant Staphylococcus aureus. *Am. J. Transl. Res.* **2022**, *14*, 3964. [PubMed]
152. Badea, I.-C.; Csaki, I.; Serban, B.-A.; Constantin, N.; Mitrica, D.; Burada, M.; Anasiei, I.; Olaru, M.T.; Ghita, A.-N.; Popescu, A.-M.J. Characterisation of a Novel Complex Concentrated Alloy for Marine Applications. *Materials* **2022**, *15*, 3345. [CrossRef] [PubMed]
153. Handler, A.M.; Fallah, M.; Pedersen, A.J.; Pedersen, G.P.; Nielsen, K.T.; Janfelt, C. MALDI mass spectrometry imaging as a complementary analytical method for improved skin distribution analysis of drug molecule and excipients. *Int. J. Pharm.* **2020**, *590*, 119949. [CrossRef] [PubMed]
154. Mulliez, M.A.; Schilling, C.; Grupp, T.M. Equivalent mechanical properties of X-ray and E-beam cross-linked vitamin E blended ultrahigh molecular weight polyethylene. *J. Biomed. Mater. Res. Part B Appl. Biomater.* **2020**, *108*, 2131–2140. [CrossRef]
155. Nazarkina, Z.K.; Chelobanov, B.P.; Kuznetsov, K.A.; Shutov, A.V.; Romanova, I.V.; Karpenko, A.A.; Laktionov, P.P. Influence of elongation of paclitaxel-eluting electrospun-produced stent coating on paclitaxel release and transport through the arterial wall after stenting. *Polymers* **2021**, *13*, 1165. [CrossRef]
156. Jana, S.; Jana, S. *Nanoengineering of Biomaterials: Drug Delivery & Biomedical Applications*; John Wiley & Sons: Hoboken, NJ, USA, 2022.
157. Podsiadły, B.; Skalski, A.; Słoma, M. Soldering of electronics components on 3D-printed conductive substrates. *Materials* **2021**, *14*, 3850. [CrossRef]
158. Okada, H. One-and three-month release injectable microspheres of the LH-RH superagonist leuprorelin acetate. *Adv. Drug Deliv. Rev.* **1997**, *28*, 43–70. [CrossRef]
159. Ullman, F.; Boutellier, R. A case study of lean drug discovery: From project driven research to innovation studios and process factories. *Drug Discov. Today* **2008**, *13*, 543–550. [CrossRef] [PubMed]
160. Costa, F.; Gumz, B. Octreotide–a review of its use in treating neuroendocrine tumours. *Eur. Endocrinol.* **2014**, *10*, 70.
161. Kane, J.M.; Eerdekens, M.; Lindenmayer, J.-P.; Keith, S.J.; Lesem, M.; Karcher, K. Long-acting injectable risperidone: Efficacy and safety of the first long-acting atypical antipsychotic. *Am. J. Psychiatry* **2003**, *160*, 1125–1132. [CrossRef] [PubMed]
162. Sun, H.; Kong, H.; Ding, H.; Xu, Q.; Zeng, J.; Jiang, F.; Yu, M.; Zhang, Y. Improving UV resistance of aramid fibers by simultaneously synthesizing TiO_2 on their surfaces and in the interfaces between fibrils/microfibrils using supercritical carbon dioxide. *Polymers* **2020**, *12*, 147. [CrossRef] [PubMed]
163. Magalhaes, S.S.; Alves, L.; Sebastiao, M.; Medronho, B.; Almeida, Z.L.; Faria, T.Q.; Brito, R.M.; Moreno, M.J.; Antunes, F.E. Effect of ethyleneoxide groups of anionic surfactants on lipase activity. *Biotechnol. Prog.* **2016**, *32*, 1276–1282. [CrossRef] [PubMed]
164. Bello, A.B.; Kim, D.; Kim, D.; Park, H.; Lee, S.-H. Engineering and functionalization of gelatin biomaterials: From cell culture to medical applications. *Tissue Eng. Part B Rev.* **2020**, *26*, 164–180. [CrossRef] [PubMed]
165. Delgado, J.F.; Peltzer, M.A.; Wagner, J.R.; Salvay, A.G. Hydration and water vapour transport properties in yeast biomass based films: A study of plasticizer content and thickness effects. *Eur. Polym. J.* **2018**, *99*, 9–17. [CrossRef]
166. Vaidya, B.; Parvathaneni, V.; Kulkarni, N.S.; Shukla, S.K.; Damon, J.K.; Sarode, A.; Kanabar, D.; Garcia, J.V.; Mitragotri, S.; Muth, A. Cyclodextrin modified erlotinib loaded PLGA nanoparticles for improved therapeutic efficacy against non-small cell lung cancer. *Int. J. Biol. Macromol.* **2019**, *122*, 338–347. [CrossRef] [PubMed]
167. Chen, H.; Cheng, J.; Ran, L.; Yu, K.; Lu, B.; Lan, G.; Dai, F.; Lu, F. An injectable self-healing hydrogel with adhesive and antibacterial properties effectively promotes wound healing. *Carbohydr. Polym.* **2018**, *201*, 522–531. [CrossRef]
168. Scharber, M.C.; Sariciftci, N.S. Efficiency of bulk-heterojunction organic solar cells. *Prog. Polym. Sci.* **2013**, *38*, 1929–1940. [CrossRef]

gels

MDPI

Article

A pH-Responsive Hydrogel for the Oral Delivery of Ursolic Acid: A Pentacyclic Triterpenoid Phytochemical

Carlos D. Gutierrez [1], Rosana L. Aranzábal [1], Ana M. Lechuga [1], Carlos A. Serrano [1], Flor Meza [2], Carlos Elvira [3], Alberto Gallardo [3] and Michael A. Ludeña [1,*]

[1] Department of Chemistry, Faculty of Chemical, Physical and Mathematical Sciences, National University of San Antonio Abad del Cusco (UNSAAC), Av. De la Cultura 733, Cusco 921, Peru; 170595@unsaac.edu.pe (C.D.G.); rosana.aranzabal@unsaac.edu.pe (R.L.A.); ana.lechuga@unsaac.edu.pe (A.M.L.); carlos.serrano@unsaac.edu.pe (C.A.S.)

[2] Technology of Materials for Environmental Remediation Group (TecMARA), Faculty of Sciences, National University of Engineering, Av. Tupac Amaru 210, Rimac 15333, Peru; flor.meza.l@uni.pe

[3] Institute of Polymer Science and Technology (ICTP-CSIC), Juan de la Cierva 3, 28006 Madrid, Spain; celvira@ictp.csic.es (C.E.); gallardo@ictp.csic.es (A.G.)

* Correspondence: michael.ludenah@unsaac.edu.pe; Tel.: +51-9633-58246

Abstract: In this study, poly(HEMA-PEGxMEM-IA) hydrogels were prepared by radical copolymerization of poly(ethylene glycol) methyl ether methacrylate (PEGxMEM), 2-hydroxyethyl methacrylate (HEMA), and itaconic acid (IA). The reaction was carried out in ethanolic solution using N,N′-methylenebisacrylamide (MBA) as a crosslinking agent and 1-hydroxycyclohexyl phenyl ketone (HCPK) as a photo-initiator. The poly(HEMA-PEGxMEM-IA) hydrogels (HGx) were evaluated as a delivery system for ursolic acid (UA), a phytochemical extracted from the plant *Clinopodium revolutum,* "flor de arena". The hydrogels were characterized by Fourier-transform infrared spectroscopy (FTIR-ATR), Raman spectroscopy, X-Ray diffraction (XRD), thermogravimetric analysis (TGA), and scanning electron microscopy (SEM). The swelling behavior was studied in buffer solutions from pH 2 to 10, specifically at pH 2.2 (gastric environment) and 7.4 (intestinal environment). It was found that the hydrogels studied showed sensitivity to pH. At pH 2.2, the degree of swelling for HG_5 and HG_9 hydrogels was 0.45 and 0.93 (g water/g hydrogel), respectively. At pH 7.4, the degree of swelling for HG_5 and HG_9 hydrogels was 1.97 and 2.64 (g water/g hydrogel), respectively. The SEM images show the variation in pore size as a function of pH, and the UA crystals in the pores of the hydrogels can also be observed. The in vitro UA release data best fit the Korsmeyer–Peppas kinetic model and the diffusion exponent indicates that the release mechanism is governed by Fickian diffusion.

Keywords: hydrogel; pH-responsive; ursolic acid; release; delivery; itaconic acid; 2-hydroxyethylmethacrylate

1. Introduction

Ursolic acid (UA) is a pentacyclic triterpene of pharmacological interest due to its various bioactive properties such as antioxidant, anti-inflammatory [1], antimicrobial [2], and anti-cancer properties [3]. This compound can be isolated from several plants such as *Rosmarinus officinalis, Malus domestica, Origanum vulgare, Salvia officinalis* [4], and *Clinopodium revolutum*, an endemic Peruvian plant commonly called "flor de arena" [5] (Figure 1). Due to the poor solubility of UA in water, the molecule has a low bioavailability, which hinders its clinical application. For this reason, studies in recent years have focused on the development of systems that transport UA to the site of absorption to improve its bioavailability [6–8]. Among these delivery systems, hydrogels are a promising approach because these polymeric materials can respond to external stimuli [9–11]. In particular, pH-responsive hydrogels have shown great potential as oral delivery systems for bioactive compounds because they respond to changes in the pH value of the gastrointestinal tract.

This means that hydrogels can be designed to retain a bioactive agent under certain conditions (e.g., in the stomach) and release it under other conditions (e.g., in the intestine) [12]. For this reason, pH-sensitive hydrogels can deliver the compound to the site of absorption and release its cargo without causing side effects [13].

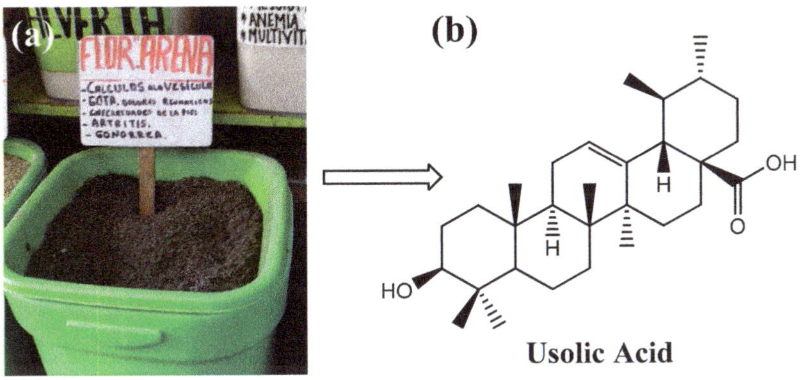

Figure 1. Commercialization of flor de arena in herb shops in Peru (**a**) and structure of ursolic acid (**b**).

Hydrogels based on poly(2-hydroxyethylmethacrylate) poly(HEMA) are of special interest because they have been used in a wide range of biomedical applications, such as contact lenses, tissue regeneration, drug delivery, wound dressings, etc. [14]. However, it is necessary to incorporate monomers with ionizable groups such as –COOH or –SO_3H to prepare pH-responsive hydrogels. Itaconic acid (IA) is an excellent choice because it has two carboxylic groups and is obtained from natural sources [15,16]. On the other hand, hydrogels based on poly(ethylene glycol) methyl methacrylate (PEGxMEM) have shown good biocompatibility, which means that they do not cause any adverse effects when in contact with any part of the human body [17–20].

The objective of this study was to prepare a hydrogel capable of transporting UA to the site of absorption (intestine) in order to increase its bioavailability and to take advantage of its full pharmacological potential. For this purpose, hydrogels based on poly(HEMA-PEGxMEM-IA) loaded with UA were prepared. The polymerization was performed by radical light curing. The hydrogels were instrumentally characterized by FTIR-ATR, RAMAN, XRD, and scanning electron microscopy (SEM). In addition, the degree of swelling of the hydrogels in water was evaluated, as well as their response to pH changes, simulating the physiological conditions of the human body. Finally, an in vitro UA release study was carried out.

Swelling analysis and SEM images showed that the hydrogels are pH sensitive, which is very useful for the delivery of active substances to a specific site such as the intestine.

2. Results and Discussion

In order to transport UA to the adsorption site and improve the bioavailability of this molecule, we selected the monomers HEMA, PEG_xMEM, and IA to prepare hydrogels (Figure 2b,c). Free radical polymerization was initiated by HCPK, and was photo-activated. These free radicals propagate with the HEMA, PEGxMEM, and IA monomers to form polymer chains. The crosslinking agent MBA facilitates the formation of chemical bonds between the polymer chains, creating a three-dimensional network (Figure 2a).

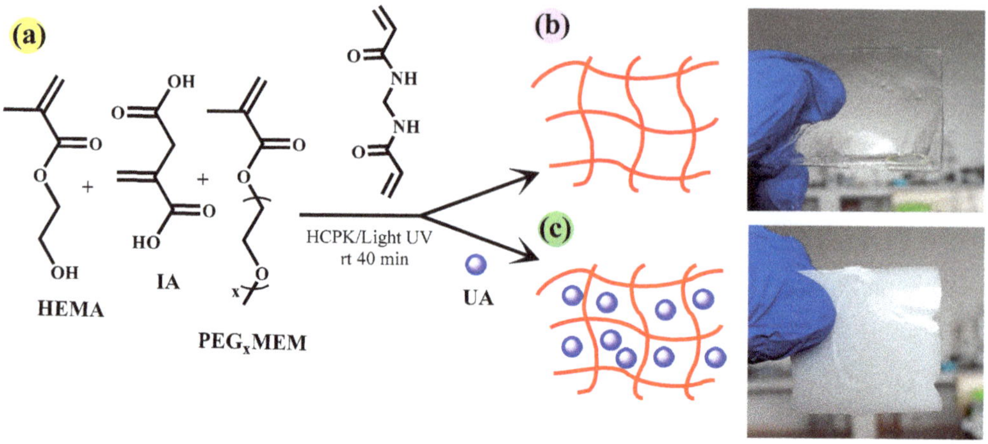

Figure 2. Monomers and crosslinking agents used to prepare the hydrogels (**a**), schematic representation of the hydrogel HG (**b**), and hydrogel loaded with UA in situ HGx-UA (**c**).

2.1. Characterizations

FT-IR spectroscopy was used to confirm the chemical composition of the prepared hydrogels (Figure 3a). Characteristic signals are observed in the spectra of the monomers HEMA, PEG_5MEM, IA, and the HG_5 hydrogel. HEMA shows peaks at 3429 cm^{-1} (–OH), between 3000 cm^{-1} and 2800 cm^{-1} (–CH, $–CH_2$, CH_3), 1716 cm^{-1} (C=O), and 1634 cm^{-1} (C=C) [21,22]. The IA monomer shows a broad band between 3230 cm^{-1} and 2750 cm^{-1} (–OH, of carboxylic acid), 2922 cm^{-1} (C–H), and 1689 cm^{-1} (C=O) [23]. In PEG_5MEM, the signals at 2873 cm^{-1}, 1689 cm^{-1}, 1634 cm^{-1}, and 1100 cm^{-1} correspond to C–H, C=O, C=C, and C–O–C groups, respectively [24]. The spectrum of the HG_5 hydrogel has peaks that are characteristic of the HEMA, PEG_5MEM, and IA monomers, except the C=C peak, indicating that these groups carry out the polymerization. Figure 3b shows the FT-IR spectra of the HGx and HGx-UA hydrogels; the characteristic UA peaks at 3420 cm^{-1} (–OH), 2975 to 2950 cm^{-1} (–CH, $–CH_2$, $–CH_3$), 1714 cm^{-1} (C=O), and 1680 cm^{-1} (C=C) are overlapped by the hydrogel signals.

RAMAN and FT-IR are complementary techniques that provide detailed information about vibrational modes. The C=C vibrations are particularly intense and well defined in RAMAN spectra [25]. For this reason, an analysis of HG_5 was carried out and compared with that of the monomer PEG_5MEM (Figure 3c). Figure 3c shows the characteristic vibrations of PEG_5MEM; the peak at 1636 cm^{-1} corresponds to the C=C group, which is absent in the HG_5 spectrum, indicating a successful polymerization through these groups and a good purification of the hydrogel to remove unreacted monomers trapped in the hydrogel matrix.

The XRD patterns of UA are found at angles of 2θ = 10.76, 14.15, 16.49, 21.9, 26.4, and 40.22 [26,27]. XRD analysis was performed for HG_5-UA and HG_9-UA hydrogels to observe the UA peaks. However, due to the amorphous nature of the hydrogels, only a broadband of 2θ = 10 to 25 was observed overlapping the crystallographic patterns of the UA crystals (Figure 3d).

The thermal stability of the HGx hydrogels was analyzed by TGA (Figure 3e,f). The TGA curves show three main stages of weight loss. The first stage of weight loss, reaching 100 °C, could be associated with water loss [28]. The second slight weight loss around 300 °C could be attributed to water loss generated by the ester formation through the carboxyl groups (–COOH) of the IA and the hydroxyl group (–OH) of the HEMA monomers [15]. The third stage corresponds to the thermal degradation of the hydrogels; the maximum degradation rate occurs at 410.5 °C and 429 °C for hydrogel HG_5 and HG_9, respectively. Since the hydrogels are intended to be used as UA transport systems, which is carried out at physiological temperature (37 °C), the prepared hydrogels will be thermally stable in this environment.

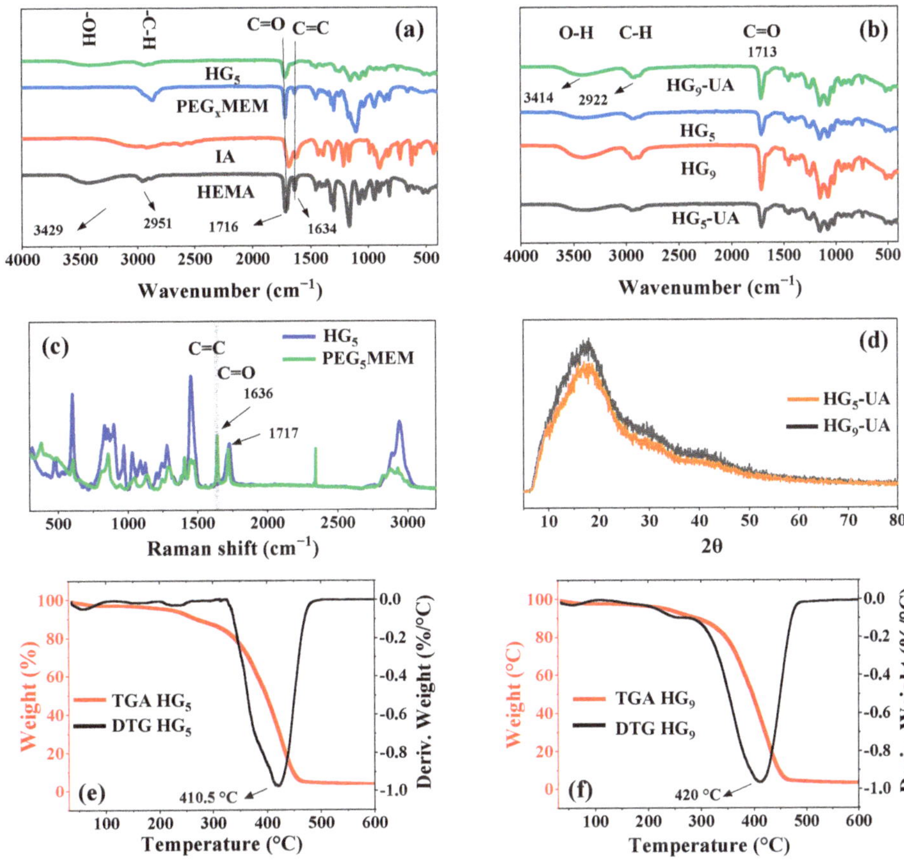

Figure 3. FT-IR spectra of HG_5 and monomers (**a**), FT-IR spectra of hydrogels (HG_5 and HG_9) and hydrogels loaded with UA (HG_5-UA and HG_9-UA) (**b**), Raman spectrum of PEG_5MEM and HG_5 (**c**), XRD analysis of HG_5-UA and HG_9-UA (**d**), TGA/DTG curves of HG_5 (**e**), and TGA/DTG curves of HG_9 (**f**).

2.2. *Swelling Behavior (q)*

The swelling behavior of HG_5 and HG_9 hydrogels in water was investigated. The degree of swelling influences the mechanical properties and the mobilization of the bioactive compound through the polymeric network [29]. Figure 4a shows the results; HG_5 and HG_9 have a q_{max} of 0.89 and 1.44 (g H_2O/g hydrogel), respectively. The degree of swelling is influenced by the inter/intramolecular hydrogen bonds between IA-IA (–COOH·····HOOC–) and IA-HEMA (–COOH·····HO–), which may be more favored in shorter polymer chains, restricting the relaxation of the polymer chains and causing a slight decrease in water absorption. In longer chains such as PEG_9MEM, there is a lower tendency to form inter/intramolecular hydrogen bonds between IA-IA (–COOH–HOOC–) and IA-HEMA (–COOH·····HO–), but a higher tendency to form IA-H_2O (–COOH·····HO–) and HEMA-H_2O (–OH·····HO–) bonds [15,30,31].

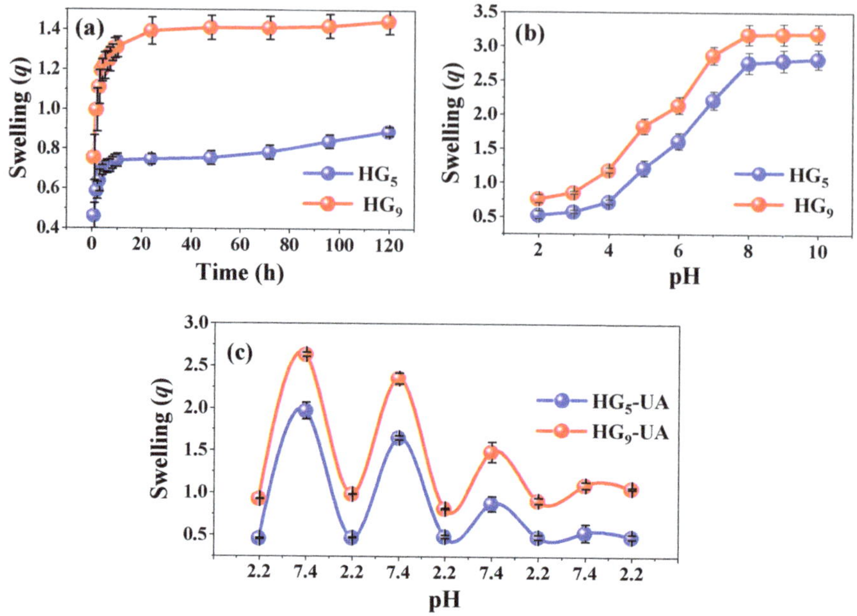

Figure 4. Swelling behavior in water (**a**), pH medium (**b**), and cyclic pH response (**c**).

The pH response of HG_5 and HG_9 hydrogels was evaluated from pH 2 to 10 at 37 °C. The swelling degree is related to the amount of ionizable carboxylic groups in the polymer network. Figure 4b shows that both HG_5 and HG_9 hydrogels respond to pH due to the dissociation of the IA carboxylic groups $pK_1 = 3.85$ and $pK_2 = 5.45$. The carboxylic groups remain protonated (–COOH) at pH values below their dissociation constants, resulting in low swelling values. However, at pH values above their dissociation constants, the carboxylic groups tend to deprotonate ($-COO^-$), becoming negatively charged and causing an electrostatic repulsion that favors the expansion of the hydrogel [32,33].

Cyclic swelling of HG_5-UA and HG_9-UA hydrogels was evaluated in buffer solutions simulating gastrointestinal conditions: pH 2.2 and 7.4 at 37 °C (Figure 4c). Figure 4c shows that in the first cycle, HG_5-UA reaches a q_{max} of 0.45 at pH 2.2 and 1.97 at pH 7.4. In the case of HG_9-UA, the q_{max} is 0.93 at pH 2.2 and 2.64 at pH 7.4. A decrease in swelling capacity after each cycle is noted, attributable to ion–dipole interactions between polymer chains [23].

2.3. SEM Characterization

Figure 5 shows the morphology of HG_5 and HG_9 hydrogels. The effect of pH on pore size is observed in both hydrogels. At pH 2.2, the pores of the hydrogels are closed, because at acidic pH levels the carboxylic groups (–COOH) of the IA are protonated and form hydrogel bonds that prevent the expansion of the hydrogel. At pH 7.4, open and evenly distributed pores are observed because at basic pH levels the carboxyl groups of the IA deprotonate ($-COO^-$), resulting in electrostatic repulse between the polymer chains, causing them to swell and expand. The porosity favors better water retention, loading, and diffusion of ursolic acid through the polymer matrix. These results are consistent with the values obtained for the swelling at different pH values since porous materials favor greater water penetration through the polymeric networks [34].

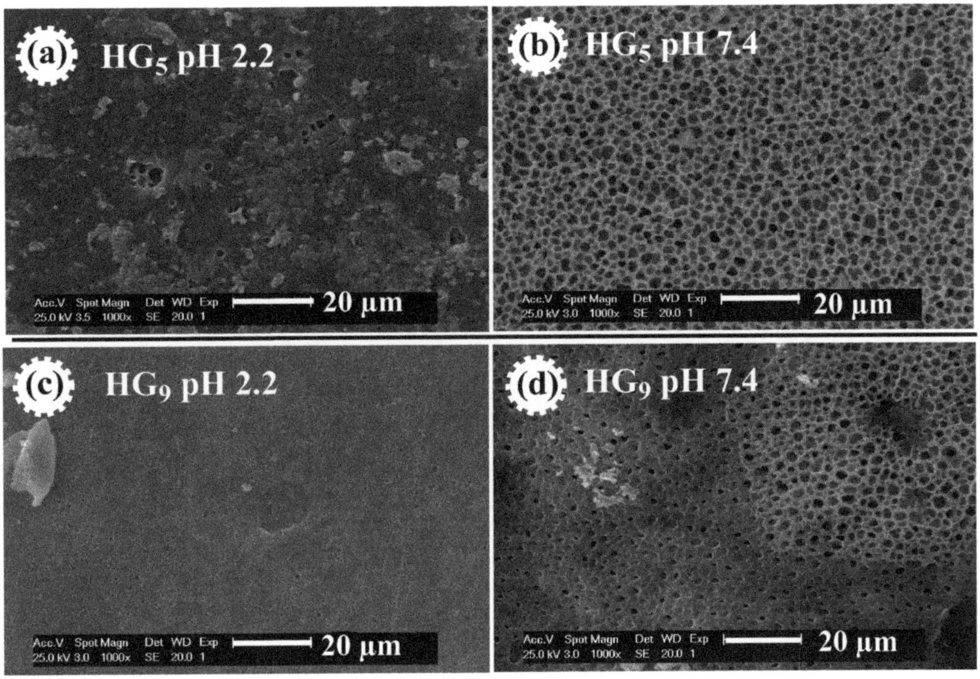

Figure 5. SEM micrographs of HG_5 hydrogel at pH 2.2 (**a**) and at pH 7.4 (**b**), and of HG_9 hydrogel at pH 2.2 (**c**) and at pH 7.4 (**d**).

Figure 6 shows SEM micrographs of HG_5 and HG_9 hydrogels at pH 7.4, where the pore size measurement performed on the hydrogel outline shows an average value of 6.96 and 10.14 µm, respectively. This could be attributed to the pore depth of the hydrogels. The pore size on the surface of HG_5 and HG_9 hydrogels is 2.15 and 1.92 µm, respectively. The larger pore depth in HG_9 compared to HG_5 also explains the higher degree of swelling of the HG_9 hydrogel.

SEM micrographs were also taken of the UA-loaded hydrogels, i.e., HG_5-UA and HG_9-UA, at pH 2.2 and 7.4 (Figure 7). Figure 7 shows the UA crystals in the pores of the hydrogels. At pH 2.2 the pores are compressed, trapping the UA crystals, which would prevent the release of UA in an acidic environment. At pH 7.4 the pores are open, which would allow the release of UA in a basic environment.

2.4. Determination of Drug Loading and Encapsulation Efficiency

Table 1 shows the drug loading content and encapsulation efficiency of the HG_5-UA and HG_9-UA hydrogels. These DLC and EE values are comparable to those reported by Das et al. [35], who achieved 3.35% loading and 55.52% encapsulation. Other authors such as Antonio et al. [36] achieved 97.47% encapsulation; Payomhom et al. [37] achieved 1.5% loading and 25% encapsulation. It has been observed that by increasing the amount of UA, the system does not gel. Attempts were made to load HG_5 and HG_9 hydrogels with UA by adsorption, but low DLC (1.45% and 1.38%) and EE (2.89% and 2.76%) values were obtained, respectively. Although experiments were also performed with solvents such as ethanol and methanol, in which UA is more soluble, low DLC and EE values were obtained. For this reason, the remaining experiments were carried out with in situ loaded hydrogel, i.e., HG_5-UA and HG_9-UA.

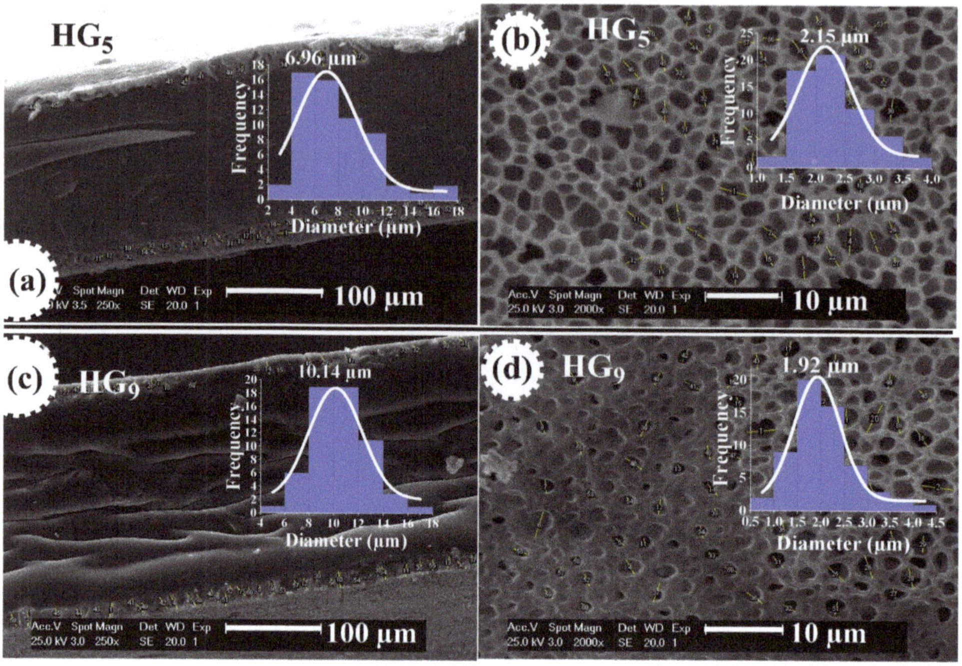

Figure 6. The pore size of HG_5 hydrogel at contour (**a**) and surface (**b**), and of HG_9 hydrogel at contour (**c**) and surface (**d**), both at pH 7.4.

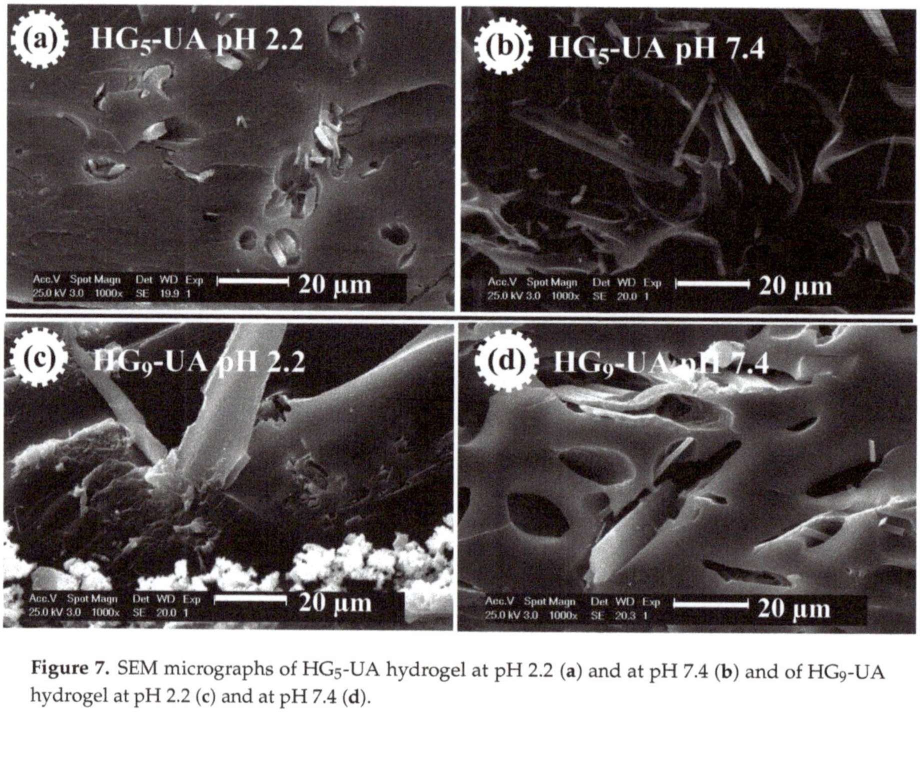

Figure 7. SEM micrographs of HG_5-UA hydrogel at pH 2.2 (**a**) and at pH 7.4 (**b**) and of HG_9-UA hydrogel at pH 2.2 (**c**) and at pH 7.4 (**d**).

Table 1. Drug loading content (DLC) and encapsulation efficiency (EE) of hydrogels.

Hydrogel	Initial UA (mg)	After Purification UA (mg)	Mass HGx (g)	DLC (%)	EE (%)
HG_5-UA	35.00	30.34	0.947	3.20	86.69
HG_9-UA	35.00	30.05	1.119	2.69	85.86

2.5. In Vitro Release of HG_5-UA and HG_9-UA

The in vitro release of UA from hydrogels was evaluated in buffer pH 2.2 (acidic environment of the stomach) and buffer pH 7.4 (basic environment of the intestine) with 3% Tween 80 at 37 °C [35]. For the application of the hydrogel as a transport system for hydrophobic bioactive compounds such as UA in the intestine, it is necessary that the hydrogel does not release its charge in an acidic medium and has a good release in a basic medium. From this point of view, the HG_5-UA and HG_9-UA hydrogels have the desired release profile (Figure 8a,b). In buffer pH 2.2, the release of UA from HG_5-UA and HG_9-UA is low due to the low degree of swelling of the hydrogels at acidic pH levels. In buffer pH 7.4, a higher amount was released due to the higher diffusion of UA from the swollen pores in basic media. Analyzing the UA release profiles for the two hydrogels, the release increases rapidly at the beginning and gradually reaches the equilibrium value in approximately 24 h. Figure 8 also shows that the percentage release with a PEG_5MEM monomer is slightly higher than with PEG_9MEM. This can be explained by the chain length as PEG_9MEM is a longer chain monomer; the UA is trapped in the matrix and diffusion is more difficult. This also explains the incomplete release of UA from the hydrogels.

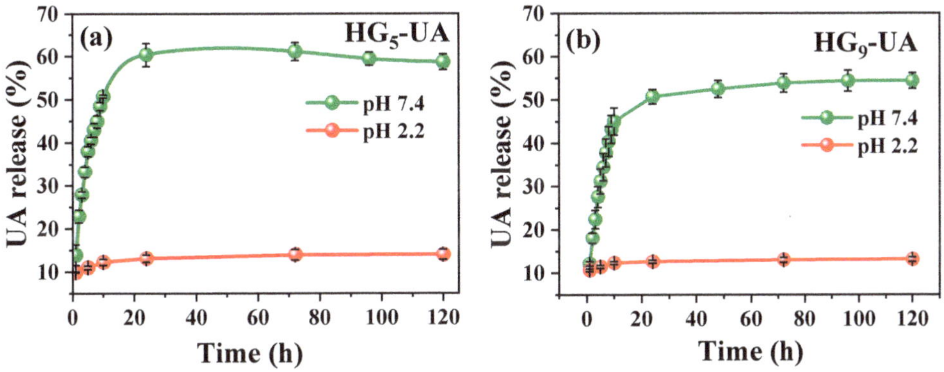

Figure 8. UA release profiles of HG_5-UA (**a**) and HG_9-UA (**b**) hydrogels at pH 2.2 and 7.4.

In order to establish the mechanism of UA release from the HG_5-UA and HG_9-UA hydrogels, the data obtained from the in vitro release were fitted to different kinetic models: zero-order, first-order, Korsmeyer–Peppas, Hixson–Crowell, and Higuchi [38]. The calculated parameters are presented in Table 2 and the sum of squared residuals (SSR), Akaike Information Criterion (AIC), and the coefficient of determination (R^2) were evaluated to identify the model that best fits the release data. The SSR, which quantifies the error between the experimental data and the values predicted by the model, is lower for the Korsmeyer–Peppas model (0.582 for HG_5-UA and 0.578 for HG_9-UA). The AIC, which balances goodness of fit with model simplicity, also showed the lowest values for the Korsmeyer–Peppas model (−40.527 for HG_5-UA and −40.619 for HG_9-UA). Furthermore, the R^2 values were 0.754 for HG_5-UA and 0.783 for HG_9-UA, indicating that the Korsmeyer–Peppas model $M_t/M_e = kt^n$ best describes the UA release mechanism from the hydrogels.

Table 2. Parameters calculated by fitting release data using various kinetic models.

		HG_5-UA			
Model	C_o	k	SSR	AIC	R^2
zero-order	36.446	0.253	1490.330	69.348	0.454
first-order	6.018	0.002	0.079	−68.548	0.520
Hixson–Crowell	-	0.006	0.709	−37.755	0.499
Higuchi	-	3.569	1089.188	64.958	0.618
Korsmeyer–Peppas	-	22.340	0.582	−40.527	0.754
		HG_9-UA			
Model	C_o	k	SSR	AIC	R^2
zero-order	30.946	0.252	1226.977	66.626	0.509
first-order	6.263	0.002	0.050	−74.927	0.584
Hixson–Crowell	-	0.006	0.487	−43.018	0.559
Higuchi	-	3.475	833.657	61.215	0.667
Korsmeyer–Peppas	-	18.359	0.578	−40.619	0.783

The value of the exponent "n" in the Korsmeyer–Peppas model is associated with the type of transport mechanism. Values of $n \leq 0.45$ indicate a predominantly Fickian diffusion-controlled release. Values of n close to 1 indicate a release controlled by polymer chain relaxation, corresponding to a zero-order kinetic model. Intermediate n values between 0.45 and 1 indicate anomalous transport where both diffusion and relaxation influence the release, which can be studied using non-Fickian diffusion [38,39]. In this study, the n values obtained were 0.256 and 0.278 for HG_5-UA and HG_9-UA, respectively, suggesting a quasi-Fickian diffusion release. This behavior is attributed to diffusion controlled mainly by the movement of the bioactive compound through the polymer matrix, which relaxes and swells in a basic environment (pH 7.4) [40].

3. Conclusions

To improve the oral bioavailability of hydrophobic phytochemicals, an approach based on the use of sensitive hydrogels is presented. The hydrophobic phytochemical UA was loaded in situ into the pH-sensitive poly(HEMA-PEG_xMEM-IA) hydrogels with an efficiency of more than 85%. From the observations of buffer swelling (pH 2.2 and 7.4) and SEM images, the hydrogels can protect UA in the stomach, where the pH is close to 2.2, and release its cargo in the intestine, where the pH is close to 7.4. The results obtained from the in vitro release under conditions simulating the gastrointestinal environment fit the Korsmeyer–Peppas kinetic model, suggesting a mechanism of diffusion through the hydrogel. Finally, this study provides relevant information for developing targeted transport systems for oral delivery of hydrophobic phytochemicals to exploit the full pharmacological potential of these molecules.

4. Materials and Methods

4.1. Materials

The main materials used for the synthesis of the hydrogel in this study were the monomers 2-hydroxyethyl methacrylate (HEMA, 97%), polyethylene glycol methyl ether methacrylate (PEG_5MEM, Mn average 300), polyethylene glycol methyl ether methacrylate (PEG_9MEM, Mn average 500), itaconic acid (IA, $\geq$ 99%), crosslinker N,N′-methylenebisacrylamide (MBA, 99%), initiator 1-hydroxycyclohexyl phenyl ketone (HCPK, 99%), and TWEEN 80. These materials were purchased from Sigma-Aldrich (St. Louis, MO, USA).

4.2. Extraction of Ursolic Acid

Ursolic acid (UA) was extracted from the medicinal plant *Clinopodium revolutum*, which is known as flor de arena in local herbal shops. The methodology was developed in a previous work [5]; 50 g of dried leaves of *Clinopodium revolutum* was macerated in 200 mL of ethanol (96%) for 24 h. Then, it was filtered and macerated again. The process was repeated three times. The ethanolic extract obtained was concentrated to dryness using a rotary evaporator, dried, and degreased with petroleum ether. The degreased extract was redissolved in 150 mL of ethanol (96%) and kept refrigerated for 24 h. The precipitate obtained was filtered and dried in an oven at 60 °C for 12 h. Crystallization was carried out in 90 mL of ethanol (96%) at 60 °C and 5 g of activated carbon was used for decolorization. The mixture was kept under constant stirring for 5 min and then filtered with a vacuum pump. The filtrate obtained was crystallized at 4 °C for 12 h. After this time, the crystals were filtered, washed with cold ethanol, and dried in an oven at 60 °C for 1 h. The extraction procedure is shown in Figure 9.

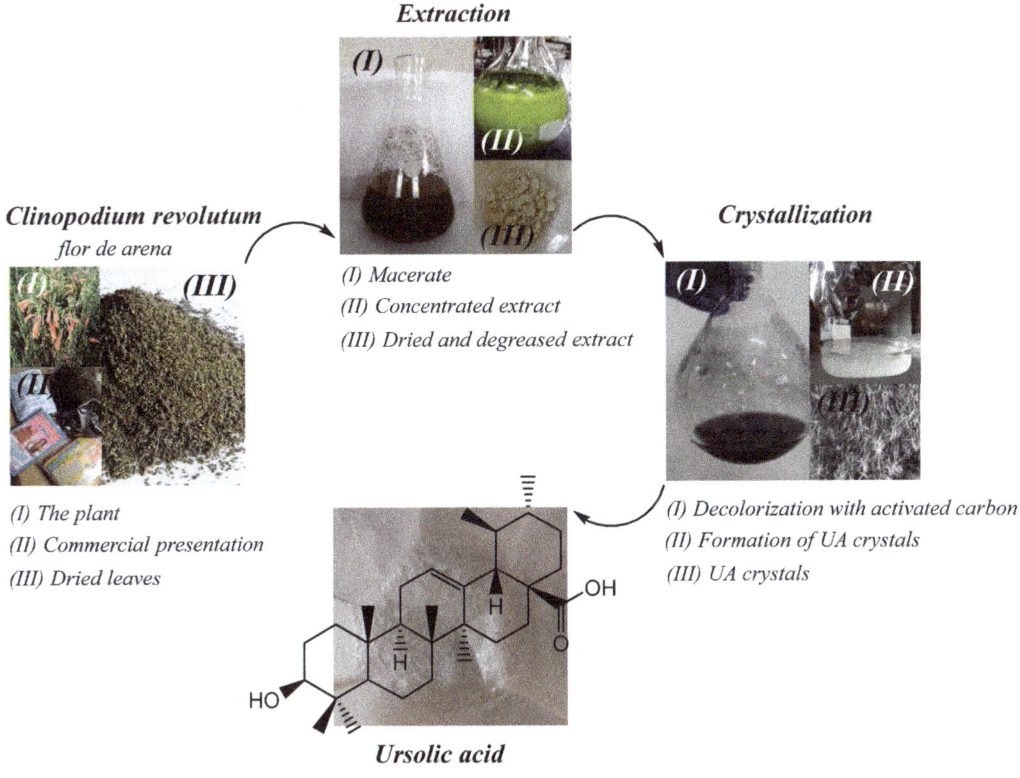

Figure 9. Process of extraction of UA from *Clinopodium revolutum*, "flor de arena".

The obtained UA crystals were analyzed by (a) UV-VIS (Thermo Scientific, Genesys 150, Waltham, MA, USA): The sample was dissolved in methanol and scanned from 200 to 750 nm. The spectrum showed a single absorption band at 210 nm, characteristic of this compound. (b) HPLC (Thermo Scientific, Ultimate 3000Thermo, Sunnyvale, CA, USA): For this analysis, a column Phenomenex RP-C18 250 × 4.6 mm and 5 μm was used. Analysis conditions were mobile phase (water/acetonitrile 2:8), flow rate 1 mL/min, isocratic, 5 μL injection, and detection at 210 nm. The chromatogram shows a peak at rt 11.30 min with a relative area of 97.52%, which corresponds to the percentage purity of the UA. (c) FTIR (Thermo, Nicolet 380, Waltham, MA, USA): The FTIR-ATR spectrum of UA crystals previously dried at 60 °C for 1 h shows characteristic peaks of this molecule at 3420 cm^{-1} (–OH), 2975 to 2950 cm^{-1} (–CH, $–CH_2$, $–CH_3$), 1714 cm^{-1} (C=O), and 1680 cm^{-1} (C=C).

An exhaustive characterization is not necessary, as it has been shown that only UA can be obtained from *Clinopodium revolutum* using the described method [5,41].

4.3. Synthesis of Hydrogels HG_x-UA

The synthesis of hydrogels based on poly(HEMA-PEGxMEM-IA) loaded in situ with UA (HGx-UA) was performed following the methodology proposed by Gallardo et al. [42], with some modifications. The monomers IA, HEMA, PEGxMEM, crosslinker MBA, and UA were mixed with 300 µL of ethanol under stirring at 40 °C for 5 min. The mixture was then bubbled with nitrogen gas for 10 min and the initiator HCPK was added. The solution was immediately injected into a 53 × 26 × 2 mm mold and placed in the photopolymerization chamber (4 watts, 365 nm) for 40 min. After this time, the hydrogels were removed from the mold and cut. Purification was performed by immersing the hydrogels in distilled water, which was renewed several times to remove unreacted substances. Finally, the hydrogels were dried at room temperature. Blank hydrogels (HG_x) were prepared similarly without the addition of UA. The feed compositions used to synthesize the hydrogels are shown in Table 3.

Table 3. Feed compositions of the poly(HEMA-PEG_xMEM-IA) hydrogels (HG_x).

Hydrogel	HEMA g (mol %)	PEG_5MEM g (mol %)	PEG_9MEM g (mol %)	IA g (mol %)	UA g	MBA g	HCPK g
HG_5-UA	0.800 (80%)	0.230 (10%)	-	0.100 (10%)	0.035	0.023	0.0156
HG_9-UA	0.800 (80%)	-	0.384 (10%)	0.100 (10%)	0.035	0.023	0.0156

4.4. Characterization

The FT-IR spectra were obtained using an FT-IR spectrometer (Perkin Elmer, Spectrum TWO, S/N 117248, Waltham, MA, USA). The samples were dried and crushed before being placed on the ATR crystal. Measurements were taken at room temperature over the range of wave numbers from 4000 to 400 cm^{-1}. A RAMAN instrument (Renishaw InVia Raman Microscope, S/N 9W596, Wotton-under-Edge, Gloucestershire, UK) was used as a complementary technique to the FTIR-ATR analysis. The hydrogels loaded with UA were analyzed using X-Ray diffraction (XRD-BRUKER D8-ADVANCE S/N 203691 SAP 604310, Karlsruhe, Germany, Cu, λ = 1.5406 Å). The hydrogels were previously dried and ground, and the analysis was performed as $2\theta = 5°–80°$. Thermogravimetric analysis (TGA) of the hydrogels was performed on a Perkin Elmer STA6000 (Waltham, MA, USA) instrument, using 10 mg of previously dried and ground hydrogels. The heating ramp was from 37 °C to 600 °C at a heating rate of 5 °C/min in an inert nitrogen gas atmosphere at a flow rate of 20 mL/min. The morphology of HG_x and HG_x-UA hydrogels was observed by scanning electron microscopy (SEM, XL30ESEM Philips, North Billerica, MA, USA). The hydrogels were previously swollen in pH 2.2 and pH 7.4 buffer at 37 °C for 24 h and then freeze-dried for 12 h. Metallization with Au/Pd alloy (80/20) was required for better observation.

4.5. Swelling Behavior (q)

The degree of hydrogel swelling (q) was determined using Equation (1). For this purpose, 20 mg of dried hydrogel (W_d) was weighed, immersed in 30 mL of water, and allowed to swell. Then, it was removed from the liquid and weighed (W_s); it is necessary to dry the surface of the hydrogel before weighing. The degree of swelling was determined every 1 h for the first 10 h, then every 24 h. This study was performed in triplicate.

$$q = \frac{W_s - W_d}{W_d} \tag{1}$$

The pH response was evaluated by determining the degree of swelling in various buffer solutions (pH 2 to 10) at 37 °C.

4.6. Drug Loading and Encapsulation Efficiency

The drug loading and encapsulation efficiency of UA were determined by a UV-VIS spectrophotometer. To determine the amount of UA entrapped in the hydrogel, the samples were first disrupted by immersing the crushed hydrogel in methanol for 24 h and then sonicated for 1 h. Briefly, 20 mg of HG_5-UA and HG_9-UA were crushed and immersed in methanol (5 mL) for 24 h, then sonicated for 1 h and their absorbance was determined at 210 nm. A calibration curve at 210 nm was previously performed with a methanol solution of UA from 5 μg/mL to 100 μg/mL.

The drug loading content (DLC) and encapsulation efficiency (EE) of ursolic acid were determined by Equations (2) and (3), respectively [35].

$$Drug\ loading\ content\ (\%) = \frac{Weight\ of\ UA\ in\ hydrogel}{weight\ of\ hydrogel} \times 100 \quad (2)$$

$$Encapsulation\ efficiency\ (\%) = \frac{Weight\ of\ UA\ in\ hydrogel}{Initial\ amount\ of\ UA} \times 100 \quad (3)$$

4.7. In Vitro Drug Release Study

In vitro release of UA from the HG_x-UA hydrogels was evaluated by immersion in buffer with Tween 80 [35]. A total of 20 mg of HG_x-UA was immersed in 5 mL of 0.1 M phosphate-buffered saline (PBS, pH 7.4) containing Tween 80 (3% v/v) at 37 °C with gentle agitation. At a predetermined time (1 h, 2 h, 3 h, 4 h, 5 h, 6 h, 7 h, 8 h, 9 h, 10 h, 24 h, 48 h, and 72 h), the hydrogels were removed and the surface was washed with water. The hydrogel was then disrupted by immersion in 5 mL of methanol for 24 h and sonication for 1 h. The absorbance of the methanol solution was recorded at 210 nm and the concentration of UA remaining in the hydrogel was determined. The amount of UA released is equal to the amount of initial UA minus the amount of UA remaining in the hydrogel.

The percentage of release was determined using Equation (4) [43].

$$\%\ release = \frac{W_t}{W_0} \times 100 \quad (4)$$

where W_t is the amount of UA released at time t and W_0 is the amount of initial hydrogel UA. The same procedure was carried out with a buffer of pH 2.2.

Author Contributions: Conceptualization, C.D.G. and M.A.L.; methodology, C.D.G., R.L.A., A.M.L., and M.A.L.; formal analysis, C.E., F.M., A.G., and M.A.L.; investigation, C.D.G. and M.A.L.; data curation, F.M., C.E., A.G., and C.A.S.; writing—original draft preparation, C.D.G. and M.A.L.; writing—review and editing, M.A.L., C.A.S., and F.M.; visualization, C.E., A.M.L., R.L.A., A.G., and M.A.L.; supervision, M.A.L.; project administration, M.A.L. All authors have read and agreed to the published version of the manuscript.

Funding: This research was funded by "CONCYTEC-PROCIENCIA under contract No. PE501085628-2023".

Institutional Review Board Statement: Not applicable.

Informed Consent Statement: Not applicable.

Data Availability Statement: The original contributions presented in the study are included in the article, further inquiries can be directed to the corresponding author.

Acknowledgments: We would like to express our sincere gratitude to Raúl Sanz for their valuable collaboration in SEM analysis, and to Isabel Muñoz for her assistance with RAMAN analysis.

Conflicts of Interest: The authors declare no conflicts of interest.

References

1. Habtemariam, S. Antioxidant and Anti-Inflammatory Mechanisms of Neuroprotection by Ursolic Acid: Addressing Brain Injury, Cerebral Ischemia, Cognition Deficit, Anxiety, and Depression. *Oxidative Med. Cell. Longev.* **2019**, *2019*, 8512048. [CrossRef] [PubMed]
2. Jyoti, M.A.; Nam, K.W.; Jang, W.S.; Kim, Y.H.; Kim, S.K.; Lee, B.E.; Song, H.Y. Antimycobacterial Activity of Methanolic Plant Extract of Artemisia Capillaris Containing Ursolic Acid and Hydroquinone against Mycobacterium Tuberculosis. *J. Infect. Chemother.* **2016**, *22*, 200–208. [CrossRef] [PubMed]
3. Iqbal, J.; Abbasi, B.A.; Ahmad, R.; Mahmood, T.; Kanwal, S.; Ali, B.; Khalil, A.T.; Shah, S.A.; Alam, M.M.; Badshah, H. Ursolic Acid a Promising Candidate in the Therapeutics of Breast Cancer: Current Status and Future Implications. *Biomed. Pharmacother.* **2018**, *108*, 752–756. [CrossRef] [PubMed]
4. Pironi, A.M.; de Araújo, P.R.; Fernandes, M.A.; Salgado, H.R.N.; Chorilli, M. Characteristics, Biological Properties and Analytical Methods of Ursolic Acid: A Review. *Crit. Rev. Anal. Chem.* **2018**, *48*, 86–93. [CrossRef]
5. Ludeña Huaman, M.A.; Tupa Quispe, A.L.; Huamán Quispe, R.I.; Serrano Flores, C.A.; Robles Caycho, J. A Simple Method to Obtain Ursolic Acid. *Results Chem.* **2021**, *3*, 100144. [CrossRef]
6. Jin, H.; Pi, J.; Yang, F.; Wu, C.; Cheng, X.; Bai, H.; Huang, D.; Jiang, J.; Cai, J.; Chen, Z.W. Ursolic Acid-Loaded Chitosan Nanoparticles Induce Potent Anti-Angiogenesis in Tumor. *Appl. Microbiol. Biotechnol.* **2016**, *100*, 6643–6652. [CrossRef]
7. Li, T.; Chen, X.; Liu, Y.; Fan, L.; Lin, L.; Xu, Y.; Chen, S.; Shao, J. PH-Sensitive Mesoporous Silica Nanoparticles Anticancer Prodrugs for Sustained Release of Ursolic Acid and the Enhanced Anti-Cancer Efficacy for Hepatocellular Carcinoma Cancer. *Eur. J. Pharm. Sci.* **2017**, *96*, 456–463. [CrossRef]
8. Shao, J.; Fang, Y.; Zhao, R.; Chen, F.; Yang, M.; Jiang, J.; Chen, Z.; Yuan, X.; Jia, L. Evolution from Small Molecule to Nano-Drug Delivery Systems: An Emerging Approach for Cancer Therapy of Ursolic Acid. *Asian J. Pharm. Sci.* **2020**, *15*, 685–700. [CrossRef]
9. Uman, S.; Dhand, A.; Burdick, J.A. Recent Advances in Shear-Thinning and Self-Healing Hydrogels for Biomedical Applications. *J. Appl. Polym. Sci.* **2020**, *137*, 48668. [CrossRef]
10. Liu, B.; Chen, K. Advances in Hydrogel-Based Drug Delivery Systems. *Gels* **2024**, *10*, 262. [CrossRef]
11. Thang, N.H.; Chien, T.B.; Cuong, D.X. Polymer-Based Hydrogels Applied in Drug Delivery: An Overview. *Gels* **2023**, *9*, 523. [CrossRef] [PubMed]
12. Yang, Z.; McClements, D.J.; Li, C.; Sang, S.; Chen, L.; Long, J.; Qiu, C.; Jin, Z. Targeted Delivery of Hydrogels in Human Gastrointestinal Tract: A Review. *Food Hydrocoll.* **2023**, *134*, 108013. [CrossRef]
13. Rizwan, M.; Yahya, R.; Hassan, A.; Yar, M.; Azzahari, A.D.; Selvanathan, V.; Sonsudin, F.; Abouloula, C.N. PH Sensitive Hydrogels in Drug Delivery: Brief History, Properties, Swelling, and Release Mechanism, Material Selection and Applications. *Polymers* **2017**, *9*, 137. [CrossRef] [PubMed]
14. Zare, M.; Bigham, A.; Zare, M.; Luo, H.; Rezvani Ghomi, E.; Ramakrishna, S. PHEMA: An Overview for Biomedical Applications. *Int. J. Mol. Sci.* **2021**, *22*, 6376. [CrossRef] [PubMed]
15. Huaman, M.A.L.; Vega-Chacón, J.; Quispe, R.I.H.; Negrón, A.C.V. Synthesis and Swelling Behaviors of Poly(2-Hydroxyethyl Methacrylate-Co-Itaconic Acid) and Poly(2-Hydroxyethyl Methacrylate-Co-Sodium Itaconate) Hydrogels as Potential Drug Carriers. *Results Chem.* **2023**, *5*, 100917. [CrossRef]
16. Teleky, B.E.; Vodnar, D.C. Recent Advances in Biotechnological Itaconic Acid Production, and Application for a Sustainable Approach. *Polymers* **2021**, *13*, 3574. [CrossRef]
17. Sano, K.; Umemoto, K.; Miura, H.; Ohno, S.; Iwata, K.; Kawakami, R.; Munekane, M.; Yamasaki, T.; Citterio, D.; Hiruta, Y.; et al. Feasibility of Using Poly[Oligo(Ethylene Glycol) Methyl Ether Methacrylate] as Tumor-Targeted Carriers of Diagnostic Drugs. *ACS Appl. Polym. Mater.* **2022**, *4*, 4734–4740. [CrossRef]
18. Suljovrujic, E.; Rogic Miladinovic, Z.; Krstic, M. Swelling Properties and Drug Release of New Biocompatible POEGOPGMA Hydrogels with VPTT near to the Human Body Temperature. *Polym. Bull.* **2021**, *78*, 2405–2425. [CrossRef]
19. Farrag, Y.; Ait Eldjoudi, D.; Farrag, M.; González-Rodríguez, M.; Ruiz-Fernández, C.; Cordero, A.; Varela-García, M.; Torrijos Pulpón, C.; Bouza, R.; Lago, F.; et al. Poly(Ethylene Glycol) Methyl Ether Methacrylate-Based Injectable Hydrogels: Swelling, Rheological, and In Vitro Biocompatibility Properties with ATDC5 Chondrogenic Lineage. *Polymers* **2023**, *15*, 4635. [CrossRef]
20. Madduma-Bandarage, U.S.K.; Madihally, S.V. Synthetic Hydrogels: Synthesis, Novel Trends, and Applications. *J. Appl. Polym. Sci.* **2021**, *138*, 50376. [CrossRef]
21. Oyarce, E.; Pizarro, G.D.C.; Oyarzún, D.P.; Zúñiga, C.; Sánchez, J.; Oyarce, E.; Pizarro, G.D.C.; Oyarzún, D.P.; Zúñiga, C.; Sánchez, J. Hydrogels based on 2-hydroxyethyl methacrylate: Synthesis, characterization and hydration capacity. *J. Chil. Chem. Soc.* **2020**, *65*, 4682–4685. [CrossRef]
22. Hsueh, Y.H.; Liaw, W.C.; Kuo, J.M.; Deng, C.S.; Wu, C.H. Hydrogel Film-Immobilized Lactobacillus Brevis RK03 for γ-Aminobutyric Acid Production. *Int. J. Mol. Sci.* **2017**, *18*, 2324. [CrossRef] [PubMed]
23. Tomić, S.L.; Babić, M.M.; Antić, K.M.; Jovašević Vuković, J.S.; Malešić, N.B.; Filipović, J.M. PH-Sensitive Hydrogels Based on (Meth)Acrylates and Itaconic Acid. *Macromol. Res.* **2014**, *22*, 1203–1213. [CrossRef]
24. Alejo, T.; Prieto, M.; García-Juan, H.; Andreu, V.; Mendoza, G.; Sebastián, V.; Arruebo, M. A Facile Method for the Controlled Polymerization of Biocompatible and Thermoresponsive Oligo(Ethylene Glycol) Methyl Ether Methacrylate Copolymers. *Polym. J.* **2018**, *50*, 203–211. [CrossRef]

25. Miloudi, L.; Bonnier, F.; Bertrand, D.; Byrne, H.J.; Perse, X.; Chourpa, I.; Munnier, E. Quantitative Analysis of Curcumin-Loaded Alginate Nanocarriers in Hydrogels Using Raman and Attenuated Total Reflection Infrared Spectroscopy. *Anal. Bioanal. Chem.* **2017**, *409*, 4593–4605. [CrossRef]
26. Antônio, E.; Antunes, O.d.R.; de Araújo, I.S.; Khalil, N.M.; Mainardes, R.M. Poly(Lactic Acid) Nanoparticles Loaded with Ursolic Acid: Characterization and in Vitro Evaluation of Radical Scavenging Activity and Cytotoxicity. *Mater. Sci. Eng. C* **2017**, *71*, 156–166. [CrossRef]
27. Qiu, L.; Zhao, X.; Zu, Y.; Zhang, Y.; Liu, Y.; Wu, W.; Li, Y. Ursolic Acid Nanoparticles for Oral Delivery Prepared by Emulsion Solvent Evaporation Method: Characterization, In Vitro Evaluation of Radical Scavenging Activity and Bioavailability. *Artif. Cells Nanomed. Biotechnol.* **2019**, *47*, 610–621. [CrossRef]
28. Huaman, M.A.L.; Manco, A.E.Q.; de Liss Meza López, F.; Carrasco, R.L.A.; Chacón, A.M.L.; Khan, S. Removal of Methylene Blue Dye from Water with Fe3O4/Poly(HEMA-Co-AMPS) Magnetic Hydrogels. *Results Chem.* **2024**, *7*, 101454. [CrossRef]
29. Chai, Q.; Jiao, Y.; Yu, X. Hydrogels for Biomedical Applications: Their Characteristics and the Mechanisms behind Them. *Gels* **2017**, *3*, 6. [CrossRef]
30. Bajpai, S.K.; Saggu, S.S. Water Uptake Behavior of Poly(Methacrylamide-co-N-vinyl-2-pyrrolidone-co-itaconic Acid) as PH-Sensitive Hydrogels: Part I. *J. Macromol. Sci. Part A Pure Appl. Chem.* **2006**, *43*, 1135–1150. [CrossRef]
31. Dobić, S.N.; Filipović, J.M.; Tomić, S.L. Synthesis and Characterization of Poly(2-Hydroxyethyl Methacrylate/Itaconic Acid/Poly(Ethylene Glycol) Dimethacrylate) Hydrogels. *Chem. Eng. J.* **2012**, *179*, 372–380. [CrossRef]
32. Tomić, S.L.; Suljovrujić, E.H.; Filipović, J.M. Biocompatible and Bioadhesive Hydrogels Based on 2-Hydroxyethyl Methacrylate, Monofunctional Poly(Alkylene Glycol)s and Itaconic Acid. *Polym. Bull.* **2006**, *57*, 691–702. [CrossRef]
33. Mahinroosta, M.; Jomeh Farsangi, Z.; Allahverdi, A.; Shakoori, Z. Hydrogels as Intelligent Materials: A Brief Review of Synthesis, Properties and Applications. *Mater. Today Chem.* **2018**, *8*, 42–55. [CrossRef]
34. Rogic Miladinovic, Z.; Micic, M.; Mrakovic, A.; Suljovrujic, E. Smart Hydrogels with Ethylene Glycol Propylene Glycol Pendant Chains. *J. Polym. Res.* **2018**, *25*, 1. [CrossRef]
35. Das, S.; Ghosh, S.; De, A.K.; Bera, T. Oral Delivery of Ursolic Acid-Loaded Nanostructured Lipid Carrier Coated with Chitosan Oligosaccharides: Development, Characterization, in Vitro and in Vivo Assessment for the Therapy of Leishmaniasis. *Int. J. Biol. Macromol.* **2017**, *102*, 996–1008. [CrossRef]
36. Antonio, E.; dos Reis Antunes Junior, O.; Marcano, R.G.D.J.V.; Diedrich, C.; da Silva Santos, J.; Machado, C.S.; Khalil, N.M.; Mainardes, R.M. Chitosan Modified Poly (Lactic Acid) Nanoparticles Increased the Ursolic Acid Oral Bioavailability. *Int. J. Biol. Macromol.* **2021**, *172*, 133–142. [CrossRef]
37. Payomhom, P.; Panyain, N.; Sakonsinsiri, C.; Wongtrakoongate, P.; Lertsuwan, K.; Pissuwan, D.; Katewongsa, K.P. Chitosan-Coated Poly(Lactic-Co-Glycolic Acid) Nanoparticles Loaded with Ursolic Acid for Breast Cancer Therapy. *ACS Appl. Nano Mater.* **2024**, *7*, 5383–5395. [CrossRef]
38. Vigata, M.; Meinert, C.; Hutmacher, D.W.; Bock, N. Hydrogels as Drug Delivery Systems: A Review of Current Characterization and Evaluation Techniques. *Pharmaceutics* **2020**, *12*, 1188. [CrossRef]
39. Altun, E.; Yuca, E.; Ekren, N.; Kalaskar, D.M.; Ficai, D.; Dolete, G.; Ficai, A.; Gunduz, O. Kinetic Release Studies of Antibiotic Patches for Local Transdermal Delivery. *Pharmaceutics* **2021**, *13*, 613. [CrossRef]
40. Alinavaz, S.; Mahdavinia, G.R.; Jafari, H.; Hazrati, M.; Akbari, A. Hydroxyapatite (HA)-Based Hybrid Bionanocomposite Hydrogels: Ciprofloxacin Delivery, Release Kinetics and Antibacterial Activity. *J. Mol. Struct.* **2021**, *1225*, 129095. [CrossRef]
41. Ludeña Huaman, M.A. Método Preparativo Para La Obtención de Ácido Ursólico a Partir de Clinopodium Revolutum. *Rev. Colomb. Química* **2018**, *47*, 10–15. [CrossRef]
42. Gallardo, A.; Lujan, N.; Reinecke, H.; García, C.; del Campo, A.; Rodriguez-Hernandez, J. Chemical and Topographical Modification of Polycarbonate Surfaces through Diffusion/Photocuring Processes of Hydrogel Precursors Based on Vinylpyrrolidone. *Langmuir* **2017**, *33*, 1614–1622. [CrossRef] [PubMed]
43. Tran Vo, T.M.; Piroonpan, T.; Preuksarattanawut, C.; Kobayashi, T.; Potiyaraj, P. Characterization of PH-Responsive High Molecular-Weight Chitosan/Poly (Vinyl Alcohol) Hydrogel Prepared by Gamma Irradiation for Localizing Drug Release. *Bioresour. Bioprocess.* **2022**, *9*, 89. [CrossRef] [PubMed]

gels

MDPI

Article

Composite Hydrogel of Polyacrylamide/Starch/Gelatin as a Novel Amoxicillin Delivery System

Yağmur Poyraz [1], Nisa Baltacı [2], Gana Hassan [2], Oubadah Alayoubi [2], Bengü Özuğur Uysal [3,*] and Önder Pekcan [3]

[1] Computational Sciences and Engineering, School of Graduate Studies, Kadir Has University, Cibali, Fatih, Istanbul 34083, Turkey
[2] Materials Science and Nanotechnology, School of Graduate Studies, Kadir Has University, Cibali, Fatih, Istanbul 34083, Turkey
[3] Faculty of Engineering and Natural Sciences, Kadir Has University, Cibali, Fatih, Istanbul 34083, Turkey; pekcan@khas.edu.tr
* Correspondence: bozugur@khas.edu.tr; Tel.: +90-2125336532

Abstract: This study investigates the development and characterization of a novel composite hydrogel composed of polyacrylamide (PAAm), starch, and gelatin for use as an amoxicillin delivery system. The optical properties, swelling behavior, and drug release profile of the composite hydrogel's were studied to evaluate its efficacy and potential applications. UV-visible spectroscopy was employed to determine the optical properties, revealing significant transparency in the visible range, which is essential for biomedical applications. The incorporation of starch and gelatin into the polyacrylamide matrix significantly enhanced the hydrogel's swelling capacity and biocompatibility. Studies on drug delivery demonstrated a sustained release profile of amoxicillin in simulated gastrointestinal fluids, which is essential for maintaining therapeutic levels for a prolonged amount of time. The results indicate that the composite hydrogel of PAAm/starch/gelatin has good swelling behavior, appealing optical characteristics, and a promising controlled drug release mechanism. These results point to this hydrogel's considerable potential as a drug delivery method, providing a viable path toward enhancing the medicinal effectiveness of amoxicillin and maybe other medications.

Keywords: polyacrylamide; gelatin; drug delivery; polymer composites

1. Introduction

The development of advanced drug delivery systems has become a critical area of study in biomedical and pharmaceutical sciences [1–4]. Conventional drug administration methods frequently have drawbacks, such as poor bioavailability, rapid degradation of active components [5], and unregulated release rates, resulting in suboptimal therapeutic outcomes [6,7]. Hydrogels have emerged as a promising class of materials for drug delivery due to their unique physicochemical properties, which include a high-water content, biocompatibility, and tunable mechanical and swelling characteristics [8–10].

Hydrogels are three-dimensional, hydrophilic polymer networks capable of absorbing significant amounts of water or biological fluids. Their ability to mimic natural tissue environments makes them highly suitable for various biomedical applications, including wound healing [11–13], tissue engineering [14–18], and controlled drug delivery [19–21]. Among the different types of hydrogels, composite hydrogels, which combine two or more polymeric materials, offer enhanced properties by leveraging the strengths of each constituent polymer [22–25].

Polyacrylamide (PAAm) is the one of most widely used hydrogels because it is inexpensive, can be formed into desired shapes, and has an excellent swelling capacity and the flexibility to match biological materials [26]. It has numerous existing and potential applications, including drug delivery systems and chemo-mechanical devices. PAAm applications have recently shifted their focus to the development of innovative polymer systems with distinct structural and functional properties. Because PAAm can be chemically infused with other elements or compounds, it has applications in wound dressing, biosensors, drug delivery, tissue regeneration, and cartilage repair [27]. The copolymerization process of hydrogel composites composed of PAAm and various reinforcing additives is also significant for their clinical applications in cell biology and drug delivery [28]. The incorporation of nanoparticles such as silicon, carbon nanotubes, gelatine, cellulose, and other materials enhances the polyacrylamide hydrogel's strength, bonding, and self-healing properties [29–34]. PAAm, a promising hosting organic matrix for composite materials, not only provides mechanical stability but also new functionalities following the incorporation of conducting materials with various structures [35–39]. Blending PAAm with different polymers, proteins, or polysaccharides has led to exceptional mechanical properties, therapeutic effects, and better biocompatibility [40–47]. Moreover, crosslinking starch with citric acid has been shown to transform the macroporous architecture of PAAm-based hydrogels, resulting in a structure that is both highly porous and interconnected [48]. The incorporation of starch into the hydrogel matrix can improve its biodegradability and enhance the mechanical properties, making the hydrogel more suitable for drug delivery applications. Starch can provide additional functional groups for crosslinking, further improving the structural integrity of the composite hydrogel [49,50]. Gelatin, a protein derived from collagen, is another natural polymer widely used in biomedical applications. It possesses excellent biocompatibility, biodegradability, and the ability to promote cell adhesion and proliferation. The inclusion of gelatin in the composite hydrogel can significantly improve its biocompatibility, making it more suitable for in vivo applications. Additionally, gelatin can enhance the hydrogel's drug loading capacity due to its affinity for various drugs, including antibiotics like amoxicillin [51–53]. Furthermore, amoxicillin plays a significant role in treating gastrointestinal infections, particularly those caused by *Helicobacter pylori*, by helping to eradicate the bacteria and reduce the risk of peptic ulcers and gastritis [54,55].

This study focuses on the development of a composite hydrogel composed of polyacrylamide, starch, and gelatin specifically designed as a novel delivery system for the antibiotic amoxicillin. The utilization of PAAm/starch/gelatin composite hydrogels as controlled release systems for amoxicillin holds significant potential for improving the therapeutic efficacy of this widely used antibiotic. By addressing the limitations of traditional drug delivery methods, such as rapid degradation and suboptimal absorption, this hydrogel system aims to enhance patient outcomes and compliance. Furthermore, the study contributes to the broader field of hydrogel-based drug delivery systems by exploring the synergistic effects of combining synthetic and natural polymers, providing insights into the design and optimization of composite hydrogels for various biomedical applications.

2. Results and Discussion

2.1. Optical Studies

The experiments were carried out using a special type of UV-vis spectrophotometer, which only measures the transmittance corresponding to one wavelength. First, the transmitted light was measured at this special wavelength during the swelling of the gels in distilled water. The absorbance values of each composite gel were calculated from the following well-known formulation [56] using measured transmittance.

$$A = 2 - \log10\ (\%T) \tag{1}$$

Here, A is the absorbance and T is the transmission (percentage transmittance). As seen in Equation (1), the absorbance has a logarithmic relationship to the transmittance.

Figure 1 depicts the absorbance behavior of PAAm/starch/gelatin composite hydrogel combinations (S1–S5) which are given in detail in Table 1. It is observed that after a certain period of time, the absorbance value decreases in an exponential decay manner and finally stabilizes. These stabilization times are different for each sample. It is obvious that as the amount of starch in the hydrogel increases (S4 and S5), it takes longer for the absorbance value to stabilize. The transparency of the PAAm/starch/gelatin composite hydrogel is an important parameter as it can influence its applicability in various biomedical fields.

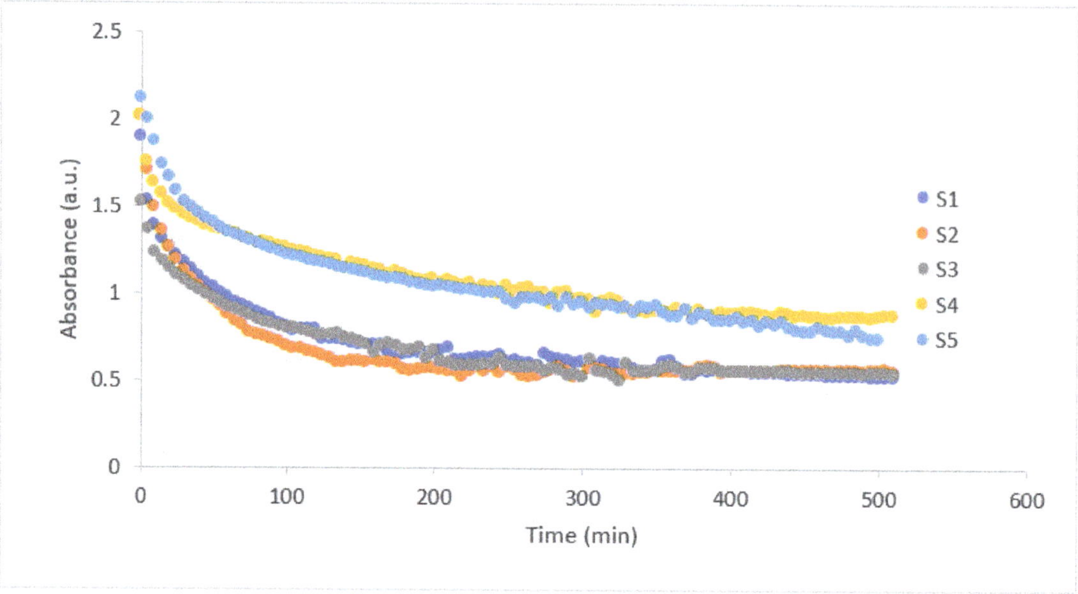

Figure 1. Absorbance versus time graph of PAAm/starch/gelatin composite hydrogels with increasing starch content from S1 to S5.

Table 1. Chemical composition (wt. %) of PAAm/starch/gelatin composite hydrogels.

	PAAm	Gelatin	Starch
S1	83.33	16.67	0.00
S2	83.33	12.50	4.17
S3	83.33	8.33	8.33
S4	83.33	4.17	12.50
S5	83.33	0.00	16.67

2.2. Swelling Behavior

The gravimetric method was used to examine the hydrogels' swelling characteristics. After the formation of gels inside the quartz cuvette, the square prism gel samples were left to dry. They were cut into three, all pieces measuring $0.6 \times 0.6 \times 0.4$ cm^3 in volume, along with their initial mass (mi), and were immersed in 2.5 mL of distilled water inside the quartz cuvette. The samples were removed from the cuvette at predefined intervals (t), weighed (mt), and then returned back to the distilled water bath inside the cuvette until their mass did not change. Table 2 gives the mass measurements using semi-dual balance before and after swelling of the gels. The mass final (mf) represents the mass of the hydrogels after the mass of the gels were constant. The swelling degree (Swelling%) at time t was calculated using the following formula [57,58]:

$$\text{Swelling\%} = \frac{\text{mt} - \text{mi}}{\text{mi}} \times 100 \quad (2)$$

As shown in Figure 2, the swelling degree of all composite gels first increased and then reached a constant point. Over time, as the interactions between polymer and solute increase, the osmotic pressure difference between gels and solutions decreases. Eventually, the rate at which aqueous solutions are absorbed continues to increase. However, as time passes on, the osmotic pressure reaches equilibrium, causing swelling to stay constant. It was observed that the equilibrium swelling degree of around 600% was reached after completely dry composite hydrogels were immersed in water for approximately 450 min. Therefore, this can be attributed to the hydrophilicity of the relevant polyacrylamide chains and the higher water retention capacity in the structure of gelatin–starch–polyacrylamide [58]. It can be seen that the swelling behavior of the hydrogels containing different amounts of starch and gelatin are similar. Accordingly, when the ratios given in Table 1 are investigated, PAAm, the main polymer, is dominant compared to the others, and it manages the entire interaction mechanism with water. The fact that the swelling degrees of all the hydrogels stabilized after almost the same period of time is proof of the dominant character of PAAm. On the other hand, it is obvious to see from S5 in Figure 2 that the starch addition promotes the swelling behavior of the gels. Moreover, the swelling test results indicate that the initial rise in swelling is due to the hydrophilic properties of starch, which enhance water uptake in the material. However, at lower starch concentrations, this effect diminishes, possibly because the starch content is too low to significantly impact the matrix, highlighting the need for further discussion on how starch concentration affects swelling behavior.

Table 2. Mass of the PAAm/starch/gelatin composite hydrogels before and after swelling. Swelling degree of the gels with different compositions.

	mi	mt	Swelling%
S1	104.66	710.60	578.9604
S2	92.34	557.20	503.4221
S3	76.56	513.57	570.8072
S4	97.25	646.19	564.4627
S5	80.60	606.80	652.8536

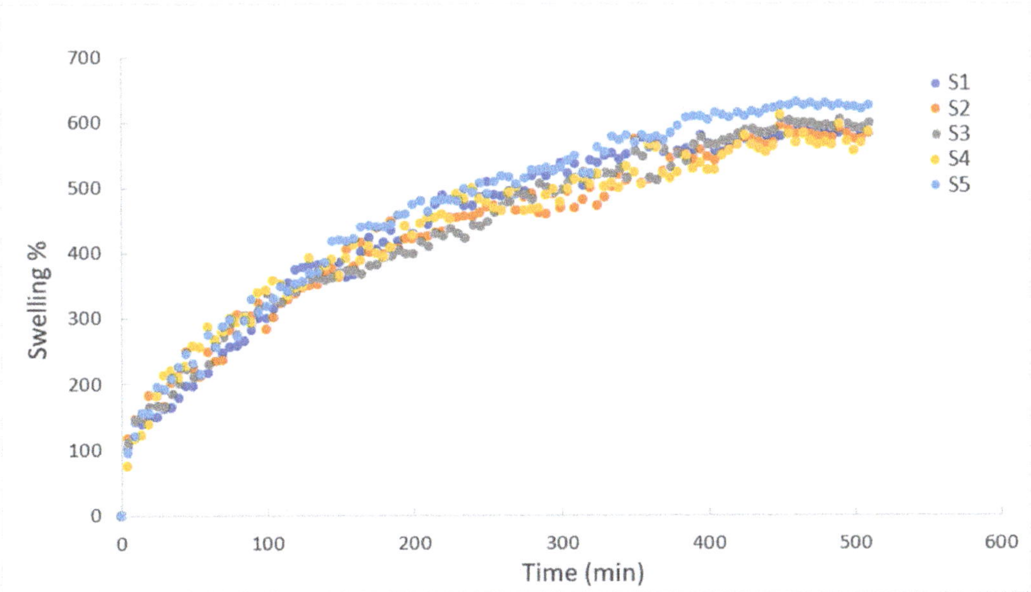

Figure 2. Swelling degree as function of time for composite hydrogels of PAAm/starch/gelatin in distilled water with different compositions.

Swelling, on the other hand, can actually be expressed as how much water diffuses into a gel. When the change in volume is considered as both bulk and shear energy, the diffusion of water into the gel and the expression of water uptake differentiate the swelling equation. In the new equation, it is not the initial gel mass that is important, but the gel mass (mf) that is fixed after swelling. In this case, the new equation can be written as follows [59,60]:

$$\left(1-\frac{\mathrm{mt}}{\mathrm{mf}}\right)=B_1\exp\left(-\frac{\mathrm{t}}{t_1}\right) \tag{3}$$

where B_1 is a parameter which is related to the longitudinal osmotic modulus, shear modulus, and geometry of the gel and it is always smaller than 1. t_1 is the relaxation time to reach the equilibrium related to the collective cooperative diffusion coefficient of the gel at the surface [59].

Alternatively, optical transmittance can also be used to study the swelling behavior. Solvent penetration into the gel, lattice heterogeneities, and solvent uptake amounts influence the transmitted light intensity, I_{tr}.

$$\left(1-\frac{\mathrm{mt}}{\mathrm{mf}}\right)=\frac{I_{tr}}{I_0} \tag{4}$$

Here, I_0 is the initial transmitted light intensity and the ratio of I_{tr}/I_0 gives the transmittance percentage value ($T\%$) divided by 100. The following relationship can be found using both Equations (3) and (4) and taking the logarithm of each side.

$$\mathrm{n}(T\%/100)=\ \ln B_1-\frac{\mathrm{t}}{t_1} \tag{5}$$

The transmittance data was obtained from the UV-vis spectrometer while the composite hydrogels were undergoing swelling, which was used to create Figure 3. These linear like ends of the graphs gives the linear regression to provide B_1 and t_1 values listed in Table 3. Those given in Table 3 are reasonable results because when the amount of starch in the composite gel increases, the shear energy of the diffusion process is very high, so the diffusion process slows down. Previously, diffusion coefficient, B_1 and t_1 values were found for disc, cylinder, and spherical PAAm gels. It has also been determined that all of these values depend on the geometry of the gel [60]. Therefore, although it would be wrong to directly compare the parameters found in the measurement results for approximately cube-shaped PAAm/starch/gelatin composite hydrogels with the results of gels with other geometries, the B_1 and t_1 values found are quite comparable to the values found by Li-Tanaka for the disk-shaped PAAm gel [60].

Table 3. The parameters calculated from the data of transmitted light measurements representing the swelling kinetics of the gels.

	B_1	t_1
S1	0.182136	935.4537
S2	0.221131	736.3770
S3	0.183599	730.4602
S4	0.066337	641.8485
S5	0.059309	464.9001

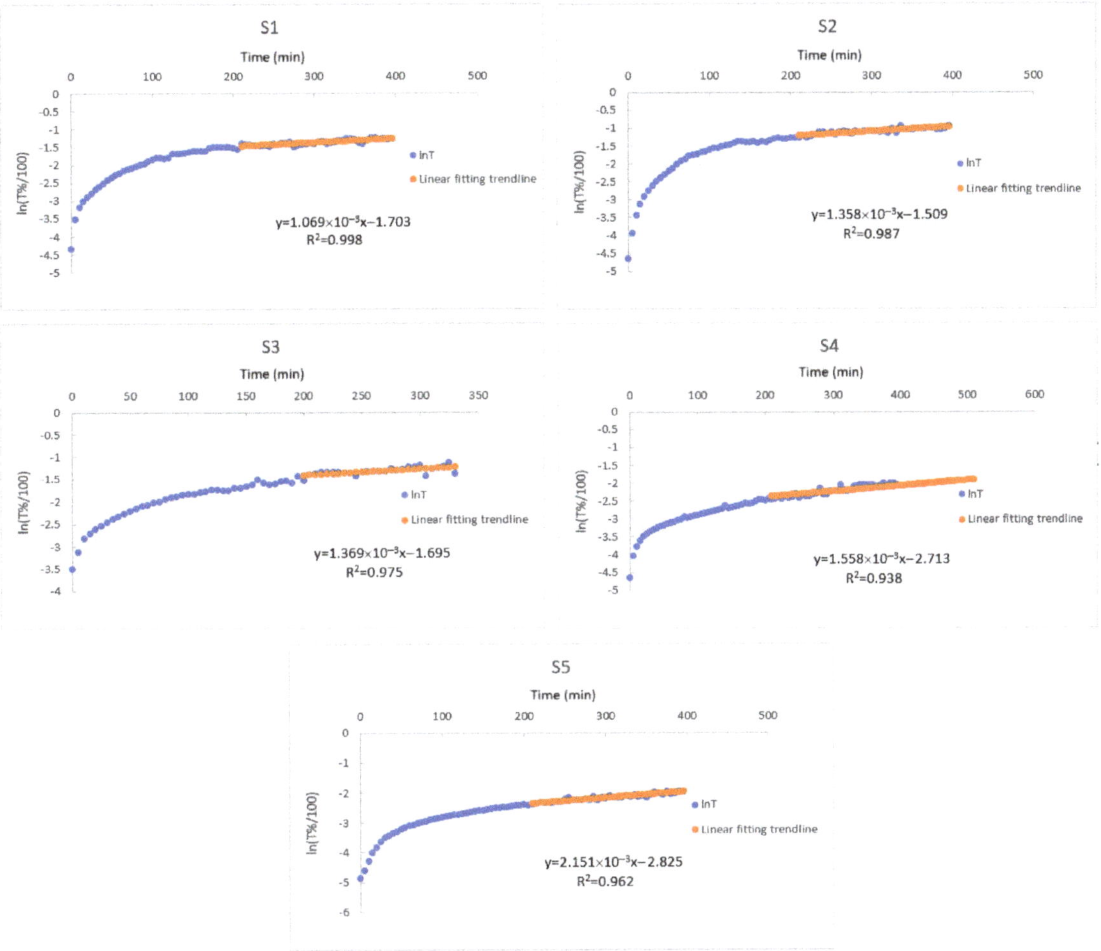

Figure 3. Plot of the natural logarithm of the transmittance data as function of time during the swelling of composite hydrogels of PAAm/starch/gelatin with different compositions (S1–S5) in distilled water.

2.3. Drug Release

To analyze the drug release properties of the gels with added amoxicillin, a fixed wavelength of 273 nm was selected. This wavelength is the calibration wavelength for amoxicillin [47]. Amoxicillin is a wide-ranging antibiotic that is effective against a range of bacterial infections. However, its therapeutic efficacy cannot be effective when it is degraded so fast in the digestive system, affecting adequate absorption when taken orally. These drawbacks can be addressed by a controlled release system, which keeps the medication from degrading and guarantees a steady release over time, preserving therapeutic drug concentrations and enhancing patient compliance. The pH environment was chosen as the same as the gastrointestinal medium (pH 3) using acetic acid and buffer solution. After amoxicillin was loaded during the gelation process, the gels were left to dry, and then the diffusion behavior of amoxicillin in the pH 3 liquid environment at room temperature was examined by a UV-vis spectrometer and transmitted light measurements at certain time intervals. The transmittance values of the liquid measured during the release of the drug were observed. Accordingly, the transmittance values of the liquid decrease over time as the drug is released into the liquid, as expected. The calculated [61] cumulative release of amoxicillin percentage graph plotted against time is presented in Figure 4. It is seen that the drug release kinetics of all composite hydrogels are similar in graphical trend due to the effect of PAAm in their content. When looked at from another perspective, it is clearly seen that the percentage release values vary according to the polymer content. Cumulative amoxicillin release percentages of composite hydrogels after 6 h are 51.575, 46.385, 41.2, 40.97, 37.4, respectively. Accordingly, as the amount of gelatin in the composite gel increases, more amount of drug can be released in a shorter time. However, due to the hydrophilic nature of starch, about 30% of the drug content is released into the environment in the first two hours of the S2, S3, and S4 composite hydrogels. The alteration in amoxicillin release behavior upon the addition of starch is primarily due to starch's hydrophilic nature, which affects the hydrogel's swelling and water absorption properties. Starch can increase the porosity of the hydrogel matrix, allowing for more water to penetrate, which accelerates the release of amoxicillin. However, at lower starch concentrations, the reduced swelling and matrix porosity may slow drug release. Starch may not chemically interact directly with the amoxicillin structure, but its physical interaction with the hydrogel network influences how the drug diffuses. The degree of crosslinking and the amount of starch added determine the balance between rapid diffusion due to swelling and controlled release due to limited matrix porosity. This variation in release profiles warrants a discussion on the role of starch concentration and its effect on hydrogel structure and drug release kinetics.

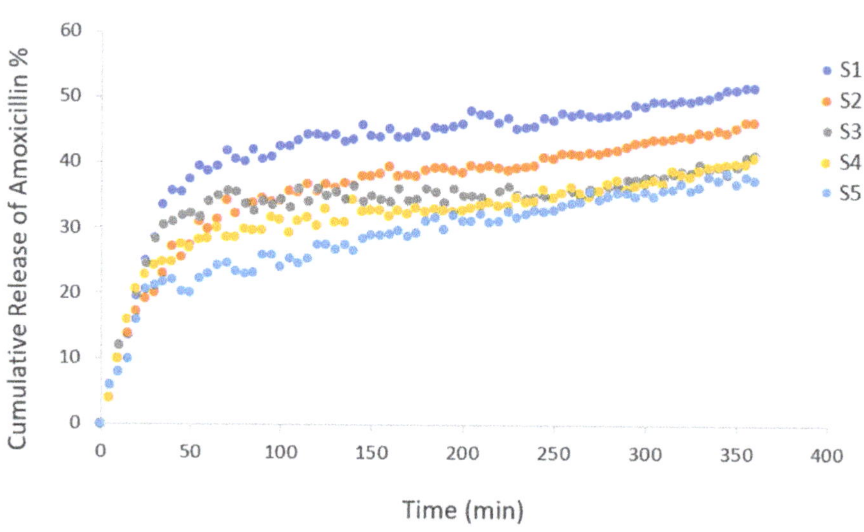

Figure 4. Plot of the cumulative release of amoxicillin from composite hydrogels PAAm/starch/gelatin with different compositions (S1–S5) in pH 3 medium. As the amount of gelatin in the composite gel increases, a greater amount of drug can be released in a shorter time. About 30% of the drug content is released into the environment in the first two hours of the S2, S3, and S4 composite hydrogels.

3. Conclusions

The advancement of composite hydrogels consisting of polyacrylamide, starch, and gelatin offers a promising controlled drug delivery system for amoxicillin. This approach proposes to improve the therapeutic efficacy of amoxicillin by addressing the drawbacks of traditional drug delivery techniques and making use of the distinctive characteristics of each polymer. Through a thorough examination of the hydrogel's optical properties, swelling behavior, and drug release profile, this research aims to provide crucial insights into its potential biomedical applications. It has been pointed out that the balanced addition of gelatin with starch, considering the swelling kinetics, offers a faster drug delivery solution in a short release time, even though only the addition of gelatin to PAAm can provide optimal release in a long-release time. These different composite hydrogels can be assessed in terms of their swelling kinetics and release characteristics based on the requirements. This study not only advances hydrogel-based drug delivery systems but also sets the stage for creating innovative composite materials for various therapeutic uses. High swelling capacity is critical for drug delivery systems because it directly influences and improves drug release from the polymer matrix, with greater swelling typically resulting in increased drug release at equilibrium.

4. Materials and Methods

4.1. Preparation of PAAm/Starch/Gelatin Composite Hydrogels

The PAAm solution was formed through a meticulously controlled free radical crosslinking copolymerization process, conducted at a stable room temperature of 22.5 °C and ambient relative humidity of 38%. Key reagents of acrylamide (AAm, Merck, Darmstadt, Germany), N,N′-Methylenebisacrylamide (BIS, Sigma-Aldrich, St. Louis, MO, USA, ABD), ammonium persulfate (APS, Sigma-Aldrich), and N,N,N′,N′-Tetramethylethylenediamine (TEMED, Sigma-Aldrich) were precisely dissolved in distilled water, employing both magnetic and mechanical stirring techniques. The methodology followed our previous research [35,37–39] and was used to prepare PAAm solutions. First, 500 mg of AAm was dissolved in 5 mL of distilled water, then 30 mg of BIS was added to the solution. TEMED was dropped into the beaker after 8 mg of APS was added to the solution. In the other beakers, 250 mg of gelatin (Sigma-Aldrich) was dissolved in 5 mL of distilled water and 125 mg of starch (food grade from local market) was mixed with 5 mL of distilled water at temperature of 80 °C. Samples S1 to S5 were prepared by varying the concentrations of starch and gelatin solutions, keeping the amount of PAAm solution constant as listed in Table 1. It was ensured that the total volume of starch and gelatin solutions was 1/5 of the volume of the PAAm solution. Distilled water with pH 7.4 was used as a solving medium. Just before the formation of the gels, the solutions were poured into the quartz cuvettes of the spectrophotometer to form a square prism shape to them (Figure 5a). After gelation occurred, the gels were carefully removed from the cuvette, divided into 3 equal parts, and left to dry at room temperature (Figure 5b). Thus, three different cube-like gels were obtained from each sample (S1–S5) for swelling and drug release measurements, thus ensuring the accuracy of the measurement results (Figure 5b,c). After the Klamox powder was used to prepare a suspension containing commercially available amoxicillin which was dissolved in 5 mL of distilled water at 60 °C, the drug was loaded by dipping the dry gels into the solution (Figure 5d). Then, the gels were cleared of excess drug and left to dry. For drug release experiments, to simulate the gastrointestinal medium, acetic acid and buffer solution was prepared at specific concentration to produce a pH 3 solution (Figure 5e).

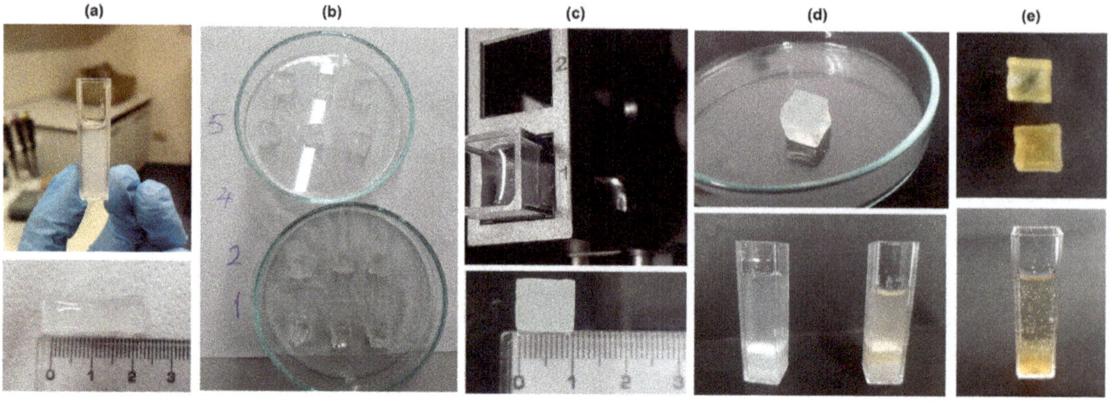

Figure 5. (**a**) ***Above:*** Sample S3 has a form of gel in the quartz cuvette. ***Below:*** After removing the gel Sample 3 from the cuvette, it has a square prism shape. (**b**) Composite hydrogels (S1, S2, S4, S5) after dividing into three. (**c**) ***Above:*** Cube shaped sample inside the distilled water in the quartz cuvette of spectrometer after drying is ready for swelling experiments. 1 and 2 show the compartments of the spectrometer cabin. ***Below:*** Swelled composite gel (S3). (**d**) ***Above:*** Swelled composite gel (S3) before drying. ***Below:*** Composite hydrogels (S2, S3) after drug loading. (**e**) ***Above:*** S2 and S3 after releasing the drug. ***Below:*** S3 after drug loading and drying inside pH 3 medium for drug release.

4.2. Characterization

All the swelling and drug release experiments were carried out using Spectro 22 UV–vis Spectrophotometer, Labomed Inc., Los Angeles, California, USA. The change in the photon transmitted light during the swelling of composite hydrogels of PAAm with various combinations of gelatin and starch was measured at $\lambda = 273$ nm wavelength. The transmittance of photon was monitored in real-time by the camera system. Swelling experiments were performed using two identical cuvettes. The dried gels were soaked in distilled water inside the cuvettes. One was put into the spectrometer cabin; the other one was put onto the desk for the gravimetric measurements. Both measurements were carried out at the same time. To perform drug release measurements, dried gels containing amoxicillin were added to acetic acid + buffer solution at pH 3 in quartz vessels and kept there. Two different experimental setups were created simultaneously. While the gels were weighed at regular intervals (5 min) with one, the intensity of the light passing through the liquid was measured by keeping the other in the spectrometer cabin (Figure 5c). A pH meter (86505 pH/mV/Cond./TDS/Temp.meter, AZ Instruments Corp., Taichung City, Taiwan) was used for swelling and drug release experiments.

4.3. Swelling Test

The swelling behavior of PAAm/starch/gelatin composite hydrogels in distilled water was studied at room temperature by gravimetric analysis. Since it is thought that the prepared gels could be used for therapeutic purposes in the future, swelling experiments were carried out in pH 7.4 environment which is close to the body fluid (intravenously via serum) because the drug delivery could be realized in the body fluid medium through these hydrogels. PAAm/starch/gelatin composite hydrogels with different compositions (S1–S5) were placed in Petri dishes for the drying process of the gels at room temperature (Figure 5b). Ten quartz cuvettes were filled with distilled water. Each hydrogel sample was soaked into the quartz cuvettes for the swelling experiments to maintain the same environment of spectrometer. Then, each was removed from the solution every 5 min and weighed on the scale and the differences in mass were recorded. When the pre-set time interval was reached, the hydrogels were taken out and the water on the surface was gently removed with filter paper. Then, the hydrogels were weighed and the change in mass after swelling was calculated. The solvent uptake percentage or swelling degree for each sample was calculated according to Equation (2) using the initial and after swelling mass of the composite hydrogels. In another approach, these can be taken as the mass of the dry state and wet state of the hydrogels [62,63]. At the same time as the swelling experiments, the other half of the hydrogel samples inside the quartz cuvettes were put in the spectrometer cabin one by one for the optical transmittance measurements. Absorbance values of the hydrogels were calculated and Figure 1 forms.

4.4. *In Vitro Drug Loading and Release Tests*

To prepare KLAMOKS ES 600 mg/42.9 mg Oral Suspension containing amoxicillin, which is actively used as an antibiotic in almost all infections of children, first enough distilled water was added to the powder medicine in the bottle, corresponding to half of the dilution line on the bottle, and the bottle was shaken well to suspend the powder. Then, the bottle had to be mixed again by adding distilled water up to the top line of the bottle. This was a dose-adjusted method used to obtain a homogeneous antibiotic solution taken orally. However, in order to fully understand the absorption of the drug in the stomach environment and to observe the role of the prepared composite hydrogels in drug release, it is necessary to add the drug during the gelation of all hydrogels and examine the drug release in a liquid medium simulating the stomach/intestines after the drying process. Therefore, the drug was loaded into the hydrogel solutions during gelation. To see the effect of starch and gelatin, all hydrogels were left to dry at room temperature of 22 °C for three days before drug loading. pH 4 standard buffer solution was added into the acetic acid solution until the pH value of the final solution was 3, and thus a solution simulating gastric fluid was prepared. Drug release experiments were then carried out alongside permeability measurements using UV–VIS spectrophotometry and the change in color was measured as evidence of detecting amoxicillin release from the cube-shaped (Figure 5d) sample into solutions. The spectroscopic method and gel weighing processes were carried out simultaneously with the same amount of hydrogel. The in vitro drug release (%) was determined from the cumulative drug release Equation (6):

$$\text{Cumulative drug release } (\%) = \sum_{t=0}^{t} \frac{M_t}{M_0} \times 100 \tag{6}$$

where M_0 is the initial amount of the drug at $t = 0$ and M_t is the cumulative amount of the drug release at time t [64].

Author Contributions: B.Ö.U. conceptualized, supervised, edited, and majorly contributed to the writing of the manuscript; Y.P. and N.B. majorly contributed to the formal analysis, validation, visualization, writing and reviewing of the original draft; G.H. and O.A. majorly contributed to the investigation, data curation, and validation of the article and partially contributed to the writing. Ö.P. majorly contributed to the reviewing and supervision of the manuscript. All authors have read and agreed to the published version of the manuscript.

Funding: This research received no external funding.

Institutional Review Board Statement: Not applicable.

Informed Consent Statement: Not applicable.

Data Availability Statement: The data that support findings of this study are available from the corresponding author upon reasonable request.

Acknowledgments: All the experiments and characterizations of this study were performed Materials Design and Innovation Laboratory (MADI LAB).

Conflicts of Interest: The authors declare no conflicts of interest.

References

1. Tiwari, G.; Tiwari, R.; Sriwastawa, B.; Bhati, L.; Pandey, S.; Pandey, P.; Bannerjee, S.K. Drug delivery systems: An updated review. *Int. J. Pharm. Investig.* **2012**, *2*, 2–11. [CrossRef] [PubMed]
2. Adepu, S.; Ramakrishna, S. Controlled Drug Delivery Systems: Current Status and Future Directions. *Molecules* **2021**, *26*, 5905. [CrossRef] [PubMed]
3. Sahu, T.; Ratre, Y.K.; Chauhan, S.; Bhaskar, L.V.K.S.; Nair, M.P.; Verma, H.K. Nanotechnology-based drug delivery system: Current strategies and emerging therapeutic potential for medical science. *J. Drug Deliv. Sci. Technol.* **2021**, *63*, 102487. [CrossRef]
4. Liu, D.; Yang, F.; Xiong, F.; Gu, N. The Smart Drug Delivery System and Its Clinical Potential. *Theranostics* **2016**, *6*, 1306–1323. [CrossRef] [PubMed]
5. Lessmann, T.; Jones, S.A.; Voigt, T.; Weisbrod, S.; Kracker, O.; Winter, S.; Zúñiga, L.A.; Stark, S.; Bisek, N.; Sprogøe, K. Degradable Hydrogel for Sustained Localized Delivery of Anti-Tumor Drugs. *J. Pharm. Sci.* **2023**, *112*, 2843–2852. [CrossRef] [PubMed]
6. Patra, J.K.; Das, G.; Fraceto, L.F.; Campos, E.V.; Rodriguez-Torres, M.D.; Acosta-Torres, L.S.; Diaz-Torres, L.A.; Grillo, R.; Swamy, M.K.; Sharma, S.; et al. Nano based drug delivery systems: Recent developments and future prospects. *J. Nanobiotechnol.* **2018**, *16*, 71. [CrossRef]
7. Hossen, S.; Hossain, M.K.; Basher, M.K.; Mia, M.N.H.; Rahman, M.T.; Uddin, M.J. Smart nanocarrier-based drug delivery systems for cancer therapy and toxicity studies: A review. *J. Adv. Res.* **2019**, *15*, 1–18. [CrossRef]
8. Cao, H.; Duan, L.; Zhang, Y.; Cao, J.; Zhang, K. Current hydrogel advances in physicochemical and biological response-driven biomedical application diversity. *Signal Transduct. Target. Ther.* **2021**, *6*, 426. [CrossRef] [PubMed]
9. Gopinath, V.; Saravanan, S.; Al-Maleki, A.R.; Ramesh, M.; Vadivelu, J. A review of natural polysaccharides for drug delivery applications: Special focus on cellulose, starch and glycogen. *Biomed. Pharmacother.* **2018**, *107*, 96–108. [CrossRef]
10. Thakur, S.; Sharma, B.; Verma, A.; Chaudhary, J.; Tamulevicius, S.; Thakur, V.K. Recent progress in sodium alginate based sustainable hydrogels for environmental applications. *J. Clean. Prod.* **2018**, *198*, 143–159. [CrossRef]
11. Liang, Y.; He, J.; Guo, B. Functional Hydrogels as Wound Dressing to Enhance Wound Healing. *ACS Nano* **2021**, *15*, 12687–12722. [CrossRef] [PubMed]
12. Chen, G.P.; Yu, Y.R.; Wu, X.W.; Wang, G.F.; Ren, J.A.; Zhao, Y.J. Bioinspired Multifunctional Hybrid Hydrogel Promotes Wound Healing. *Adv. Funct. Mater.* **2018**, *28*, 1801386. [CrossRef]
13. Luo, Y.; Diao, H.; Xia, S.; Dong, L.; Chen, J.; Zhang, J. A physiologically active polysaccharide hydrogel promotes wound healing. *J. Biomed. Mater. Res. A* **2010**, *94A*, 193–204. [CrossRef]
14. Lee, K.Y.; Mooney, D.J. Hydrogels for tissue engineering. *Chem. Rev.* **2001**, *101*, 1869–1880. [CrossRef] [PubMed]
15. Drury, J.L.; Mooney, D.J. Hydrogels for tissue engineering: Scaffold design variables and applications. *Biomaterials* **2003**, *24*, 4337–4351. [CrossRef]
16. Nguyen, K.T.; West, J.L. Photopolymerizable hydrogels for tissue engineering applications. *Biomaterials* **2002**, *23*, 4307–4314. [CrossRef]
17. Khademhosseini, A.; Langer, R. Microengineered hydrogels for tissue engineering. *Biomaterials* **2007**, *28*, 5087–5092. [CrossRef]
18. Mantha, S.; Pillai, S.; Khayambashi, P.; Upadhyay, A.; Zhang, Y.; Tao, O.; Pham, H.M.; Tran, S.D. Smart hydrogels in tissue engineering and regenerative medicine. *Materials* **2019**, *12*, 3323. [CrossRef]
19. Li, J.; Mooney, D.J. Designing hydrogels for controlled drug delivery. *Nat. Rev. Mater.* **2016**, *1*, 16071. [CrossRef]
20. Ganji, F.; Vasheghani-Farahani, E. Hydrogels in controlled drug delivery systems. *Iran. Polym. J.* **2009**, *18*, 63–88.
21. Gupta, P.; Vermani, K.; Garg, S. Hydrogels: From controlled release to pH-responsive drug delivery. *Drug Discov. Today* **2002**, *7*, 569–579. [CrossRef] [PubMed]
22. Dhand, A.P.; Galarraga, J.H.; Burdick, J.A. Enhancing biopolymer hydrogel functionality through interpenetrating networks. *Trends Biotechnol.* **2021**, *39*, 519–538. [CrossRef] [PubMed]
23. Chimene, D.; Kaunas, R.; Gaharwar, A.K. Hydrogel bioink reinforcement for additive manufacturing: A focused review of emerging strategies. *Adv. Mater.* **2020**, *32*, 1902026. [CrossRef] [PubMed]
24. Thang, N.H.; Chien, T.B.; Cuong, D.X. Polymer-based hydrogels applied in drug delivery: An overview. *Gels* **2023**, *9*, 523. [CrossRef] [PubMed]
25. Tozzi, G.; De Mori, A.; Oliveira, A.; Roldo, M. Composite hydrogels for bone regeneration. *Materials* **2016**, *9*, 267. [CrossRef]
26. Byron, M.L.; Variano, E.A. Refractive-index-matched hydrogel materials for measuring flow-structure interactions. *Exp. Fluids* **2013**, *54*, 1456. [CrossRef]
27. Chen, X.; Yan, H.; Bao, C.; Zhu, Q.; Liu, Z.; Wen, Y.; Li, Z.; Zhang, T.; Lin, Q. Fabrication and evaluation of homogeneous alginate/polyacrylamide–chitosan–gelatin composite hydrogel scaffolds based on the interpenetrating networks for tissue engineering. *Polym. Eng. Sci.* **2022**, *62*, 116–128. [CrossRef]
28. Kalshetti, P.P.; Rajendra, V.B.; Dixit, D.N.; Parekh, P.P. Hydrogels as a drug delivery system and applications: A review. *Int. J. Pharm. Pharm. Sci.* **2012**, *4*, 1–7.
29. Voronova, M.I.; Surov, O.V.; Afineevskii, A.V.; Zakharov, A.G. Properties of polyacrylamide composites reinforced by cellulose nanocrystals. *Heliyon* **2020**, *6*, e05529. [CrossRef]
30. Rukmanikrishnan, B.; Ramalingam, S.; Lee, J. Quaternary ammonium silane-reinforced agar/polyacrylamide composites for packaging applications. *Int. J. Biol. Macromol.* **2021**, *182*, 1301–1309. [CrossRef]

31. Yang, R.M.; Liu, Y.H.; Dong, G.X.; Zhao, D.J. Fabrication and properties of composites of linear polyacrylamide and functionalized carbon nanotubes. *Adv. Mater. Res.* **2014**, *936*, 12–16. [CrossRef]
32. Kausar, A. Properties of polyacrylamide and functional multi-walled carbon nanotube composite. *Am. J. Nanosci. Nanotechnol. Res.* **2016**, *4*, 1–8.
33. Narimani, A.; Kordnejad, F.; Kaur, P.; Bazgir, S.; Hemmati, M.; Duong, A. Rheological and thermal stability of interpenetrating polymer network hydrogel based on polyacrylamide/hydroxypropyl guar reinforced with graphene oxide for application in oil recovery. *J. Polym. Eng.* **2021**, *41*, 788–798. [CrossRef]
34. Awasthi, S.; Gaur, J.K.; Bobji, M.S.; Srivastava, C. Nanoparticle-reinforced polyacrylamide hydrogel composites for clinical applications: A review. *J. Mater. Sci.* **2022**, *57*, 8041–8063. [CrossRef]
35. Özuğur Uysal, B.; Evingür, G.A.; Pekcan, Ö. Polyacrylamide mediated polyvinylpyrrolidone composites incorporated with aligned molybdenum disulfide. *J. Appl. Polym. Sci.* **2022**, *139*, 52061. [CrossRef]
36. Evingür, G.A.; Sağlam, N.A.; Çimen, B.; Özuğur Uysal, B.; Pekcan, Ö. The WS_2 dependence on the elasticity and optical band gap energies of swollen PAAm composites. *J. Compos. Mater.* **2021**, *55*, 71–76. [CrossRef]
37. Nayır, Ş.; Kıvrak, S.; Kara, İ.; Özuğur Uysal, B.; Pekcan, Ö. Tungsten disulfide (WS_2) doped polyacrylamide (PAAm) composites: Gelation and optical studies. *Optik* **2021**, *245*, 167673. [CrossRef]
38. Özuğur Uysal, B.; Nayır, Ş.; Açba, M.; Çıtır, B.; Durmaz, S.; Koçoğlu, Ş.; Yıldız, E.; Pekcan, Ö. 2D materials (WS_2, MoS_2, $MoSe_2$) enhanced polyacrylamide gels for multi-functional applications. *Gels* **2022**, *8*, 465. [CrossRef]
39. Kalaycıoğlu, Z.; Özuğur Uysal, B.; Pekcan, Ö.; Erim, F.B. Efficient photocatalytic degradation of methylene blue dye from aqueous solution with cerium oxide nanoparticles and graphene oxide doped polyacrylamide. *ACS Omega* **2023**, *8*, 13004–13015. [CrossRef] [PubMed]
40. Xue, H.; Hu, L.; Xiong, Y.; Zhu, X.; Wei, C.; Cao, F.; Zhou, W.; Sun, Y.; Endo, Y.; Liu, M.; et al. Quaternized chitosan-Matrigel polyacrylamide hydrogels as wound dressing for wound repair and regeneration. *Carbohydr. Polym.* **2019**, *226*, 115302. [CrossRef]
41. Pérez-Martínez, C.J.; Chávez, S.D.; del Castillo-Castro, T.; Ceniceros, T.E.; Castillo-Ortega, M.M.; Rodríguez-Félix, D.E.; Ruiz, J.C. Electroconductive nanocomposite hydrogel for pulsatile drug release. *React. Funct. Polym.* **2016**, *100*, 12–17. [CrossRef]
42. Yang, Z.; Peng, H.; Wang, W.; Liu, T. Crystallization behavior of poly(ε-caprolactone)/layered double hydroxide nanocomposites. *J. Appl. Polym. Sci.* **2010**, *116*, 2658–2667. [CrossRef]
43. Mandal, B.B.; Kapoor, S.; Kundu, S.C. Silk fibroin/polyacrylamide semi-interpenetrating network hydrogels for controlled drug release. *Biomaterials* **2009**, *30*, 2826–2836. [CrossRef] [PubMed]
44. Miranda, M.E.; Marcolla, C.; Rodrígues, C.A.; Wilhelm, H.M.; Sierakowski, M.R.; Bresolin, T.M.; de Freitas, R.A. Chitosan and N-carboxymethylchitosan: I. The role of N-carboxymethylation of chitosan in the thermal stability and dynamic mechanical properties of its films. *Polym. Int.* **2006**, *55*, 961–969. [CrossRef]
45. Wang, J.; Zhou, X.; Xiao, H. Structure and properties of cellulose/poly(N-isopropylacrylamide) hydrogels prepared by SIPN strategy. *Carbohydr. Polym.* **2013**, *94*, 749–754. [CrossRef]
46. Elvira, C.; Mano, J.F.; San Román, J.; Reis, R.L. Starch-based biodegradable hydrogels with potential biomedical applications as drug delivery systems. *Biomaterials* **2002**, *23*, 1955–1966. [CrossRef] [PubMed]
47. Torres-Figueroa, A.V.; Pérez-Martínez, C.J.; Castillo-Castro, T.D.; Bolado-Martínez, E.; Corella-Madueño, M.A.; García-Alegría, A.M.; Lara-Ceniceros, T.E.; Armenta-Villegas, L. Composite hydrogel of poly(acrylamide) and starch as potential system for controlled release of amoxicillin and inhibition of bacterial growth. *J. Chem.* **2020**, *2020*, 5860487. [CrossRef]
48. Kavousi, F.; Nikfarjam, N. Highly interconnected microporous structures made from starch nanoparticle-stabilized medium internal phase emulsion polymerization for use in cell culture. *Polymer* **2019**, *180*, 121744. [CrossRef]
49. Pushpamalar, J.; Veeramachineni, A.K.; Owh, C.; Loh, X.J. Biodegradable polysaccharides for controlled drug delivery. *ChemPlusChem* **2016**, *81*, 504–514. [CrossRef]
50. Lee, C.S.; Hwang, H.S. Starch-based hydrogels as a drug delivery system in biomedical applications. *Gels* **2023**, *9*, 951. [CrossRef]
51. Mir, A.; Kumar, A.; Alam, J.; Riaz, U. Synthesis and characterization of pH-responsive conducting polymer/Na-alginate/gelatin-based composite hydrogels for sustained release of amoxicillin drug. *Int. J. Biol. Macromol.* **2023**, *252*, 126015. [CrossRef] [PubMed]
52. Gholamali, I.; Yadollahi, M. Bio-nanocomposite polymer hydrogels containing nanoparticles for drug delivery: A review. *Regen. Eng. Transl. Med.* **2021**, *7*, 129–146. [CrossRef]
53. Hakim, L.K.; Yazdanian, M.; Alam, M.; Abbasi, K.; Tebyaniyan, H.; Tahmasebi, E.; Yazdanian, A. Biocompatible and biomaterials application in drug delivery system in oral cavity. *Evid.-Based Complement. Altern. Med.* **2021**, *2021*, 9011226. [CrossRef] [PubMed]
54. Chey, W.D.; Leontiadis, G.I.; Howden, C.W.; Moss, S.F. ACG Clinical Guideline: Treatment of Helicobacter pylori infection. *Am. J. Gastroenterol.* **2017**, *112*, 212–239. [CrossRef] [PubMed]
55. Fallone, C.A.; Moss, S.F.; Malfertheiner, P. Helicobacter pylori infection: Guidelines for management. *Gut* **2020**, *69*, 2093–2100. [CrossRef]
56. International Union of Pure and Applied Chemistry-IUPAC. *Compendium of Chemical Terminology*, 2nd ed.; The "Gold Book"; McNaught, A.D., Wilkinson, A., Eds.; Blackwell Scientific Publications: Oxford, UK, 2019. [CrossRef]
57. Claus, J.; Brietzke, A.; Lehnert, C.; Oschatz, S.; Grabow, N.; Kragl, U. Swelling characteristics and biocompatibility of ionic liquid based hydrogels for biomedical applications. *PLoS ONE* **2020**, *15*, 0231421. [CrossRef]

58. Saber-Samandari, S.; Gazi, M.; Yilmaz, E. UV-induced synthesis of chitosan-g-polyacrylamide semi-IPN superabsorbent hydrogels. *Polym. Bull.* **2012**, *68*, 1623–1639. [CrossRef]
59. Pekcan, O.; Kara, S. Photon transmission technique for monitoring formation and swelling of polyacrylamide gels. *Polym.-Plast. Technol. Eng.* **2002**, *41*, 573–588. [CrossRef]
60. Li, Y.; Tanaka, T. Kinetics of swelling and shrinking of gels. *J. Chem. Phys.* **1990**, *92*, 1365–1370. [CrossRef]
61. Xu, L.; Qiu, L.; Sheng, Y.; Sun, Y.; Deng, L.; Li, X.; Bradley, M.; Zhang, R. Biodegradable pH-responsive hydrogels for controlled dual-drug release. *J. Mater. Chem. B* **2018**, *6*, 510–517. [CrossRef]
62. Li, L.; Zhao, J.; Sun, Y.; Yu, F.; Ma, J. Ionically cross-linked sodium alginate/κ-carrageenan double-network gel beads with low-swelling, enhanced mechanical properties, and excellent adsorption performance. *Chem. Eng. J.* **2019**, *372*, 1091–1103. [CrossRef]
63. Mirza, S.; Jolly, R.; Zia, I.; Umar, M.S.; Owais, M.; Shakir, M. Bioactive gum arabic/κ-carrageenan-incorporated nano-hydroxyapatite nanocomposites and their relative biological functionalities in bone tissue engineering. *ACS Omega* **2020**, *5*, 11279–11290. [CrossRef] [PubMed]
64. Singh, P.; Verma, C.; Mukhopadhyay, S.; Gupta, A.; Gupta, B. Preparation of thyme oil-loaded κ-carrageenan-polyethylene glycol hydrogel membranes as wound care system. *Int. J. Pharm.* **2022**, *618*, 121661. [CrossRef] [PubMed]

gels

MDPI

Article

Photopolymerization of Chlorpromazine-Loaded Gelatin Methacryloyl Hydrogels: Characterization and Antimicrobial Applications

Tatiana Tozar [1,*,†], Simona Nistorescu [1,2,†], Gratiela Gradisteanu Pircalabioru [3,4], Mihai Boni [1,*] and Angela Staicu [1,*]

1 Laser Department, National Institute for Laser, Plasma and Radiation Physics, 409 Atomistilor, Magurele, 077125 Ilfov, Romania
2 Department of Biochemistry and Molecular Biology, Faculty of Biology, University of Bucharest, 91–95 Splaiul Independentei, 050095 Bucharest, Romania
3 Research Institute of the University of Bucharest (ICUB), University of Bucharest, 050095 Bucharest, Romania; gratiela.gradisteanu@icub.unibuc.ro
4 Academy of Romanian Scientists, Ilfov Street 3, 050054 Bucharest, Romania
* Correspondence: tatiana.alexandru@inflpr.ro (T.T.); mihai.boni@inflpr.ro (M.B.); angela.staicu@inflpr.ro (A.S.); Tel.: +40-21-457-5739 (T.T. & M.B. & A.S.)
† These authors contributed equally to this work.

Abstract: This study investigates the synthesis, characterization, and antimicrobial properties of hydrogels synthesized through the UV-pulsed laser photopolymerization of a polymer–photoinitiator–chlorpromazine mixture. Chlorpromazine was used for its known enhanced antimicrobial properties when exposed to UV laser radiation. The hydrogel was formed from a mixture containing 0.05% Irgacure 2959, 10% gelatin methacryloyl, and various concentrations of chlorpromazine (1, 2, and 4 mg/mL). Laser-induced fluorescence spectroscopy was employed to monitor the photoinduced changes of chlorpromazine and Irgacure 2959 during hydrogel formation, providing insight into the photodegradation dynamics. FTIR spectroscopy confirmed the incorporation of irradiated chlorpromazine within the hydrogel matrix, while the release profiles of chlorpromazine showed sustained release only in hydrogels containing 1 mg/mL of CPZ. The hydrogel showed significant antimicrobial activity against MRSA bacteria when compared to that of penicillin. These findings highlight the potential of CPZ loaded during the photopolymerization process into hydrogels as effective antimicrobial agents with sustained release properties, making them suitable for combating resistant bacterial strains.

Keywords: Irgacure 2959; gelatin methacryloyl; chlorpromazine; photopolymerization

1. Introduction

Chlorpromazine (CPZ) is a well-known antipsychotic drug belonging to the phenothiazine class. Beyond its primary use in psychiatry, CPZ has demonstrated significant antimicrobial properties against a variety of pathogens, including bacteria [1,2], fungi [3,4], and mycobacteria [5].

The antimicrobial effect of CPZ irradiated with a 266 nm laser beam has been studied, revealing significant improvements in its antibacterial properties. When CPZ is exposed to a 266 nm laser beam, it undergoes photochemical reactions that produce new species with potent antimicrobial activities [2,6]. These new products exhibit increased efficacy against various bacterial strains, including Gram-positive and Gram-negative bacteria. For instance, prolonged irradiation of CPZ significantly enhances its antibacterial activity against *Staphylococcus aureus* and *Escherichia coli*, although it does not affect their efflux pumps [7]. Additionally, the irradiated CPZ shows antimicrobial and antibiofilm activities against several Gram-positive bacteria, including methicillin-resistant *Staphylococcus aureus*

(MRSA) and *Enterococcus* species, by inhibiting efflux pump activity and inducing cellular membrane lesions [2]. Moreover, the products formed during irradiation also demonstrated activity against mycobacteria, including multidrug-resistant tuberculosis strains, with lower cytotoxicity compared to the unirradiated compound [8]. These studies show that CPZ irradiation with pulsed laser radiation could be a promising approach to improve current antimicrobial treatments and combat antibiotic resistance [6,9].

Hydrogels represent an important progression in drug delivery system development [10]. Their customizable properties, biocompatibility, and ability to provide controlled and continuous release of therapeutic agents make them invaluable in biomedical applications [11].

Photopolymerization is a widely used technique for forming hydrogels, particularly in biomedical applications, where gelatin methacryloyl (GelMa) is a popular choice of material due to its biocompatibility and tunable mechanical properties. Photopolymerization uses UV or visible light to dissociate a co-initiator/photoinitiator into radicals that trigger the bonding of monomers or macromers into a crosslinked network, which forms the hydrogel [12]. The type of light source and photoinitiator needs to be selected accordingly because it impacts the efficiency, cytocompatibility, and mechanical properties of the resulting hydrogels [13–15]. This technique is widely used in tissue engineering, drug delivery, and the fabrication of microfluidic devices due to its ability to provide precise spatial and temporal control over the polymerization process [16]. This can be achieved by adjusting the light intensity, exposure time, or photoinitiator concentration [13,17]. Photopolymerization, which typically involves the use of a photoinitiator, such as Irgacure 2959, initiates the crosslinking of GelMa upon exposure to UV light [10,18]. Irgacure 2959 is able to reduce the curing time of hydrogels and allows faster photo-crosslinking [10,19]. Additionally, it shows improved mechanical properties, such as compressive modulus and stability, which help to maintain the integrity of the hydrogel [20,21], and it is considered biocompatible [22]. GelMa hydrogels formed through photopolymerization using Irgacure 2959 have been extensively used in various biomedical applications, including tissue engineering [23], wound healing [24], and drug delivery [10,25].

In our previous studies, Tozar et al. [10] presented the synthesis and characterization of hydrogels obtained after the irradiation of various Irgacure 2959 concentrations and GelMa at 10% w/v up to 30 min with a 266 nm pulsed laser beam at different energies (0.25, 0.45, 0.75, and 1 mJ). Considering the unreacted Irgacure, swelling behavior, drug release profile, and transparency of the hydrogels, the optimal conditions for hydrogel synthesis were a beam energy of 0.75 mJ and exposure time of 1 min. The end goal of the study was to assess the potential of the obtained GelMa hydrogels as drug delivery systems for irradiated CPZ. A volume of 2 mg/mL solution of CPZ (concentration 2 mg/mL) was previously and separately irradiated (energy 6.5 mJ and time period of 30 min), and loaded afterward into already formed GelMa hydrogels. The irradiation conditions for CPZ were chosen in accordance with Tozar et al. [2], where the 30 min irradiated CPZ presented the best irradiation condition in terms of antimicrobial activity. Consequently, the GelMa hydrogel loaded with CPZ (irradiated independently) was shown to be effective against *Staphylococcus aureus* ATCC 25923 and MRSA.

In contrast, the present study aims to uses the same conditions for GelMa hydrogel synthesis (266 nm laser beam, 0.7 mJ energy) while incorporating the irradiation of CPZ directly during the photopolymerization process of the GelMa hydrogels. By irradiating GelMa–Irgacure 2959–CPZ mixtures with a 266 nm laser at 0.7 mJ and for up to 5 min, the active CPZ photoproducts are directly formed during the photopolymerization process within a GelMa hydrogel matrix. The irradiation time was increased up to 5 min to address the simultaneous absorption of 266 nm radiation by both CPZ and Irgacure, as it is possible that longer exposure times might be necessary for proper hydrogel formation. This approach allows direct encapsulation of the drug into the delivery system and can increase the overall efficacy of the drug delivery system by ensuring that the CPZ photoproducts are uniformly distributed within the hydrogel matrix. In this way, hydrogels can protect the CPZ photoproducts from degradation, ensuring their stability and potency over time.

2. Results and Discussion

Three concentrations of CPZ (1, 2, and 4 mg/mL), together with Irgacure 2959 (0.05% v/w) and GelMa (10% v/w), were chosen to evaluate the effects of various CPZ concentrations on the photopolymerization process and the antimicrobial properties of the resulting hydrogels. This approach allows the determination of the optimal concentration for maximum antimicrobial efficacy while maintaining the structural integrity of the hydrogel. To simplify the terminology used in this paper, Irgacure 2959 at a concentration of 0.05% will be referred to as Irgacure, and GelMa at a concentration of 10% will be referred to as GelMa. The following formulations are named as follows: Irgacure 0.05%–GelMa 10%–CPZ 1 mg/mL hydrogel will be referred to as hydrogel 1, Irgacure 0.05%–GelMa 10%–CPZ 2 mg/mL hydrogel will be referred to as hydrogel 2, and Irgacure 0.05%–GelMa 10%–CPZ 4 mg/mL hydrogel will be referred to as hydrogel 4.

A volume of 35 μL from each solution was placed into a mold and exposed to a 266 nm laser beam (10 Hz repetition rate). The laser beam diameter was adjusted to match the mold's inner diameter (0.7 cm), and a beam energy of 0.75 mJ (intensity of 19.7 mW/cm^2) was used. The solutions were irradiated for 1 min and 5 min, delivering a total dose of 1.18 J/cm^2 and 5.91 J/cm^2, respectively.

2.1. Absorption Spectroscopy Analysis

The absorption spectra of CPZ solutions at the three different concentrations after the irradiation with 266 nm laser beams at 0.75 mJ up to 5 min in the 35 μL molds are shown in Figure 1. The absorption spectrum of unirradiated CPZ was characterized by an absorption band with a maximum at 266 nm. Upon irradiation, the absorption spectrum underwent significant changes only for the 1 mg/mL CPZ solution, where the absorbance began to decrease during irradiation by 30%, and the absorption maximum shifted to longer wavelengths, from 266 nm to 270 nm. This indicates molecular changes in the CPZ molecule due to photochemical reactions induced by the laser irradiation. For the 2 and 4 mg/mL CPZ solutions, there was only a decrease in absorbance (25% for 2 mg/mL, 21.43% for 4 mg/mL), with changes being more pronounced for the 2 mg/mL CPZ solution, suggesting a slower photodegradation of the CPZ molecule at higher concentrations.

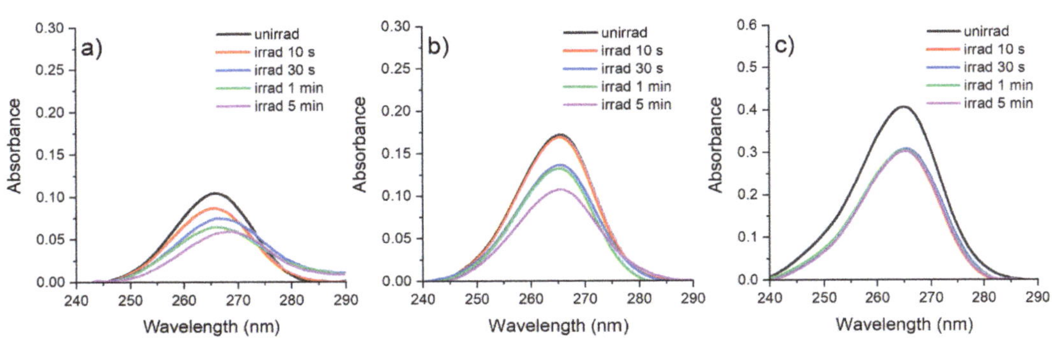

Figure 1. Absorption spectra for CPZ solutions after exposure to 266 nm laser radiation at 0.75 mJ for 5 min at concentrations of (**a**) 1 mg/mL, (**b**) 2 mg/mL, and (**c**) 4 mg/mL.

Altogether, the absorption spectra showed that the laser-induced photodegradation of CPZ was concentration-dependent, with more substantial photochemical changes occurring at lower concentrations, where the newly formed photoproducts had different absorption characteristics. CPZ is known to undergo several photochemical reactions under UV light [6,26,27], leading to several photoproducts such as CPZ sulfoxide (oxidation of the sulfur atom), desmethyl CPZ (loss of a methyl group from the nitrogen atom), CPZ radical cations (formation of a radical cation through one-electron oxidation, or amino derivatives (hydrolysis of the amide bond leading to various amino derivatives). These photoproducts exhibit different absorption characteristics, typically shifting towards longer wavelengths due to the formation of new conjugated molecules or functional groups [28].

2.2. Laser-Induced Fluoresce Analysis

The laser-induced fluorescence (LIF) spectra and fluorescence kinetics profiles for CPZ solutions at concentrations of 1, 2, and 4 mg/mL irradiated with 266 nm for 5 min at energy of 0.75 mJ are shown in Figure 2. The fluorescence kinetics profile was obtained from the LIF spectrum, recorded every 5 s, and represents the fluorescence intensity of the fluorescence peak. The solution of 1 mg/mL CPZ showed a peak at 465 nm. An increase in fluorescence intensity with increasing CPZ concentration was observed. For CPZ 2 mg/mL and 4 mg/mL, it was noted that in the first 10 s, the fluorescence intensity was similar, indicating that for CPZ 4 mg/mL there was significant absorption of the excitation beam and/or re-absorption of the emission by the sample. At higher concentrations, fluorophore aggregation or re-absorption often occurs, which causes the fluorescence spectrum shape to differ from that of a diluted sample, along with nonlinear concentration behavior [29]. This leads to self-quenching due to proximity interactions, reducing quantum yield and altering fluorescence intensity.

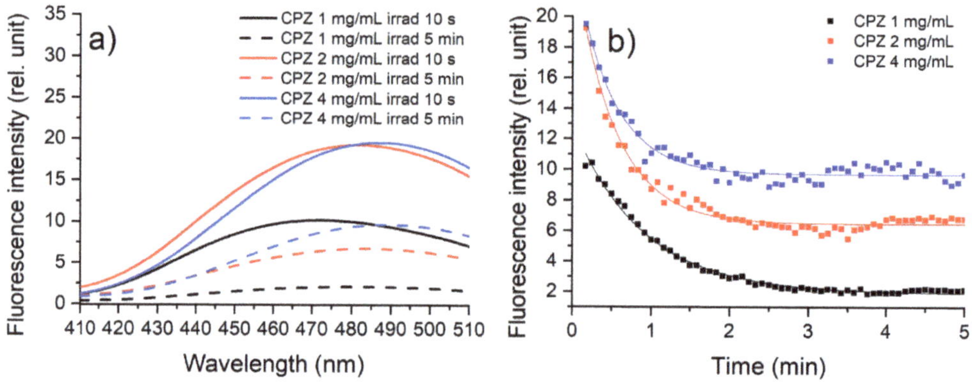

Figure 2. (**a**) LIF spectra of CPZ solutions at concentrations of 1, 2, and 4 mg/mL irradiated with 266 nm for 5 min at an energy of 0.75 mJ; (**b**) fluorescence kinetics profiles for CPZ solutions at concentrations of 1, 2, and 4 mg/mL irradiated with 266 nm for 5 min at an energy of 0.75 mJ.

During irradiation, a decrease in fluorescence intensity was observed for all samples (Figure 2b): for 3 min in the case of CPZ 1 mg/mL, 2 min for CPZ 2 mg/mL, and 1.5 min for CPZ 4 mg/mL, after which the intensity remained constant. As CPZ was exposed to radiation, it degraded, leading to a decrease in fluorescence intensity over time. Monitoring this decrease can give insights into the extent and kinetics of photodegradation. Correspondingly, as the concentration of CPZ increased, the wavelength shifted to longer wavelengths, being consistent across both irradiation times (10 s and 5 min). When evaluating the influence of irradiation time, for each concentration, the wavelength was redshifted after 5 min compared to that of 10 s. This indicated that prolonged irradiation further shifts the wavelength, possibly due to increased photodegradation effects or other molecular interactions that occur over time. The intensity of 2 mg/mL CPZ was almost the same as that of 4 mg/mL CPZ when irradiated for 10 s, with a redshift in wavelength for the higher concentration. The redshift of the wavelength with the higher concentration was likely due to the inner filter effect [30], where reabsorption of emitted light causes the observed emission to shift to longer wavelengths.

In Figure 2b, it can be observed that by increasing the concentration of CPZ from 1 to 4 mg/mL, the fluorescence exhibited an increase in intensity for the entire duration of the irradiation process. This was due to the larger number of fluorescent molecules available at higher concentrations, which could absorb more excitation light. The faster decay in fluorescence intensity at lower concentrations suggested that these solutions are more susceptible to photodegradation, possibly due to a higher light dose per number of molecules. Overall, the fluorescence kinetic profiles indicated that the photodegradation rate was inversely related to the concentration of CPZ.

Further, the LIF spectra were registered during hydrogel formation and analyzed to elucidate how laser radiation influences the production of photoproducts and the photopolymerization process. Additionally, for comparison, the LIF spectra for Irgacure, the Irgacure–GelMa mixture, and Irgacure–CPZ (1 mg/mL, 2 mg/mL, and 4 mg/mL) mixtures were measured, and are presented together with hydrogel spectra in Figure 3 for exposures to laser irradiation of 10 s, 1 min, and 5 min. The hydrogel LIF spectra showed the characteristic bands of CPZ and Irgacure, and a new band with intensity maximum at 380 nm.

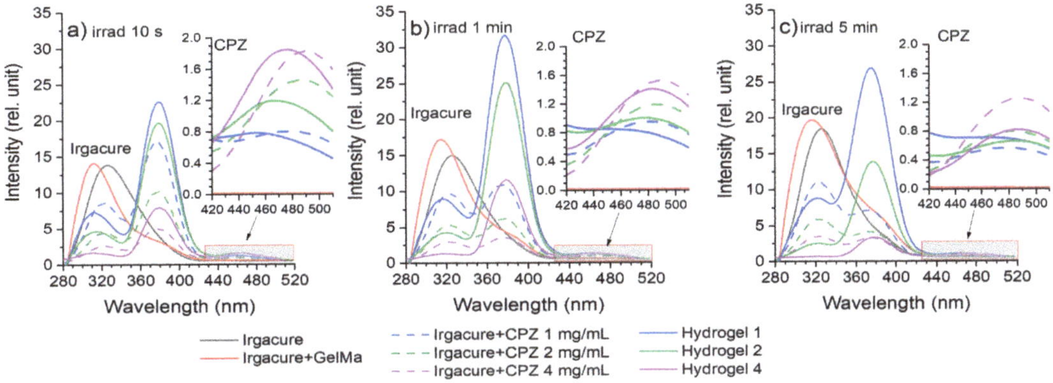

Figure 3. LIF spectra of hydrogels and their constituents recorded following laser irradiation for (**a**) 10 s, (**b**) 1 min, and (**c**) 5 min.

Irgacure, for an irradiation time of 10 s (Figure 3a), in Irgacure bare solution, exhibited a peak around 330 nm. When Irgacure was mixed with GelMa, the LIF spectrum showed a blue shift of the Irgacure peak position compared to that of Irgacure alone, with slightly higher intensity, probably due to the viscosity of GelMa. As irradiation time increased (1 min—Figure 3b, and 5 min—Figure 3c), Irgacure peak fluorescence intensity increased for both Irgacure and Irgacure–GelMa solutions, with a slight red shift observed for the peak of the Irgacure–GelMa solution. The increased fluorescence under continuous UV irradiation can be attributed to photo-transformation into benzoyl and alkyl radicals [31] or conformational changes, which are species with a higher fluorescence quantum yield.

When Irgacure was mixed with CPZ, the spectrum combined the emission characteristics of both Irgacure (330 nm) and CPZ (470 nm), along with the formation of a new peak at 380 nm. The new peak at 380 nm was not observed previously by Tozar et al. [10] for Irgacure–GelMa, and probably originated from photochemical-induced reactions between CPZ and Irgacure, and the formation of new chemical species or complexes as a result of laser irradiation. For the Irgacure–CPZ solutions, the Irgacure peak intensity decreased with increasing CPZ concentrations (Figures 3a–c and 4). As the concentration of CPZ increases, there are more CPZ molecules that absorb the excitation light, reducing the available excitation light for Irgacure and thereby lowering its fluorescence intensity. In contrast, at the same CZP concentration, the Irgacure peak intensity increased with longer exposure times, similar to the behavior observed in the Irgacure solution when irradiated alone. As expected, the smallest increase in Irgacure fluorescence intensity as a function of irradiation time was observed when Irgacure was mixed with CPZ 4 mg/mL due to the quenching effect of CPZ molecules on Irgacure fluorescence.

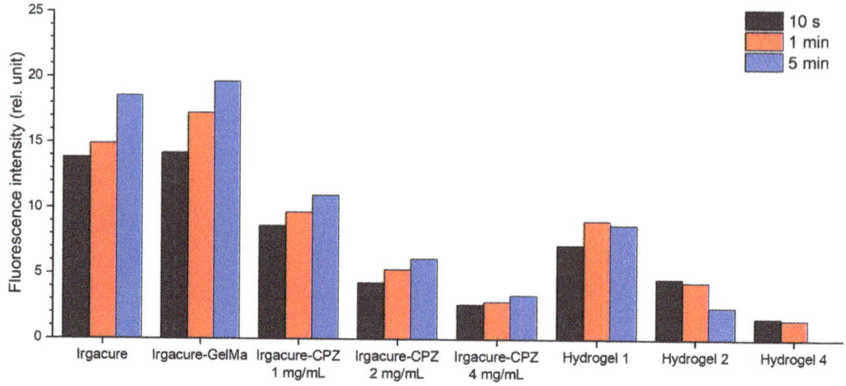

Figure 4. Fluorescence intensity variation of the Irgacure emission peak (330 nm) when Irgacure was exposed to a 266 nm laser beam in different formulations.

Considering the evolution of the Irgacure peak as a function of CPZ concentration and irradiation time (Figure 4), the Irgacure fluorescence intensity in the hydrogels exhibited a similar pattern with Irgacure–CPZ solutions, but showed a different trend when the exposure time was taken into account. In hydrogel 1, the Irgacure fluorescence intensity increased up to 1 min of irradiation, followed by a slight decrease at 5 min. For hydrogel 2 and hydrogel 4, the intensity of the Irgacure peak decreased continuously throughout the irradiation period, until it disappeared completely for hydrogel 4. The lower Irgacure peak intensity in hydrogels when compared with that of Irgacure–CPZ solution demonstrated consumption of Irgacure in the photo-crosslinking process. The same trend was observed when compared with Irgacure–GelMa. In this respect, the presence of CPZ in the hydrogel introduced competing photochemical and quenching effects that reduced the fluorescence of Irgacure with increasing irradiation time.

For the CPZ peak at 470 nm, at an irradiation time of 10 s (Figure 3a), the spectra of GelMa–CPZ solutions exhibited an increase in fluorescence intensity with increasing CPZ concentrations. With increasing exposure times (Figure 3b,c), CPZ fluorescence intensity decreased across all the CPZ concentrations used (Figure 5). This showed that CPZ is photodegraded into photoproducts despite the viscous medium created by GelMa.

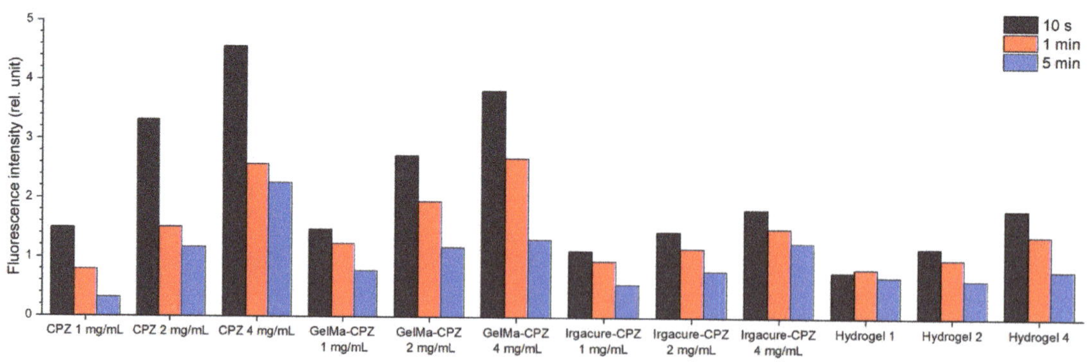

Figure 5. Fluorescence intensity variation of the CPZ emission peak (470 nm) when CPZ was exposed to a 266 nm laser beam in different formulations.

The fluorescence intensity of the CPZ peak in the GelMa–CPZ solutions exhibited a similar pattern of changes with irradiation time as CPZ alone (Figure 5). However, due to the GelMa matrix, the degradation rate was slowed down, indicating that the overall photodegradation process of CPZ was altered. Further, the fluorescence intensity of the CPZ peak from Irgacure–CPZ formulations (1, 2, and 4 mg/mL) was lower compared to the corresponding concentrations of CPZ alone. This indicates that the presence of Irgacure reduced the fluorescence of CPZ, thus also slowing the photodegradation process, because Irgacure itself absorbed the 266 nm laser beams. The smallest fluorescence intensity of the CPZ peak was also observed in the hydrogel LIF spectra. Since the hydrogel precursor solution consisted of a mixture of GelMa, Irgacure, and CPZ, the fluorescence emission of CPZ was influenced by the interactions with both GelMa and Irgacure. Irgacure competed with CPZ for the absorption of 266 nm photons, while GelMa formed a matrix that encapsulated the photoproducts generated from the irradiated CPZ.

When analyzing the band with a maximum at 380 nm (Figure 6), one can observe that, for the Irgacure-CPZ solution with an increase in laser exposure, the fluorescence intensity followed a similar pattern to that of the CPZ peak (Figure 5) from the same solution, where the fluorescence intensity decreased with longer exposure time. This peak was not present when CPZ and Irgacure were evaluated independently (Figure 3a–c), supporting the hypothesis that the 380 nm peak arises from interactions between CPZ and Irgacure. This behavior suggests that the formation of the compound with a peak at 380 nm was closely linked to CPZ's photochemical dynamics. In contrast, the fluorescence intensity of the Irgacure peak (Figure 4) increased with irradiation time in the same formulation.

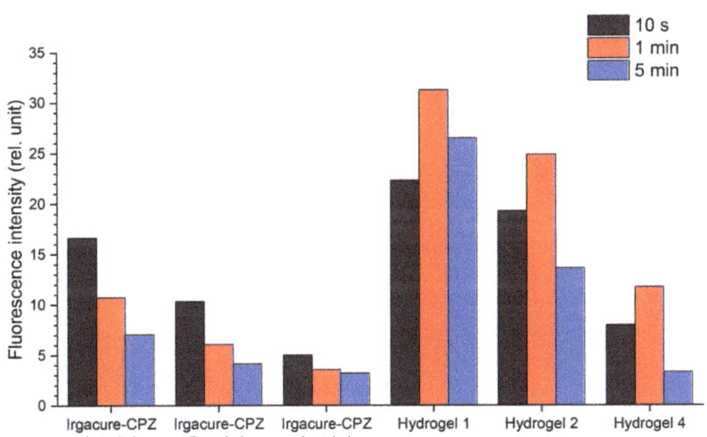

Figure 6. Fluorescence intensity variation of compounds with an emission peak at 380 nm when CPZ and Irgacure were exposed to a 266 nm laser beam in different formulations.

Instead, in the hydrogel formulations, the 380 nm fluorescence peak intensity decreased with increasing CPZ concentrations (Figure 6). This behavior was similar to the evolution of the Irgacure peak in the same formulations, confirming that the compound with a peak at 380 nm was also like the photochemical dynamics of Irgacure, as it was consumed during hydrogel photopolymerization. In addition, the shoulder that appears in the LIF spectra Irgacure–GelMa solution irradiated for 5 min (Figure 3b) demonstrated that a by-product of irradiated Irgacure could be involved in the formation of a 380 nm compound. When comparing the irradiation times, it was observed that the 380 nm peak intensity increased in the first 1 min of exposure, followed by a decrease until the end of the irradiation period. This trend was observed both in the hydrogel (the 380 nm peak investigated) and the Irgacure–CPZ solution (Irgacure peak investigated) only when a 1 mg/mL CPZ concentration was used. These observations highlight how photodegradation, particularly of CPZ, played a critical role in changing the fluorescence dynamics, influencing the relative intensities of the Irgacure and 380 nm peaks over time, and consequently the photopolymerization processes and hydrogel formation.

Figure 7 shows the fluorescence kinetics profiles of Irgacure (330 nm peak), CPZ (470 nm), and the compound with a peak at 380 nm, when CPZ concentration was varied (1, 2, and 4 mg/mL) in formulations such as Irgacure–CPZ solutions and the precursor solution of Irgacure–GelMa–CPZ. When exposed to laser radiation, this precursor solution starts to photopolymerize the GelMa into hydrogel and to transform CPZ into photoproducts in the same time. The fluorescence kinetic profiles represent the fluorescence intensity measured in real time during the irradiation process. In the Irgacure–CPZ solution, the fluorescence intensity of Irgacure and 380 nm peaks increased at the beginning of the irradiation, then decreased, followed by its stabilization. The maximum fluorescence intensity for both Irgacure and the 380 nm peaks occurred at the same times across all initial CPZ concentrations: 25 s for Irgacure and 15 s for the 380 nm peaks. For the CPZ peak, the time required to reach the peak fluorescence intensity was reached after 20 s for CPZ at 1 mg/mL and after 35 s for CPZ at 2 mg/mL. For the initial CPZ concentration of 4 mg/mL in the Irgacure–CPZ solution, from the beginning of irradiation the CPZ peak showed a decrease in fluorescence intensity.

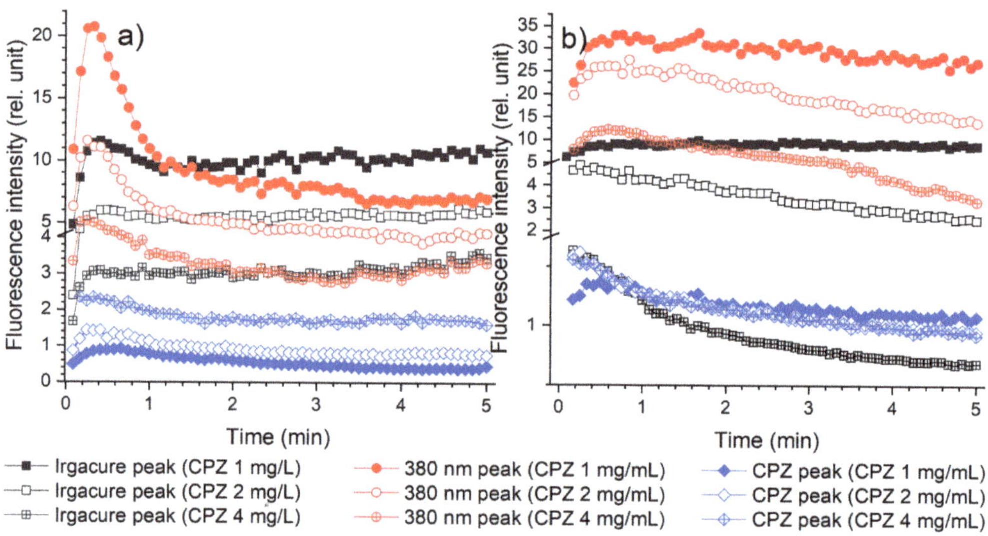

Figure 7. The fluorescence kinetics profile of Irgacure (330 nm peak), CPZ (470 nm), and the compound with a peak at 380 nm in formulations having concentrations of CPZ of 1, 2 and 4 mg/mL in (**a**) Irgacure–CPZ solutions and (**b**) precursor solutions of Irgacure–GelMa–CPZ, which lead to hydrogel photopolymerization; all the samples were irradiated for 5 min with a 266 nm pulsed laser beams at energy of 0.75 mJ.

When comparing the CPZ fluorescence peaks, at different initial CPZ concentrations in the Irgacure–CPZ solution (Figure 7a—in blue), it was observed that, for the entire irradiation period, the fluorescence intensity had higher values with increasing CPZ concentration. When analyzing the impact of irradiation time, for initial CPZ concentrations of 1 mg/mL and 2 mg/mL, the CPZ fluorescence initially increased, followed by a decay in intensity. The intensity decay occurred at a higher rate for the 1 mg/mL concentration, indicating a faster photodegradation of CPZ at lower concentration. In contrast, for the Irgacure–CPZ solution with an initial CPZ concentration of 4 mg/mL, there was no initial increase in CPZ fluorescence. Instead, a continuous decrease in fluorescence intensity was observed, but at a slower decay rate compared to the 1 mg/mL and 2 mg/mL concentrations. This suggests a slower photodegradation process due to the higher number of CPZ molecules. Regarding the stabilization times, as the dynamic equilibrium between the processes that influence fluorescence was reached, the time for stabilization became shorter with the increase in the initial CPZ concentration: 275 s for 1 mg/mL, 225 s for 2 mg/mL, and 200 s for 4 mg/mL. These processes could include photodegradation, self-quenching, or complex formation [32–34]. The behavior of the stabilization time is due to the high molecular density of CPZ molecules, which enhanced the energy transfer efficiency, leading to faster quenching of excited states and stabilization of fluorescence [35,36].

When comparing the influence of the initial CPZ concentration on Irgacure fluorescence peaks, in the Irgacure–CPZ solution (Figure 7a—in black), it was observed that the overall fluorescence intensity decreased with increasing CPZ concentration. When analyzing the impact of irradiation time, for all initial CPZ concentrations, Irgacure fluorescence initially increased up to 25 s, followed by an intensity decay. The intensity decay occurred at a higher rate for a 1 mg/mL concentration than a 2 mg/mL CPZ concentration, indicating a faster photodegradation of Irgacure. A faster degradation of Irgacure is transposed in a faster photopolymerization of GelMa hydrogels, as the radicals formed during irradiation bind the polymer chains. In contrast, for the Irgacure–CPZ solution with an initial CPZ concentration of 4 mg/mL, a stable Irgacure fluorescence intensity was observed until 200 s, followed by a rapid increase in its intensity. This behavior, combined with the observation that the CPZ peak in the Irgacure–CPZ (4 mg/mL) solution decreased in intensity up to 200 s before stabilizing, suggests that during the first 200 s, the primary process occurring is the photodegradation of CPZ. After 200 s, the increase in fluorescence indicates that the photodegradation of Irgacure becomes the dominant process.

When examining the influence of initial CPZ concentration on the 380 nm fluorescence peaks in the Irgacure–CPZ solution (Figure 7a—in red), it was observed that the overall fluorescence intensity decreased as the CPZ concentration increased. When analyzing the impact of irradiation time, for all initial CPZ concentrations, the 380 nm peak fluorescence initially increased up to 15 s, followed by a decay in intensity. As the initial CPZ concentration increased, the decay rate of the 380 nm peak slowed down due to increased interactions among CPZ molecules. It appears that 200 s was also a significant point for the 380 nm peak in the Irgacure–CPZ (4 mg/mL) solution, as the fluorescence intensity decreased up to 200 s and then began to increase, confirming its existence was linked to both CPZ and Irgacure.

Further, the fluorescence intensity of the same peaks was investigated during the photopolymerization of hydrogel 1, hydrogel 2, and hydrogel 3, and their fluorescence kinetics are shown in Figure 7b.

During the crosslinking of hydrogels 1, 2, and 4, the Irgacure peak (Figure 7b—in black) showed a decrease in overall fluorescence intensity as the initial CPZ concentration increased. In hydrogel 1 (CPZ 1 mg/mL), the fluorescence intensity of Irgacure increased during the first 65 s of irradiation before stabilizing, which is significantly longer compared to the behavior observed in the solutions, i.e., 25 s. In contrast, in hydrogel 2 (CPZ 2 mg/mL) and hydrogel 4 (CPZ 4 mg/mL), the fluorescence intensity of the Irgacure peak began to decrease from the beginning of irradiation, with a fluorescence intensity of the Irgacure peak in hydrogel 2 displaying a faster decay rate than that in hydrogel 4.

For the CPZ peak in hydrogel 1, the fluorescence intensity increased during the first 20 s, then gradually decreased until the end of irradiation. In hydrogels 2 and 4, the CPZ peak fluorescence showed a continuous decline starting from the beginning of irradiation. This behavior is similar to what is observed in the Irgacure–CPZ solution (Figure 7a), but only at a concentration of 4 mg/mL CPZ. The fluorescence decay rate of the CPZ peak is faster in hydrogel 2 compared to hydrogel 4 for up to 150 s of laser exposure, but after this time, the intensities follow a similar trend.

When examining the influence of the initial CPZ concentration on the 380 nm fluorescence peak in the hydrogels (Figure 7b—in red), it was observed that the kinetic fluorescence profile exhibits lower intensities for the entire irradiation time as the CPZ concentration is increased. Independent of the initial CPZ concentration, the 380 nm peak fluorescence increased for the first 40 s of irradiation, followed by a decay. As the CPZ concentration increased from 1 mg/mL to 2 mg/mL, the decay rate of the 380 nm peak was higher. In hydrogel 4 (CPZ 4 mg/mL), the decay rate of the 380 nm fluorescence peak was similar to that observed in hydrogel 2 (CPZ 2 mg/mL) up to 150 s.

The presence of GelMa in the hydrogels introduced additional processes such as crosslinking and photopolymerization, which directly affect the fluorescence kinetics. These processes are absent in Irgacure–CPZ solutions, leading to distinct kinetic profiles between the two environments. In the absence of GelMa, solutions show fluorescence profiles influenced by irradiation and consequent photodegradation. The kinetic profiles represent a combination of direct chemical interactions and structural transformations. The hydrogel matrix limits molecular movement and alter the fluorescence response. The presence of GelMa leads to immediate involvement in polymerization reactions, thus altering the fluorescence profile as crosslinking competes with photodegradation. In solutions, the fluorescence intensity of the Irgacure and 380 nm peaks initially increases, followed by a decline and stabilization, indicating that both peaks are affected by the irradiation and chemical interactions occurring in the solution phase. In hydrogels, the fluorescence intensity of these peaks continuously decreases without significant initial increases. The initial increase in the 380 nm peak observed in solutions indicated the involvement of Irgacure and CPZ, whereas in hydrogels, this increase was smaller because Irgacure was also used in the crosslinking and polymerization reactions that dominated the environment. Moreover, slower decay rates at higher CPZ concentrations were seen in both environments, but hydrogels maintained a generally lower fluorescence due to ongoing photopolymerization.

2.3. FTIR Analysis

Further, the overall composition of the samples was examined using FTIR absorption spectroscopy. The IR spectra of the dried hydrogels were recorded in attenuated total reflection mode in the spectral range of 1800–700 cm^{-1} and are presented in Figure 8. These spectra are compared with those of GelMa powder, the 2 mg/mL CPZ dissolved in ultrapure water solution irradiated for 30 min used by Tozar et al. [2], and the Irgacure 0.05% solution irradiated for 1 min. The comparison with the CPZ solution irradiated for 30 min was made to assess whether the photodegradation necessary for achieving the best antimicrobial effect was adequately achieved during the shorter irradiation time used in the hydrogel formation. Additionally, the FTIR spectrum of hydrogels 1, 2, and 4 was compared with that of Irgacure–GelMa (the hydrogel without CPZ), represented by the green line in Figure 8, to determine if the crosslinking density was significantly affected by CPZ.

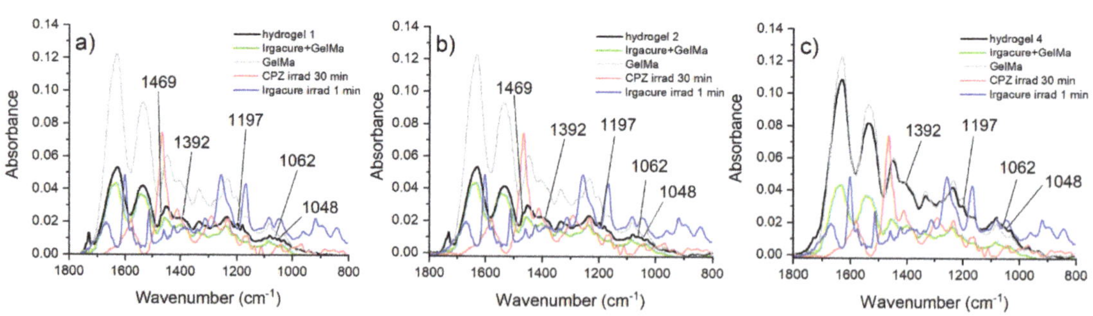

Figure 8. The IR spectra of the Irgacure 0.05%–GelMa 10%–CPZ hydrogels, where the CPZ concentration was (**a**) 1 mg/mL, (**b**) 2 mg/mL, and (**c**) 4 mg/mL.

The IR spectra of the dried hydrogels show a major influence of GelMa, with most of the IR bands of GelMa being present: 1630 cm^{-1}—stretching vibration C=O (amide I), 1544 cm^{-1}—deformation vibration of C–N–H, 1237 cm^{-1}—deformation vibration N-H (amide II), 1450 cm^{-1}—deformation vibration C–H, and 1335 cm^{-1}—C–N stretching vibration within amide III [10]. The consistent peak positions around 1630 cm^{-1} suggested that the overall crosslinking density of GelMa did not change significantly with CPZ addition. Thus, the FTIR spectrum of hydrogels 1, 2, and 4 showed the presence of the main functional groups of Irgacure–GelMa, indicating the preservation of expected physical characteristics. The IR bands corresponding to the 2 mg/mL CPZ solution irradiated for 30 min can also be observed in the IR spectra of the hydrogels at 1469 cm^{-1} (C–H stretching vibration, CH_2), 1392 cm^{-1} (C–H deformation vibration, CH_3), 1197 cm^{-1} (S–O bond stretching vibration, sulfoxide group), 1062 cm^{-1} (in-plane C–H shear deformation vibration), and 1048 cm^{-1} (C–O stretching vibration, phenol group), suggesting the generation of CPZ photoproducts containing phenol and sulfoxide groups. These results mean that the CPZ hydrogels contain the active photoproducts that proved to have antibacterial efficacity in the previous studies [2].

2.4. Hydrogel Release Behavior

The loaded hydrogels were dehydrated before use. Six different hydrogels containing CPZ at 1, 2, and 4 mg/mL were obtained after exposure to a 266 nm laser beam for 1 min and 5 min. They were immersed in 1 mL PBS (phosphate-buffered saline) and incubated at 37 °C for various times (2, 4, 8, 24, 48, and 84 h). To determine the concentration in mg/mL of irradiated CPZ released in the PBS, it is necessary to have a calibration curve with various known concentrations of irradiated CPZ. However, the calibration curve of CPZ irradiated during the hydrogel crosslinking process cannot be obtained, because the specific photoproducts formed during irradiation cannot be directly quantified. As an alternative, the released irradiated CPZ is instead reported based on its absorbance measured at 266 nm (Figure 9). The swelling ratio of these hydrogels could not be determined because, upon immersion in water, the hydrogels immediately began releasing irradiated CPZ, making it impossible to determine their swollen weight.

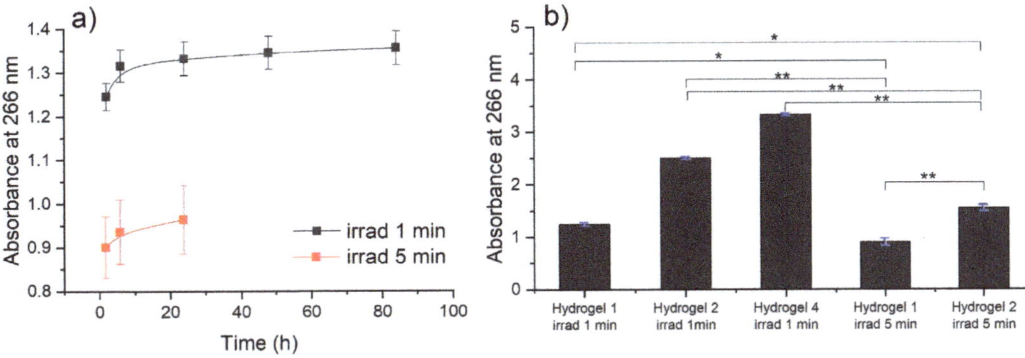

Figure 9. (**a**) Release profiles over time of irradiated CPZ from hydrogel 1 (CPZ 1 mg/mL) photopolymerized for 1 min and 5 min. (**b**) Released irradiated CPZ from hydrogels 1, 2, and 4 within the first 2 h; results are expressed as mean ± standard error from three independent experiments; the data points were analyzed using a *t*-test, showing a statistical significance of $p < 0.001$ between the groups, except for ** $p < 0.01$ and * $p < 0.05$.

The release curves of irradiated CPZ demonstrate how the release behavior varies depending on the initial CPZ concentration (1, 2, and 4 mg/mL) and the irradiation duration (1 or 5 min). Among all the hydrogels, only hydrogel 1 (initial CPZ concentration of 1 mg/mL) when exposed to laser radiation for 1 min released irradiated CPZ for periods longer than 24 h (Figure 9a). Hydrogel 1 irradiated for 5 min released irradiated CPZ within only the first 24 h. The rest of the hydrogels, namely, hydrogel 2 (CPZ 2 mg/mL) and hydrogel 4 (CPZ 4 mg/mL), irradiated for both 1 and 5 min, released irradiated CPZ only in the first 2 h. As expected, hydrogel 2 and hydrogel 4 released a higher amount of irradiated CPZ within the first 2 h compared to hydrogel 1 (Figure 9b) due to higher initial concentrations of CPZ. In addition, after 2 h, structural alterations in hydrogels 2 and 4 were observed. This behavior suggested that the structural composition of the hydrogel matrix, influenced by the initial CPZ concentration, played a crucial role in its release behavior.

Moreover, the hydrogels irradiated for longer periods (5 min) showed a lower release compared to those irradiated for shorter durations (1 min). This suggests that the lower release observed in the hydrogels irradiated for 5 min is due to over-crosslinking of the GelMa matrix, resulting in a stiffer structure that more effectively encapsulates the drug, thereby slowing down its release [37,38]. At the same time, it is important to note that longer irradiation significantly affects the photodegradation of CPZ, leading to the destruction of CPZ molecules and their photoproducts, making their detection impossible. These observations highlight the need for careful optimization of irradiation time to balance hydrogel crosslinking and drug release efficiency, ensuring the desired outcome.

2.5. Antimicrobial Activity

The antimicrobial activity of the hydrogels was studied on methicillin-resistant *Staphylococcus aureus* (MRSA) using the disc diffusion method and the colony-forming unit (CFU) determination method. The disc diffusion method indicates the susceptibility of the bacterial strain to the loaded hydrogels through the appearance of an inhibition zone (inhibition area) around the hydrogels [39,40]. Figure 10 presents the antimicrobial effects in the form of inhibition zones and inhibition areas for the hydrogels 1, 2, and 4 containing 1, 2, and 4 mg/mL initial CPZ concentrations. Figure 10a) shows the image with the zone of inhibition for irradiated CPZ released from hydrogel 1 (CPZ 1 mg/mL), hydrogel 2 (CPZ 2 mg/mL), and hydrogel 4 (CPZ 2 mg/mL) obtained by 1 min irradiation of Irgacure–GelMa–CPZ (1, 2, and 4 mg/mL) mixtures and compares them with the control hydrogels (Irgacure–GelMa). The inhibition areas from Figure 10b were extracted from Figure 10a using ImageJ software (version 1.54g). The hydrogels were produced through photopolymerization with irradiation times of 1 min and 5 min. For the hydrogel without CPZ, compared to that formed from the irradiation of the Irgacure–GelMa mixture, no inhibition zone was observed (Figure 10a).

The results indicated that the hydrogels containing higher CPZ concentrations (2 mg/mL and 4 mg/mL) showed significantly larger zones of inhibition compared to the 1 mg/mL CPZ hydrogels, reflecting enhanced antimicrobial efficacy against MRSA. Thus, higher drug loading was directly correlated with increased antimicrobial potency. Despite the higher antimicrobial activity, the release behavior of these hydrogels indicated that hydrogels with 2 mg/mL and 4 mg/mL CPZ concentrations primarily released their drug content within the first 2 h. This rapid release pattern occurred due to structural alterations in the hydrogel, which contributed to the large initial inhibition zones but limited the potential for sustained antibacterial effects.

Hydrogels irradiated for 5 min showed smaller inhibition zones compared to those irradiated for 1 min across all CPZ concentrations. This can be attributed to enhanced crosslinking of the hydrogel matrix, which restricts irradiated CPZ release, and the extensive photodegradation of CPZ, reducing its antimicrobial efficacy.

Further, the CFU method validates the antibacterial effect of the drug-loaded hydrogels in the formation of microbial biofilms [41,42]. The antibacterial effect of hydrogels 1, 2, and 4 was compared with that of a control and penicillin hydrogels. The control hydrogel was the hydrogel formed during the photopolymerization of the Irgacure–GelMa mixture, and the penicillin hydrogel was the control hydrogel loaded with penicillin. In this respect, the adherence of MRSA bacteria to hydrogel 1 resulting from 1 min and 5 min irradiation was assessed using the viable cell count method after 24 and 48 h incubation periods (Figure 11). These hydrogels demonstrated nearly complete inhibition of MRSA colonies after 24 h of treatment. The drastic reduction in the number of bacterial colonies suggested that these hydrogels are highly effective in preventing MRSA adhesion and proliferation during the initial period of exposure. After 48 h, the CPZ hydrogel irradiated for 1 min maintained a very low CFU count, whereas the hydrogel irradiated for 5 min did not release any CPZ after 24 h and was not taken into consideration. Despite this, both hydrogels were far more effective than penicillin and the control hydrogels.

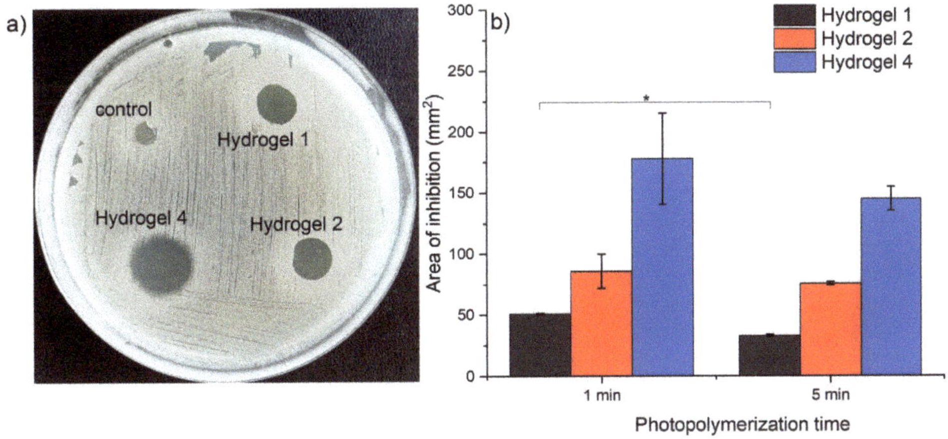

Figure 10. (**a**) Image of inhibition zones for irradiated CPZ released from the control hydrogel, hydrogel 1, hydrogel 2, and hydrogel 4 obtained by 1 min irradiation; the hydrogels were incubated for 18 h at 37 °C together with MRSA. (**b**) Areas of inhibition of irradiated CPZ released from hydrogel 1, hydrogel 2, and hydrogel 4 obtained by 1 min and 5 min irradiation; the areas were extracted from the zone of inhibition images using ImageJ; results are expressed as mean ± standard error from three independent experiments; the data points were analyzed using a *t*-test, showing a statistical significance only between hydrogel 1 resulted from 1 min and 5 min irradiation for * $p < 0.05$.

Hydrogels resulting from 1 min laser irradiation showed better performance, maintaining lower CFU counts than those irradiated for 5 min. This aligns with previous observations that shorter irradiation times maintained a better crosslinked structure that optimized the release of CPZ, sustaining its antimicrobial action. The CFU data correlated well with disc diffusion method results, suggesting that 1 mg/mL CPZ hydrogels showed sustained antimicrobial activity over time, even though their inhibition zones were smaller compared to the ones with higher CPZ concentrations. This sustained release helps maintain low bacterial counts over extended periods, making them suitable for longer-term antimicrobial applications.

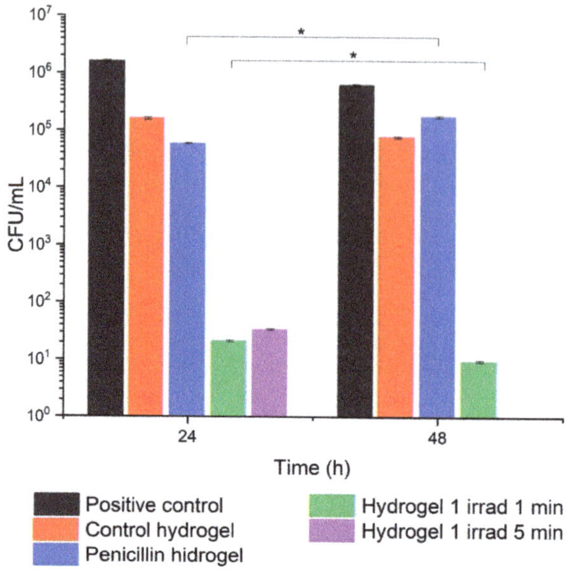

Figure 11. Colony-forming unit (CFU) analysis of MRSA after 24 and 48 h treatment with hydrogels with 1 mg/mL CPZresulted from 1 min and 5 min exposure to laser radiation; the positive control was represented by pure bacterial culture in the absence of hydrogels, the control hydrogels represented hydrogel formed during the photopolymerization of Irgacure–GelMa mixture, and penicillin hydrogel was the control hydrogel loaded with penicillin; results are expressed as mean ± standard error from three independent experiments; the data points were analyzed using a *t*-test, showing a statistical significance between 24 and 48 h for hydrogel 1 and hydrogel loaded with penicillin for * $p < 0.05$.

3. Conclusions

This study evaluated both the impact of CPZ at concentrations of 1, 2, and 4 mg/mL on the photopolymerization of hydrogels, and the capability of the hydrogel to have a prolonged and controlled release of the drug and the capability to form antimicrobial photoproducts of CPZ during the same crosslinking process. The assessment focused on absorption spectroscopy, LIF spectra, fluorescence kinetics, FTIR spectra, drug release behavior, and antimicrobial efficiency against MRSA, highlighting that 1 mg/mL concentration is optimal.

The absorption spectra showed that 1 mg/mL CPZ suffered changes in its absorption spectrum upon irradiation with a 266 nm laser beam, indicating photochemical changes. In contrast, 2 mg/mL and 4 mg/mL CPZ exhibited smaller reductions in absorbance and slower photodegradation. The LIF spectra and fluorescence kinetics showed that higher concentrations quench the fluorescence signal due to aggregation and reabsorption effects, also reducing the photodegradation of CPZ. Moreover, the fluorescence decay curves demonstrated that CPZ at the 1 mg/mL concentration displayed the fastest decay, suggesting significant photochemical transformation, which is beneficial for enhancing antimicrobial efficacy. Thus, real-time fluorescence monitoring can provide immediate feedback on the polymerization process, enabling adjustments to UV exposure, light intensity, or component photodegradation. Moreover, the identification of induction periods and stabilization points from direct comparisons of fluorescence profiles helps adjust the photopolymerization conditions for optimal hydrogel formation. Further, the hydrogel showed sustained release only for 1 mg/mL CPZ and a 1 min irradiation time for the photopolymerization process. This prolonged release enhanced the antimicrobial effect against MRSA when compared with that of hydrogel loaded with penicillin. These insights underscore the importance of hydrogel formulation in optimizing the stability, performance, and therapeutic efficacy of irradiated CPZ for antimicrobial applications.

4. Materials and Methods

Irgacure 2959 (2-hydroxy-1-[4-(2-hydroxyethoxy) phenyl]-2-methyl-1-propanone), purchased from Sigma-Aldrich (St. Louis, MO, USA), was dissolved in ultrapure water at a concentration of 0.05% *w*/*v*. Gelatin methacryloyl (GelMA), with a gel strength of 300 g bloom and an 80% degree of substitution, was obtained from Sigma-Aldrich and prepared at a concertation of 10% *w*/*v* using ultrapure water as solvent. Chlorpromazine hydrochloride (CPZ, purity of ≥98), was purchased from Sigma-Aldrich and dissolved in ultrapure water. Penicillin G sodium 1,000,000 UI from Antibiotice (Iasi, Romania), used at a concentration of 2 mg/mL, was loaded into the hydrogel resulting from the photopolymerization of the Irgacure–GelMa mixture. This was used as a negative control to compare its antimicrobial activity with that of hydrogels formed during this study. All the powders were used as received without any further purification.

Irgacure 2959 (0.05%)–GelMA (10%) solution was mixed using a magnetic stirrer at 200 rpm for 30 min at a temperature of 70 °C to ensure proper dissolution of each component. Three different concentrations of CPZ (1 mg/mL, 2 mg/mL, and 4 mg/mL) were used together with an Irgacure 2959 (0.05%)–GelMA (10%) mixture to synthesize the hydrogels. All three formulations were tested to determine the optimal concentration of CPZ to obtain the best antimicrobial efficacy while maintaining the structural integrity of the hydrogel. A volume of 35 μL of Irgacure 2959 (0.05%)–GelMA (10%)–CPZ (1 mg/mL, 2 mg/mL, and 4 mg/mL) mixture was placed in a mold and exposed to pulsed laser radiation to obtain the photopolymerization of hydrogels.

The irradiation source was a Continuum Nd laser (10 Hz, 6 ns FWHM) emitting at 266 nm. The solutions were exposed to 266 nm for 1 min and 5 min at a beam energy of 0.75 mJ (I = 19.7 mW/cm^2). The mold was 3D-printed from polylactic acid and had an inner diameter of 0.7 cm and a height of 0.1 cm. The diameter of the laser beam was adjusted using dielectric mirrors, lenses, and diaphragms to match the diameter of the mold.

The hydrogels were removed from the mold and immersed in ultrapure water (3 mL) at room temperature to remove precursor residues and to achieve absorption equilibrium (detection of unreacted compounds). They were then dried in a desiccator for 24 h and stored in a desiccator at 4 °C in the dark.

The hydrogels were evaluated using UV-Vis and FTIR absorption spectroscopy, and laser-induced fluorescence spectroscopy. The laser-induced fluorescence (LIF) signal was collected using an optical fiber (M93L02, Thorlabs, core diameter 1500 μm) positioned at 45° to the incident beam and was recorded using a SpectraPro SP-2750 spectrograph (Acton Research, Czerny-Turner configuration, Trenton, NJ, USA) coupled with a PIMAX 1024RB ICCD camera (Princeton Instruments, Trenton, NJ, USA). A Perkin Elmer spectrophotometer (Waltham, MA, USA), model Lambda 950, was used to record absorption spectra with a resolution of 1 nm. The optical path of the spectrophotometric cell used was 0.01 mm. The Nicolet iS50 FTIR spectrometer (Thermo Fisher Scientific, Waltham, MA, USA) was used to record the IR spectra of the aqueous solutions, dried hydrogels, and powder forms. The IR spectra of the solution samples were recorded in transmittance mode between 1800 and 700 cm^{-1}, at a resolution of 4 cm^{-1} and an average of 32 spectra. The dried hydrogels and powder form samples were measured in attenuated total refraction mode, equipped with a ZnSe crystal, in the spectral range of 1800–700 cm^{-1}, with a resolution of 4 cm^{-1} and an average of 16 spectra.

The antimicrobial activity of the hydrogels loaded with CPZ irradiated during the photopolymerization process was investigated on methicillin-resistant *Staphylococcus aureus* (MRSA) by the disk diffusion method [39,40] and viable cell count method [41,42]. The disk diffusion method was conducted by inoculating with a bacteria suspension on the surface of the agar plate. Afterward, instead of a disc, the hydrogels were directly applied to the agar plate and incubated together at 37 °C for 18 h. The hydrogels were in direct contact with the bacterial culture. The susceptibility of the bacterial isolates to each hydrogel was subsequently quantified by measuring the inhibition zone areas using ImageJ software. Further, the viable cell count method was used to determine the bacterial adherence to the hydrogels. A bacterial suspension of 10^6 CFU/mL was prepared in phosphate buffer solution (PBS). In this assay, both positive and negative controls were included to ensure the validity of the results. Two positive controls were used, one represented by pure bacterial culture in the absence of hydrogels, and the other represented by hydrogel formed during the photopolymerization of Irgacure–GelMa mixture and named the control hydrogel. The negative control was a penicillin hydrogel, represented by a control hydrogel loaded with penicillin. The control hydrogel, hydrogel loaded with penicillin, and the hydrogels with 1, 2, and 4 gm/mL CPZ were incubated at 37 °C for 24 and 48 h together with 1 mL of bacterial suspension. Following that, the hydrogels with attached bacteria were extracted, immersed in 1 mL PBS, and vortexed. Serial dilutions of the samples were plated onto Plate Count Agar and incubated overnight at 37 °C. The bacterial quantity in the initial sample was determined by counting the colonies on the plates and factoring in the dilution ratio.

Author Contributions: Conceptualization, T.T., M.B. and A.S.; Data curation, T.T., S.N. and M.B.; Formal analysis, T.T., S.N. and M.B.; Funding acquisition, T.T.; Investigation, T.T., S.N. and M.B.; Methodology, T.T., S.N., G.G.P. and M.B.; Project administration, T.T. and A.S.; Resources, T.T. and A.S.; Software, T.T., S.N. and M.B.; Supervision, G.G.P. and A.S.; Validation, T.T.; Visualization, T.T.; Writing—original draft, T.T.; Writing—review and editing, M.B. and A.S. All authors have read and agreed to the published version of the manuscript.

Funding: This research was funded by the Ministry of Research, Innovation and Digitization, project number PN-III-P1-1.1-PD-2019-1117 and Romanian National Nucleu Program LAPLAS VII–contract no. 30N/2023.

Institutional Review Board Statement: Not applicable.

Informed Consent Statement: Not applicable.

Data Availability Statement: All data and materials are available on request from the corresponding author.

Conflicts of Interest: The authors declare no conflicts of interest.

References

1. Ordway, D.; Viveiros, M.; Leandro, C.; Amaral, L.; Arroz, M.J.; Molnar, J.; Kristiansen, J.E. Chlorpromazine Has Intracellular Killing Activity against Phagocytosed Staphylococcus Aureus at Clinical Concentrations. *J. Infect. Chemother.* **2002**, *8*, 227–231. [CrossRef] [PubMed]
2. Tozar, T.; Nastasa, V.; Stoicu, A.; Chifiriuc, M.C.; Popa, M.; Kamerzan, C.; Pascu, M.L. In Vitro Antimicrobial Efficacy of Laser Exposed Chlorpromazine against Gram-Positive Bacteria in Planktonic and Biofilm Growth State. *Microb. Pathog.* **2019**, *129*, 250–256. [CrossRef] [PubMed]
3. Wood, N.C.; Nugent, K.M. Inhibitory Effects of Chlorpromazine on Candida Species. *Antimicrob Agents Chemother* **1985**, *27*, 692–694. [CrossRef] [PubMed]
4. Vitale, R.G.; Afeltra, J.; Meis, J.F.G.M.; Verweij, P.E. Activity and Post Antifungal Effect of Chlorpromazine and Trifluopherazine against *Aspergillus, Scedosporium* and Zygomycetes. *Mycoses* **2007**, *50*, 270–276. [CrossRef] [PubMed]
5. Crowle, A.J.; Douvas, G.S.; May, M.H. Chlorpromazine: A Drug Potentially Useful for Treating Mycobacterial Infections. *Chemotherapy* **1992**, *38*, 410–419. [CrossRef] [PubMed]
6. Alexandru, T.; Staicu, A.; Pascu, A.; Radu, E.; Stoicu, A.; Nastasa, V.; Dinache, A.; Boni, M.; Amaral, L.; Pascu, M.L. Characterization of Mixtures of Compounds Produced in Chlorpromazine Aqueous Solutions by Ultraviolet Laser Irradiation: Their Applications in Antimicrobial Assays. *J. Biomed. Opt.* **2014**, *20*, 051002. [CrossRef]
7. Alexandru, T.; Armada, A.; Danko, B.; Hunyadi, A.; Militaru, A.; Boni, M.; Nastasa, V.; Martins, A.; Viveiros, M.; Pascu, M.; et al. Biological Evaluation of Products Formed from the Irradiation of Chlorpromazine with a 266 nm Laser Beam. *Biochem. Pharmacol.* **2013**, *2*, 109. [CrossRef]
8. Armada, A.M.; Alexandru, T.; Machado, D.; Danko, B.; Hunyadi, A.; Dinache, A.; Nastasa, V.; Boni, M.; Ramos, J.; Viveiros, M.; et al. The In Vitro Activity of Products Formed from Exposure of Chlorpromazine to a 266nm LASER Beam Against Species of Mycobacteria of Human Interest. *In Vivo* **2013**, *27*, 605–610.
9. Nistorescu, S.; Gradisteanu Pircalabioru, G.; Udrea, A.-M.; Simon, Á.; Pascu, M.; Chifiriuc, M.-C. Laser-Irradiated Chlorpromazine as a Potent Anti-Biofilm Agent for Coating of Biomedical Devices. *Coatings* **2020**, *10*, 1230. [CrossRef]

10. Tozar, T.; Nistorescu, S.; Boni, M.; Gradisteanu Pircalabioru, G.; Negut, I.; Staicu, A. Pulsed Laser Photo-Crosslinking of Gelatin Methacryloyl Hydrogels for the Controlled Delivery of Chlorpromazine to Combat Antimicrobial Resistance. *Pharmaceutics* **2022**, *14*, 2121. [CrossRef]
11. Li, J.; Mooney, D.J. Designing Hydrogels for Controlled Drug Delivery. *Nat. Rev. Mater.* **2016**, *1*, 16071. [CrossRef] [PubMed]
12. Bahney, C.; Lujan, T.; Hsu, C.; Bottlang, M.; West, J.; Johnstone, B. Visible Light Photoinitiation of Mesenchymal Stem Cell-Laden Bioresponsive Hydrogels. *Eur. Cell. Mater.* **2011**, *22*, 43–55. [CrossRef] [PubMed]
13. Mironi-Harpaz, I.; Wang, D.Y.; Venkatraman, S.; Seliktar, D. Photopolymerization of Cell-Encapsulating Hydrogels: Crosslinking Efficiency versus Cytotoxicity. *Acta Biomater.* **2012**, *8*, 1838–1848. [CrossRef] [PubMed]
14. Ki, C.S.; Shih, H.; Lin, C.-C. Facile Preparation of Photodegradable Hydrogels by Photopolymerization. *Polymer* **2013**, *54*, 2115–2122. [CrossRef] [PubMed]
15. Shih, H.; Greene, T.; Korc, M.; Lin, C.-C. Modular and Adaptable Tumor Niche Prepared from Visible Light Initiated Thiol-Norbornene Photopolymerization. *Biomacromolecules* **2016**, *17*, 3872–3882. [CrossRef]
16. Baroli, B. Photopolymerization of Biomaterials: Issues and Potentialities in Drug Delivery, Tissue Engineering, and Cell Encapsulation Applications. *J. Chem. Tech. Biotech.* **2006**, *81*, 491–499. [CrossRef]
17. Wiley, K.L.; Ovadia, E.M.; Calo, C.J.; Huber, R.E.; Kloxin, A.M. Rate-Based Approach for Controlling the Mechanical Properties of 'Thiol–Ene' Hydrogels Formed with Visible Light. *Polym. Chem.* **2019**, *10*, 4428–4440. [CrossRef]
18. O'Connell, C.D.; Zhang, B.; Onofrillo, C.; Duchi, S.; Blanchard, R.; Quigley, A.; Bourke, J.; Gambhir, S.; Kapsa, R.; Di Bella, C.; et al. Tailoring the Mechanical Properties of Gelatin Methacryloyl Hydrogels through Manipulation of the Photocrosslinking Conditions. *Soft Matter* **2018**, *14*, 2142–2151. [CrossRef] [PubMed]
19. Han, W.T.; Jang, T.; Chen, S.; Chong, L.S.H.; Jung, H.-D.; Song, J. Improved Cell Viability for Large-Scale Biofabrication with Photo-Crosslinkable Hydrogel Systems through a Dual-Photoinitiator Approach. *Biomater. Sci.* **2020**, *8*, 450–461. [CrossRef]
20. Aubry, B.; Dumur, F.; Lansalot, M.; Bourgeat-Lami, E.; Lacôte, E.; Lalevée, J. Development of Water-Soluble Type I Photoinitiators for Hydrogel Synthesis. *Macromol* **2022**, *2*, 131–140. [CrossRef]
21. Nguyen, T.; Watkins, K.E.; Kishore, V. Photochemically Crosslinked Cell-laden Methacrylated Collagen Hydrogels with High Cell Viability and Functionality. *J. Biomed. Mater. Res.* **2019**, *107*, 1541–1550. [CrossRef] [PubMed]
22. Fedorovich, N.E.; Oudshoorn, M.H.; Van Geemen, D.; Hennink, W.E.; Alblas, J.; Dhert, W.J.A. The Effect of Photopolymerization on Stem Cells Embedded in Hydrogels. *Biomaterials* **2009**, *30*, 344–353. [CrossRef] [PubMed]
23. Goto, R.; Nishida, E.; Kobayashi, S.; Aino, M.; Ohno, T.; Iwamura, Y.; Kikuchi, T.; Hayashi, J.; Yamamoto, G.; Asakura, M.; et al. Gelatin Methacryloyl–Riboflavin (GelMA–RF) Hydrogels for Bone Regeneration. *Int. J. Mol. Sci.* **2021**, *22*, 1635. [CrossRef] [PubMed]
24. Montazerian, H.; Baidya, A.; Haghniaz, R.; Davoodi, E.; Ahadian, S.; Annabi, N.; Khademhosseini, A.; Weiss, P.S. Stretchable and Bioadhesive Gelatin Methacryloyl-Based Hydrogels Enabled by in Situ Dopamine Polymerization. *ACS Appl. Mater. Interfaces* **2021**, *13*, 40290–40301. [CrossRef] [PubMed]
25. Yue, K.; Trujillo-de Santiago, G.; Alvarez, M.M.; Tamayol, A.; Annabi, N.; Khademhosseini, A. Synthesis, Properties, and Biomedical Applications of Gelatin Methacryloyl (GelMA) Hydrogels. *Biomaterials* **2015**, *73*, 254–271. [CrossRef]
26. De Mol, N.J.; Busker, R.W. Irreversible Binding of the Chlorpromazine Radical Cation and of Photoactivated Chlorpromazine to Biological Macromolecules. *Chem.-Biol. Interact.* **1984**, *52*, 79–92. [CrossRef]
27. Chignell, C.F.; Motten, A.G.; Buettner, G.R. Photoinduced Free Radicals from Chlorpromazine and Related Phenothiazines: Relationship to Phenothiazine-Induced Photosensitization. *Environ. Health Perspect.* **1985**, *64*, 103–110. [CrossRef]
28. Chanana, G.; Batra, K. Investigating Functional Performance and Substituent Effect in Modelling Molecular Structure, UV-Visible Spectra, and Optical Properties of D-π-A Conjugated Organic Dye Molecules: A DFT and TD-DFT Study. *J. Mol. Model.* **2021**, *27*, 229. [CrossRef]
29. Bae, W.; Yoon, T.-Y.; Jeong, C. Direct Evaluation of Self-Quenching Behavior of Fluorophores at High Concentrations Using an Evanescent Field. *PLoS ONE* **2021**, *16*, e0247326. [CrossRef]
30. Chen, S.; Yu, Y.-L.; Wang, J.-H. Inner Filter Effect-Based Fluorescent Sensing Systems: A Review. *Anal. Chim. Acta* **2018**, *999*, 13–26. [CrossRef]
31. Liu, M.; Li, M.-D.; Xue, J.; Phillips, D.L. Time-Resolved Spectroscopic and Density Functional Theory Study of the Photochemistry of Irgacure-2959 in an Aqueous Solution. *J. Phys. Chem. A* **2014**, *118*, 8701–8707. [CrossRef] [PubMed]
32. Hübner, C.G.; Renn, A.; Renge, I.; Wild, U.P. Direct Observation of the Triplet Lifetime Quenching of Single Dye Molecules by Molecular Oxygen. *J. Chem. Phys.* **2001**, *115*, 9619–9622. [CrossRef]
33. Souza, G.A.; Cordeiro, D.S.; Ernter, T.D.M. Steady-State and Fluorescence Lifetime Quenching of Self-Assembled Diphenylalanine/Coumarin Nanostructures as a Method to Determine Dissolved O_2 in Water. *Adv. Nat. Sci.* **2023**, *14*, 015011. [CrossRef]
34. Guerret-Legras, L.; Audibert, J.; Gonzalez-Ojeda, I.M.; Dubacheva, G.; Clavier, G.; Miomandre, F. Time-Resolved Fluorescence Microscopy Combined with Scanning Electrochemical Microscopy: A New Way to Visualize Photo-Induced Electron Transfer Quenching with an Electrofluorochromic Probe. *J. Phys. Chem. C* **2020**, *124*, 23938–23948. [CrossRef]
35. Jamorski Jödicke, C.; Lüthi, H.P. Time-Dependent Density Functional Theory (TDDFT) Study of the Excited Charge-Transfer State Formation of a Series of Aromatic Donor−acceptor Systems. *J. Am. Chem. Soc.* **2003**, *125*, 252–264. [CrossRef]
36. Anger, P.; Bharadwaj, P.; Novotny, L. Enhancement and Quenching of Single-Molecule Fluorescence. *Phys. Rev. Lett.* **2006**, *96*, 113002. [CrossRef]

37. Chansoria, P.; Asif, S.; Polkoff, K.; Chung, J.; Piedrahita, J.A.; Shirwaiker, R.A. Characterizing the Effects of Synergistic Thermal and Photo-Cross-Linking during Biofabrication on the Structural and Functional Properties of Gelatin Methacryloyl (Gelma) Hydrogels. *ACS Biomater. Sci. Eng.* **2021**, *7*, 5175–5188. [CrossRef]
38. Deng, J.; Pan, J.; Yu, L.; Wang, Y.; Zhang, W.; Huang, W.; Fan, Y.; Liu, Y. The Effects of Irradiation Time on Gelatin Methacrylate Hydrogels Used for Bone Tissue Engineering. *J. Biomater. Tissue Eng.* **2022**, *12*, 192–198. [CrossRef]
39. Brown, D.F.; Kothari, D. Comparison of Antibiotic Discs from Different Sources. *J. Clin. Pathol.* **1975**, *28*, 779–783. [CrossRef]
40. Bauer, A.W. Single-Disk Antibiotic-Sensitivity Testing of Staphylococci: An Analysis of Technique and Results. *AMA Arch. Intern. Med.* **1959**, *104*, 208. [CrossRef]
41. Dutta, D.; Willcox, M. A Laboratory Assessment of Factors That Affect Bacterial Adhesion to Contact Lenses. *Biology* **2013**, *2*, 1268–1281. [CrossRef] [PubMed]
42. Lima, M.; Teixeira-Santos, R.; Gomes, L.C.; Faria, S.I.; Valcarcel, J.; Vázquez, J.A.; Cerqueira, M.A.; Pastrana, L.; Bourbon, A.I.; Mergulhão, F.J. Development of Chitosan-Based Surfaces to Prevent Single- and Dual-Species Biofilms of Staphylococcus Aureus and Pseudomonas Aeruginosa. *Molecules* **2021**, *26*, 4378. [CrossRef] [PubMed]

gels

Article

Development, Optimization, and Evaluation of New Gel Formulations with Cyclodextrin Complexes and Volatile Oils with Antimicrobial Activity

Alina Ionela Stancu [1], Eliza Oprea [2,*], Lia Mara Dițu [2,3], Anton Ficai [1,4,5,*], Cornelia-Ioana Ilie [1,5], Irinel Adriana Badea [6], Mihaela Buleandra [6], Oana Brîncoveanu [7], Mihaela Violeta Ghica [8,9], Ionela Avram [3,10], Cristina Elena Dinu Pîrvu [8,9] and Magdalena Mititelu [11]

1 Department Science and Engineering of Oxide Materials and Nanomaterials, Faculty of Chemical Engineering and Biotechnology, National University of Science and Technology Politehnica Bucharest, 1–7 Polizu Street, 011061 Bucharest, Romania; alina.stancu1995@gmail.com (A.I.S.)
2 Department of Botany and Microbiology, Faculty of Biology, University of Bucharest, Portocalilor 1-3, 060101 Bucharest, Romania; lia-mara.ditu@bio.unibuc.ro
3 MICROGEN Research Centre, Faculty of Biology, University of Bucharest, Portocalilor 1-3, 060101 Bucharest, Romania; ionela.sarbu@bio.unibuc.ro
4 Academy of Romanian Scientists, Ilfov Street 1-3, 050045 Bucharest, Romania
5 National Centre for Micro and Nanomaterials and National Centre for Food Safety, National University of Science and Technology Politehnica Bucharest, 060042 Bucharest, Romania
6 Department of Analytical Chemistry and Physical Chemistry, Faculty of Chemistry, University of Bucharest, 90–92 Panduri Street, 050663 Bucharest, Romania; irinel.badea@chimie.unibuc.ro (I.A.B.); mihaela.buleandra@g.unibuc.ro (M.B.)
7 National Institute for Research and Development in Microtechnologies, 126A Erou Iancu Nicolae Street, 077190 Bucharest, Romania; oana.brincoveanu@imt.ro
8 Department of Physical and Colloidal Chemistry, Faculty of Pharmacy, University of Medicine and Pharmacy Carol Davila, 6 Traian Vuia Street, 020956 Bucharest, Romania; mihaela.ghica@umfcd.ro (M.V.G.); cristina.dinu@umfcd.ro (C.E.D.P.)
9 Innovative Therapeutic Structures Research and Development Centre (InnoTher), University of Medicine and Pharmacy Carol Davila, 6 Traian Vuia Street, 020956 Bucharest, Romania
10 Department of Genetics, Faculty of Biology, University of Bucharest, Portocalilor 1-3, 060101 Bucharest, Romania
11 Department of Clinical Laboratory and Food Safety, Faculty of Pharmacy, University of Medicine and Pharmacy Carol Davila, 6 Traian Vuia Street, 020956 Bucharest, Romania; magdalena.mititelu@umfcd.ro
* Correspondence: eliza.oprea@g.unibuc.ro (E.O.); anton.ficai@upb.ro (A.F.)

Abstract: This study aimed to develop and evaluate hydrogels containing a cyclodextrin complex with clove essential oil and other free volatile oils with antimicrobial properties (tea tree and rosemary essential oils), focusing on their pharmaco-technical and rheological characteristics. The formulations varied in the Carbopol 940 (a hydrophilic polymer) and volatile oils' concentrations. Rheological analysis indicated that the gels displayed pseudoplastic behavior, with the flow index (n) values below 1, ensuring appropriate consistency and handling. The results showed that increasing the Carbopol concentration significantly enhanced the yield stress, consistency index, and viscosity, with gel B, containing 1% Carbopol, 1.5% tea tree essential oil, and 1.5% rosemary essential oil, demonstrating optimal stability and rheological properties. At the same time, the concentration of volatile oils was found to modulate the gels' flow parameters, but their effect was less pronounced than that of the gel-forming polymer. Antimicrobial testing revealed that both gel B and gel E (containing 1% Carbopol, 2% tea tree essential oil, and 2% rosemary essential oil) exhibited antimicrobial activity against Gram-positive, Gram-negative bacteria, and *Candida* spp., with gel E showing superior efficacy against *Candida tropicalis*. The antimicrobial effects were likely influenced by the higher concentrations of tea tree and rosemary essential oils in gel E. Overall, the study demonstrates that the concentration of Carbopol 940 primarily determines the gel's rheological behavior, while volatile oil concentration modulates antimicrobial effectiveness.

Keywords: antimicrobial agents; β-cyclodextrin complex; volatile oils; hydrogels

1. Introduction

Hydrogels are aqueous or hydro-glycerinated gels in which macromolecules form a three-dimensional network comprising the entire liquid phase. The active substances could be easily released if not integrated into or bound to this polymer network. The pores in the gel network allow relatively free diffusion of molecules of active substances with not too large dimensions. Consistency is chosen depending on the mode of administration, the climatic conditions endured by the preparations, and the nature of the active principles, which can change the viscosity of the gel base, acting on the polymer bonds [1–3]. The growing demand for developing new hydrogels is mainly due to their wide range of applications, namely hygiene and personal care products, pharmaceuticals and cosmetics, food and agriculture, and more recently, tissue engineering or regenerative medicine. The use of hydrogels is based on the following advantages: they are washable, are preferred for people with oily skin, for the treatment of eye diseases and the treatment of hairy regions or mucous membranes, have good skin tolerance, the drug absorptions from these bases are superior to fatty bases, they are compatible with many active substances, however, taking into account the ionic character of both the ointment bases and the incorporated active substances [4–6]. Nevertheless, some disadvantages can be mentioned, such as rapid water loss and susceptibility to microbial invasion, which requires the mandatory addition of preservatives.

Antimicrobial hydrogels and essential oils in topical formulations have been widely studied, but challenges such as stability, bioavailability, and efficacy in long-term use need more studies. Recent studies have explored the development of advanced antimicrobial hydrogels, yet issues with the stability and effectiveness of essential oils, particularly their rapid degradation or volatility, limit their potential for sustained therapeutic effects. For instance, according to recent findings, hydrogels formulated with cyclodextrin complexes demonstrate enhanced stability and controlled release of bioactive agents, making them promising for biomedical applications. Specifically, carbopol-based hydrogels with cyclodextrin complexes have shown improved drug delivery performance due to their capacity to form inclusion complexes with diverse compounds, such as eugenol [7], thymol [8], clotrimazole [9], etc.

Additionally, a recent study highlighted essential oils' role in enhancing hydrogel antimicrobial properties. Still, these oils are prone to degradation and require encapsulation or stabilization to prolong their activity [10].

Furthermore, cyclodextrins based hydrogels have gained special attention due to their properties (extended polymeric network, dynamic stiffness like an extracellular matrix, biocompatibility, etc.) and their potential for biomedical applications [11]. Moreover, adding essential oils with antimicrobial properties in such formulations enhances their wound-healing properties, which could be more potent than conventional antimicrobial drugs [12,13].

Hydrophilic gels are obtained from colloidal macromolecules, which have the property of soaking with water or other hydrophilic solvents by absorption. Carbopol is an active acrylic acid polymer anionic that forms a low-density white powder and gels in concentrations ranging from 0.5 to 1.5% [14].

Carbopol can be used to process non-greasy ointments, is easily washable, stable, non-irritating to the skin, and has rapid release. Several varieties of Carbopol are known: 940, 974, and ULTREZ 10. To obtain the hydrogel, the Carbopol is dispersed under stirring in a preservative solution, left to hydrate, and then neutralized with a base (sodium, potassium, triethanolamine hydroxides), when the acid polymer passes into a soluble state. This is the mixed slowly and completed with preservative solution. Formulation characteristics, including viscosity, elasticity, and rheology, are the most important factors in semisolid preparation development and the final behavior of semisolid preparations [15].

One of the major advantages of topical administration for the local action of a drug substance is the avoidance of side effects at the systemic level. Macromolecular agents forming semisolid structures of the carbomer type are polymers of acrylic acid, depending on the sort of different molecular weights and degrees of crosslinking. The assigned role is usually correlated with local skin or mucous applications. The emulsifier's role is mentioned less and is associated with low concentration levels (0.1–0.5%). This aspect was considered when selecting the composition of emulsions containing volatile oils. Outstanding biocompatibility is doubled by adequate microstructure control through quality attributes such as pH value or neutralizing agent used (hydroxide alkaline or ethanolamine derivative) [16,17].

This study focused on the development and comprehensive evaluation of hydrogels formulated with a cyclodextrin complex containing clove essential oil (CO), as well as hydrogels incorporating free volatile oils such as tea tree and rosemary, known for their antimicrobial properties. The research aimed to assess the pharmaco-technical properties of these hydrogels, including their stability, texture, ease of application, and rheological behavior, which is crucial for understanding the flow and deformation characteristics of the gels. By combining these natural antimicrobial agents with cyclodextrin, the study sought to enhance the stability and effectiveness of the volatile oils, leading to innovative topical formulations with improved therapeutic potential.

2. Results and Discussion

2.1. GC-MS Analysis

The chemical composition of *Melaleuca alternifolia* (tea tree) essential oil by GC-MS is presented in Table 1.

Table 1. The chemical composition of *Melaleuca alternifolia* essential oil.

Compounds	KI *	t_R (min) **	Relative Area (%)
α-Pinene	930	6.01	1.02
Sabinene (β-Thujene)	969	6.72	0.72
β-Pinene	982	6.95	0.45
α-Phellandrene	997	7.23	0.27
α-Terpinene	1009	7.44	10.85
p-Cymene	1017	7.58	2.63
Eucalyptol	1026	7.73	3.76
γ-Terpinene	1051	8.17	18.77
α-Terpinolene	1078	8.64	3.43
trans-Sabinene hydrate	1090	8.84	0.15
cis-2-p-Menthen-1-ol	1113	9.21	0.43
Borneol	1162	9.99	0.01
Terpinen-4-ol	1175	10.20	f36.32
α-Terpineol	1183	10.32	2.63
cis-Piperitol	1197	10.54	0.17
Geraniol	1238	11.15	0.01
δ-Elemene	1324	12.39	0.06
α-Cubebene	1336	12.55	0.09
Eugenol	1344	12.66	0.08
α-Copaene	1364	12.94	0.28
Methyleugenol	1384	13.23	0.09
α-Gurjunene	1398	13.42	0.75
β-Caryophyllene	1409	13.56	0.41
γ-Elemene	1430	13.82	1.95
Alloaromadendrene	1454	14.11	0.75
γ-Muurolene	1463	14.22	0.91
β-Guaiene	1480	14.43	0.53
α-Muurolene	1490	14.56	3.88
γ-Cadinene	1512	14.82	3.48
δ-Cadinene	1523	14.95	0.38
Spathulenol	1574	15.56	0.27
Globulol	1582	15.65	0.71
Viridiflorol	1590	15.75	0.63
Rosifoliol	1597	15.84	0.15
Ledol	1601	15.88	0.10
Cubenol	1614	16.12	0.55
epi-Cubenol	1621	16.25	0.15
τ-Cadinol	1623	16.29	0.45
Total			98.27

* KI-Kovats Index, ** t_R—retention time.

The chemical composition of *Rosmarinus officinalis* (rosemary) essential oil by GC-MS is shown in Table 2.

Table 2. The chemical composition of *Rosmarinus officinalis* essential oil.

Compounds	KI *	t_R (min) **	Relative Area (%)
α-Pinene	932	6.03	11.83
Camphene	946	6.29	3.93
Sabinene (β-Thujene)	973	6.79	4.10
β-Pinene	982	6.96	0.71
α-Phellandrene	998	7.26	0.11
p-Cymene	1011	7.48	0.03
Eucalyptol	1030	7.80	49.70
γ-Terpinene	1049	8.14	0.52
cis-Sabinene hydrate	1060	8.33	0.04
α-Terpinolene	1078	8.64	0.35
Linalool	1087	8.79	0.63
endo-Fenchol	1107	9.12	0.03
α-Campholenal	1116	9.26	0.04
Camphor	1143	9.69	14.12
Borneol	1161	9.98	3.36
Terpinen-4-ol	1169	10.10	0.56
α-Terpineol	1183	10.32	2.00
Myrtenol	1189	10.41	0.04
Verbenone	1204	10.65	0.01
cis-Carveol	1208	10.71	0.01
Thymol	1271	11.62	0.02
Bornyl acetate	1275	11.68	0.75
Carvacrol	1287	11.86	0.02
Eugenol	1344	12.66	0.02
α-Ylangene	1359	12.88	0.03
α-Copaene	1364	12.94	0.02
Methyleugenol	1389	13.29	0.03
β-Caryophyllene	1412	13.60	5.80
β-Ylangene	1418	13.67	0.05
α-Guaiene	1431	13.83	0.03
Aromadendrene	1439	13.93	0.03
α-Humulene	1446	14.01	0.42
γ-Muurolene	1465	14.25	0.04
α-Muurolene	1491	14.57	0.15
γ-Cadinene	1511	14.81	0.03
α-Calacorene	1535	15.10	0.01
Caryophyllene oxide	1582	15.65	0.24
Methyl jasmonate	1621	16.26	0.04
Total			99.84

* KI-Kovats Index, ** t_R—retention time.

GC-MS analysis showed that the most abundant constituent of the *Melaleuca alternifolia* volatile oil is terpinen-4-ol (36.32%), followed by γ-terpinene (18.85%) and α-terpinene (10.85%). A study from 2019 [18] confirmed that these three components are the major constituents of the tea tree essential oil (TTO), taking into account small variations of percentages.

For *Rosmarinus officinalis*, the most abundant component of the volatile oil (RO) is eucalyptol (49.70%), followed by camphor (14.12%), α-pinene (11.83%), and β-caryophyllene (5.80%). The literature data confirm the results obtained. Studies [19,20] conducted on volatile oil hydrodistilled from different parts of *Rosmarinus officinalis* L. also showed that the major component of the oil is eucalyptol, followed by α-pinene and camphor. Furthermore, significant amounts of borneol, camphene, and verbenone were found.

2.2. Gels Characteristics

Carbopol is a widely used polymer in hydrogel formulations due to its excellent gelling properties, ease of use, and biocompatibility. The 0.5–1.5% concentration range is commonly employed in pharmaceutical and cosmetic formulations to achieve optimal gel viscosity, texture, and stability. In particular, a concentration of 1% is often chosen as it offers a balance between effective gel formation and ease of application without being overly dense or challenging to spread. The literature frequently cites 1% Carbopol as a standard concentration that forms a stable and easily applicable hydrogel. Studies have demonstrated that at this concentration, Carbopol provides sufficient viscosity and structure to support the incorporation of active substances while maintaining a smooth texture suitable for topical applications [21]. Higher concentrations, such as 2%, are sometimes used when a firmer gel consistency is required or when higher viscosities are necessary for a specific delivery route (e.g., localized skin application). However, excessively high concentrations can result in too thick or difficult to spread gels, thus limiting patient compliance [22]. In addition, volatile oils such as tea tree, rosemary, and clove are known for their antimicrobial properties and are often used in topical formulations. The concentration of these oils in a formulation is critical to balancing efficacy with potential skin irritation. A concentration of 2% essential oil is commonly employed in topical formulations, providing potent antimicrobial activity while minimizing the irritation risk. According to studies on essential oil-based hydrogels, concentrations in the range of 1–3% are optimal for achieving therapeutic benefits without overwhelming the formulation with too much oil, which could affect the stability or texture of the gel [23]. Additionally, studies on wound healing formulations often recommend using essential oils at concentrations around 2% to ensure both efficacy and patient comfort [24]. Furthermore, combining different volatile oils at this concentration generates synergistic antimicrobial effects without increasing the risk of adverse reactions or compromising the overall gel structure.

Preliminary experiments involved testing various Carbopol and essential oils concentrations to determine the optimal formulation. These tests have guided the decision to use 1% Carbopol and 2% essential oils, as they produced hydrogels with suitable rheological properties, ease of application, and antimicrobial potential.

TTO is well known for its potent antimicrobial and antifungal properties and has been extensively studied for its biocompatibility in topical applications. Many studies show it is safe for humans when used in concentrations up to 5%. The TTO used in this study at 2% concentration aligns with established safe concentrations, allowing the oil to exert its antimicrobial effects without posing significant toxicity risks [25].

RO contains compounds like carnosic acid and rosmarinic acid, which are known for their antioxidant, antimicrobial, and anti-inflammatory properties. It has been used in various cosmetic and medicinal formulations and is considered biocompatible for topical applications. Studies have demonstrated that RO is well tolerated by the skin at concentrations typically used in therapeutic products (1–2%). It has also been shown to enhance wound healing and reduce skin irritation, making it a suitable choice for incorporation into hydrogels [26].

The TTO, CO, and RO selection considered the synergistic antimicrobial activity, which can enhance the overall therapeutic outcome while allowing for lower concentrations of each oil. This reduces the likelihood of adverse reactions associated with higher concentrations of a single oil. At the same time, combining these essential oils leverages their complementary properties: analgesic and anti-inflammatory benefits (CO), broad-spectrum antimicrobial activity (TTO), and wound healing and antioxidant protection (RO). The combined use of these oils ensures a balanced formulation that maximizes therapeutic benefits while minimizing toxicity risks [27].

Gels containing RO loaded into lipid nanoparticles (containing 3% RO *w/w*) increased skin hydration and elasticity compared to gels containing free RO in human volunteers [28].

Regarding biocompatibility, eugenol is known to promote wound healing and has been used historically in dental care due to its ability to reduce pain and inflammation. This main active compound from CO has been shown to have good biocompatibility when used in appropriate concentrations for topical applications. Research has demonstrated that low concentrations of CO (1–3%) in topical formulations are generally safe and well tolerated, although higher concentrations may cause skin irritation [29]. Therefore, the study uses CO at controlled concentrations to ensure formula efficacy and safety.

RO is considered non-toxic when used in topical formulations at concentrations typically below 5%. Higher concentrations can irritate, but its incorporation at 2% in the study's hydrogel formulation is consistent with safety recommendations. Rosemary essential oil (RO) is also less likely to cause allergic reactions than other essential oils, enhancing its suitability for sensitive or damaged skin [28]. In addition, gels containing RO loaded into lipid nanoparticles (containing 3% RO *w*/*w*) increased skin hydration and elasticity compared to gels containing free RO in human volunteers [28]. This study suggested that gel formulations are indicated for treating various surface cutaneous alterations.

TTO is generally considered safe for topical use in 1–5% concentrations, but it can be toxic if ingested or applied at very high concentrations. Prolonged exposure to high concentrations of TTO can lead to allergic reactions or skin sensitization in some individuals. The concentration chosen in this study (2%) is below the toxicity threshold and aligns with the safe use guidelines for maintaining efficacy without causing adverse effects [30]. Moreover, the chitosan/polyvinyl alcohol films containing 1.0 and 1.5% of TTO showed signs of reabsorption comparable to those of porcine collagen, indicating that the oil's incorporation promotes more significant reabsorption and biocompatibility, stimulating a more substantial interaction with phagocytic cells [31].

Considering that it is essential to know aspects related to toxicity in order to develop a pharmaceutical product, TTO, RO, and CO were chosen as bioactive components of the formulations for their low toxicity and antimicrobial activity against various bacterial strains. These two properties being supported by both the literature data and the results presented further in this study.

Thus, studies conducted on Winstar rats demonstrate that the LD_{50} is greater than 2.000 mg/kg of body weight in the case of RO and between 1.9–2.6 mL/kg in the case of TTO when administrated orally [30,32], while CO toxicity against albino rats led to a LD_{50} value of 3597.5 mg/kg [33].

The characteristics of the gel samples are presented in Tables 3 and 4.

Table 3. Gel characteristics.

Characteristic	Formula A	Formula B	Formula C
Initial macroscopic characteristics	appearance: homogenous; color: yellowish; smell: specific	appearance: homogenous; color: yellowish; smell: specific	appearance: homogenous; color: yellowish; smell: specific
Macroscopic characteristics after 60 days	appearance: homogenous; color: yellowish smell: specific	appearance: homogenous; color: yellowish; smell: specific	appearance: homogenous; color: yellowish; smell: specific
Initial pH	6.50	6.00	6.70
pH after 60 days	6.40	6.60	6.60

Table 4. Gel characteristics.

Characteristic	Formula D	Formula E	Formula F
Initial macroscopic characteristics	appearance: homogenous; color: yellowish; smell: specific	appearance: homogenous; color: yellowish; smell: specific	appearance: homogenous; color: yellowish; smell: specific
Macroscopic characteristics after 60 days	appearance: homogenous; color: yellowish smell: specific	appearance: homogenous; color: yellowish; smell: specific	appearance: homogenous; color: yellowish; smell: specific
Initial pH	6.70	6.60	6.40
pH after 60 days	6.70	6.50	6.30

The data from Tables 3 and 4 show that the gels are homogenous. All gels presented good stability by maintaining a homogenous appearance at 2 °C and 40 °C, even after 30 days. A concentration in volatile oils over 8% produces an un-homogenous appearance, and the formulas become unstable.

As observed in Figure 1, the analysis of the spreading area of the gels revealed significant variations attributable to differences in their consistency. The experimental data demonstrated that all the prepared formulations were stable and homogeneous, displaying good consistency and a spreading capacity that remained within desirable limits over time. Notably, formulations B, E, and F exhibited the highest values for spreading area, indicating superior spread ability, which is an important characteristic for topical applications. The stability and rheological studies further highlighted the robustness and optimal rheological properties of formula B. Specifically, formula B demonstrated excellent stability, maintaining its structural integrity and performance over time. Its optimal rheological characteristics, such as viscosity and flow behavior, make it particularly suitable for applications where consistent texture and ease of application are essential. Given these promising results, the concentration of carbopol in formula B, which was set at 1%, has been strategically chosen to enhance the incorporation of volatile oils. This adjustment aims to capitalize on the formula's stability and spreading capacity, allowing for an increased concentration of active ingredients without compromising the gel's consistency or performance. The combination of high spreading area values and excellent stability underscores the potential of formula B as an ideal candidate for further development, particularly in formulations requiring a higher load of volatile oils for enhanced therapeutic efficacy.

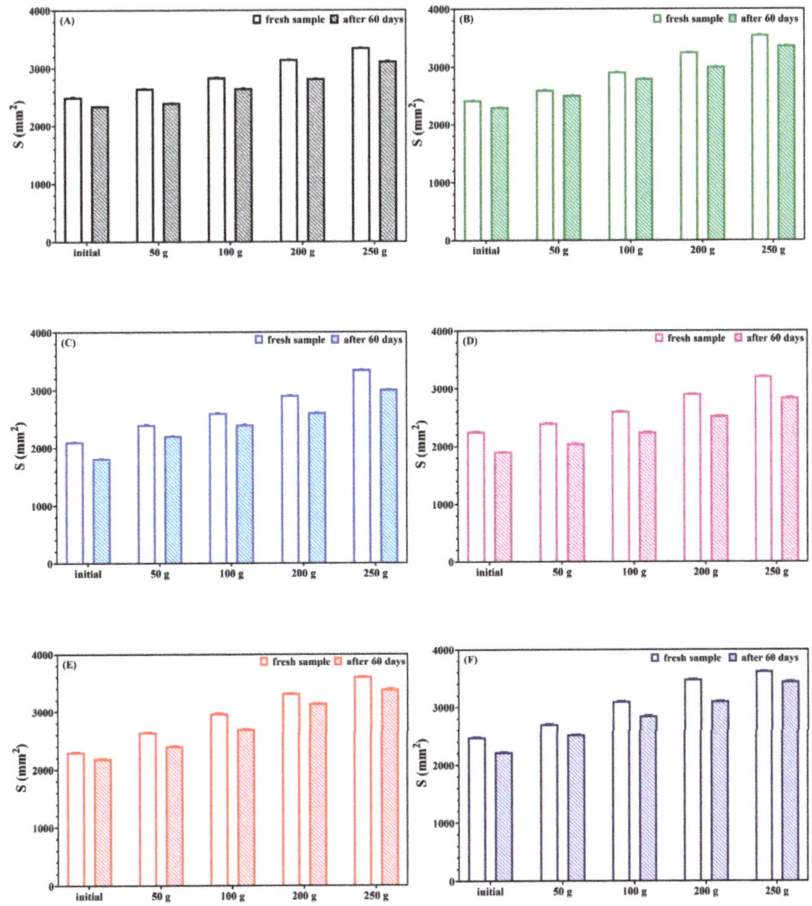

Figure 1. Spreading area function of the applied mass for samples. (**A–F**) represent the gel formulas A, B, C, D, E, and F. The differences between samples (fresh vs. 60 days) for each formula were statistically analyzed using one-way ANOVA and Tukey's multiple comparisons test. The resulting data were statistically significant ($p < 0.05$).

2.3. Rheological Data

For each carbopol gel, an upward rheogram was obtained by plotting the shear stress versus shear rate (Figure 2).

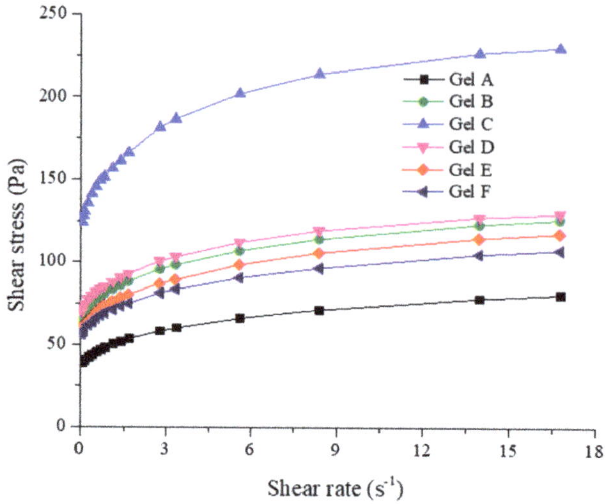

Figure 2. The upward rheograms for carbopol gels were analyzed at 33 °C.

As can be seen from Figure 2, all formulations presented similar shapes of flow profiles with a shear stress increase for the shear rate increase, indicating a non-Newtonian behavior.

The gels' rheological characteristics were evaluated using different models (Equations (1)–(4)), described in the Materials and Methods Section. There are two main indicators used to investigate the goodness of fit for different rheological models: the determination coefficient R^2 and the adjusted R squared. The adjusted R^2 takes into account the complexity of the model and provides a more accurate reflection of the model's performance compared to the standard R^2. This metric penalizes models for having unnecessary parameters, making it useful for comparing models with different numbers of predictors: Herschel-Bulkley model has three parameters compared to Bingham, Casson, and Ostawld-de-Waele. Which involves two parameters. The values of R^2 and adjusted R squared of all formulations are presented in Table 5.

Table 5. The determination coefficients, adjusted R^2, and AIC_c values for different rheological models tested at 33 °C.

Gel/Rheological Model	Casson			Bingham			Ostwald-de Waele			Herschel-Bulkley		
	R^2	Adj R^2	AIC_c	R^2	Adj R^2	AIC_c	R^2	Adj R^2	AIC_c	R^2	Adj R^2	AIC_c
Formula A	0.9733	0.9715	33.29	0.8766	0.8684	59.29	0.9790	0.9776	29.16	0.9981	0.9978	−7.961
Formula B	0.9648	0.9624	50.01	0.8556	0.8460	74.01	0.9847	0.9837	35.85	0.9986	0.9984	−1.536
Formula C	0.9473	0.9437	77.29	0.8230	0.8112	97.87	0.9862	0.9853	54.51	0.9947	0.9939	41.870
Formula D	0.9605	0.9578	51.98	0.8462	0.8360	75.07	0.9832	0.9821	37.45	0.9969	0.9964	12.390
Formula E	0.9676	0.9654	47.99	0.8632	0.8541	72.47	0.9833	0.9822	36.73	0.9983	0.9981	1.090
Formula F	0.9672	0.9650	43.43	0.8603	0.8510	68.05	0.9840	0.9830	31.19	0.9990	0.9989	−12.980

As can be remarked from Table 5, the R^2 values of the Herschel-Bulkey model (Equation (4)) best fitted the experimental data, due to the highest R^2 values ranging from 0.9947 and 0.9990 and the adjusted R squared, from 0.9939 to 0.9989. The Herschel-Bulkley model showed the highest R^2 and adjusted R^2 values compared to the other three models, suggesting that this rheological model is considered the best to fit the experimental data, taking into account the model complexity.

The models ranking based on accuracy alone involving the comparison of determination coefficients (R^2) values is not enough because the variability of the model is not included. Thus, alongside R^2 and adjusted R^2, the model comparison and assessment were realized with the application of the Akaike Information Criterion (AIC), which estimates not only the goodness of fit, but also model variability [34]. In this study, we used the small-sample corrected AICc because the number of points was small. Therefore, the rheological model that best represents statistically the drug mechanism is the model with the lowest values of AICc [35]. According to Table 5, the lowest AICc values are recorded for Herschel-Bulkley model, which is considered to be the best model to fit the data, considering its complexity. Correlating the highest R^2 and adjusted R^2 values, and the smallest AICc values, we selected the best rheological model to fit the data which is represented by the Herschel-Bulkley model.

The flow parameters specific to the above model along with the viscosity recorded at 0.3 rpm, are given in Table 6.

Table 6. Herschel-Bulkey model flow parameters obtained through stationary shear analysis at 33 ± 0.1 °C for the designed carbopol gels.

Gel/ Flow Parameters	Yield Stress (Pa) (τ_0—Pa)	Consistency Index (K—Pa·s^n)	Flow Index (n)	Viscosity at 0.30 rpm ($\eta_{0.3}$—Pa·s)	
				Initial	After 60 Days
Formula A	29.518	20.021	0.34	489.20	472.10
Formula B	48.333	34.938	0.29	822.90	710.20
Formula C	80.150	76.884	0.25	1553.00	1432.80
Formula D	51.397	36.334	0.28	871.90	760.30
Formula E	43.268	31.869	0.31	738.10	682.00
Formula F	41.732	28.915	0.30	698.80	536.40

It can be noticed that the value of the flow index (n) is smaller than 1, indicating a pseudoplastic behavior that ensures suitable gels' manipulation and administration.

According to Table 6, the influence of composition, varying in terms of both volatile oils and carbopol concentrations, is reflected in parameters specific to the Herschel-Bulkey model and on viscosity at 0.30 rpm.

For Serie A-B-C, the concentration of gel-forming polymer is the critical ingredient affecting the rheological characteristics of the designed gels. Thus, the increase in carbopol concentration determines a significant increase of the yield stress (τ_0), consistency index (K) and viscosity at 0.30 rpm ($\eta_{0.3}$). Compared to gel A (with lower carbopol concentration), the yield stress is 1.64 times higher for gel B (with medium carbopol concentration) and 2.72 times higher for gel C (with high carbopol concentration). For a carbopol concentration varying from lower to high level, the consistency index increases 3.84 times, while the viscosity at 0.30 rpm has a 3.17 times increase. Gel B's parameters K and $\eta_{0.3}$ are about 2.20 and, respectively, 1.89 times smaller than gel C, while compared to gel A, the parameters K and $\eta_{0.3}$ values are about 1.70 times higher.

For the Serie B-D-E-F, the variation of volatile oils concentration is the main factor influencing the flow parameters. All carbopol gels yield stress, consistency index, and viscosity decrease about 1.25 times when the concentration of the volatile oil varies between the minimum (2%) and maximum level (5%).

The results show that the concentration of gel-forming polymer has a stronger influence on the flow parameters, while adding essential oils modulates the gel's rheological behavior. According to the rheological data, formulations B and E were considered the best, and the morphological and biological properties will be assessed only for these two gels. Gel B, containing 1% Carbopol, 1.5% TTO, and 1.5% RO, displayed a balanced pseudoplastic behavior with appropriate consistency and handling characteristics, making it easy to apply and spread, essential for topical treatments. The formulation showed excellent stability, maintaining its structural integrity over time. Gel E, formulated with 1% Carbopol, 2% TTO, and 2% RO, also demonstrated rheological characteristics and stability over time superior to the other formulations; in addition, it has the advantage of an increased concentration of volatile oils with a positive impact on the antimicrobial potential. Although the effect of the volatile oils on flow parameters was less pronounced than that of the gel-forming polymer, Gel E still maintained desirable rheological characteristics, ensuring ease of application and user comfort.

2.4. Scanning Electron Microscopy

Scanning electron microscopy (SEM) was employed to obtain detailed images of gels B and E, which were identified as the optimal formulations based on their superior rheological properties. These images provided valuable insights into the microstructure of the gels, revealing the surface morphology and the distribution of the encapsulated compounds within the hydrogel matrix. The analysis of gels B and E through SEM helped to understand how the structural characteristics of these formulations contribute to their stability, texture, and overall performance, supporting their selection as the most promising candidates for further development in topical applications.

As revealed by SEM, the structural characteristics of gels B and E play an important role in determining their stability, texture, and overall performance, which are key factors in their selection as promising candidates for topical applications. The SEM images (Figures 3 and 4) detailed these gels' microarchitecture, highlighting the gel matrix's uniformity and homogeneity. This uniform distribution of encapsulated compounds is essential for maintaining the stability of the active ingredients, as it prevents their premature release and degradation. Additionally, the fine, interconnected network observed in the gel structure contributes to its desirable texture, ensuring a smooth and consistent application on the skin. This structural integrity also enhances the gel's ability to retain its shape and resist deformation under stress, which is critical for maintaining its rheological properties over time. The stability of the gel matrix ensures that the active ingredients are effectively preserved and delivered, while the appropriate texture promotes ease of application and user comfort. Furthermore, the well-organized microstructure facilitates a controlled and sustained release of the encapsulated compounds, which is particularly important for maintaining the antimicrobial efficacy of the gels over extended periods. This controlled release mechanism not only improves the therapeutic effectiveness of the gels but also minimizes potential side effects associated with the rapid release of active ingredients.

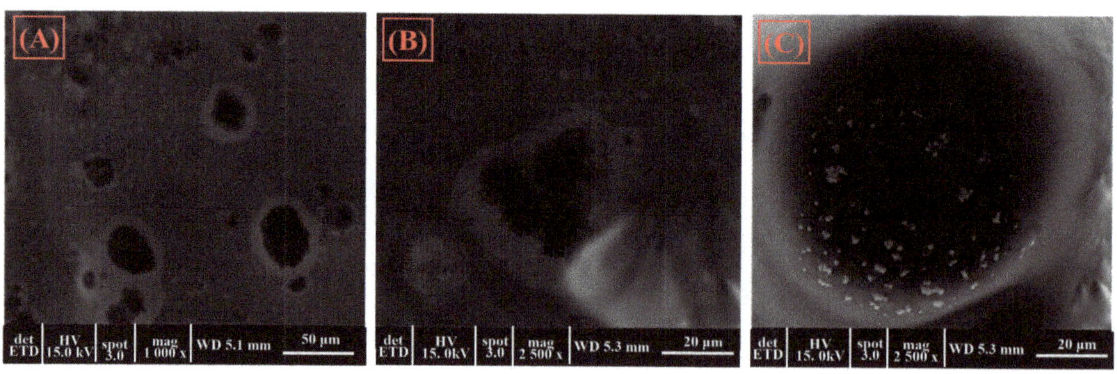

Figure 3. SEM images for the gel B at 1000× magnification (**A**) and 2500× magnification (**B**,**C**).

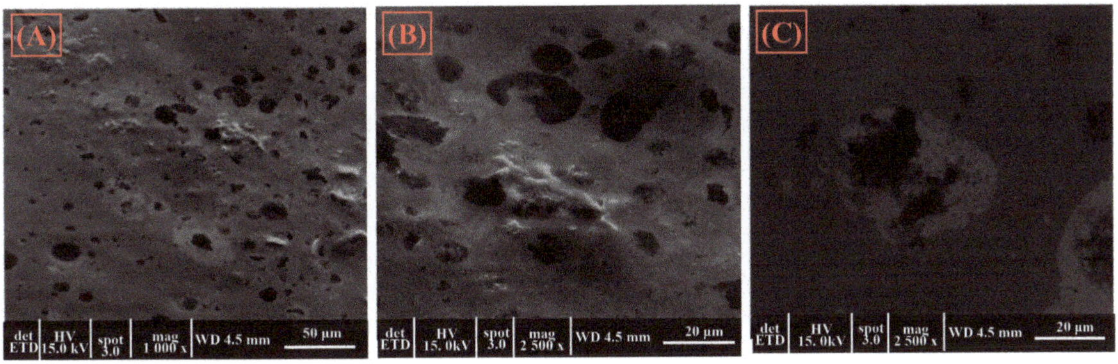

Figure 4. SEM images for the gel E at 1000× magnification (**A**) and 2500× magnification (**B**,**C**).

Overall, the structural characteristics of gels B and E, including their homogeneous distribution, stable matrix, and favorable texture, make them highly suitable for further development as topical formulations. These properties support their potential for enhanced stability, effective delivery of active compounds, and improved patient compliance, positioning them as leading candidates for innovative and effective topical therapies.

2.5. Antimicrobial Activity

2.5.1. Qualitative Assessment of the Antimicrobial Activity

Antimicrobial activity was qualitatively evaluated by determining the growth inhibition zone diameters (GIZD) that appeared around the spot (Table 7).

Table 7. The influence of developed pharmaceutical formulations on selected pathogenic strains.

Strains	Samples											
	GB	B	E	CO	RO	TTO	UA	Complex	UA:CO	UA:RO	UA:TTO	DMSO
Gram-positive bacteria												
E. faecalis ATCC 29212	-	+	+	+++	+++	+++	+++	+++	+++	+++	+++	-
S. aureus ATCC 25923	-	+	+	+++	+	+	++	+++	++	+++	+++	-
Gram-negative bacteria												
E. coli ATCC 25922	+	+	+	++	++	++	++	++	++	++	++	-
E. coli 135	-	++	++	++	-	-	++	++	++	++	++	-
E. coli ESBL	-	++	++	++	++	++	++	++	++	++	++	-
E. coli 2425	+	++	+	++	++	++	++	++	++	++	++	-
E. coli 5075	-	++	++	+++	+++	+++	+++	+++	+++	+++	+++	-
P. aeruginosa ATCC 27853	-	+	++	+++	+++	+++	+++	+++	+++	+++	+++	-
Yeasts												
C. albicans ATCC 10231	-	++	++	+	+	++	++	++	++	++	++	-
C. albicans 5316	-	++	++	+++	+++	+++	+++	+++	+++	+++	+++	-
C. albicans 5319	-	+	+	+++	+++	+++	+	+	+++	+++	+++	+
C. albicans 5325	-	++	+	+++	+++	+++	+++	+++	+++	+++	+++	-
C. albicans 5328	-	++	++	++	++	++	++	++	++	+++	++	-
C. krusei 5299	-	++	++	++	++	++	++	++	++	++	++	-
C. krusei 5343	-	+	++	+	+	++	++	++	++	++	++	-
C. glabrata 5328	-	+	+	+	+	+	++	-	++	++	++	-
C. parapsilosis ATCC 22019	-	++	++	++	++	++	+++	+++	+++	+++	+++	-
C. parapsilosis 514	-	+	+	++	++	++	++	++	+++	+++	+++	+
C. tropicalis 5770	-	++	++	++	+	++	++	++	++	++	++	-

GB = gel base; B = formula B; E = formula E; CO = clove essential oil; RO = Rosemary essential oil; TTO = tea tree essential oil; UA = Usnic acid; Complex = Cyclodextrin complex with CO. (-)/pale green is represented by the absence of the inhibition; (+)/light green = GIZD ≤ 5 mm; (++)/green = GIZD between 5 and 10 mm; (+++)/forest green = GIZD between 10 and 18 mm. The significant impact of the formulas and their bioactive compounds on each microbial strain was statistically analyzed using one-way ANOVA and Tukey's multiple comparisons test. The differences between groups were statistically significant ($p < 0.05$).

Following the qualitative assessment of the antimicrobial activity, it can be seen that both the gels and the components had a variable antimicrobial effect on all the tested strains. Larger growth inhibition zone diameters of the same strains were obtained for the gel components compared to the inhibition diameters obtained for the gels. These results were expected considering that one of the reasons for incorporating the bioactive components into the polymeric matrix was their gradual release, thus ensuring a prolonged effect.

For some strains (*S. aureus* 14, *S. aureus* 20, *S. aureus* 25, *S. aureus* 30, *S. aureus* 34, *S. aureus* 38, *S. aureus* 540) the growth inhibition was observed through the lower density of bacterial colonies compared to the areas where the test product was not applied. However, the inhibition diameter of bacterial growth could not be measured. Therefore, quantitative testing was performed to quantify the growth inhibition activity against these strains.

2.5.2. Quantitative Assessment of the Antimicrobial Activity

The quantitative assessment of antimicrobial activity involves establishing the minimum inhibitory concentration (MIC), the lowest concentration of the antimicrobial agent that prevents the visible growth of a microorganism. The MIC results are presented in Figure 5 for gels B and E, and Figure 6 displays the MIC results for their components.

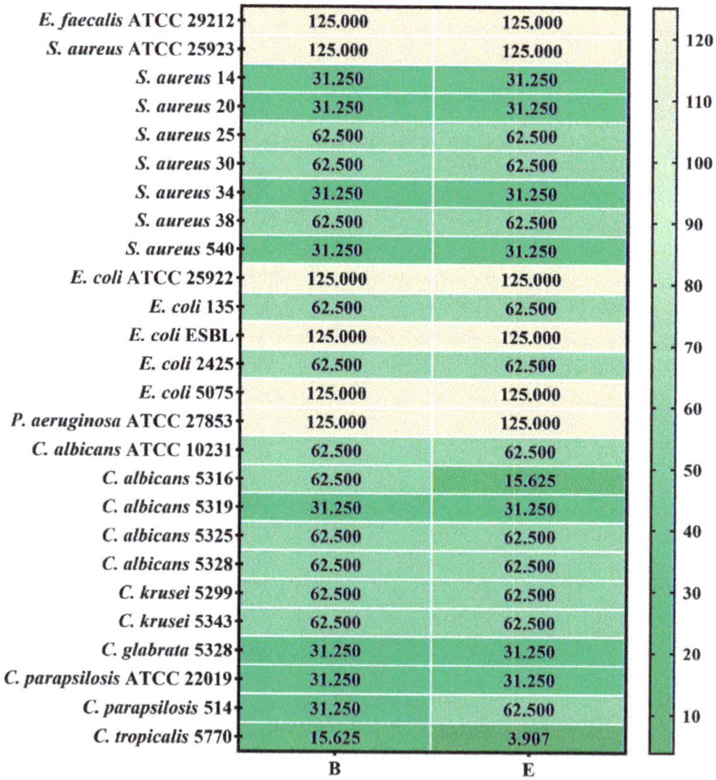

Figure 5. Heatmap of MIC values (mg/mL) for gels B and E. The scale bar displays the variations in the sensitivity of the strains from the highest (green forest) to the lowest (light vanilla). Legend: GB = gel base; B = formula B; E = formula E; CO = clove essential oil; RO = Rosemary essential oil; TTO = tea tree essential oil; UA = Usnic acid; Complex = Cyclodextrin complex with CO. The influence of the formulas B and E on each microbial strain was statistically analyzed using one-way ANOVA and Tukey's multiple comparisons test. The data results were statistically significant ($p < 0.05$).

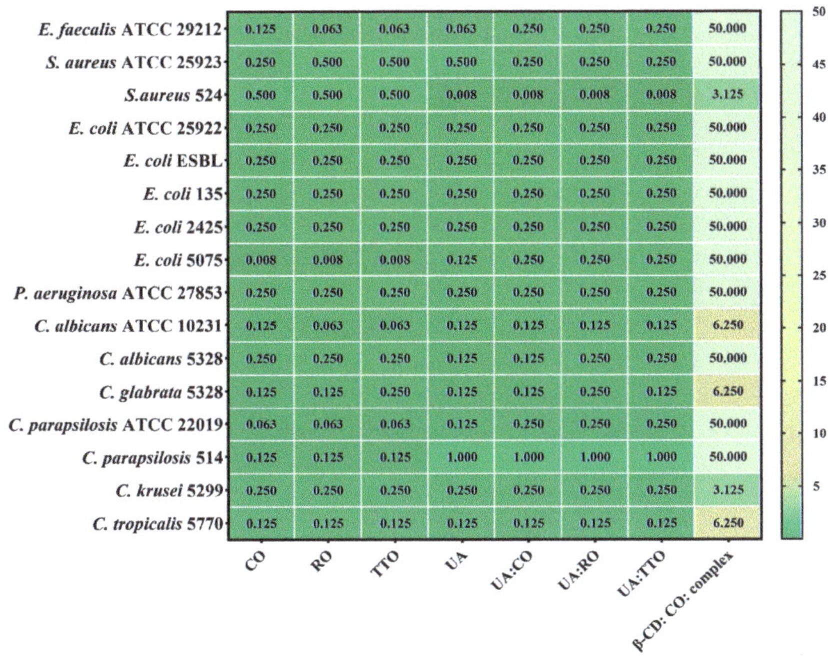

Figure 6. Heatmap of bioactive components' MIC values (mg/mL) from gel formulations. Legend: Clove essential oil = CO; Rosemary essential oil = RO; tea tree essential oil = TTO; Usnic acid = UA; complex = Cyclodextrin complex with CO; β-CD = β-Cyclodextrin. The scale bar displays the variations in the sensitivity of the strains from the highest (green forest) to the lowest (light vanilla). The influence of the bioactive compounds on each microbial strain was statistically analyzed using one-way ANOVA and Tukey's multiple comparisons test. The data results were statistically significant ($p < 0.05$).

The data obtained demonstrated that both gel formulations exhibited antimicrobial activity against Gram-positive bacteria, Gram-negative bacteria, and yeasts from *Candida* spp., cultured from standardized ATCC strains or isolated from biological samples (Table 7). Although the antimicrobial activities of the two formulations (B and E) were generally comparable, specific differences were evident. The MICs ranged from 31.250 to 125.000 mg/mL for bacterial strains and from 3.907 to 62.500 mg/mL for yeasts. Both formulations showed similar activity, but formulation E exhibited superior efficacy against *C. tropicalis* 5770, with a MIC as low as 3.907 mg/mL, compared to formulation B, which had a MIC of 15.625 mg/mL. This enhanced activity in formulation E is likely due to its higher content of TTO and RO, known for their potent antimicrobial properties (Figures 5 and 6). Despite the differences, the similar antimicrobial activity observed against the other microbial strains may be attributed to the identical concentration of Carbopol 940 in both formulations, as well as the similar inclusion of the cyclodextrin complex. These factors could result in comparable release kinetics of the bioactive compounds, thus leading to similar levels of antimicrobial effectiveness [36]. These results encouraged us to continue testing the gels using a larger number of bacterial strains isolated from the clinic.

2.5.3. Semiquantitative Assessment of the Microbial Adherence to the Inert Substratum

The semiquantitative assessment of microbial adherence to the inert substratum involved evaluating the microorganisms' ability to attach and form biofilms on non-biological surfaces used to mimic medical devices or other non-living materials [37]. The minimum biofilm eradication concentration (MBEC) is critical in evaluating antimicrobial agents' effectiveness, mainly when dealing with biofilm-associated infections that are challenging to treat. In our study on hydrogels containing cyclodextrin complexes with volatile oils, MBEC plays a vital role in determining the lowest concentration of the formulation needed to eradicate biofilms formed by pathogens completely. Biofilms provide a protective barrier for microorganisms, making them more resistant to treatment than planktonic (free-floating) bacteria. By assessing MBEC, the study offers new insights into the real-world efficacy of these hydrogels against resilient biofilm-forming pathogens, ensuring that the formulations are effective against free-floating microbes (sometimes resistant strains) and capable of penetrating and eradicating biofilms.

The MBEC results are presented in Figure 7 for gels B and E, and Figure 8 displays the MBEC results for their components.

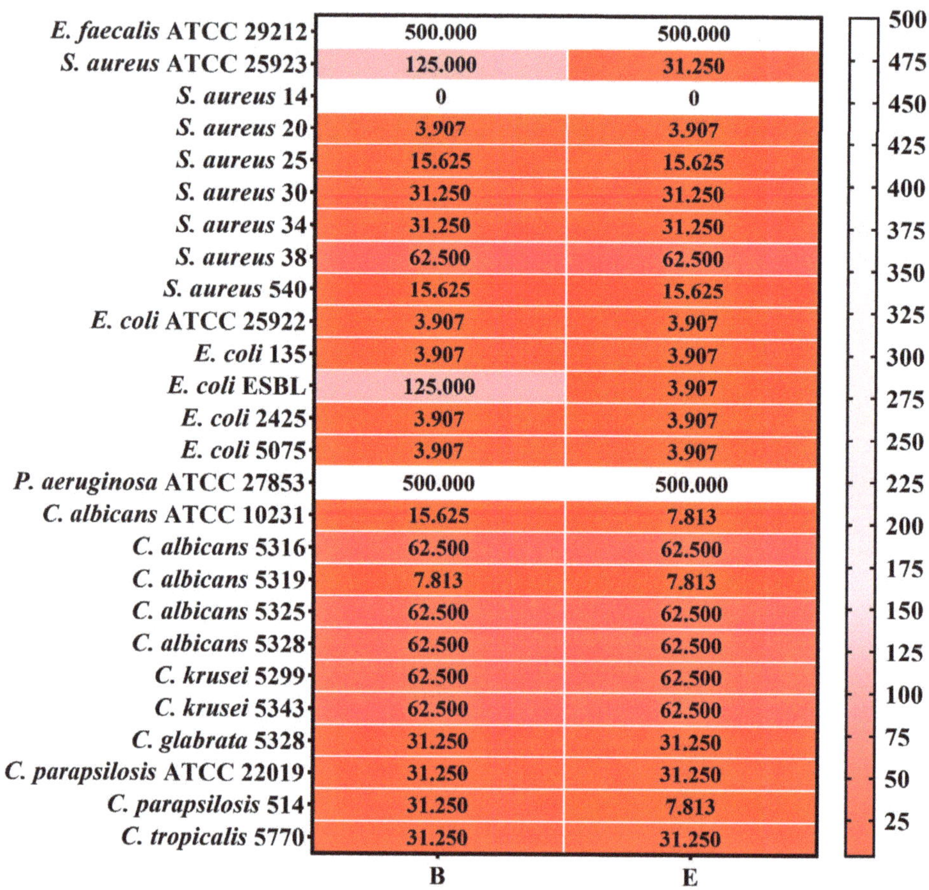

Figure 7. Heatmap of MBEC values (mg/mL) for gel formulations B and E. The scale bar displays the variations in the sensitivity of the strains from the highest (intense red) to the lowest (light red). Legend: B = gel formulation B; E = gel formulation E. The scale bar displays the variations in the sensitivity of the strains from the highest (intense red) to the lowest (white). The influence of the formulas B and E on the adherence of each microbial strain tested was statistically analyzed using one-way ANOVA and Tukey's multiple comparisons test. The data results were statistically significant ($p < 0.05$).

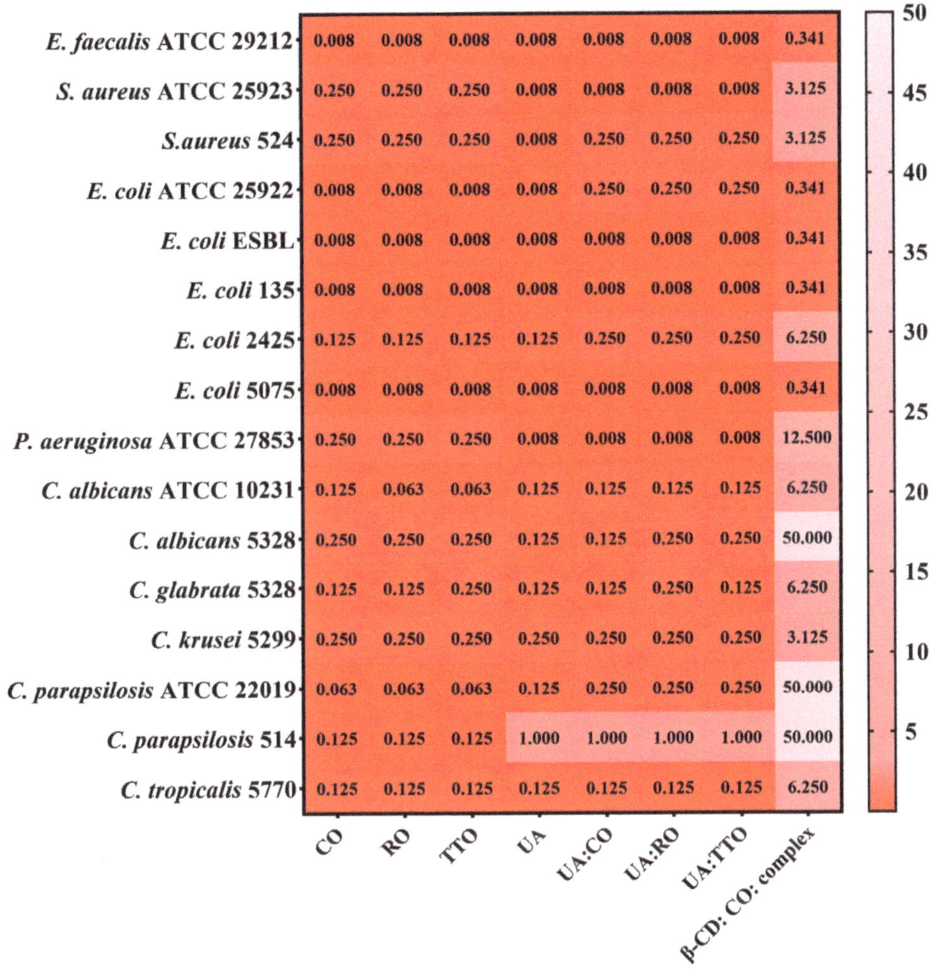

Figure 8. Heatmap of MBEC values (mg/mL) for bioactive components from gel formulations. Legend: Clove essential oil = CO; Rosemary essential oil = RO; Tea tree essential oil = TTO; Usnic acid = UA; Complex = Cyclodextrin complex with CO; β-CD = β-Cyclodextrin. The scale bar displays the variations in the sensitivity of the strains from the highest (intense red) to the lowest (white). The influence of the bioactive compounds on each microbial strain' adherence was statistically analyzed using one-way ANOVA and Tukey's multiple comparisons test. The data results were statistically significant ($p < 0.05$).

However, by evaluating microbial adherence to an inert substrate, neither formulation significantly affected the *S. aureus* 14 clinical strain. Additionally, higher concentrations of both products were required to inhibit microbial adherence in the cases of *E. faecalis* ATCC 29212 and *P. aeruginosa* ATCC 27853, indicating that while the gels are effective in inhibiting microbial growth, their impact on microbial adherence may be limited and strain-specific (Figures 7 and 8).

The literature data confirm the inhibitory effect of tea tree, rosemary, and clove essential oils against the growth of bacterial and yeast strains. These oils are suitable especially for wound infections produced by *S. aureus*, *S. epidermidis*, *S. pyogenes*, *E. faecalis*, *E. coli*, *C. albicans* [38–41].

In a study from 2012, Sienkiewicz et al. [42] demonstrated the antimicrobial activity of RO on *E. coli* (ESBL) clinical strains isolated from the abdominal cavity. Additional studies have shown the antibacterial properties of RO against *E. coli, Bacillus cereus, S. aureus, Clostridium perfringens, Aeromonas hydrophila,* and *Salmonella choleraesuis* [43]. On the other hand, Fabio et al. [44] reported that RO and CO exhibit antibacterial effects against various microorganisms responsible for respiratory infections isolated from some clinical samples. These include both antibiotic-sensitive and antibiotic-resistant strains such (*S. agalactiae, S. pyogenes, S. pneumoniae, S. aureus, Klebsiella pneumoniae* and *Stenotrophomonas maltophilia*).

Studies have also shown that TTO has the ability to inhibit the growth of some bacterial strains susceptible to antibiotic resistance (*E. coli* strain AG100 and *S. aureus* NCTC 8325) by increasing membrane permeability and inhibiting respiration in microbial cells. Furthermore, some studies mention the ability of Carbopol® Ultrez hydrogels with TTO nanoemulsions and nanocapsules improve wound healing and possess an antiedematogenic effect [45].

The antimicrobial activity of TTO and CO was also highlighted by Altaf et al. [46], who incorporated them into PVA/starch hydrogels.

In addition to the fact that *in vitro* antibacterial analysis of TTO-loaded hydrogels (using the disc diffusion method) demonstrated good antibacterial activity against *E. coli* and multi-resistant *S. aureus* (MRSA), they also have the capacity to accelerate the process of wound healing. However, it was not more effective than CO-loaded hydrogels [46].

The antimicrobial efficacy of the volatile oils against bacterial strains and yeasts may be attributed to the synergistic effects of their various constituents within the volatile fraction, rather than the influence of any single component. For instance, a study on the antimicrobial activity of terpinen-4-ol (the primary constituent of TTO) showed that *S. aureus* strains isolated from biological samples (nasal and oropharyngeal secretions) are sensitive. Furthermore, terpinen-4-ol demonstrated a significant ability to prevent the biofilm formation of these strains by targeting the penicillin-binding protein 2a [47]. Likewise, Zhang et al. [48] demonstrated that terpinen-4-ol affected the cell membrane and wall of *Streptococcus agalactiae* by increasing the cell membrane permeability and by releasing lactate dehydrogenase. Another study indicated that components of the TTO (terpinen-4-ol, α-terpineol, terpinolene, linalool, cineole, α-terpinene, γ-terpinene) had variable actions against *B. subtilis, C. albicans, Bacteroides fragilis, Clostridium perfringens, E. faecalis, E. coli, Lactobacillus acidophilus, Moraxella catarrhalis, Mycobacterium smegmatis, Serratia marcescens* and *S. aureus*) [49].

Eucalyptol, the significant component of RO, is also known as an antimicrobial agent and has attracted considerable interest for its potential to reduce antibiotic resistance. Studies have shown that it is effective against Gram-positive strains (*S. aureus* and *B. subtilis*), Gram-negative strains (*E. coli* and *P. aeruginosa*) and yeasts (*C. albicans* and *C. glabrata*) [50–56]. The primary mechanism of action of eucalyptol is based on the disruption of membrane integrity, alteration of surface charge, and generation of reactive oxygen species (ROS)/oxidative stress [57]. Also, eucalyptol is capable of downregulating genes related to carbohydrate metabolism and membrane proteins at the mRNA level. Moreover, at the fungal level, eucalyptol downregulated ergosterol biosynthetic genes, inhibited biofilm formation, generated ROS, caused cell cycle arrest at the G1/S phase, and altered the mitochondrial membrane [58].

The main component of CO, eugenol, has been reported in the literature as both a bactericidal and bacteriostatic agent, also possessing antifungal properties. The antimicrobial mechanism of action of eugenol has been attributed to the free OH group in its molecular structure. Moreover, eugenol damages the cytoplasmatic membrane and generates the leakage of intracellular components [59]. It has shown inhibitory effects on the growth of several strains, including *E. faecalis, S. pyogenes, S. aureus, S. pneumoniae, Salmonella choleraesuis, Yersinia enterocolitica, Helicobacter pylori, P. aeruginosa, E. coli* [60–63]. The antifungal activity of eugenol has also been reported against *C. albicans, C. tropicalis,* and *C. krusei* [63–65].

Moreover, it is well known that usnic acid exhibits antimicrobial activity. In a 2007 study, Elo et al. [66] examined the in vitro antimicrobial activity of usnic acid and its sodium salt against clinical isolates of vancomycin-resistant enterococci (VRE) and methicillin-resistant *S. aureus* (MRSA). The results showed that usnic acid, particularly its sodium salt, exhibited strong antimicrobial activity against all tested clinical isolates. In addition, *Vibrio harveyi* and *B. subtilis* have been found to be sensitive to usnic acid at various concentrations [67]. The growth inhibition of *C. orthopsilosis* and *C. parapsilosis* strains, and *C. albicans* biofilms demonstrates that usnic acid can be a good candidate for formulating pharmaceutical products for treating candidiasis [68,69].

It can also be observed that the bioactive components have both MIC and MBEC values lower when they were tested as such compared to the gels in which they were incorporated. This aspect highlights the ability of the carbopol matrix to gradually release the volatiles compounds from the TTO and RO as the first antimicrobial barrier, as well as the gradual release of the CO from the complex and then its delivery into the biological environment. This data focus attention to the potential of the gels to provide antimicrobial protection for a period greater than 24 h.

2.6. Cytotoxic Activity

The impact of pharmaceutical formulations B, E, and the gel base (GB) on cell viability and proliferation of the Human Colorectal Adenocarcinoma Cell Line (ATCC HTB-38) was assessed using the MTT assay (Figure 9).

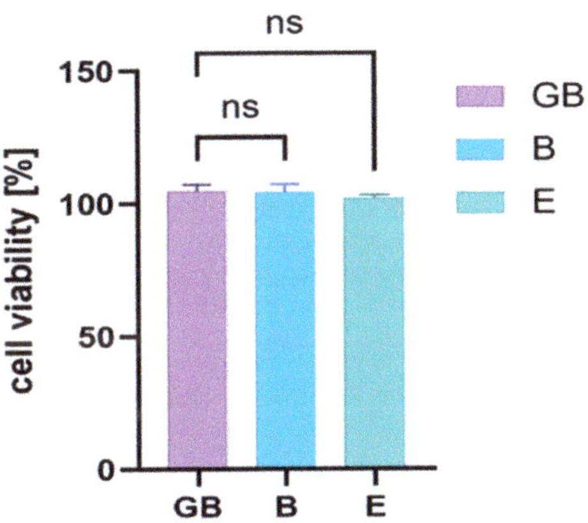

Figure 9. The gels' effect on the viability of the antitumoral cells. Legend: GB = gel base; B = formula B; E = formula E; ns = not significant. The gels' influence was statistically analyzed using two-way ANOVA followed by Dunnett's multiple comparisons tests, which did not reveal statistically significant correlations.

The essential oil components added to GB did not modify HTB-38 tumoral cell proliferation in the 1% concentration gels tested. On the other part, values close to 100% indicate that most cells survived the treatment with the respective gels, and their cytotoxicity is relatively low at the 1% concentration, where no statistically significant changes are observed.

Other types of complex BCD-based also proved to be non-toxic [70]. Toxicity studies on a curcumin-loaded hydrogel with formulation materials based on 2-hydroxypropyl-β-CD, sodium alginate, and chitosan designed for wound dressing materials with antimicrobial activity, tested on NCTC clone 929 cells and normal human dermal fibroblasts, showed the hydrogel was non-toxic.

A doxorubicin-loaded hydrogel containing β-CD and agarose did not exhibit toxicity toward HEK-293 (Human Embryonic Kidney) and HeLa cells [71].

Otherwise, the majority of the inclusion complexes of LCEO (*Litsea cubeba* essential oil) into β-CD (β-cyclodextrin) exhibited antitumor activity against the tumor (HT-29 and HeLa) and non-tumor (Vero) cell lines by MTT assay [72].

3. Conclusions

The composition of the designed gels influences the flow parameters, which is more evident for the carbopol concentration variation. All hydrogels exhibited non-Newtonian pseudoplastic behavior with yield stress. The rheological evaluation is paramount for a complex physico-chemical evaluation of semisolid dosage forms, providing valuable information concerning their fabrication technology, quality and stability control during preservation, and therapeutical activity. This study developed and evaluated hydrogels containing a cyclodextrin complex with CO alongside TTO and RO, focusing on their pharmaco-technical and rheological properties. The results demonstrate that the concentration of Carbopol 940 is the primary factor influencing the gels' rheological behavior, with a higher concentration leading to increased yield stress, consistency index, and viscosity. Formula B, containing 1% Carbopol, 1.5% TTO, and 1.5% RO, exhibited optimal stability and rheological properties, making it suitable for practical application. In contrast, Formula E, with the same Carbopol concentration but higher amounts of TTO (2%) and RO (2%), displayed superior antimicrobial efficacy, particularly against *Candida tropicalis*. This enhanced activity is attributed to the increased levels of free volatile oils. The study underscores the importance of balancing the polymer and volatile oil concentrations to optimize the hydrogels' physical properties and antimicrobial effectiveness, highlighting their potential for medical and cosmetic applications. Based on this study, the proof of concept was laid down and further studies will be done for a complete characterization considering the desired pharmaceutical and therapeutic applications.

The current focus on topical applications could be expanded to explore other therapeutic areas, such as mucosal drug delivery, ophthalmic formulations, or vaginal/rectal delivery. Hydrogels are ideal candidates for these applications due to their ability to adhere to mucosal surfaces and provide localized drug delivery with minimal systemic absorption. Research into biodegradable hydrogels for tissue engineering or regenerative medicine could also be an important future direction, exploring how these formulations can serve as scaffolds for cell growth or as delivery vehicles for growth factors and stem cells in tissue repair.

To fully unlock the potential of these hydrogels in pharmaceutical and therapeutic applications, future research should focus on more advanced characterization methods that assess drug release behavior, biocompatibility, therapeutic efficacy, and mechanical properties under conditions mimicking their intended use. Such studies will significantly enhance the clinical relevance of the findings and open up broader opportunities for the application of these hydrogels in medicine and healthcare.

4. Materials and Methods

4.1. GC-MS Analysis

The chemical composition of essential oils from *Melaleuca alternifolia* (tea tree) and *Rosmarinus officinalis* (rosemary) was analyzed using a Focus gas paired with a Polaris Q ion trap mass spectrometer and a Triplus autosampler (Thermo Fisher Scientific, Waltham, MA, USA). The system utilized a DB-5MS capillary column (25 m length, 0.25 mm diameter, and 0.25 μm film thickness). The temperature program for the oven started at 60 °C for 3 min, increased at a rate of 10 °C per minute up to 200 °C (held for 2 min), and then further increased at 12 °C per minute to a final temperature of 240 °C. Helium was used as the carrier gas with a flow rate of 1 mL/min. The ion source and interface temperatures were set to 200 °C and 250 °C, respectively, with the mass spectrometer operating in electron impact mode at 70 eV. Detection was carried out within an m/z range of 35–300, and the mass spectrometer was run in full-scan mode. Chromatogram analysis was performed using X calibur software 4.3 (Thermo Fisher Scientific, Waltham, MA, USA)., supported by the NIST 11 database for compound identification. An alkane standard solution for GC (C8-C20 in hexane, Sigma-Aldrich, Darmstadt, Germany) was used to determine Kovats indices (KIs), the percentage composition of the identified compounds being calculated from the total ion chromatogram based on GC peak areas.

The oil samples were diluted with hexane to volume ratio 1:10.

4.2. Formulation of Hydrogels

The objective of this study was the development and pharmaco-technical characterization, especially rheological, of volatile oil-based hydrogels. For the formulation of gels with antimicrobial action, two levels of variation of the composition were chosen: the concentration of hydrophilic polymer (Carbopol 940, Sigma-Aldrich, Darmstadt, Germany) in the gel base (Table 8) and the concentration of volatile oils in the final formula (Table 9).

Table 8. Gels' compositions.

Components	Formula A	Formula B	Formula C
Carbopol 940	0.8 g	1 g	1.2 g
Glycerin	5 g	5 g	5 g
Triethanolamine	q.s.	q.s.	q.s.
Cyclodextrin complex with clove essential oil	1 g	1 g	1 g
Usnic acid	0.5 g	0.5 g	0.5 g
Tea tree essential oil	1.5 g	1.5 g	1.5 g
Rosemary essential oil	1.5 g	1.5 g	1.5 g
Purified water	until 100 g	until 100 g	until 100 g

Table 9. Gels' compositions.

Components	Formula D	Formula E	Formula F
Carbopol 940	1 g	1 g	1 g
Glycerin	5 g	5 g	5 g
Triethanolamine	q.s.	q.s.	q.s.
Cyclodextrin complex with clove essential oil	1 g	1 g	1 g
Usnic acid	0.5 g	0.5 g	0.5 g
Tea tree essential oil	1 g	2 g	2.5 g
Rosemary essential oil	1 g	2 g	2.5 g
Purified water	until 100 g	until 100 g	until 100 g

For the preparation of semisolid hydrogel pharmaceutical forms, the polyacrylic type network (Carbopol 940, corresponding to a final concentration of 0.8, 1, respectively, 1.2%) was hydrated using 75% of the amount of purified water provided in the formula for at least 24 h in the presence of glycerin (purity over 99%; Glycerin from Merck, Darmstadt, Germany) used as a dispersing agent. Triethanolamine (purity over 99%; Triethanolamine from Carl Roth GmbH + Co. KG., Karlsruhe, Germany) was used for neutralization at the end of this interval (Table 8). The remaining amount of water was dispersed with cyclodextrin complex with CO (synthesized in the laboratory) and added to the semisolid matrix generated by hydration of the hydrophilic polymer under intense stirring (2000 rpm for 10 min, using a turbine stirrer in a Heidolph RZR 2020, Heidolph Instruments GmbH and Co. KG, Schwabach, Germany). Finally, the usnic acid (purity over 98%; from Merck, Darmstadt, Germany) was mixed with the volatile oils and added to the semisolid matrix under stirring until complete homogenization. The volatile oils used to prepare gels are organic products from Mayam, with a quality certificate (certified by Ecocert Greenlife according to the Ecocert/Cosmos standard). The TTO and RO have antimicrobial action and ensure good preservation of the gels.

In the second case, gels with Carbopol 940 1% were made in which the concentration of volatile oils represented 2%, 4%, and 5% in the total mass of the preparations (Table 9). Purified water (conductivity below 0.05 μS/cm) was obtained in a system Evoqua Ultra Clear TP ED ultrapure water system, Evoqua, Berlin, Germany. The remaining reagents used were purity analytical (Merck, Darmstadt, Germany).

Carbopol 940 is a polymer of carboxyvinyl that appears as a white, light powder, partially soluble in water, and soluble in solutions of alkaline hydroxides and amines. Glycerol is a syrupy liquid, clear, colorless, odorless and sweet in taste. It is hygroscopic, miscible with alcohol and water, and insoluble in fatty and volatile oils.

Due to the strong hydrophilic character of carbopol, it tends to form agglomerations that are difficult to disperse later when introduced into water, so the carbopol is slowly introduced into water and under continuous agitation. Stirring is continued until an opalescent dispersion is obtained without agglomeration. The soaking stand can be extended up to 24 h, during which time any air incorporated during stirring is removed. When triethanolamine is added, the acid groups of carbopol are neutralized, simultaneously with its dissolution in water and gelation of the dispersion.

The spreading capacity of the gel formulations was measured 48 h after preparation by measuring the spreading diameter of 1 g of the gel between two 20 × 20 cm glass plates after 1 min. The mass of the upper plate was standardized at 125 g. Weighs of 50 g, 100 g, 200 g and 250 g were subsequently placed over the sample at 1 min. intervals. The spreading areas reached by the sample were measured in millimeters in the vertical and horizontal axes.

The results were expressed in terms of the spreading area as a function of the applied mass according to the following equation:

$S_i = d_i^2\ (\pi/4)$, in which S_i is the spreading area (mm^2) resulting from the applied mass i (g) and d_i^2 is the mean diameter (mm) reached by the sample [73].

The gels were also submitted to some control tests to determine their characteristics and stability:

- The determination of the appearance was made by examination with the magnifying glass (4.5×) of a sample stretched by a thin layer on a microscopic blade;
- The determination of the main characteristics was made according to Romanian Pharmacopoeia Xth edition [74];
- pH was determined after the gel samples were suitably processed, respectively after the dispersion of samples in water (1:5), followed by the measuring of the pH of an aqueous phase, as follows: 25 mL of distilled water were added to 5 g sample and the mixture was stirred into an Erlenmeyer glass with cork heating on the water bath at 60 °C for 10 min. After cooling on the watery phase, the pH was determined with Radelkis pH meter (Radelkis Ktsz.; Budapest; Hungary);
- The determination of the viscosity was performed with a rotational Brookfield LFV viscometer (AMETEK Brookfield, Middleboro, MA, USA);
- The stability was performed by maintaining the samples at 2 °C and 40 °C: 5 g of sample were introduced into a weighing ampoule with a lid, and then, the ampoule was maintained for 8 h at mentioned temperatures. Then, the appearance of the sample was examined.

The gels' compositions were presented in Tables 8 and 9, and gel base (GB) is considered the formulation without bioactive compounds (cyclodextrin complex with volatile oil, usnic acid, or volatile oils).

4.3. Rheological Analysis and Data Modeling

The rheological behavior of the designed carbopol gels was evaluated through stationary shear analysis at 33 °C ± 0.1 °C (to simulate the skin temperature), using a rotational viscometer Multi-Visc Rheometer (Fungilab, Madrid, Spain). The measuring system was equipped with a ThermoHaake P5 Ultrathermostat to maintain constant the sample temperature during the experiment. Our previous works detailed the operating conditions [75,76].

Briefly, after mechanical and thermal equilibration, the gels were sheared at a shear rate specific to the TR 10 standard spindle, from 0.08 to 16.8 s^{-1}, corresponding to a rotational speed between 0.30 and 60 rpm. The shear stress as a function of shear rate upward rheograms was obtained. The rheological data were further analyzed by applying different shear stress (τ) versus shear rate ($\dot{\gamma}$) models as follows: Bingham (Equation (1)), Casson (Equation (2)), Ostwald-de Waele (Equation (3)) and Herschel-Bulkley (Equation (4)):

$$\tau = \tau_0 + \eta \cdot \dot{\gamma} \quad (1)$$

$$\tau^{0.5} = \tau_0{}^{0.5} + \eta^{0.5} \cdot \dot{\gamma}^{0.5} \quad (2)$$

$$\tau = K \cdot \dot{\gamma}^{n} \quad (3)$$

$$\tau = \tau_0 + K \cdot \dot{\gamma}^{n} \quad (4)$$

where η is plastic viscosity (Pa·s), τ_0—yield stress (Pa), K—consistency index (Pa·s^n), and n—flow index (dimensionless) [76–78]. The flow parameters were determined using Table Curve 2D software 5.1, Systat Software (Palo Alto, CA, USA).

4.4. SEM Analysis

Surface morphology of the samples was obtained using an FEI Nova NanoSEM 630 scanning electron microscope (Nanotech, Tokyo, Japan) with a TLD (Through-Lens-Detector), at an acceleration voltage of 5 kV and a working distance of 4.7 mm.

4.5. Antimicrobial Activity

The antimicrobial assessments were performed with standard strains (*Enterococcus faecalis* ATCC 29212, *Staphylococcus aureus* ATCC 25923, *Escherichia coli* ATCC 25922, *Pseudomonas aeruginosa* ATCC 27853, *Candida albicans* ATCC 10231, and *Candida parapsilosis* ATCC 22019. In addition, clinically isolated strains from skin and mucous infections (*Staphylococcus aureus* 14, *Staphylococcus aureus* 20, *Staphylococcus aureus* 25, *Staphylococcus aureus* 30, *Staphylococcus aureus* 34, *Staphylococcus aureus* 38, *Staphylococcus aureus* 540, *Escherichia coli* 135, *Escherichia coli* 2425, *Escherichia coli* 5075, *Escherichia coli* ESBL, *Candida albicans* 5316, *Candida albicans* 5319, *Candida albicans* 5325, *Candida albicans* 5328, *Candida krusei* 5299, *Candida krusei* 5343, *Candida glabrata* 5328, *Candida parapsilosis* 514 and *Candida tropicalis* 5770) were also used. All strains tested are provided from the Microorganisms Collection of the Department of Microbiology, Faculty of Biology and Research Institute of the University of Bucharest.

4.5.1. Qualitative Assay of the Antimicrobial Activity

The inhibitory effects of the gels were assessed using a spot diffusion method and according to the Clinical Laboratory Standards Institute [79,80]. Bacterial and yeast suspensions (1.5×10^8 CFU/mL and 3×10^8 CFU/mL, respectively) were obtained from 24 h cultures on Nutrient Broth No. 2 (NB) and Sabouraud Glucose Agar with chloramphenicol (Sab) medium. Petri plates with the specific media were seeded with inoculums, and each 20 µL of each sample was spotted. The negative control was considered the sterile medium, and the positive control was the NB/Sab medium inoculated with microbial suspensions. After diffusion, the dishes were incubated at 37 °C for 24 h for bacteria and 48 h for yeast strains.

4.5.2. Quantitative Assay of the Antimicrobial Activity

The minimum inhibitory concentration (MIC) assessment was performed using an adapted binary serial microdilution standard assay in liquid media utilizing 96-well microtiter plates. From each sample, serial two-fold micro-dilutions were realized in 150 µL of corresponding broth medium seeded with the standard inoculum. The microtiter plates were incubated at 37 °C for 24 h. Visual and spectrophotometric analyses determined the

MIC values by measuring the absorbance at 620 nm via the BIOTEK SYNERGY-HTX ELISA multi-mode reader (Winooski, VT, USA) [79].

4.5.3. Semiquantitative Assessment of the Microbial Adherence to the Inert Substratum

The biofilm development on the inert substratum was assessed utilizing the same serial two-fold microdilution method. Following 24 h of incubation, the medium from microtiter plates (containing binary dilutions of the samples) was removed, the wells were washed three times with sterile physiological buffer saline, and the bacterial cells adhered to the walls were fixed with methanol (5 min) and tinted with 1% crystal violet (15 min). The stained biofilm was resuspended with 33% acetic acid, and the absorbance was measured at 490 nm [79].

4.6. Cytotoxic Activity

The cytotoxicity of the gels was assessed by determining the viability of a Human Colorectal Adenocarcinoma Cell Line (ATCC HTB-38) using the MTT assay (Sigma, Santa Clara, CA, USA). HTB-38 cells were cultured in RPMI 1640 medium (Lonza, Basel, Switzerland) supplemented with 10% fetal bovine serum (FBS) and Pen-Strep (Biochrom, Berlin, Germany) in 96-well polystyrene plates. The cells were incubated at 37 °C in a 5% CO_2 environment until they reached 70% confluence (passage 48). The medium was then removed, and the cells were exposed to 100 µL of RPMI 1640 medium containing 10% FBS, Pen-Strep, and the gel samples for 24 h under the same conditions. After incubation, the medium and biomaterials were removed, and the cells were washed twice with warm PBS before being treated with 100 µg/mL MTT solution for 4 h at 37 °C in a 5% CO_2 atmosphere. Following incubation, the dye was dissolved in dimethyl sulfoxide (DMSO), and absorbance was measured at 540 nm using a Synergy HTX spectrophotometer (Agilent Technology Biotek, Santa Clara, CA, USA).

4.7. β-cyclodextrin-Eugenia caryophyllata Volatile Oil Complex Preparation

The encapsulation of *Eugenia caryophyllata* (clove) volatile oil was achieved through a methodical process to ensure optimal inclusion within the β-cyclodextrin matrix. Initially, β-cyclodextrin was dissolved in a water/ethanol solution (3:1/*v*:*v*), providing an appropriate medium for the complexation process. The volatile oil was then gradually introduced to the solution at room temperature, maintaining constant stirring to promote uniform dispersion and interaction between the cyclodextrin and the oil. The mixture adhered to a precise mass ratio of 4:1/*w*:*w* (β-cyclodextrin/volatile oil), a ratio selected to maximize encapsulation efficiency while preserving the stability of the complex. Following the formation of a homogeneous suspension, the mixture underwent lyophilization—a freeze-drying process that gently removed the solvent without compromising the integrity of the encapsulated oil. This method yielded a dry, stable complex in powder form, suitable for further application in various pharmaceutical formulations [81–83].

4.8. β-cyclodextrin-Eugenia caryophyllata Volatile Oil Complex Characteristics

The β-cyclodextrin-*Eugenia caryophyllata* (clove) volatile oil complex was successfully obtained as a compact white powder with a distinctive clove-like aroma, indicating the presence of the encapsulated volatile oil. The encapsulation efficiency was notably high (83.35%), which corresponding to approximately 170 mg of volatile oil per gram of the complex, reflecting the effectiveness of the β-cyclodextrin in trapping the volatile components. This encapsulation is essential for protecting the oil's active compounds from degradation, enhancing their stability, and potentially improving their bioavailability in subsequent applications. The detailed analysis and comprehensive characterization of this complex, including its physicochemical properties, thermal stability, and potential interactions within the matrix, will be thoroughly explored in a forthcoming publication, which constitutes the second part of this study.

4.9. Statistical Analysis

The data results were statistically analyzed with GraphPad Prism 10.3 from GraphPad Software, San Diego, CA, USA. All experiments were performed in three independent determinations. The results are expressed as ±SD (standard deviation) and analyzed using a one-way analysis of variance followed by a multiple comparisons assay agreeing to the experiment method. The differences between groups/samples were considered statistically significant when the p-value was <0.05.

Author Contributions: Conceptualization, A.I.S. and A.F.; methodology, E.O. and A.F.; software, M.B.; validation, C.-I.I., L.M.D., I.A.B. and M.M.; formal analysis, M.B., O.B., M.V.G., C.E.D.P., A.I.S. and I.A.; investigation, C.-I.I., L.M.D., I.A.B. and M.M.; resources, M.V.G. and C.E.D.P.; data curation, I.A.; writing—original draft preparation, E.O., A.I.S., M.M. and A.F.; writing—review and editing, E.O. and A.F.; visualization, M.M.; supervision, E.O.; project administration, A.I.S. and A.F.; funding acquisition, M.M. All authors have read and agreed to the published version of the manuscript.

Funding: This research received no external funding.

Institutional Review Board Statement: Not applicable.

Informed Consent Statement: Not applicable.

Data Availability Statement: The original contributions presented in the study are included in the article; further inquiries can be directed to the corresponding author.

Acknowledgments: This scientific paper was financially supported by the University of Medicine and Pharmacy Carol Davila through contract CNFIS-FDI-2024-F-0570. We acknowledge the support of the project CNFIS-FDI-2024-F-0484 INOVEX: Supporting the Development of New Competencies and Innovative Tools for Excellence in Interdisciplinary Research at the University of Bucharest.

Conflicts of Interest: The authors declare no conflicts of interest.

References

1. Slater, J. The Effects of Co-Solvent Levels and Neutralisation on the Rheology of Carbopol Gels. In *Third European Rheology Conference and Golden Jubilee Meeting of the British Society of Rheology*; Oliver, D.R., Ed.; Springer: Dordrecht, The Netherlands, 1990; pp. 453–455.
2. Islam, M.T.; Rodríguez-Hornedo, N.; Ciotti, S.; Ackermann, C. Rheological Characterization of Topical Carbomer Gels Neutralized to Different pH. *Pharm. Res.* **2004**, *21*, 1192–1199. [CrossRef] [PubMed]
3. Kim, J.-Y.; Song, J.-Y.; Lee, E.-J.; Park, S.-K. Rheological properties and microstructures of Carbopol gel network system. *Colloid Polym. Sci.* **2003**, *281*, 614–623. [CrossRef]
4. Laxton, P.B.; Berg, J.C. Gel trapping of dense colloids. *J. Colloid Interface Sci.* **2005**, *285*, 152–157. [CrossRef] [PubMed]
5. Oppong, F.K.; Rubatat, L.; Frisken, B.J.; Bailey, A.E.; de Bruyn, J.R. Microrheology and structure of a yield-stress polymer gel. *Phys. Rev. E* **2006**, *73*, 041405. [CrossRef] [PubMed]
6. Piau, J.M. Carbopol gels: Elastoviscoplastic and slippery glasses made of individual swollen sponges. *J. Non-Newton. Fluid Mech.* **2007**, *144*, 1–29. [CrossRef]
7. Garg, A.; Gupta, B.; Prakash, R.; Singh, S. Preparation and Characterization of Hydroxypropyl-b-Cyclodextrin Inclusion Complex of Eugenol: Differential Pulse Voltammetry and 1H-NMR. *Chem. Pharm. Bull.* **2010**, *58*, 1313–1319. [CrossRef]
8. Garg, A.; Ahmad, J.; Hassan, M.Z. Inclusion complex of thymol and hydroxypropyl-β-cyclodextrin (HP-β-CD) in polymeric hydrogel for topical application: Physicochemical characterization, molecular docking, and stability evaluation. *J. Drug Deliv. Sci. Technol.* **2021**, *64*, 102609. [CrossRef]
9. Bilensoy, E.; Rouf, M.A.; Vural, I.; Hincal, A.A. Thermosensitive vaginal gel formulation for the controlled release of clotrimazole via complexation to beta-cyclodextrin. *J. Control Release* **2006**, *116*, e107–e109. [CrossRef]
10. Joita, F.A.; Oprea, E.; Musuc, A.M.; Mititelu, M.; Marinescu, F.; Lupuliasa, D.; Hincu, L.; Rosca, A.C.; Boroghina, S.C.; Popescu, I.A. Development of antimicrobial hydrogels using alginate-chitosan matrix enhanced with essential oils. *Farmacia* **2024**, *72*, 906–916.
11. Jain, M.; Nowak, B.P.; Ravoo, B.J. Supramolecular Hydrogels Based on Cyclodextrins: Progress and Perspectives. *Chemnanomat* **2022**, *8*, e202200077. [CrossRef]
12. Bendi, A.; Jafar Ahamed, A.; Jaison Jose, T.; Raghav, N.; Mujafarkani, N.; Atri, S. Synthesis, Characterization, and biological evaluation of a novel PTF terpolymer and its copper Polychelate: Antibacterial and antifungal efficacy. *J. Mol. Liq.* **2024**, *408*, 125403. [CrossRef]
13. Carvalho-Silva, J.M.; Gaspar, C.S.; Dos Reis, A.C.; Teixeira, A.B.V. Denture stomatitis: Treatment with antimicrobial drugs or antifungal gels? A systematic review of clinical trials. *J. Prosthet. Dent.* 2024; *in press*.

14. Aher, S.D.; Banerjee, S.K.; Gadhave, M.V.; Gaikwad, D.D. Emulgels—A New Dosage Form for Topical Drug Delivery. *Int. J. Inst. Pharm. Life Sci.* **2013**, *3*, 1–10.
15. Preeti, B.; Gnanaranjan, G. Emulgel—A Novel Formulation Approach for Topical Delivery of Hydrophobic Drugs. *Int. Res. J. Pharm.* **2013**, *4*, 12–16.
16. Baibhav, J.; Gurpreet, S.; Seema, S.; Vikas, S. Emulgel: A comprehensive review on the recent advances in topical drug delivery. *Int. Res. J. Pharm.* **2011**, *2*, 66–70.
17. Kumar, D.; Singh, J.; Antil, M.; Kumar, V. Emulgel-Novel Topical Drug Delivery System—A comprehensive review. *Int. J. Pharm. Sci. Res.* **2016**, *7*, 4733–4742.
18. Elmi, A.; Ventrella, D.; Barone, F.; Carnevali, G.; Filippini, G.; Pisi, A.; Benvenuti, S.; Scozzoli, M.; Bacci, M.L. In Vitro Effects of Tea Tree Oil (*Melaleuca alternifolia* Essential Oil) and its Principal Component Terpinen-4-ol on Swine Spermatozoa. *Molecules* **2019**, *24*, 1071. [CrossRef]
19. Zaouali, Y.; Bouzaine, T.; Boussaid, M. Essential oils composition in two *Rosmarinus officinalis* L. varieties and incidence for antimicrobial and antioxidant activities. *Food Chem. Toxicol.* **2010**, *48*, 3144–3152. [CrossRef]
20. Hudaib, M.M.; Tawaha, K.A.; Hudaib, H.S.; Battah, A.H. Chemical Composition of Volatile Oil from the Aerial Parts of *Rosmarinus officinalis* L. Grown in Jordan. *J. Essent. Oil Bear. Plants* **2015**, *18*, 1282–1286. [CrossRef]
21. Varges, P.R.; Costa, C.M.; Fonseca, B.S.; Naccache, M.F.; De Souza Mendes, P. Rheological Characterization of Carbopol® Dispersions in Water and in Water/Glycerol Solutions. *Fluids* **2019**, *4*, 3. [CrossRef]
22. Zheng, Y.; Ouyang, W.Q.; Wei, Y.P.; Syed, S.F.; Hao, C.S.; Wang, B.Z.; Shang, Y.H. Effects of Carbopol® 934 proportion on nanoemulsion gel for topical and transdermal drug delivery: A skin permeation study. *Int. J. Nanomed.* **2016**, *11*, 5971–5987. [CrossRef]
23. Bassole, I.H.; Juliani, H.R. Essential oils in combination and their antimicrobial properties. *Molecules* **2012**, *17*, 3989–4006. [CrossRef] [PubMed]
24. Alven, S.; Peter, S.; Aderibigbe, B.A. Polymer-Based Hydrogels Enriched with Essential Oils: A Promising Approach for the Treatment of Infected Wounds. *Polymers* **2022**, *14*, 3772. [CrossRef]
25. Hammer, K.A.; Carson, C.F.; Riley, T.V. Antimicrobial activity of essential oils and other plant extracts. *J. Appl. Microbiol.* **1999**, *86*, 985–990. [CrossRef] [PubMed]
26. Li Pomi, F.; Papa, V.; Borgia, F.; Vaccaro, M.; Allegra, A.; Cicero, N.; Gangemi, S. *Rosmarinus officinalis* and Skin: Antioxidant Activity and Possible Therapeutical Role in Cutaneous Diseases. *Antioxidants* **2023**, *12*, 680. [CrossRef] [PubMed]
27. Puvaca, N.; Milenkovic, J.; Galonja Coghill, T.; Bursic, V.; Petrovic, A.; Tanaskovic, S.; Pelic, M.; Ljubojevic Pelic, D.; Miljkovic, T. Antimicrobial Activity of Selected Essential Oils against Selected Pathogenic Bacteria: In Vitro Study. *Antioxidants* **2021**, *10*, 546. [CrossRef]
28. Montenegro, L.; Pasquinucci, L.; Zappala, A.; Chiechio, S.; Turnaturi, R.; Parenti, C. Rosemary Essential Oil-Loaded Lipid Nanoparticles: In Vivo Topical Activity from Gel Vehicles. *Pharmaceutics* **2017**, *9*, 48. [CrossRef]
29. Prashar, A.; Locke, I.C.; Evans, C.S. Cytotoxicity of clove (*Syzygium aromaticum*) oil and its major components to human skin cells. *Cell Prolif.* **2006**, *39*, 241–248. [CrossRef] [PubMed]
30. Hammer, K.A.; Carson, C.F.; Riley, T.V.; Nielsen, J.B. A review of the toxicity of *Melaleuca alternifolia* (tea tree) oil. *Food Chem. Toxicol.* **2006**, *44*, 616–625. [CrossRef]
31. Castro, J.I.; Valencia-Llano, C.H.; Valencia Zapata, M.E.; Restrepo, Y.J.; Mina Hernandez, J.H.; Navia-Porras, D.P.; Valencia, Y.; Valencia, C.; Grande-Tovar, C.D. Chitosan/Polyvinyl Alcohol/Tea Tree Essential Oil Composite Films for Biomedical Applications. *Polymers* **2021**, *13*, 3753. [CrossRef]
32. Anadon, A.; Martinez-Larranaga, M.R.; Martinez, M.A.; Ares, I.; Garcia-Risco, M.R.; Senorans, F.J.; Reglero, G. Acute oral safety study of rosemary extracts in rats. *J. Food Prot.* **2008**, *71*, 790–795. [CrossRef]
33. Shalaby, S.E.M.; El-Din, M.M.; Mettwally, M.; Abo-Donia, S.A.; Attia, Z.A. Toxicological Affects of Essential Oils from Eucalyptus *Eucalyptus globules* and Clove *Eugenia caryophyllus* on Albino Rats. *Pol. J. Environ. Stud.* **2011**, *20*, 429–434.
34. Saffron, C.M.; Park, J.-H.; Dale, B.E.; Voice, T.C. Kinetics of Contaminant Desorption from Soil: Comparison of Model Formulations Using the Akaike Information Criterion. *Environ. Sci. Technol.* **2006**, *40*, 7662–7667. [CrossRef] [PubMed]
35. Romero, A.I.; Villegas, M.; Cid, A.G.; Parentis, M.L.; Gonzo, E.E.; Bermudez, J.M. Validation of kinetic modeling of progesterone release from polymeric membranes. *Asian J. Pharm. Sci.* **2018**, *13*, 54–62. [CrossRef] [PubMed]
36. Boczar, D.; Michalska, K. Cyclodextrin Inclusion Complexes with Antibiotics and Antibacterial Agents as Drug-Delivery Systems—A Pharmaceutical Perspective. *Pharmaceutics* **2022**, *14*, 1389. [CrossRef] [PubMed]
37. Wilson, C.; Lukowicz, R.; Merchant, S.; Valquier-Flynn, H.; Caballero, J.; Sandoval, J.; Okuom, M.; Huber, C.; Brooks, T.D.; Wilson, E.; et al. Quantitative and Qualitative Assessment Methods for Biofilm Growth: A Mini-review. *Res. Rev. J. Eng. Technol.* **2017**, *4*, 1–25.
38. Abers, M.; Schroeder, S.; Goelz, L.; Sulser, A.; St Rose, T.; Puchalski, K.; Langland, J. Antimicrobial activity of the volatile substances from essential oils. *BMC Complement. Med. Ther.* **2021**, *21*, 124. [CrossRef]
39. López, P.; Sánchez, C.; Batlle, R.; Nerín, C. Solid- and Vapor-Phase Antimicrobial Activities of Six Essential Oils: Susceptibility of Selected Foodborne Bacterial and Fungal Strains. *J. Agric. Food Chem.* **2005**, *53*, 6939–6946. [CrossRef]

40. Tornuk, F.; Cankurt, H.; Ozturk, I.; Sagdic, O.; Bayram, O.; Yetim, H. Efficacy of various plant hydrosols as natural food sanitizers in reducing *Escherichia coli* O157:H7 and *Salmonella typhimurium* on fresh cut carrots and apples. *Int. J. Food Microbiol.* **2011**, *148*, 30–35. [CrossRef]
41. Cox, S.D.; Mann, C.M.; Markham, J.L.; Gustafson, J.E.; Warmington, J.R.; Wyllie, S.G. Determining the Antimicrobial Actions of Tea Tree Oil. *Molecules* **2001**, *6*, 87–91. [CrossRef]
42. Sienkiewicz, M.; Lysakowska, M.; Pastuszka, M.; Bienias, W.; Kowalczyk, E. The potential of use basil and rosemary essential oils as effective antibacterial agents. *Molecules* **2013**, *18*, 9334–9351. [CrossRef]
43. Burt, S. Essential oils: Their antibacterial properties and potential applications in foods—A review. *Int. J. Food Microbiol.* **2004**, *94*, 223–253. [CrossRef] [PubMed]
44. Fabio, A.; Cermelli, C.; Fabio, G.; Nicoletti, P.; Quaglio, P. Screening of the antibacterial effects of a variety of essential oils on microorganisms responsible for respiratory infections. *Phytother. Res.* **2007**, *21*, 374–377. [CrossRef] [PubMed]
45. Flores, F.C.; Lima, J.A.d.; Silva, C.R.d.; Benvegnú, D.; Ferreira, J.; Burger, M.E.; Beck, R.C.R.; Rolim, C.M.B.; Rocha, M.I.U.M.; da Veiga, M.L.; et al. Hydrogels Containing Nanocapsules and Nanoemulsions of Tea Tree Oil Provide Antiedematogenic Effect and Improved Skin Wound Healing. *J. Nanosci. Nanotechnol.* **2015**, *15*, 800–809. [CrossRef] [PubMed]
46. Altaf, F.; Niazi, M.B.K.; Jahan, Z.; Ahmad, T.; Akram, M.A.; Safdar, A.; Butt, M.S.; Noor, T.; Sher, F. Synthesis and Characterization of PVA/Starch Hydrogel Membranes Incorporating Essential Oils Aimed to be Used in Wound Dressing Applications. *J. Polym. Environ.* **2020**, *29*, 156–174. [CrossRef]
47. Cordeiro, L.; Figueiredo, P.; Souza, H.; Sousa, A.; Andrade-Junior, F.; Medeiros, D.; Nobrega, J.; Silva, D.; Martins, E.; Barbosa-Filho, J.; et al. Terpinen-4-ol as an Antibacterial and Antibiofilm Agent against *Staphylococcus aureus*. *Int. J. Mol. Sci.* **2020**, *21*, 4531. [CrossRef] [PubMed]
48. Zhang, Y.; Feng, R.; Li, L.; Zhou, X.; Li, Z.; Jia, R.; Song, X.; Zou, Y.; Yin, L.; He, C.; et al. The Antibacterial Mechanism of Terpinen-4-ol against *Streptococcus agalactiae*. *Curr. Microbiol.* **2018**, *75*, 1214–1220. [CrossRef]
49. Carson, C.F.; Riley, T.V. Antimicrobial activity of the major components of the essential oil of *Melaleuca alternifolia*. *J. Appl. Bacteriol.* **1995**, *78*, 264–269. [CrossRef]
50. Shahina, Z.; Al Homsi, R.; Price, J.D.W.; Whiteway, M.; Sultana, T.; Dahms, T.E.S. Rosemary essential oil and its components 1,8-cineole and alpha-pinene induce ROS-dependent lethality and ROS-independent virulence inhibition in *Candida albicans*. *PLoS ONE* **2022**, *17*, e0277097. [CrossRef]
51. Guzzo, F.; Scognamiglio, M.; Fiorentino, A.; Buommino, E.; D'Abrosca, B. Plant Derived Natural Products against *Pseudomonas aeruginosa* and *Staphylococcus aureus*: Antibiofilm Activity and Molecular Mechanisms. *Molecules* **2020**, *25*, 5024. [CrossRef]
52. Farhanghi, A.; Aliakbarlu, J.; Tajik, H.; Mortazavi, N.; Manafi, L.; Jalilzadeh-Amin, G. Antibacterial interactions of pulegone and 1,8-cineole with monolaurin ornisin against *Staphylococcus aureus*. *Food Sci. Nutr.* **2022**, *10*, 2659–2666. [CrossRef]
53. Kifer, D.; Muzinic, V.; Klaric, M.S. Antimicrobial potency of single and combined mupirocin and monoterpenes, thymol, menthol and 1,8-cineole against *Staphylococcus aureus* planktonic and biofilm growth. *J. Antibiot.* **2016**, *69*, 689–696. [CrossRef]
54. Ojeda-Sana, A.M.; van Baren, C.M.; Elechosa, M.A.; Juárez, M.A.; Moreno, S. New insights into antibacterial and antioxidant activities of rosemary essential oils and their main components. *Food Control* **2013**, *31*, 189–195. [CrossRef]
55. Akhmouch, A.A.; Hriouech, S.; Mzabi, A.; Tanghort, M.; Chefchaou, H.; Remmal, A.; Chami, N. Synergistic Action of AMX Associated with 1,8-Cineole and Its Effect on the ESBL Enzymatic Resistance Mechanism. *Antibiotics* **2022**, *11*, 1002. [CrossRef]
56. Merghni, A.; Noumi, E.; Hadded, O.; Dridi, N.; Panwar, H.; Ceylan, O.; Mastouri, M.; Snoussi, M. Assessment of the antibiofilm and antiquorum sensing activities of Eucalyptus globulus essential oil and its main component 1,8-cineole against methicillin-resistant *Staphylococcus aureus* strains. *Microb. Pathog.* **2018**, *118*, 74–80. [CrossRef]
57. Merghni, A.; Belmamoun, A.R.; Urcan, A.C.; Bobis, O.; Lassoued, M.A. 1,8-Cineol (Eucalyptol) Disrupts Membrane Integrity and Induces Oxidative Stress in Methicillin-Resistant *Staphylococcus aureus*. *Antioxidants* **2023**, *12*, 1388. [CrossRef] [PubMed]
58. Hoch, C.C.; Petry, J.; Griesbaum, L.; Weiser, T.; Werner, K.; Ploch, M.; Verschoor, A.; Multhoff, G.; Bashiri Dezfouli, A.; Wollenberg, B. 1,8-cineole (eucalyptol): A versatile phytochemical with therapeutic applications across multiple diseases. *Biomed. Pharmacother.* **2023**, *167*, 115467. [CrossRef] [PubMed]
59. Ulanowska, M.; Olas, B. Biological Properties and Prospects for the Application of Eugenol—A Review. *Int. J. Mol. Sci.* **2021**, *22*, 3671. [CrossRef]
60. Marchese, A.; Barbieri, R.; Coppo, E.; Orhan, I.E.; Daglia, M.; Nabavi, S.F.; Izadi, M.; Abdollahi, M.; Nabavi, S.M.; Ajami, M. Antimicrobial activity of eugenol and essential oils containing eugenol: A mechanistic viewpoint. *Crit. Rev. Microbiol.* **2017**, *43*, 668–689. [CrossRef]
61. Hyldgaard, M.; Mygind, T.; Meyer, R.L. Essential oils in food preservation: Mode of action, synergies, and interactions with food matrix components. *Front. Microbiol.* **2012**, *3*, 12. [CrossRef]
62. Devi, K.P.; Nisha, S.A.; Sakthivel, R.; Pandian, S.K. Eugenol (an essential oil of clove) acts as an antibacterial agent against *Salmonella typhi* by disrupting the cellular membrane. *J. Ethnopharmacol.* **2010**, *130*, 107–115. [CrossRef]
63. Nisar, M.F.; Khadim, M.; Rafiq, M.; Chen, J.; Yang, Y.; Wan, C.C. Pharmacological Properties and Health Benefits of Eugenol: A Comprehensive Review. *Oxidative Med. Cell. Longev.* **2021**, *2021*, 1–14. [CrossRef]
64. Zore, G.B.; Thakre, A.D.; Jadhav, S.; Karuppayil, S.M. Terpenoids inhibit *Candida albicans* growth by affecting membrane integrity and arrest of cell cycle. *Phytomedicine* **2011**, *18*, 1181–1190. [CrossRef]

65. Ahmad, A.; Khan, A.; Khan, L.A.; Manzoor, N. In vitro synergy of eugenol and methyleugenol with fluconazole against clinical *Candida* isolates. *J. Med. Microbiol.* **2010**, *59*, 1178–1184. [CrossRef] [PubMed]
66. Elo, H.; Matikainen, J.; Pelttari, E. Potent activity of the lichen antibiotic (+)-usnic acid against clinical isolates of vancomycin-resistant enterococci and methicillin-resistant *Staphylococcus aureus. Naturwissenschaften* **2007**, *94*, 465–468. [CrossRef] [PubMed]
67. Maciag-Dorszynska, M.; Wegrzyn, G.; Guzow-Krzeminska, B. Antibacterial activity of lichen secondary metabolite usnic acid is primarily caused by inhibition of RNA and DNA synthesis. *Fems Microbiol. Lett.* **2014**, *353*, 57–62. [CrossRef] [PubMed]
68. Pires, R.H.; Lucarini, R.; Mendes-Giannini, M.J. Effect of usnic acid on *Candida orthopsilosis* and *C. parapsilosis. Antimicrob. Agents Chemother.* **2012**, *56*, 595–597. [CrossRef]
69. Nithyanand, P.; Beema Shafreen, R.M.; Muthamil, S.; Karutha Pandian, S. Usnic acid inhibits biofilm formation and virulent morphological traits of *Candida albicans. Microbiol. Res.* **2015**, *179*, 20–28. [CrossRef] [PubMed]
70. Kiti, K.; Suwantong, O. Bilayer wound dressing based on sodium alginate incorporated with curcumin-beta-cyclodextrin inclusion complex/chitosan hydrogel. *Int. J. Biol. Macromol.* **2020**, *164*, 4113–4124. [CrossRef]
71. Kim, C.; Jeong, D.; Kim, S.; Kim, Y.; Jung, S. Cyclodextrin functionalized agarose gel with low gelling temperature for controlled drug delivery systems. *Carbohydr. Polym.* **2019**, *222*, 115011. [CrossRef]
72. Pante, G.C.; Castro, J.C.; Lini, R.S.; Romoli, J.C.Z.; Pires, T.Y.; Garcia, F.P.; Nakamura, C.V.; Mulati, A.C.N.; Matioli, G.; Machinski Junior, M. Inclusion Complexes of *Litsea cubeba* (Lour.) Pers Essential Oil into beta-Cyclodextrin: Preparation, Physicochemical Characterization, Cytotoxicity and Antifungal Activity. *Molecules* **2024**, *29*, 1626. [CrossRef]
73. Atyim, P.; Olah, N.K.; Osser, G.; Toma, C.C.; Morgovan, C.; Atyim, E. Practical Investigation of Gels Containing Aristolochia (*Aristolochia Clematitis)* Extract. *Stud. Univ. Babes-Bolyai Chem.* **2017**, *62*, 153–164. [CrossRef]
74. *Romanian Farmacopeia*, Xth ed.; Editura Medicala: Bucharest, Romania, 1998; p. 1316.
75. Ghica, M.V.; Albu, M.G.; Dinu-Pirvu, C.; Moisescu, S. In vitro Kinetic Release and Flow Behaviour of Some Collagen-Minocycline Topical Hydrogels. *Rev. Chim.* **2012**, *63*, 929–935.
76. Ghica, M.V.; Hirjau, M.; Lupuleasa, D.; Dinu-Pirvu, C.E. Flow and Thixotropic Parameters for Rheological Characterization of Hydrogels. *Molecules* **2016**, *21*, 786. [CrossRef] [PubMed]
77. Păunica-Panea, G.; Ficai, A.; Marin, M.M.; Marin, Ş.; Albu, M.G.; Constantin, V.D.; Dinu-Pîrvu, C.; Vuluga, Z.; Corobea, M.C.; Ghica, M.V. New Collagen-Dextran-Zinc Oxide Composites for Wound Dressing. *J. Nanomater.* **2016**, *2016*, 1–7. [CrossRef]
78. Puri, A.; Nguyen, H.X.; Banga, A.K. Microneedle-mediated intradermal delivery of epigallocatechin-3-gallate. *Int. J. Cosmet. Sci.* **2016**, *38*, 512–523. [CrossRef]
79. Ilie, C.I.; Spoiala, A.; Geana, E.I.; Chircov, C.; Ficai, A.; Ditu, L.M.; Oprea, E. Bee Bread: A Promising Source of Bioactive Compounds with Antioxidant Properties-First Report on Some Antimicrobial Features. *Antioxidants* **2024**, *13*, 353. [CrossRef]
80. *CLSI Supplement M100*; Performance Standards for Antimicrobial Susceptibility Testing. Clinical and Laboratory Standards Institute: Wayne, PA, USA, 2021; pp. 1–352.
81. Wu, K.; Zhang, T.; Chai, X.; Duan, X.; He, D.; Yu, H.; Liu, X.; Tao, Z. Encapsulation Efficiency and Functional Stability of Cinnamon Essential Oil in Modified Beta-Cyclodextrins: In Vitro and In Silico Evidence. *Foods* **2022**, *12*, 45. [CrossRef]
82. Devrnja, N.; Andelkovic, B.; Ljujic, J.; Cosic, T.; Stupar, S.; Milutinovic, M.; Savic, J. Encapsulation of Fennel and Basil Essential Oils in beta-Cyclodextrin for Novel Biopesticide Formulation. *Biomolecules* **2024**, *14*, 353. [CrossRef]
83. Alizadeh, N.; Nazari, F. Thymol essential oil/β-cyclodextrin inclusion complex into chitosan nanoparticles: Improvement of thymol properties in vitro studies. *J. Mol. Liq.* **2022**, *346*, 118250. [CrossRef]

gels

MDPI

Review

Hydrogel-Forming Microneedles in the Management of Dermal Disorders Through a Non-Invasive Process: A Review

Popat Mohite [1], Abhijeet Puri [1], Shubham Munde [1], Nitin Ade [1], Ashwini Kumar [2], Pensak Jantrawut [3], Sudarshan Singh [3,4,*] and Chuda Chittasupho [3,*]

1 AETs St. John Institute of Pharmacy and Research, Palghar 401404, Maharashtra, India; mohitepb@gmail.com (P.M.); abhijeetp@sjipr.edu.in (A.P.); shubhamvmunde@gmail.com (S.M.); nitinade2@gmail.com (N.A.)

2 Research and Development Cell, School of Engineering and Technology, Manav Rachna International Institute of Research and Studies, Faridabad 121003, Haryana, India; drashwinikumar.research@gmail.com

3 Faculty of Pharmacy, Chiang Mai University, Chiang Mai 50200, Thailand; pensak.j@cmu.ac.th

4 Office of Research Administration, Chiang Mai University, Chiang Mai 50200, Thailand

* Correspondence: sudarshan.s@cmu.ac.th or sudarshansingh83@hotmail.com (S.S.); chuda.c@cmu.ac.th (C.C.)

Abstract: Microneedle (MN) technology has emerged as a promising approach for delivering therapeutic agents to the skin, offering significant potential in treating various dermal conditions. Among these technologies, hydrogel-forming microneedles (HFMNs) represent a transformative advancement in the management of dermal diseases through non-invasive drug delivery. These innovative devices consist of micrometer-sized needles made of native or crosslinked hydrophilic polymers, capable of penetrating the stratum corneum without damaging underlying tissues. Upon insertion, HFMNs rapidly absorb interstitial fluid, swelling to form a hydrogel conduit that enables the efficient transport of therapeutic agents directly into the dermal microcirculation. The non-invasive nature of HFMNs enhances patient compliance by eliminating the pain and discomfort associated with traditional hypodermic needles. This technology allows for the delivery of a wide range of drugs, including macromolecules and biomacromolecules, which are often difficult to administer dermally due to their size and polarity. Moreover, HFMNs provide controlled and regulated release profiles, enabling sustained therapeutic effects while minimizing systemic side effects. Additionally, HFMNs can be used for both drug delivery and real-time interstitial fluid monitoring, offering valuable insights into disease states and treatment responses. This dual functionality positions HFMNs as a versatile dermatology tool capable of effectively addressing various dermal complications. This review explores the potential use of polymeric biomaterials in HFMN fabrication and their application in treating major dermal disorders, such as acne, psoriasis, and other skin conditions. Furthermore, the review highlights the non-invasive nature of MN-based treatments, underscoring their potential to reduce patient discomfort and improve treatment adherence, as supported by the recent literature.

Keywords: biocompatible; biodegradable; dermal disease; hydrogel; microneedles; non-invasive

1. Introduction

The skin is the body's largest and most versatile organ, providing essential protection, regulating temperature, and enabling sensory perception. It prevents water loss and blocks the entry of toxic compounds, allergens, irritants, and microbes [1]. Most dermatological disorders affect the skin's first viable tissue layer, which can be impacted by various diseases and conditions, each with distinct causes and treatment approaches. The causes of skin disorders may include genetic factors, immune system disorders, illnesses affecting the thyroid or kidneys, diabetes, and infections from viruses, fungi, or bacteria trapped in hair follicles and skin pores. Other sources include a weakened immune system, contact with irritants or allergenic chemicals, exposure to infected individuals, and microorganisms, parasites, or fungi living on the skin [1]. A common dermal disorder is acne, which is caused by the blockage of hair follicles and is typically managed with topical treatments or medications [2]. Treatments for eczema, also known as atopic dermatitis, include topical steroids and moisturizers. This condition is characterized by itchy, inflamed areas of skin, often triggered by environmental factors and genetic predisposition [3]. Another common dermal condition is psoriasis, an autoimmune disease that leads to scaly patches and accelerated skin cell turnover [4,5]. It can be managed with topical medications, systemic treatments, or phototherapy [6]. Topical drug delivery effectively addresses superficial infections and disorders. However, for deep dermal therapeutic activity, drug permeation is a critical factor that must be considered. Therefore, developing an effective and safe delivery system is essential for treating a variety of skin conditions [7].

Liposomes and nanoparticles, developed using polymeric matrices, have shown significant efficacy in overcoming the skin barrier and facilitating drug absorption through the skin while allowing for controlled and prolonged medication release [8–10]. While these formulations address the challenges of targeted drug delivery systems, they have drawbacks, including a limited understanding of penetration mechanisms, scalability issues, and difficulty in regulating deeper drug penetration [11]. Novel methods have been reported to enhance drug permeability through the skin layers. Various physical approaches include hypodermic needles, iontophoresis, electrophoresis, and ablation. However, each method comes with its own advantages and disadvantages [12,13]. These methods may lead to skin allergies and irritation, require qualified personnel, and involve cost considerations. Additionally, they can compromise the skin's natural barrier function over an extended period [14,15]. Microneedle (MN) technology presents a promising drug delivery method that can penetrate the skin with minimal discomfort [12]. Microneedles can create transient microchannels, allowing for the delivery of therapies that are unsuitable for transdermal or intradermal administration due to their large macromolecular size. Additionally, these small arrays of needles can also be used to diagnose infectious diseases [13]. Microneedles are self-managing devices capable of identifying biomarkers from the interstitial fluid of the skin in a minimally invasive manner, facilitating illness detection. These tiny, one-millimeter-diameter structures can access the dermal layers without touching blood vessels or pain-sensing neurons, offering painless, non-invasive, and controlled drug delivery for treating dermal disorders and infections. Microneedles effectively transfer molecules across the skin barrier, making hypodermic needle injections less uncomfortable. Furthermore, this non-invasive device reduces the risk of spreading blood-borne infectious diseases and minimizes damage from needle sticks [16]. Microneedles can be fabricated from various materials and are classified into several types: solid microneedles (MNs), coated microneedles, hollow microneedles, dissolving microneedles, and hydrogel-forming microneedles (HFMNs) [17].

Hydrogel-forming microneedles, an intriguing category of microneedles first reported in 2012, consist of swellable polymers, specifically crosslinked hydrogels such as chitosan, hyaluronic acid, sodium alginate, and poly(vinyl alcohol). These materials enable the sustained delivery of drugs over extended periods by either incorporating the drug into the polymer structure during preparation or by loading the drug into a separate reservoir and attaching it to the HFMNs [18–21]. Compared to conventional microneedles (MNs), hydrogel-forming microneedles (HFMNs) offer several advantages and represent a significant advancement in the field of dermal drug administration [22]. These cutting-edge tools combine the benefits of hydrogels with advanced technology, enhancing performance and broadening applications, particularly in the management of skin disorders. Conventional microneedles, made from silicon, polymers, or metals, primarily function by creating microconduits in the skin to facilitate the transport of medicinal substances. While traditional microneedles are effective, they have drawbacks, including the potential for irritation or skin damage due to their rigidity [23]. Typically, conventional microneedles rely on diffuse release or passive diffusion to administer medications, which can be ineffective and occasionally result in suboptimal therapeutic outcomes. In contrast, hydrogel-forming microneedles represent a paradigm shift due to their unique features and functionalities.

Generally composed of hydrophilic and biocompatible polymers that swell in the presence of moisture, such as skin interstitial fluid, hydrogel microneedles are increasingly utilized in medical applications [24]. Thus, due to their ability to swell, hydrogel microneedles can form a gel-like matrix that penetrates the skin and serves as a reservoir for regulated drug delivery [25]. Comparing this method to conventional microneedles reveals several advantages, including enhanced comfort and reduced invasiveness. Additionally, hydrogel microneedles are softer and more flexible than standard materials, offering greater adaptability and comfort at the administration site [26]. In addition to treating skin conditions, hydrogel-forming microneedles (HFMNs) have been investigated for their potential to deliver biopharmaceuticals, gene therapies, and vaccines [27,28]. Hydrogel-forming microneedles offer several advantages over injections and invasive procedures. They are easy to administer, minimizing discomfort and anxiety associated with injections, particularly for patients who fear needles or require frequent dosing. Moreover, the familiarity and simplicity of using a pill or applying a patch can enhance patient acceptance of non-invasive methods, as individuals are generally more inclined to embrace these approaches.

Hydrogel-forming microneedles offer several benefits. The hydrogel matrix enables controlled and sustained release, providing a non-invasive alternative to injections. HFMNs have successfully delivered various drugs and therapeutic agents, including insulin, for managing diabetes [29]. Metformin has been delivered using hydrogel-forming microneedles (HFMNs) to provide sustained release, thereby enhancing patient compliance compared to traditional oral administration [29]. Moreover, hydrogel-forming microneedles (HFMNs) have been utilized to deliver vaccines, including those for influenza and hepatitis B, by targeting immune cells in the skin, which enhances immune responses [30]. Additionally, hydrogel-forming microneedles (HFMNs) have been used for the localized delivery of doxorubicin, a chemotherapeutic agent, directly to skin tumors, improving treatment efficacy while minimizing systemic side effects [31]. HFMNs have been used to deliver corticosteroids, such as dexamethasone, for treating inflammatory skin conditions like eczema and psoriasis, providing targeted delivery while reducing systemic effects [32]. However, several issues still need to be addressed, including potential biosafety concerns associated with long-term use, challenges in industrial production, and sterilization. The development of hydrogel materials that are both cost-effective and durable is essential for their widespread application. Additionally, further research is required to ensure the stability of the medication within the hydrogel matrix and to achieve reliable and consistent drug release [33]. Future developments are likely to focus on refining hydrogel compositions, exploring new production methods, and enhancing the overall functionality and applicability of hydrogel-forming microneedles (HFMNs). This review aims to provide a comprehensive analysis of HFMNs and their applications in managing skin disorders, addressing existing knowledge gaps. Additionally, it summarizes the fundamental principles underlying HFMNs, including structural and material composition, as well as an assessment of evaluation studies that confirm the integrity of HFMNs' therapeutic applications.

2. Dermal Drug Delivery: A Versatile Approach for Skin-Targeted Therapies

Dermal drug delivery is a versatile method suitable for various formulations and applications. Its localized nature and reduced systemic side effects make it an attractive option for many medical conditions, especially those affecting the skin or requiring targeted treatment [34]. Human skin is the largest and most versatile organ in the body. It serves as a protective barrier, regulating temperature and sensory perception. The skin prevents water loss and protects against the potential penetration of toxic compounds, allergens, irritants, and microbes. Additionally, it functions as a complex physical barrier against ultraviolet radiation and particulate matter from the external environment [35]. The skin comprises three essential layers: the outermost epidermis, the dermis, and the subcutaneous tissue or hypodermis. The epidermis consists of five layers, with the topmost layer, the stratum corneum (SC), responsible for the skin's barrier properties. The dermis contains connective tissues, blood vessels, lymphatic vessels, nerve endings, hair follicles, sebaceous glands, and eccrine glands. The subcutaneous tissue is composed of adipose cells and provides insulation to the body (Figure 1). The outer layer of the epidermis, known as the SC, acts as a barrier that restricts the penetration of molecules larger than 500 Da. The stratum corneum mainly consists of corneocytes surrounded by hydrophobic lipid layers that are approximately 10–20 μm thick. Beneath the SC lies the viable epidermis, composed of keratinocytes, melanocytes, Merkel cells, and Langerhans cells, with a thickness of 50–100 μm. Most dermatological disorders occur in this first viable tissue layer of the skin [36]. Skin-associated disorders, such as chronic wounds, psoriasis, eczema, acne, hyperpigmentation, skin aging, and vitiligo, affect millions of people worldwide [37]. Wound healing is often associated with common terms such as "scab", which refers to a hard covering of dried blood that forms over a wound to protect the area as it heals, and "fibrotic skin", a pathological condition characterized by excessive accumulation of fibrous connective tissue in the skin, primarily within the dermis. Additionally, "epithelial hypertrophy" describes the abnormal increase in the size or number of epithelial layers. This condition can occur in various tissues and is often a response to chronic irritation, inflammation, or injury.

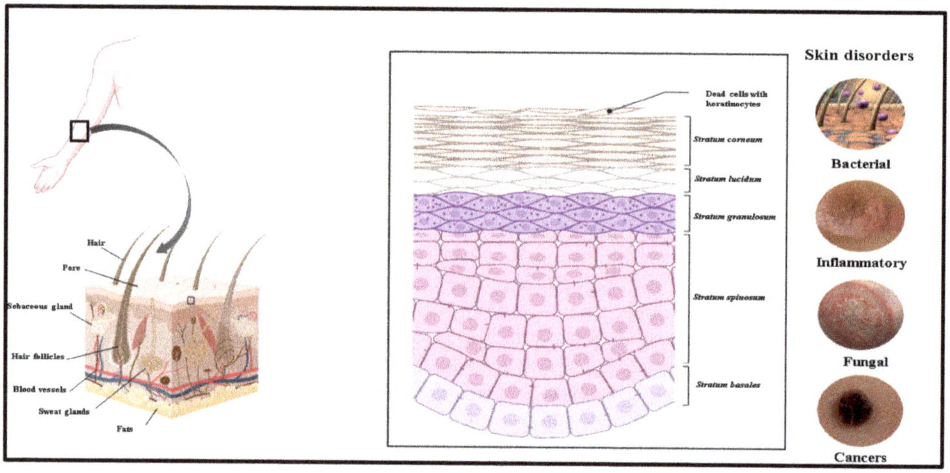

Figure 1. Illustration for anatomy of skin and related disorders. (The figure was created based on the authors' own ideas using BioRender: ScientificImage and Illustration Software. Version 04).

Traditional dermal treatments typically involve topical or systemic therapies, which can be invasive or less effective. Non-invasive drug delivery systems, such as hydrogel-forming microneedles (MNs), offer promising alternatives by delivering targeted therapies directly to the affected skin layers. Chronic wounds and conditions such as diabetic ulcers, psoriasis, eczema, acne, hyperpigmentation, skin aging, and vitiligo can be effectively treated using MNs [38]. These microneedles (MNs) can deliver therapeutic agents such as growth factors, antimicrobial agents, and cytokines directly to the wound site, enhancing healing and reducing infection risks. Conditions like psoriasis, eczema, and atopic dermatitis can be effectively treated using hydrogel-forming microneedles (HFMNs) that deliver therapeutics such as corticosteroids or moisturizers directly into the affected skin layers, improving treatment efficacy while minimizing side effects. Additionally, hyperpigmentation disorders like melasma and age spots can be addressed with skin-brightening agents like vitamin C or kojic acid delivered directly to the epidermal–dermal layers, leading to improved pigmentation treatments and a more uniform skin tone. Furthermore, drug delivery for vaccines can benefit from HFMNs by stimulating robust immune responses while providing a more comfortable experience. In dermatological cancer treatments, HFMNs can deliver chemotherapeutic agents or immune modulators directly to cancerous lesions, enhancing treatment efficacy and minimizing systemic side effects.

3. Hydrogel-Forming Microneedles: A Promising Alternative for Controlled and Targeted Drug Delivery

The unique properties of the skin make the microneedle (MN) delivery system a promising alternative to conventional drug delivery methods. Its defensive, inflammatory, and immunological characteristics contribute to this potential. Among various dermal drug delivery techniques, the MN-mediated system is defined as the non-invasive delivery of medications through the skin, and it has garnered significant attention from research institutions and companies alike [39]. These micron-scale needles have been shown to penetrate the skin through the stratum corneum (SC) into the viable epidermis while avoiding nerve fibers and blood vessels, which are primarily located in the dermal layer [40]. Moreover, these microneedles (MNs) are smaller and shorter than traditional hypodermic needles, making them less painful as they penetrate only the outer layer of the skin (the epidermis) and sometimes the upper layer of the dermis. This limited penetration activates fewer pain receptors, resulting in a sensation akin to a light prick or slight pressure. Additionally, MNs can be designed for quick insertion, minimizing discomfort duration and making the application less intrusive than that of a slower hypodermic needle. MNs are versatile, innovative devices available in various shapes, sizes, and materials, making them suitable for a wide range of applications. They can be designed to detect, diagnose, and treat numerous conditions by efficiently delivering vaccines, nanoparticles, proteins, antibodies, and drugs of varying molecular weights. These therapeutics or carriers can be precisely loaded into MNs to target specific skin layers, effectively reaching immune cells such as neutrophils, Langerhans cells, and dendritic cells, thereby promoting a robust immunological response [41]. Traditional microneedles (MNs) are categorized into four basic types based on their mechanisms: solid, coated, dissolving, and hollow (Figure 2). Each type offers specific benefits, such as controlled drug release or enhanced drug stability.

Hydrogel-forming microneedles represent an innovative advancement in microneedle (MN) technology, with the potential to address several limitations commonly associated with traditional MNs. These include significantly reduced drug-loading capacity, challenges in achieving precise drug coating, and difficulties in controlling the rate and extent of drug release [42]. These microneedles (MNs) are fabricated from biocompatible, water-responsive polymeric materials that form a gel upon insertion into the skin. Once inserted, hydrogel-forming microneedles (HFMNs) absorb surrounding fluids, causing them to swell and create microchannels in the skin. This process allows for controlled and sustained drug release while maintaining the needle's structure, effectively providing a pathway for the medication to penetrate deeper into the dermal layers [43]. Their unique ability to hydrate and form a gel ensures efficient, regulated drug diffusion, particularly for hydrophilic compounds, without leaving any residual material in the skin after removal [33]. These controlled or regulated release mechanisms involve the absorption and swelling of drug molecules by body fluids, forming a gel-like layer that modulates drug diffusion. Some HFMNs also incorporate erosion-based mechanisms, wherein the matrix degrades over time, allowing for controlled drug release. Additionally, certain HFMNs can be designed to respond to specific environmental conditions, such as changes in pH or temperature, further regulating the release profile. The controlled release offers several therapeutic advantages, including improved bioavailability, reduced side effects, dosing flexibility, targeted delivery, and enhanced patient compliance. It can also decrease dosing frequency, particularly for chronic conditions, and simplify medication regimens through extended-release formulations. Overall, controlled release can improve the effectiveness of HFMNs in maintaining therapeutic levels and ensuring patient adherence. Moreover, HFMNs can deliver macromolecules with enhanced therapeutic efficacy when applied topically. The hydrogel matrix allows for sustained and controlled drug release, maintaining therapeutic levels over an extended period. This minimizes systemic side effects, which is especially beneficial for biomacromolecules that may cause adverse effects if absorbed into the bloodstream.

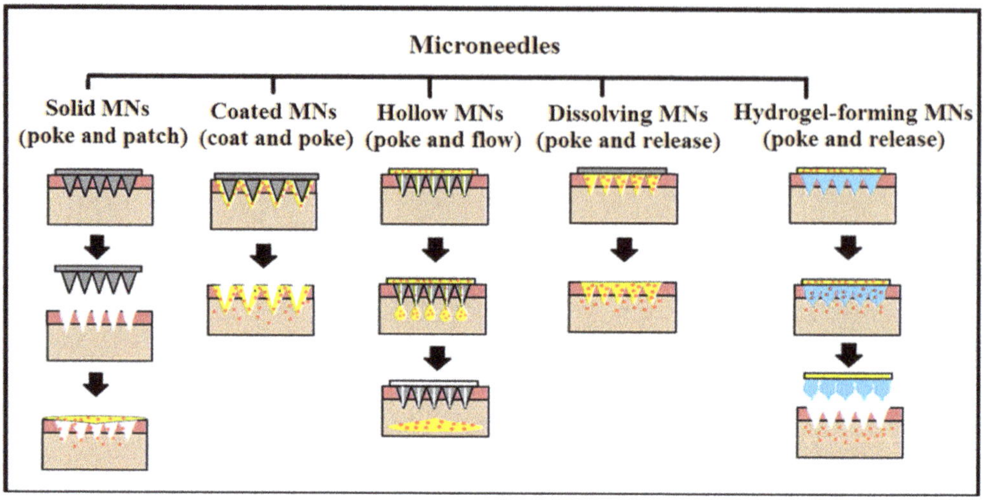

Figure 2. The drug delivery mechanism of solid microneedles (solid MNs), coated microneedles (coated MNs), hollow microneedles (hollow MNs), dissolving microneedles (dissolving MNs), and hydrogel-forming microneedles (hydrogel-forming MNs). Reproduced with permission from [44] under CC BY 4.0.

Hydrogel-forming microneedles (HFMNs) are integrated systems composed of two main components: an array of microneedles made from crosslinked polymers and a drug reservoir. This design enhances skin penetration, enabling deeper drug delivery into the dermis for localized treatment of various skin conditions. HFMNs are minimally invasive, resulting in less pain and discomfort compared to traditional delivery methods, which in turn improves patient compliance. The hydrogel matrix within HFMNs allows for controlled drug release, thereby enhancing therapeutic effects and prolonging the drug's availability at the target site. By delivering drugs directly to the action site, HFMNs reduce systemic exposure, minimizing absorption and associated side effects, and thereby improving the overall safety profile of the treatment. Typically, the polymers used in HFMNs are hydrocolloids, such as cellulosic or cellulose derivatives, which can absorb significant amounts of interstitial fluid and swell upon insertion into the skin. Once the microneedles are inserted, they absorb interstitial fluid, creating a swollen polymeric matrix rich in capillaries. This process generates continuous microchannels that connect the drug reservoir to the surrounding tissue, facilitating enhanced drug delivery. The swollen matrix acts as a membrane that controls the drug release rate. After the drug delivery is complete, the empty microneedles can be removed from the skin without leaving any polymeric residue, providing greater flexibility in terms of shape and size. Additionally, the density of the hydrogel matrix can be adjusted to achieve specific drug release rates. However, despite their advantages, HFMNs may experience limitations, such as poor mechanical strength and physical stability, which could affect their performance and durability in practical applications [44].

Hydrogel-forming microneedles (HFMNs) significantly enhance patient compliance due to their reduced pain, ease of self-administration, and quick application. Their minimally invasive design makes them more comfortable compared to traditional injections, which encourages regular use among patients. HFMNs can be conveniently applied at home, removing the need for professional assistance, which is particularly beneficial for those with chronic conditions requiring frequent treatments. The fast application process typically takes only a few minutes, allowing patients to seamlessly integrate HFMNs into their daily routines with minimal disruption. The design features of HFMNs, including smaller tip diameters, lower tip angles, and higher tip height-to-width ratios, contribute to successful skin penetration. In studies comparing different base geometries of microneedles, it was found that HFMNs with triangular and square bases achieved greater penetration depths (340 μm and 343 μm, respectively) than those with hexagonal bases (197 μm). Specifically, the average penetration distance from the microneedle base plate to the stratum corneum was measured to be 660 μm for the triangle base, 657 μm for the square base, and 803 μm for the hexagonal base, indicating that the geometric design plays a crucial role in the effectiveness of drug delivery through the skin. This improved penetration capability further underscores the advantages of HFMNs in facilitating efficient and effective transdermal drug delivery [45]. A summary of design considerations is presented in Table 1 and Figure 3.

Table 1. Various parameters that need to be considered while fabricating HFMNs. Reproduced with permission from [42] under CC BY 4.0.

Parameters	Size and Dimension
Length (*L*)	Vary between 500 and 800 μm depending on applicability
Diameter of needle base (*Db*)	Vary between 150 and 300 μm depending on applicability
Tip diameter (*Dt*)	<15 μm
Internal spacing (center to center) (IS_1)	Vary between 400 and 450 μm depending on applicability
Interneedle spacing (edge to edge) (IS_2)	Vary between 50 and 150 μm depending on applicability
Array size	Vary between 1 × 9 and 19 × 19 depending on applicability

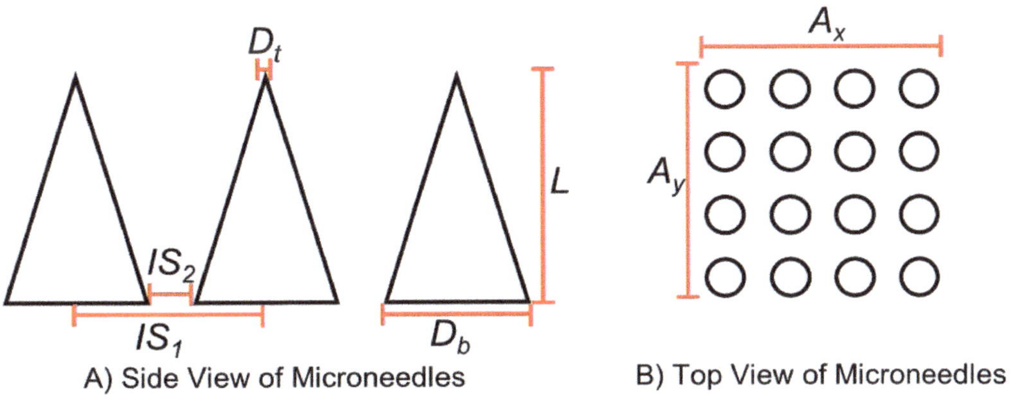

Figure 3. (**A**,**B**) Illustration showing the different dimensions taken into consideration for microneedle arrays. Reproduced with permission from [42] under CC BY 4.0.

4. Fabrication Methods for Hydrogel-Forming Microneedle Arrays

4.1. Polymeric Materials Used in the Fabrication of Hydrogel-Forming Microneedles

Microneedles (MNs) function by penetrating the protective layers of human skin or mucosa, making it crucial that the materials used are biocompatible. Generally, hydrogels are biocompatible and can be used without causing harm or discomfort to the user. Several polymers employed in the fabrication of hydrogel-forming microneedles (HFMNs) have been extensively explored and tested for medical and dermatological applications, demonstrating essential properties such as biocompatibility and biodegradability. Figure 4 illustrates the benefits and drawbacks of various polymers used to fabricate MNs.

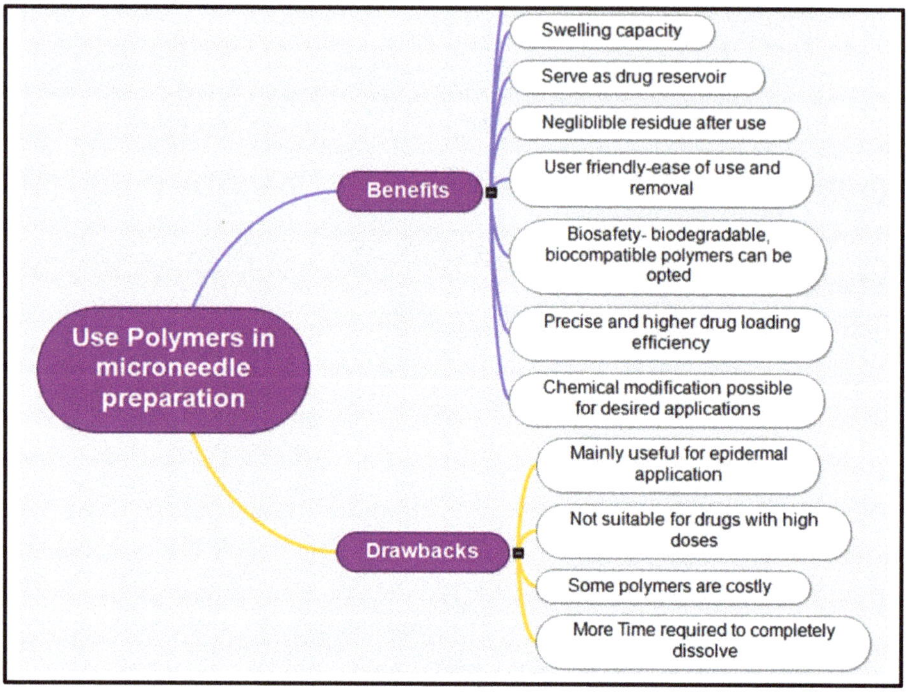

Figure 4. Benefits and drawbacks of polymeric MNs. Reproduced from [45] under CCBY 3.0.

4.1.1. Natural Polymers Fabricated Hydrogel-Forming Microneedles

Biocompatible polymeric materials derived from natural sources that can form hydrogels are commonly utilized in the fabrication of microneedles (MNs). In carbohydrate-based MNs, natural polysaccharides such as chitosan, cellulose, and starch are used to develop the hydrogel matrix. Protein-based MNs often incorporate gelatin or silk fibroin as the matrix-forming components. These MNs are characterized by their biocompatibility, biodegradability, and non-toxicity, exhibiting properties such as swelling capacity. Natural polymer-based hydrogel MNs have demonstrated promising results in drug delivery, wound healing, and dermal vaccination applications [46].

Chitosan and Chitosan Derivatives

Chitosan (CH) is an alkaline copolymer of glucosamine and N-acetylglucosamine derived from chitin, which originates from lower organisms such as certain algae, fungi, invertebrates, insects, and crustaceans [47]. This material is valued for its excellent biocompatibility, biodegradability, and antimicrobial properties, making it a key component in food and biomedical engineering. Chitosan derivatives are also extensively used in the fabrication of various drug delivery systems, cosmetics, and water treatment applications due to their enhanced water solubility and antibacterial activity, which result from the effective interaction of carboxymethyl groups with water and their natural biocompatibility [48].

Chitosan-based HFMNs have been investigated for transmucosal vaccine delivery, including through the mouth and nasal passages. In a study by Bobbala and Hook, an antigen was delivered using chitosan-based HFMNs to the oral mucosa in a rat model, resulting in a robust immune response. This finding suggests that HFMNs could be a viable method for oral vaccine delivery [49]. In Haojie Wei's study, HFMNs were fabricated using chitosan and pullulan to enhance dermal drug delivery. The research involved two types of hydrogels: carboxymethyl chitosan–silk fibroin and oxidized pullulan, noted for their excellent swelling and water retention capabilities. These hydrogels were used to develop MNs loaded with *Salvia miltiorrhiza*, named HFMNs-1 (prepared using chitosan) and HFMNs-2 (prepared using pullulan). The results showed that HFMNs-1 had excellent mechanical properties and allowed for rapid drug release when applied to newborn porcine skin. These findings highlight the potential of natural polymer-based hydrogel MNs for effective, painless, and biocompatible dermal drug delivery [50].

Hyaluronic Acid

Hyaluronic acid (HA) is a glycosaminoglycan found in epithelial and dermal layers, as well as in connective tissue. Approximately 50% of the body's total HA is located in the skin. The body degrades about one-third of its HA daily, replacing it with newly synthesized HA. Under normal physiological conditions, HA is converted to its more hydrophilic sodium salt form. Moreover, due to the numerous hydroxyl groups, HA can retain up to 1000 times its weight in water. This exceptional water-holding capacity supports various physiological functions and homeostatic processes in the body. HA-based microneedles (HA-MNs) are known for their high biocompatibility and resistance to deformation, and they are commonly used in skincare products [51].

Additionally, HA-based microneedles (HA-MNs) are robust enough to penetrate the skin effectively, dissolve quickly, and release drugs or active ingredients within a controlled, short time frame. The fabrication of HA-MNs does not require heating or organic solvents, which helps preserve and maintain the stability of heat-sensitive or chemically unstable agents, such as insulin [52]. Moreover, hyaluronic acid (HA) of varying molecular weights can impact the skin differently. High-molecular-weight HA has anti-aging effects, forms a protective film on the skin's surface, and retains moisture, whereas medium-molecular-weight and low-molecular-weight HA can penetrate deeper into the skin, providing moisturizing benefits. Due to these advantageous properties, HA is a compelling choice as a base material for dermal delivery of active ingredients via microneedles (MNs) [53].

Sodium Alginate

Sodium alginate is a linear polysaccharide extracted from brown algae. It consists of 1,4-β-d-mannuronic (M) and α-L-guluronic (G) acids in varying proportions, resulting in a highly viscous aqueous solution. Due to its abundance of carboxyl and hydroxyl groups, sodium alginate exhibits significant chemical activity and can quickly form a hydrogel with a three-dimensional network structure. It is non-toxic, odorless, and known for its excellent biocompatibility and environmental friendliness. Sodium alginate has been safely used in dental applications, such as impression materials, since the 1950s. Additionally, sodium alginate and its derivatives are readily available, cost-effective, and renewable [54].

A study by Atefeh Malek-Khatab developed a new approach to treating acne using sodium alginate and gelatin microneedle (MN) patches loaded with clindamycin. The study focused on developing MNs with varying concentrations of clindamycin hydrochloride (6, 8, and 10 μmol/L) and assessed their mechanical strength, density, and drug release behavior. The results indicated that the addition of gelatin enhanced the mechanical properties and density of the MNs, while the concentration of clindamycin influenced the drug release profile. The MNs successfully penetrated pig cadaver skin and inhibited the growth of Cutibacterium acnes without harming normal human dermal fibroblast cells, suggesting a practical option for treating acne [53].

4.1.2. Synthetic Polymers Fabricated Hydrogel-Forming Microneedles

Microneedles (MNs) fabricated using synthetic polymers offer advantages in controlled drug delivery due to their ability to dissolve or swell in response to moisture or heat. This responsiveness allows for the precise release of medications or other therapeutic agents into the body. Compared to natural polymer-based MNs, those made from synthetic polymers typically exhibit more consistent and robust mechanical properties, enhancing their overall effectiveness and reliability. Furthermore, synthetic polymers can be tailored to achieve specific characteristics, such as adjustable degradation rates, which adds flexibility to their applications in drug delivery systems.

Poly(vinyl) Alcohol

Poly(vinyl) alcohol is a water-soluble, polar synthetic polymer known for its excellent biocompatibility and biodegradability, along with its inherent non-toxicity and favorable mechanical properties. Poly(vinyl) alcohol can be crosslinked either chemically or physically to fabricate hydrogels. Additionally, due to their wound-healing capabilities, which involve the upregulation of transforming growth factor beta, poly(vinyl) alcohol hydrogels are frequently employed as matrix materials in wound dressings [55]. Samant and Prausnitz demonstrated the capability of crosslinked poly(vinyl) alcohol HFMNs to extract interstitial fluid. In their study, the HFMNs achieved an extraction rate of 0.0030 μL per MN volume after 12 h of use on porcine skin, compared to a 0.0039 μL extraction rate using micropores after just 20 min. These findings further validated that crosslinked poly(vinyl) alcohol, when used alone without additional polymers, exhibits a slower swelling rate [56]. In another study, Tang et al. modified a 10 wt. % poly(vinyl) alcohol formulation by incorporating Cy5.5 and poly(ethylene glycol) methyl ether amine. This modification enhanced both the water solubility and water retention of the HFMNs. In addition, the inclusion of Cy5.5, a commonly used dye, facilitated the fluorescence-based detection of the HFMNs during application [57].

Methacrylate-Based Hyaluronic Acid

Chemical modification of HA with methacrylic acid (MA) yields methacrylate-based hyaluronic acid (HAMA). This modification results in a composite-based hydrogel characterized by a continuous three-dimensional network structure, which imparts excellent swelling properties, mechanical strength, and drug-loading capacity. The HAMA hydrogel maintains high stability under simulated human physiological conditions (pH 7.4) [58]. Xu et al. utilized HAMA to develop an HFMN patch for managing diabetic ulcers. This HFMN patch, which incorporates platelet-derived growth factor D and human adipose-derived stem cells, was tested in a diabetic mouse model and demonstrated efficacy in promoting angiogenesis and enhancing wound healing [59].

Gantrez S-97

Grantrez S-97 is a versatile hydrophilic polymer primarily composed of methyl vinyl ether and maleic anhydride. Its structure includes vicinal dicarboxylic acid functionalities, which enhance its chelating properties for metal ions such as iron, magnesium, zinc, and calcium. Moreover, this polymer is recognized for its unique properties, making it suitable for various applications, particularly in the pharmaceuticals, personal care, and food industries. A study reported by the Donnelly group using Grantrez S-97, PEG, and sodium bicarbonate demonstrated robust and effective penetration with extensively swellable HFMNs [60].

4.2. Techniques Involved in the Fabrication of Hydrogel-Forming Microneedle Arrays

Hydrogel-forming microneedles can be easily fabricated using various methods, depending on the hydrogel-forming polymeric materials and the crosslinking mechanisms employed [61]. As outlined in the previous subsections, the materials include both natural and synthetic polymers. These polymers can undergo physical crosslinking, electrostatic interactions, or chemical crosslinking to form hydrogels, which are subsequently shaped into microneedle patches, as described in this section.

The fabrication of hydrogel-forming microneedles (HFMNs) is a detailed process involving several steps: mold development, hydrogel formulation, casting, and post-fabrication treatments. First, an MN-shaped mold is precisely created using advanced photolithography or micro-molding techniques. Next, biocompatible polymeric materials are carefully mixed with a suitable crosslinking agent to form a customized hydrogel. This hydrogel is then poured or injected into the mold cavities, with vacuum or centrifugation employed to eliminate any air bubbles. Afterward, the hydrogel is crosslinked, either chemically or physically, to ensure uniformity and structural integrity. Finally, post-fabrication treatments, such as dehydration, sterilization, and surface modifications, are applied to enhance drug loading, release properties, and mechanical strength [62,63]. Figure 5 illustrates a generalized technique for fabricating microneedles (MNs) using a poloxamer solution through a cold method. Researchers developed a sustained dermal drug delivery system utilizing thermoresponsive poloxamers, which formed depots within the skin micropores after MN application. The optimized MN arrays demonstrated good mechanical strength and sustained drug release for 96 h. This sustained release was further confirmed by confocal microscopy, which revealed a higher fluorescence intensity of fluorescein sodium within the skin tissue [64].

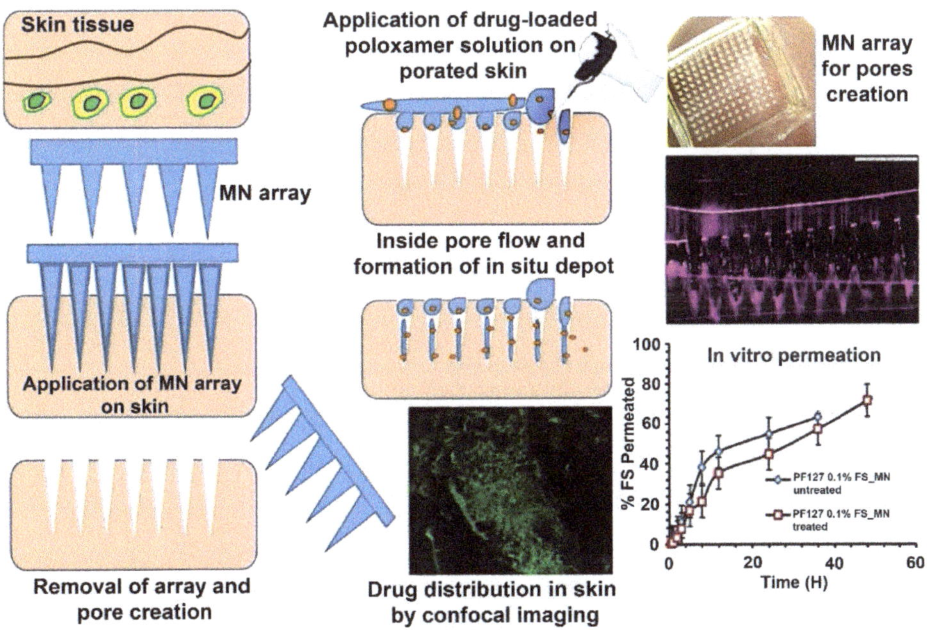

Figure 5. Illustration for development of in situ depot-forming MNs using poloxamer gels. Transition is loaded into the MN pores, and in situ gels are developed at body temperature. Reproduced with permission from [64] under CCBY.

4.2.1. Casting

Casting is a widely used method for developing hydrogel-forming microneedles (HFMNs). The process begins with creating a master mold in the desired MN shape using photolithography or microfabrication techniques. A hydrogel solution, containing water-soluble monomers, catalysts, and active ingredients, is then poured into this mold. Solidification occurs through crosslinking, typically achieved by UV exposure, heat, or a chemical agent. Once solidified, the MNs are extracted from the mold. The casting technique allows for the production of MNs with intricate shapes and sizes that can be tailored for specific applications. It also facilitates the incorporation of bioactive agents, such as drugs, peptides, or growth factors, into the hydrogel, enabling controlled release upon skin insertion. This method is favored for its simplicity, cost-effectiveness, and scalability, making it suitable for a variety of biomedical applications [65]. However, casting presents several challenges, including limited control over microneedle geometry, the risk of air bubble formation, and difficulties in achieving uniform consistency [63].

4.2.2. Electrospinning

Electrospinning employs a high-voltage electric field to draw a biodegradable polymer solution, such as poly(vinyl) alcohol, into a thin jet. As the jet moves toward a collector, the solvent evaporates, causing the polymer to solidify into a fibrous mat. Hydrogel-forming microneedles (HFMNs) are subsequently created by coating these fibers with poly(vinyl) pyrrolidone or hyaluronic acid (HA). By adjusting parameters such as voltage, flow rate, and the distance between the needle and collector, microneedles of various shapes and sizes can be produced [50,66]. MNs produced through electrospinning have a high aspect ratio, meaning their length is significantly greater than their width, which enhances skin penetration efficiency. Additionally, the electrospun polymer allows for controlled release of drugs or active agents, as manufacturers can fine-tune the diameter, length, and porous structure of the MNs by adjusting the electrospinning parameters. However, the electrospinning process is relatively complex and requires specialized equipment [67].

4.2.3. Micro-Molding Method

Micro-molding is a widely used method for preparing hydrogel-forming microneedles (HFMNs). Typically, polydimethylsiloxane (PDMS) casts are created by casting around a solid master template and curing at 70 °C for two hours. This process produces a negative micro-mold that can be reused to quickly fabricate multiple arrays of HFMNs, making it ideal for optimizing various parameters. In drug delivery applications, a two-step fabrication process is often employed, concentrating active ingredients at the tips of the HFMNs to enhance release efficiency [68]. Donnelly et al. employed laser machining controlled by a galvanometer and guided by pre-designed computer-aided designs to produce micro-molds. Their approach demonstrated the feasibility of producing and reusing these micro-molds for HFMN manufacturing, facilitating the development of specialized molds. In another study, Lutton et al. utilized injection molding to fabricate micro-molds. In their method, metal microneedle master templates were placed in an injection molding machine, where pre-mixed silicone elastomer was injected into the molds and subsequently cured to form the micro-molds [69].

Both casting and micro-molding techniques play crucial roles in the development of microneedles, each offering unique benefits that cater to different aspects of drug delivery technology. Table 2 summarizes the differences between these two techniques.

Table 2. Summary of the differences between casting and micro-molding techniques in the development of MNs.

Microneedles Through Casting Technique	Microneedles Through Micro-Molding Technique
Pouring liquid into molds	Developing a negative mold
A broad range of materials is utilized	Specialized polymeric materials are utilized
Moderate precision is observed	High precision is observed
Relative process is faster for large scale-up	Slower but scalable in fabrication
Flexible in design	High accuracy in clinical use

4.2.4. Solution-Cast Micro-Molding in the Fabrication of MNs

Solution-casting micro-molding is a notable method for fabricating hydrogel-forming microneedles (HFMNs), combining the advantages of both solution-casting and micro-molding techniques. This method is particularly effective for developing microneedles that can deliver drugs dermally while maintaining the properties of hydrogels, such as biocompatibility and controlled release. Smith et al. developed microneedles using the solution-cast micro-molding technique (vac-and-fill) with polymers such as polyvinyl pyrrolidone (either 20% or 40%) and hydroxyethyl cellulose with glycerol. This simple and cost-effective micro-molding technique eliminates air entrapment and bubble formation, which can reduce the reproducibility of the method [70]. However, while solution-cast micro-molding offers numerous benefits, challenges include ensuring adequate mechanical strength for effective skin penetration and maintaining stability during storage and use.

4.2.5. Additive Manufacturing in the Fabrication of MNs

Additive manufacturing, commonly known as 3D printing, has revolutionized the fabrication of microneedles (MNs), offering significant advantages over traditional manufacturing methods. This technology enables the development of customizable, complex MN arrays that can be tailored to specific applications in drug delivery. As technology advances, the integration of additive manufacturing techniques is likely to enhance the functionality and applicability of MNs in various biomedical fields. The inks used for hydrogel-forming MNs typically consist of polymers that can form hydrogels upon application, combined with other additives to enhance performance. Examples of these inks include dextran, hyaluronic acid, chitin, chitosan, methacrylate gelatin, Gantrez, alginate, poly(vinyl alcohol), poly(cyclopentyl methacrylate), polystyrene-block-poly(acrylic acid) (PSPAA), polylactic acid, poly(methyl methacrylate) (PMMA), polystyrene, and polycaprolactone [45]. Hydrogel-forming microneedles (MNs) are widely used due to their biocompatibility and swelling properties. The concentration of bio-ink used for these MNs is determined by several factors, including mechanical strength, swelling properties, biocompatibility, drug loading and release, crosslinking density, viscosity and printability, degradation rate, and penetration depth [45]. Baramee et al. investigated four different needle shapes: a pyramidal shape over a long cube, a cone mounted over a cylinder, a pyramidal shape, and a conical shape, using computer-aided design with varied compensated bases. The printed MN molds were developed using polylactic acid resin, and MN patches were further fabricated using hydroxypropyl methylcellulose and polyvinyl pyrrolidone. The results of tests for printing parameters (curing time, printing angle, and anti-aliasing), physical appearance, mechanical properties, and skin insertion ability revealed better physicochemical properties for the pyramidal shape over a long cube and the cone mounted over a cylinder compared to the pyramidal and conical shapes. This suggests that 3D-printed construct MNs could serve as an excellent alternative to conventional mold-based MNs [71]. In another study, Baramee et al. suggested that a 3D-printed MN construct could serve as an alternative to MNs prepared using conventional techniques by fabricating lidocaine HCl-loaded MNs for a faster onset of anesthetic action. Furthermore, this 3D construct was fortified with Oryza sativa L extract complex, demonstrating enhanced skin penetration via the transfollicular route, along with safety and efficacy for the management of keratinocytes [72].

4.3. Evaluation Methods for Hydrogel-Forming Microneedle Arrays

The materials, designs, and preparation methods are vital parameters that determine the properties of hydrogel-forming microneedles (HFMNs). Effective targeted delivery relies on optimal characteristics such as mechanical strength, biocompatibility, flexibility, hardness, degradability, skin permeation, and release kinetics of HFMNs. Additionally, factors like length and geometry, array configuration, coating options, and fabrication techniques—including micro-molding, 3D printing, and laser ablation—collectively contribute to the successful application of microneedles in drug delivery. Comprehensive evaluations necessary for microneedles encompass rheological characteristics of polymers, sol–gel transition properties, polymer–drug–polymer compatibility, morphology analysis, in vitro and ex vivo skin-swelling indices, water content, mechanical strength, insertion force over the skin, depth of penetration, in vitro permeation studies, and both in vitro and in vivo drug release assessments, as well as histopathology studies.

Rheological analysis of polymeric materials is crucial in developing and optimizing hydrogel-forming microneedles (HFMNs) as it provides essential information about the flow and deformation characteristics of polymeric hydrogels. These properties are pivotal in determining the suitability of hydrogels for microneedle fabrication and functionality. HFMNs utilize hydrogels that swell in moisture, making them ideal for dermal drug delivery. Consequently, key parameters such as viscosity (measured using a rheometer), elasticity, gelation kinetics, and swelling behavior are typically analyzed prior to HFMN development. This analysis ensures that the microneedles are effective, reliable, and suitable for their intended applications. As advancements in hydrogel technology continue, rheological analysis remains an essential tool for guiding the development of innovative and high-performance HFMNs [64].

Studies on drug–polymer compatibility are crucial for the development of hydrogel-forming microneedles (HFMNs). By examining the interactions between pharmaceuticals and the polymeric matrix, researchers can ensure the stability, effectiveness, and reliability of microneedle systems. This research focuses on evaluating the compatibility between therapeutic agents and the polymeric matrix used in hydrogels to guarantee effective drug delivery and optimal performance of the microneedle systems. Maintaining the therapeutic efficacy of medications is essential, as drug stability within hydrogel matrices can be compromised by incompatibility. Incompatible drug–polymer interactions may lead to a gradual deterioration or loss of drug potency, affect the chemical structure, or induce degradation, ultimately impacting the drug's effectiveness. Additionally, the compatibility of the drug and polymer significantly influences the controlled release of the therapeutic agent. Various spectroscopic methods, including Fourier-transform infrared spectroscopy (FTIR) and nuclear magnetic resonance spectroscopy (NMR), as well as chromatographic techniques such as advanced high-performance liquid chromatography (HPLC), are employed to assess drug–polymer compatibility [48,73,74].

The transition of a material from a liquid (sol) phase to a gel (solid) phase is referred to as the sol–gel transition. This fundamental phenomenon is observed in polymeric and colloidal systems and is crucial for various applications, including drug delivery, materials science, and biological processes [75]. The development of enhanced delivery systems and various applications relies heavily on the texture, mechanical strength, and release characteristics of hydrogel systems, all of which are influenced by the sol–gel transition properties. Hydrogel-forming microneedles (HFMNs) utilize hydrogels that undergo this transition to create a stable three-dimensional network, facilitating effective drug delivery. Therefore, evaluating sol–gel properties is of prime importance. Various methods have been reported for this evaluation, including rheological measurements, microscopy, mechanical testing, swelling assessments, degradation studies, and biocompatibility analyses [64,76].

Morphological examination of hydrogel-forming microneedles (MNs) is essential for understanding their structural integrity, functionality, and performance in applications. These tiny needles, designed to penetrate the skin's outer layer, rely on hydrogel materials for effective delivery. Analyzing the morphology of MNs aids in comprehending their architecture, enhancing functionality, and ensuring efficacy in drug delivery and diagnostics. This evaluation confirms that MNs maintain their shape and mechanical strength during and after insertion into the skin. It also ensures that the MNs possess consistent dimensions, which is crucial for reproducibility and effectiveness. Additionally, morphological analysis assesses swelling behavior. Various methods, such as field emission scanning electron microscopy (FESEM) and transmission electron microscopy (TEM), are utilized to analyze the structure of MNs [61,77]. Figure 6 illustrates a scanning electron microscopy (SEM) image of microneedles (MNs) fabricated using polydimethylsiloxane (PDMS) miniature round molds. Each mold has a diameter of 17.5 mm, with a spacing of 700 μm between the centers of adjacent needle tips. The needle tips feature a bottom diameter of 270 μm and a height of 500 μm. The hydrogel-forming microneedles (HFMNs) are fortified with vascular endothelial growth factor and ritlecitinib to promote the proliferation and development of hair follicle cells, thereby enhancing angiogenesis [78].

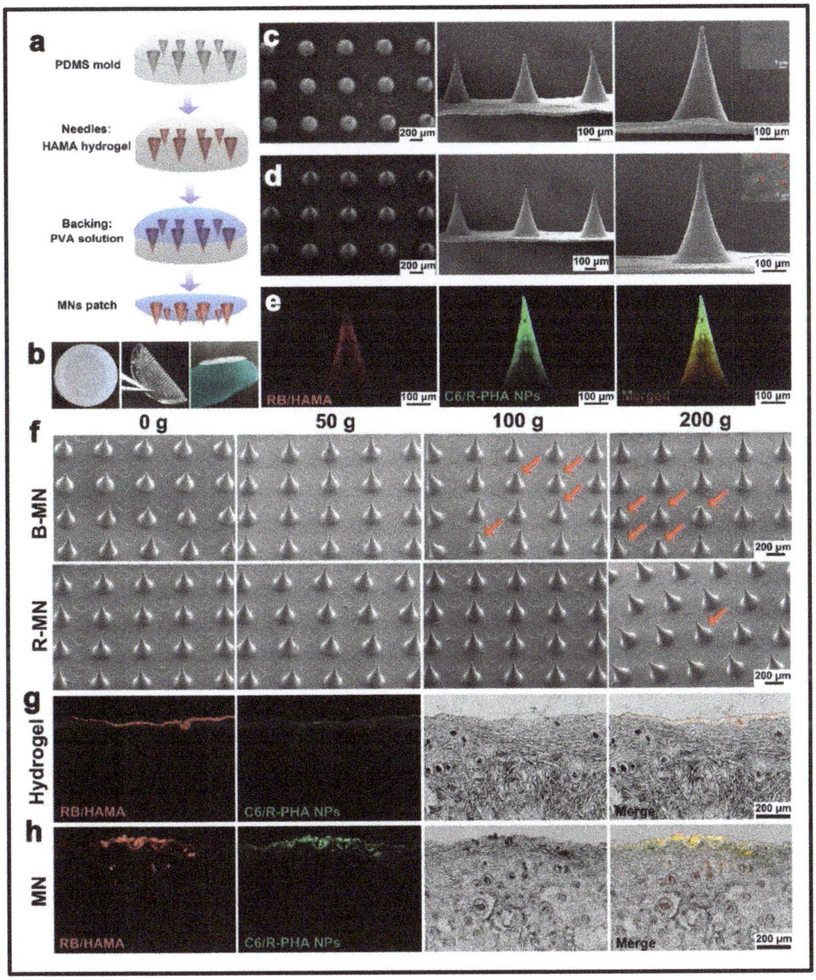

Figure 6. Illustrations of the fabrication process of HAMA-MNs (**a**) in PDMS mold (**b**). Scanning electron microscopy images of the blank HAMA hydrogel-forming microneedle (B-MN) patch (**c**), ritlecitinib–polyhydroxyalkanoate (R-PHA) NP-loaded HAMA-HFMN (R-MN) patch (**d**). Fluorescence microscopy images of the R-PHA NP-loaded HAMA-HFMNs (containing RB-labeled HAMA and coumarin 6-labeled R-PHA NPs) (**e**). Morphological changes in B-MN (blank HAMA-HFMN group) and R-MN (R-PHA NP-loaded HAMA-HFMN groups) after loading different mass weights (0, 50, 100, and 200 g) for 5 min (**f**). Representative fluorescence images of skin sections 24 h after topical application of fluorescence HAMA hydrogel (**g**) and fluorescence MNs (**h**), containing rhodamine B-labeled HAMA and coumarin 6-labeled R-PHA NPs. Reproduced with permission from [79] under CCBY-4.0.

One of the essential aspects of hydrogel-forming microneedle (HFMN) performance is the interaction with the skin, particularly regarding swelling behavior. Swelling studies are crucial for understanding how hydrogel MNs absorb interstitial fluid, expand, and release drugs [80]. Swelling behavior directly affects the release kinetics of therapeutic agents, and the extent of swelling influences the penetrability of microneedles (MNs) into the skin. To evaluate the swelling efficacy of the hydrogel-forming microneedle (HFMN) array, it is placed in contact with water and assessed at specific time intervals. Another method involves an ex vivo study using porcine skin, where the subcutaneous layer is removed. The HFMN patches are punctured into the isolated skin and then removed at designated time intervals to measure base-width capacity. Additionally, swelling is further tested concerning the water insolubility of HFMNs by placing the MNs in contact with water, followed by drying at 90 °C to compare the initial and final weights [81] (Figure 7).

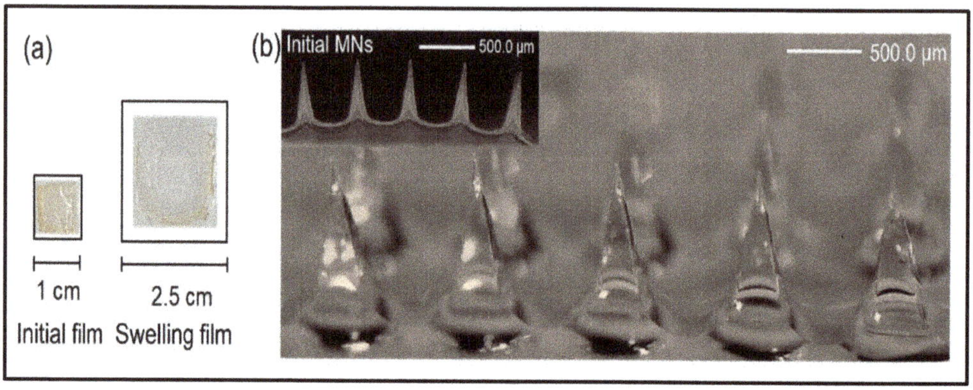

Figure 7. Swelling degree illustration for HFMNs in a comparative evaluation from the top view (**a**) and front view (**b**). Reproduced from [81] under CCBY-4.0.

Furthermore, the water content of hydrogel-forming microneedles (HFMNs) is crucial for their development and application, particularly in drug delivery and diagnostic systems. Water content influences various properties of hydrogels, including swelling behavior, mechanical characteristics, drug release rates, and overall stability. Therefore, accurate measurement and control of water content are essential to ensure the optimal performance and safety of microneedles. Swelling behavior significantly affects the effectiveness of hydrogels within microneedles, as higher water content typically results in more pronounced swelling. Mechanical properties also impact the ease of insertion and stability of microneedles. Additionally, appropriate water content can influence penetration and insertion, drug delivery efficiency, shelf life, and stability. By effectively managing these aspects, researchers and manufacturers can enhance the functionality and reliability of microneedle systems, ensuring effective performance and improved outcomes in medicinal applications.

For hydrogel-forming microneedles (HFMNs), mechanical strength is a crucial factor that impacts skin insertion, drug distribution, and overall durability. The primary objective of the mechanical assessment is to evaluate the resilience of microneedles to forces that could cause deformation, fracture, or failure. Key parameters in assessing mechanical strength include hardness, tensile strength, and fracture resistance. The mechanical strength of HFMNs is influenced by several factors, such as the composition of the polymeric hydrogel, manufacturing processes, and environmental conditions. Hardness measures a material's resistance to indentation and abrasion, ensuring structural integrity and wear resistance during insertion and drug delivery. In contrast, tensile strength assesses the durability and flexibility of the material, while fracture resistance indicates its ability to withstand crack propagation and breakage under stress. Hydrogel composition and crosslinking density are also significant, with higher polymer concentrations typically enhancing strength. Additionally, manufacturing processes, including molding precision and drying conditions, can affect mechanical properties. Environmental factors, such as moisture and temperature variations, further influence these properties. Adhering to testing standards and implementing rigorous quality control measures are essential for optimizing microneedle design and performance [81,82].

Systems such as universal testing machines and custom force sensors are commonly employed to measure insertion force for microneedles (MNs). Various factors influence the required force, including MN design, geometry, needle tip shape, hydrogel properties, skin characteristics, hydration levels, and insertion speed. Evaluating comfort and user experience is critical, as lower insertion forces are generally associated with reduced discomfort for patients. Adherence to standardized testing protocols ensures consistency and reliability in measuring insertion force. By optimizing these parameters and following established testing guidelines, researchers and manufacturers can enhance MN performance, improve patient comfort, and ensure effective application in medical and diagnostic fields [83]. In a study conducted by Dawud et al. on hydrogel-forming microneedles (HFMNs) featuring programmed mesophase transitions for controlled drug delivery, the insertion force was tested on chicken skin at a vertical insertion rate of 1 mm/min until a desired normal force of 20 N was achieved. Following this, a dwell time of 30 s was maintained under the loaded state. The results indicated that an average insertion force of approximately 100 mN per needle was required when tested through a Parafilm skin-simulating model, as illustrated in Figure 8 [84].

The depth of penetration of hydrogel-forming microneedles (HFMNs) into the skin is critical for effective drug delivery and diagnostic applications. Evaluating this depth is essential to determine the effectiveness and safety of microneedles in accessing the targeted layers of the skin [85]. Various measurement techniques are utilized to assess the depth of penetration of hydrogel-forming microneedles (HFMNs), including optical microscopy, histological analysis, advanced imaging techniques, and mechanical testing. Factors influencing penetration depth encompass microneedle design, hydrogel properties, skin characteristics, and insertion conditions. Generally, microneedles with longer lengths and larger diameters tend to achieve deeper penetration, while sharper tips enhance effectiveness [86]. For effective penetration, hydrogels with high swelling behavior and mechanical properties must be optimized. Skin characteristics, including thickness, elasticity, and the speed and pressure of injection, significantly influence penetration depth. Establishing evaluation protocols is crucial for obtaining reliable results in depth penetration studies. Standardized testing environments, which include consistent skin types, hydration levels, and insertion speeds, help ensure accurate and reproducible measurements. Safety considerations involve assessing potential tissue damage or irritation caused by microneedles during penetration. Histological analysis can identify adverse effects on skin tissues, while risk assessments evaluate the potential impacts of penetration depth on overall skin health and device performance [87]. Yu and colleagues developed layered dissolving microneedles (MNs) fortified with the immunosuppressant tacrolimus and diclofenac to alleviate skin and joint lesions in psoriatic arthritis. They tested the insertion depth on full-thickness rat skin using a force of 30 N for 5 min. Optical coherence tomography images, as shown in Figures 8 and 9, indicated an insertion depth of approximately 300 μm through a 100 μm Parafilm layer covering the skin. Furthermore, the puncture hole ratio revealed a remarkable 100% pore creation, confirming that the thicknesses of the stratum corneum (SC), viable epidermis, and dermis are 10–20 μm, 50–100 μm, and 1–3 mm, respectively. This suggests that the fabricated HFMNs can effectively penetrate and deliver the loaded drug to deeper sites [78].

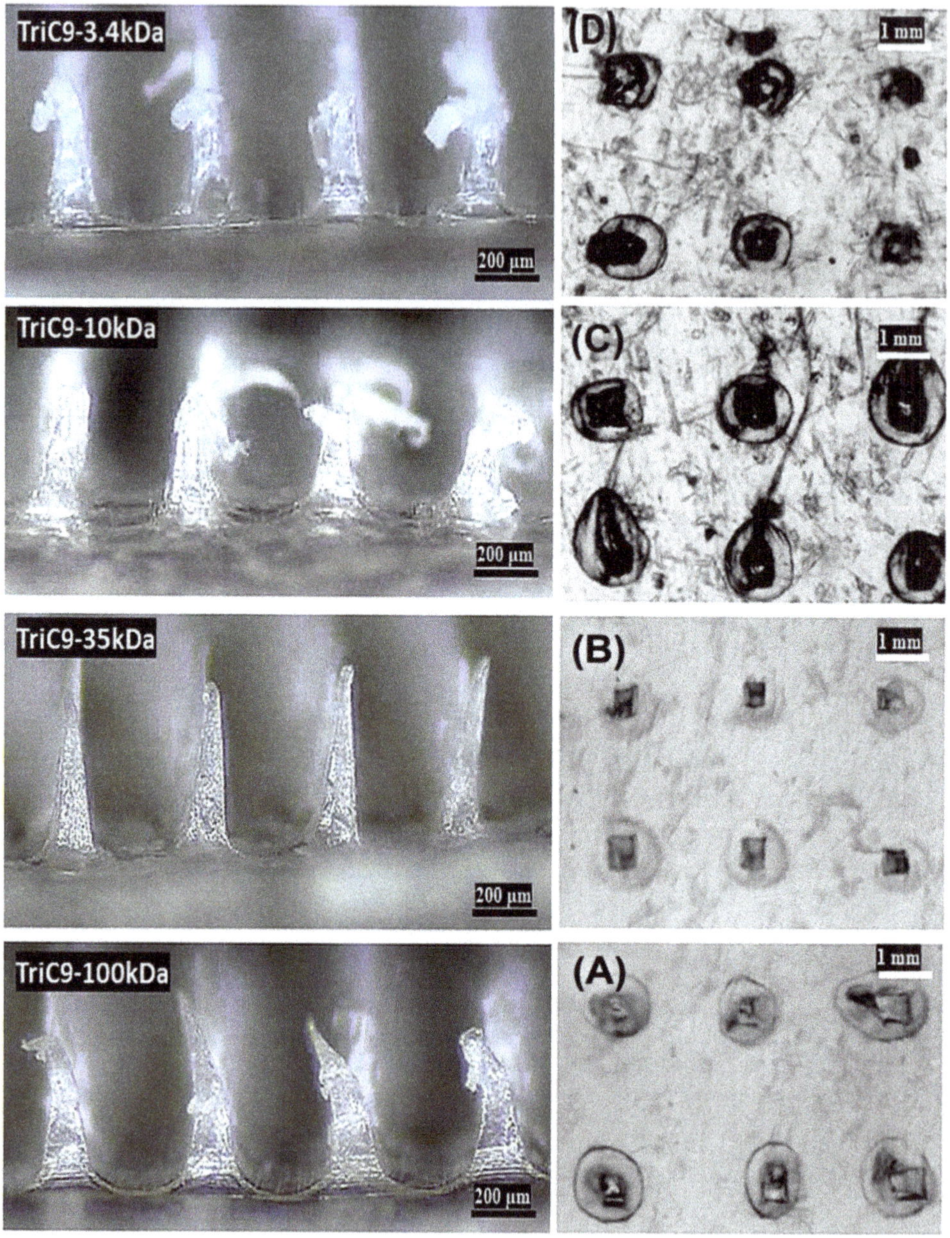

Figure 8. Insertion test in the Parafilm skin-simulant model. Percentage of holes created in the first two Parafilm layers by the MNs (**A**), height of MNs post-insertion to Parafilm layers (**B**), MN bending after insertion into the Parafilm layer (**C**), and the holes observed on the first layer by each MN patch (**D**). Reproduced with permission from [84] under CCBY-4.0.

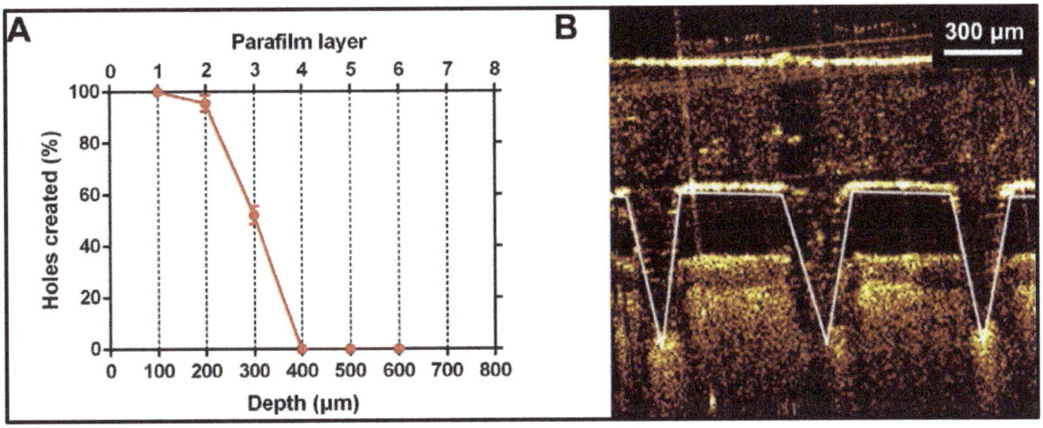

Figure 9. Illustration for insertion depth of MNs in (**A**) an artificial membrane and (**B**) rat skin using optical microscopy. Reproduced with permission from [78] under CCBY-NC-ND 4.0.

To understand how a drug is released from microneedles (MNs) over time, evaluating drug release profiles is essential. Typically, in vitro release experiments are conducted to assess the release profile, followed by fitting the data to various kinetic models, such as zero-order, first-order, Higuchi, and Korsmeyer–Peppas [43]. Furthermore, in vitro permeation studies are crucial for evaluating the effectiveness of hydrogel-forming microneedles (HFMNs) in delivering therapeutic agents across the skin. These studies provide insights into drug transport, formulation optimization, and safety compliance. The study involves several key components and procedures, including the selection of skin models, experimental setups, preparation of MNs, application to skin, and subsequent collection and analysis of data. While human skin is typically preferred due to its relevance to human applications, ethical concerns and availability may limit its use. Franz diffusion assembly is commonly employed to investigate drug diffusion across skin or membrane samples, utilizing either animal or synthetic membranes. The procedure includes loading the drug into the hydrogel matrix, curing the MNs, and ensuring they are adequately hydrated before application [88]. The application duration of hydrogel-forming microneedles (HFMNs) is optimized based on the type of microneedles used and the therapeutic requirements. Samples from the receptor compartment are collected at various intervals and analyzed to determine drug concentration. Understanding these methodologies and key parameters is essential for ensuring that MNs meet the required efficacy and safety standards. In vitro permeation studies are critical for evaluating the drug delivery capabilities of HFMNs and their effectiveness in clinical applications. Key parameters such as permeation rate, flux, lag time, and cumulative permeation provide valuable insights into the performance of the MNs. Factors influencing permeation include MN design, hydrogel properties, drug characteristics, and skin conditions. Generally, longer or sharper MNs achieve better permeation, while hydrogels with optimal properties facilitate effective drug delivery. Additionally, drug properties—such as solubility and molecular size—impact delivery efficacy, and skin characteristics—like thickness and hydration—can affect drug permeability. Pre-existing skin conditions or treatments may also influence permeation results, as can application parameters such as duration and pressure. Consistent application techniques are essential for obtaining reliable and reproducible results [61,88].

Histopathological studies are essential for assessing the safety and effectiveness of hydrogel-forming microneedles (HFMNs). These studies analyze tissue responses at a microscopic level to identify potential damage, irritation, or adverse effects. Understanding the results is crucial for ensuring that MNs are safe for use and perform as intended without causing significant harm to the skin. This detailed examination offers valuable insights into the biocompatibility and overall safety profile of MNs. Histopathology studies are vital for several reasons: they help elucidate the skin's reaction to MNs, identify any inflammatory responses, and detect cellular damage or structural changes that may occur following MN application. Furthermore, these studies ensure biocompatibility by assessing whether the MNs and their components are compatible with skin tissues and do not induce harmful reactions [89]. Key parameters evaluated during histopathology studies include inflammation, cellular damage, structural changes, and the healing response. Several factors can influence the outcomes of these studies, such as microneedle design and properties, application parameters, the type and condition of the skin model used, and the duration of the study. Specifically, the design of the microneedles, along with how they are applied, significantly impacts the histopathological results, highlighting the importance of these variables in assessing the safety and efficacy of microneedle applications [90]. Ripolin et al. developed hydrogel-forming microneedles (HFMNs) fortified with alendronic acid and risedronate sodium to enhance the management of osteoporosis. In vivo testing on osteoporotic female Sprague Dawley rats demonstrated that the HFMNs significantly improved mean serum bone alkaline phosphatase levels, bone volume, and porosity compared to untreated bilateral ovariectomy controls. Furthermore, photomicrographs, as shown in Figure 10, revealed the active presence of inflammatory cells in the epidermis and dermis of animals treated with the microarray patch. Notably, the alendronic acid formulation exhibited more pronounced visible skin reactions and a greater presence of inflammatory cells in the dermis compared to the risedronate formulation [91].

Lastly, biocompatibility is a crucial evaluation parameter for hydrogel-forming microneedles (HFMNs), as it determines their safety and efficacy in medical applications. This assessment ensures that microneedles do not provoke harmful immune responses, cytotoxic effects, or other negative interactions with tissues. Evaluating biocompatibility is essential for confirming that HFMNs can be safely integrated into clinical settings without compromising patient health [92]. Biocompatibility is essential for several reasons, including safety, regulatory compliance, and effectiveness. To assess biocompatibility, various testing methods are employed, such as in vitro and in vivo tests, histopathological analyses, clinical studies, and long-term safety monitoring. These evaluations ensure that hydrogel-forming microneedles (HFMNs) interact safely with biological tissues and maintain their intended therapeutic effects without causing adverse reactions [92]. Key biocompatibility parameters for hydrogel-forming microneedles (HFMNs) include cytotoxicity, skin irritation, sensitization, inflammatory response, and the healing and repair processes. Several factors influence biocompatibility, such as material composition, microneedle design, application parameters, skin characteristics, and the testing methods employed. Material composition encompasses hydrogel properties, additives, and potential contaminants. Additionally, MN design, injection depth and pressure, duration of contact, and specific skin characteristics all play significant roles in determining the overall biocompatibility of the device [93]. Microneedle design, including factors such as size, shape, and surface properties, significantly impacts tissue penetration and the subsequent biological response. Application parameters, including injection depth, pressure, duration of contact, and specific skin characteristics, also play critical roles in determining biocompatibility. These elements collectively influence how the microneedles interact with the skin, affecting both safety and efficacy [94].

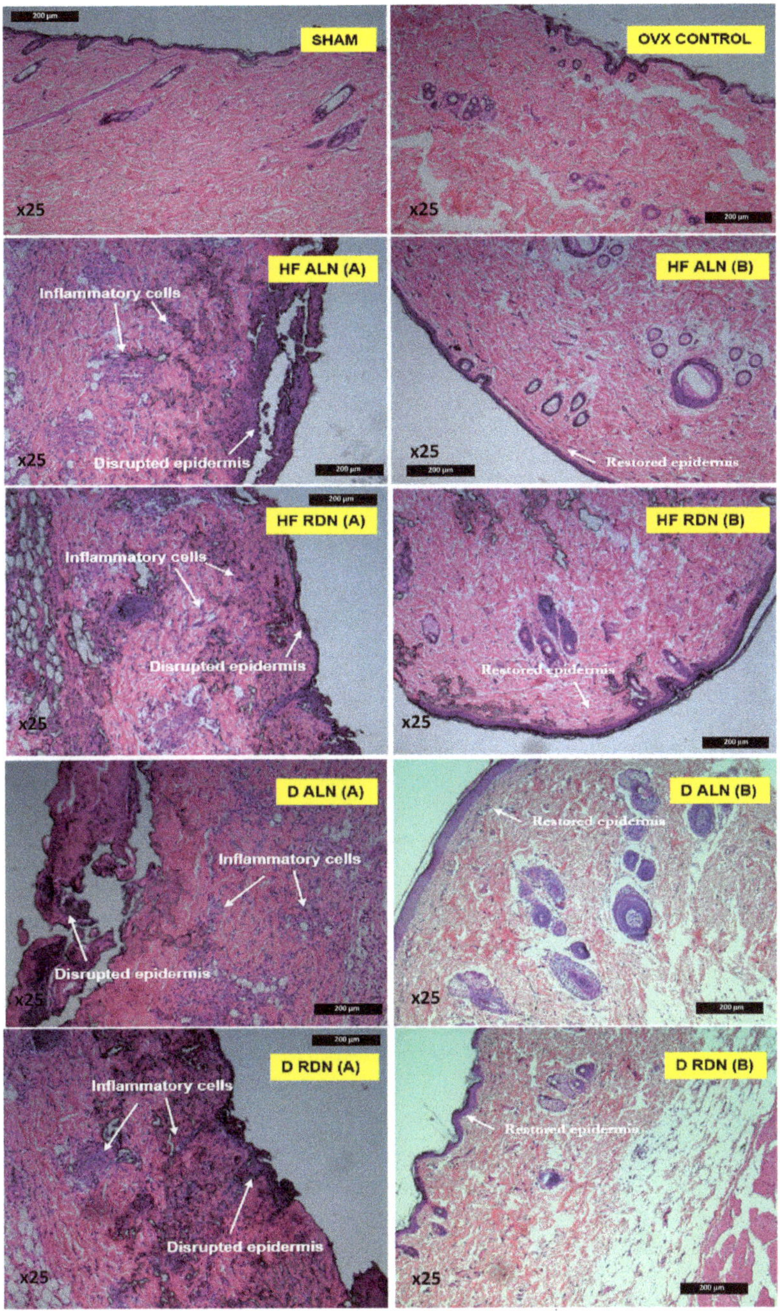

Figure 10. Annotated histological slides of SHAM and ovariectomy (OVX) control skin samples, as well as (**A**) regions of active inflammation for each MAP cohort, i.e., alendronic acid and risedronate sodium (RDN) [95] and (**B**) skin restoration images for post-application. Reproduced with permission from [96] under CCBY-4.0.

5. Application of Hydrogel-Forming Microneedles

In the realm of nanotechnology-enabled dermal drug delivery, hydrogel and in situ gel-forming microneedles (MNs) represent cutting-edge alternatives with significant potential for treating various skin-related conditions. These advanced MN systems enable controlled, precise, and efficient drug administration to specific skin layers, thereby enhancing therapeutic outcomes and reducing systemic side effects. HFMNs are designed to penetrate the stratum corneum and deliver therapeutic agents into the viable epidermis and dermis, offering promising applications for managing a range of skin-associated diseases. By targeting these layers directly, hydrogel and in situ gel-forming MNs improve the effectiveness of treatments while minimizing adverse systemic effects.

Naser and co-workers developed poly(ethylene glycol)-based hydrogel-forming microneedles (HFMNs) utilizing a solid dispersion reservoir to deliver a micro-depot of atorvastatin (see Figure 11). The study revealed that approximately 2.05 mg of the drug was released from the dispersion over a 24 h period through an ex vivo diffusion compartment, maintaining therapeutic concentrations of over 20 ng/mL for up to 14 days. This indicates a tenfold increase in systemic exposure levels, which could enhance patient compliance significantly [97]. In another study, Courtenay et al. developed hydrogel-forming microneedles (HFMNs) for esketamine to address challenges associated with parental administration. Analysis of blood plasma samples revealed enhanced permeation of esketamine, demonstrating concentrations exceeding the required therapeutic range of 0.15 to 0.3 μg/mL over a 24 h period [98]. Turner et al. developed an array of hydrogel-forming microneedles (HFMNs) for the controlled delivery of amoxicillin and vancomycin. Their evaluation demonstrated potent antimicrobial activity against *Escherichia coli* and *Staphylococcus aureus*, highlighting HFMNs as a promising alternative to conventional formulations [99]. Jadach et al. fabricated an array of hydrogel-forming microneedles (HFMNs) coated with clotrimazole to treat fungal infections caused by skin mycosis. Their findings revealed that the application of clotrimazole effectively inhibited the growth of *Candida albicans*, as demonstrated by the suspension-plate technique. Additionally, the microneedles coated with clotrimazole dissolved in hydrogel exhibited superior antifungal action compared to conventional formulations [96]. Abraham et al. prepared hydrogel-forming microneedles (HFMNs) composed of rifampicin. Their findings revealed a dermal permeation profile that demonstrated approximately 500 μg of rifampicin penetration, along with a four-fold increase in rifampicin deposition (around 80 μg) within the skin layers. This study suggests that smart films can serve as innovative drug reservoirs for HFMNs, enhancing drug loading and diffusion characteristics through the hydrogel matrix [100].

Tekko et al. developed a hydrogel-forming microneedle (HFMN) array for the delivery of methotrexate, targeting arthritis treatment. The study found that the HFMNs exhibited mild swelling characteristics alongside acceptable mechanical strength, demonstrating effective insertion into excised newborn pig skin. The patch-like reservoir was loaded with a high dose of methotrexate (150.3 $\pm$ 5.3 μg/mg) without causing precipitation. An ex vivo study indicated that the integrated patch delivered methotrexate at a steady-state flow rate of 506.8 $\pm$ 136.9 $\mu g/cm^2/h$ [101]. In another study, Yadav et al. fabricated super swelling hydrogel-forming microneedles (HFMNs) for the delivery of ibuprofen sodium. In vitro diffusion experiments conducted over excised pig skin demonstrated the release of approximately 20% of the loaded ibuprofen sodium from the lyophilized wafer within 24 h. The findings suggest that enhancing drug transport through the skin can be achieved by increasing the solubility of ibuprofen sodium in the reservoir [102]. Mahfufah et al. developed a hydrogel-forming microneedle (HFMN) system for the delivery of albendazole to treat parasitic infections. Investigations into skin integrity showed no alterations due to the penetration of HFMNs into the skin. Furthermore, ex vivo permeation tests utilizing a polyethylene glycol (PEG) reservoir demonstrated a penetration of 4584.43 $\pm$ 26.61 $\mu g/cm^2$ of albendazole into the skin [103]. Yi et al. developed HFMNs of GelMa encapsulated with quercetin to evaluate wound healing activity. It was demonstrated that quercetin HMNs aided in wound healing in both in vitro and in vivo settings, encouraging the production of collagen and neo-angiogenesis while decreasing oxidative stress. As a result, increased vascularization and collagen production were observed, suggesting that the given HFMN array can promote wound healing (Figure 12) [104]. Yao et al. developed an HFMN array patch loaded with stem cell-derived mitochondrial extracellular vesicles to improve wound healing. Metformin was used to enhance mitochondrial biogenesis. The findings reveal that the array patch enhances the healing process in in vivo examinations [105].

Interstitial fluid is used as an alternative to blood for quantifying the exogenous content administered; however, current strategies require sophisticated instruments that consume both time and resources for patients. Recent studies have demonstrated that MNs are a potential substitute for these methods. Li et al. developed surface-enhanced Raman spectroscopy MNs fortified with dye and mitoxantrone. In contrast, a gold–silver substrate with a hydrogel coating was used to compare painless, real-time analysis of drugs in dermal interstitial fluid after intravenous injection. The pharmacokinetic data suggested that mitoxantrone concentration was comparable in blood and dermal interstitial fluid, although the concentration of mitoxantrone in dermal interstitial fluid was 2–3 orders of magnitude lower than in blood, providing insightful information into the potential of dermal interstitial fluid as an alternative to blood for in vivo drug detection [106]. In another study, Razzaghi and co-workers developed MNs made of polyethylene glycol diacrylate as a device that acts as a biomarker in interstitial skin fluid within minutes of insertion, successfully managing metabolic disorders [107].

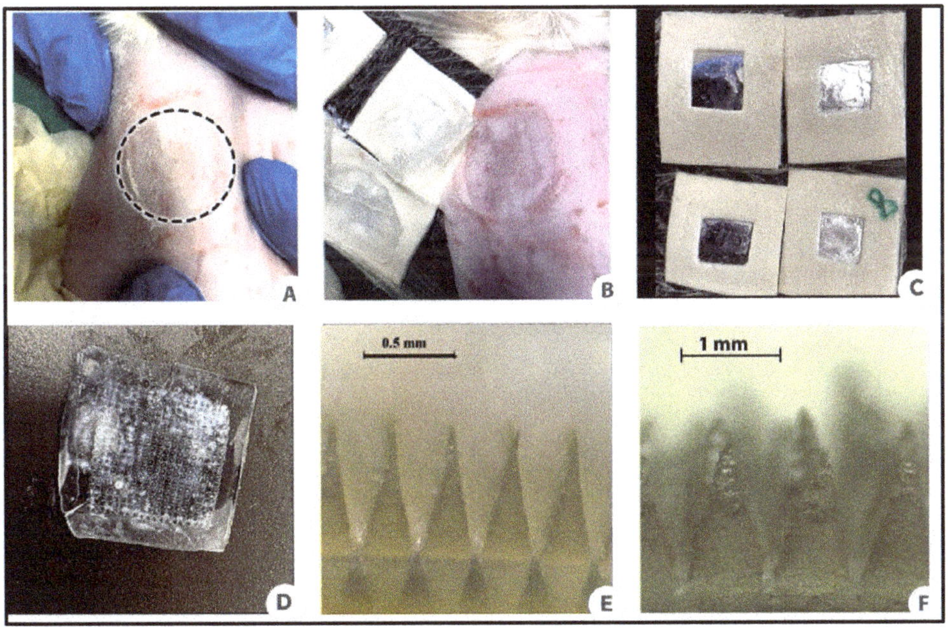

Figure 11. Macroscopic illustration captured after 24 h of HFMN applications and immediately upon HFMN removal, site of application of HFMNs (**A**), easy removal of swollen HFMNs in intact form (**B**), backing adhesive layer, where the reservoirs were inserted before their application (**C**), swollen HFMNs after removal from skin and backing layer (**D**), microscopic image of HFMNs prior to insertion into skin at scale bar of 0.5 mm (**E**), and microscopic images after insertion at scale bar of 1.0 mm (**F**). Reproduced with permission from [97] under CC BY 4.0.

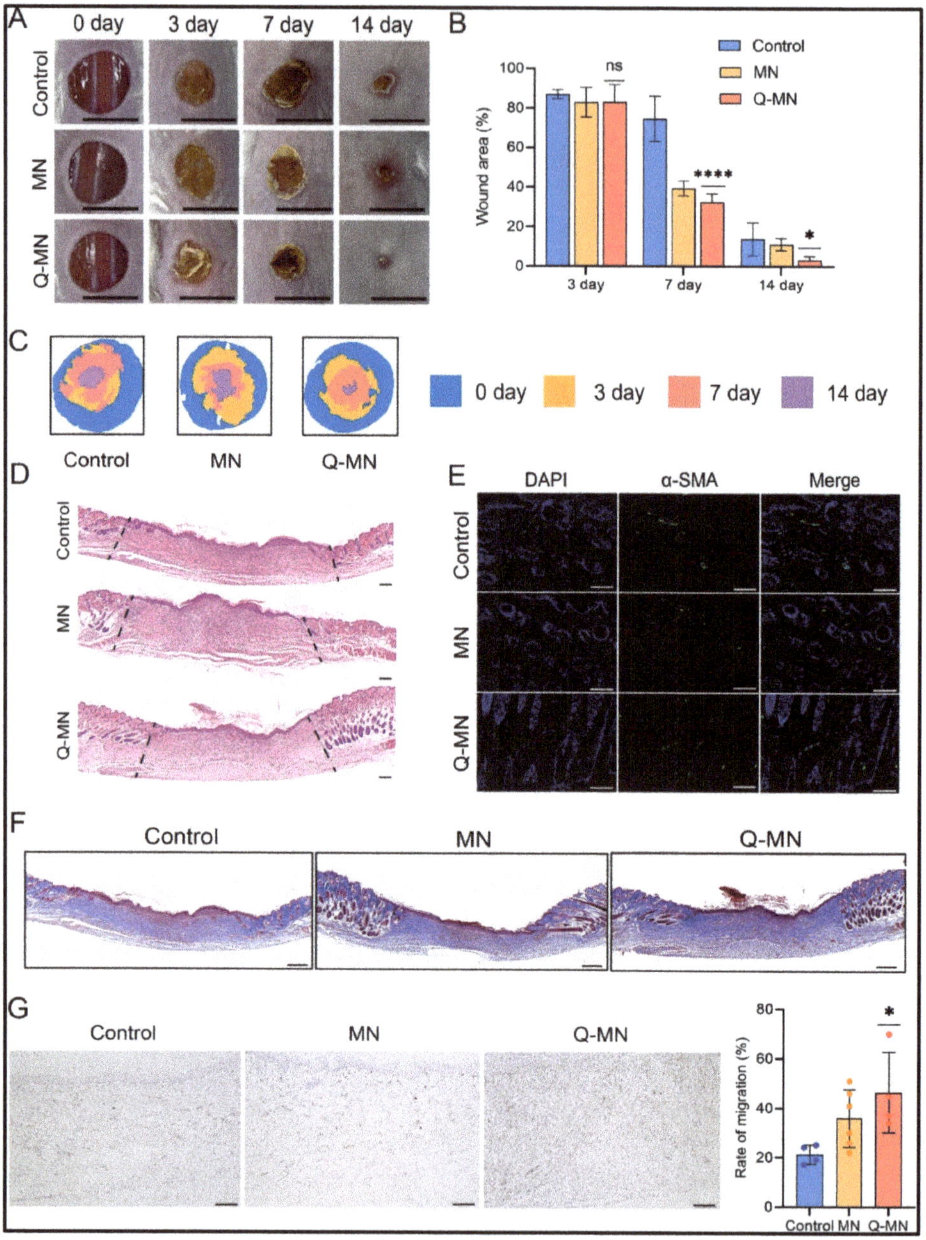

Figure 12. The illustration for wound healing progression activity. Microscopic image of wound in 3 groups (control, MN, and quercetin-loaded MN) at various time intervals in days (**A**), statistical representation of wound healing data (%) observed at various time intervals in days (**B**), wound healing progression representation (**C**), histo-morphological staining of wound tissue representation (**D**), immunofluorescence staining of wound tissue using α-SMA (**E**), Masson staining of wound tissue obtained on day 14 (**F**), neovascularization of wound at day 14 (scale bar of 30 μm) (**G**). Reproduced with permission from [104] under CC BY-NC-ND 4.0. * $p < 0.05$, **** $p < 0.0001$, ns, not significant.

6. Clinical Updates and Challenges

Hydrogel-forming microneedles are emerging as a promising technology in the management of dermal disorders, particularly for drug delivery and patient monitoring. Recent advancements have highlighted their potential to enhance dermal drug delivery, minimize invasiveness, and improve patient compliance. Kasasbeh and co-workers conducted a clinical study involving repeated applications of an HFMN array made from a copolymer of vinyl ether and maleic acid crosslinked with polyethylene glycol. The findings revealed that, upon repeated application, no visible quantity of polymer was observed; however, some patients experienced mild erythema, which resolved within 7 days, confirming patient compliance with fewer or no side effects from the HFMNs [108]. In another study conducted by Donnelly and co-workers on HFMNs for enhanced dermal drug delivery, gamma-sterilized HFMNs were applied to the ventral forearm skin of six healthy human volunteers, aged between 23 and 31 years (three men and three women), who had no prior skin issues. Pain scores were recorded immediately after application of the patch, concluding that no adverse effects were observed after 24 h [23].

Hydrogel-forming microneedles (HFMNs) for dermal drug delivery face challenges related to manufacturing scalability, regulatory approval, patient acceptance, efficacy and dosage control, storage stability, integration with existing therapies, and cost-effectiveness. Advanced manufacturing methods, such as 3D printing and microfabrication, can enhance scalability and uniformity, while early collaboration with regulatory bodies can streamline the approval process. Patient education through clinical trials and public outreach can increase acceptance. Tailoring formulations and dosing strategies to specific populations can ensure consistent drug delivery and therapeutic effectiveness. Stability issues may be mitigated through research into more durable hydrogel compositions. Integrating HFMNs with existing treatments may require updates to clinical practices, supported by guidelines and evidence of efficacy. Cost challenges, particularly in resource-limited settings, could be addressed through cost-reduction strategies in manufacturing and partnerships with healthcare providers for initial subsidies. By focusing on these areas—research, regulatory alignment, patient education, and manufacturing innovations—HFMNs could become more widely adopted in dermal drug delivery.

As a potential advancement in dermal medication delivery, HFMNs have been utilized in both cosmetic applications and the management of chronic illnesses. However, to fully realize their potential, several obstacles must be addressed [21]. These challenges include regulatory compliance, skin variability, medication delivery efficiency, biocompatibility and safety, manufacturing and scalability, as well as environmental and sustainability concerns. Cost is a significant obstacle, and successful manufacturing and scalability depend on precise control over the hydrogel characteristics, size, and geometry of the microneedles. Long-term safety data are essential to prevent issues such as persistent inflammation, allergic reactions, or skin degeneration, making biocompatibility and safety critical considerations. Skin variability also affects performance, highlighting the need for regulated release and medication stability for effective drug administration. Moreover, regulatory approval processes can be complex, with local standards for quality, safety, and efficacy varying significantly [31].

7. Conclusions and Future Perspectives

Hydrogel-forming microneedles are gaining traction in the field of dermatology due to their innovative approach to managing dermal disorders. Hydrogel-forming microneedles enhance drug delivery by providing sustained release of therapeutic agents, making them a game changer in managing skin diseases. This innovative approach addresses the limitations of traditional dermal systems. The efficacy and safety of these microneedles have been improved through advanced fabrication techniques and the use of polymeric materials. Nevertheless, challenges remain that need to be addressed. More robust clinical data are required to validate their efficacy and safety across different patient groups.

Artificial intelligence, on the other hand, has shown tremendous potential in the design of precise drug-delivery systems, increasingly playing a pivotal role in the development of HFMNs by enhancing their design, fabrication, and applications. The integration of machine learning and artificial intelligence technologies facilitates more efficient and innovative approaches to microneedle development. AI can further assist in the fabrication of microneedles through predictive modeling, selecting optimal materials, and utilizing the best-fit techniques in HFMN development.

Hydrogel-forming microneedles (HFMNs) are advancing rapidly in material innovation and application. Biodegradable hydrogels are being developed to reduce environmental impact and enhance patient safety. Composite materials, including nanoparticles and fibers, are boosting mechanical strength and drug-loading capabilities. The application range for HFMNs is expanding to areas such as vaccine delivery, chronic disease management, cosmetic treatments, and integration with digital health. Smart delivery systems now incorporate sensors and microelectronics, enabling real-time monitoring and feedback. Telehealth applications allow for easy sample collection and remote monitoring. Additionally, new regulatory pathways are establishing clearer guidelines and standards for microneedle development and testing. These advances promise to improve the functionality, safety, and application scope of HFMNs in medicine and cosmetics.

Future research should focus on optimizing the design and materials of microneedles, exploring their applications in a broader range of skin conditions, and improving their biocompatibility and user comfort. Moreover, advancements in nanotechnology and material science could further revolutionize this field, leading to even more effective and patient-friendly drug delivery systems. As these technologies continue to progress, they have the potential to significantly enhance the quality of life of individuals with various skin disorders.

Author Contributions: Conceptualization, S.S., P.M., and C.C.; methodology, A.P., S.M., and N.A; software, P.J. and A.K.; validation, P.J., S.S., and C.C.; formal analysis, A.K.; investigation, S.M. and N.A.; resources, S.S.; data curation, S.M. and N.A.; writing—original draft preparation, S.M. and N.A.; writing—review and editing, S.S.; visualization, A.K.; supervision, S.S., P.M., and C.C.; project administration, S.S. All authors have read and agreed to the published version of the manuscript.

Funding: This research received no external funding.

Institutional Review Board Statement: Not applicable.

Informed Consent Statement: Not applicable.

Data Availability Statement: Data can be made available on request to corresponding authors.

Acknowledgments: This work was partially supported by CMU Proactive Researcher Scheme (2023), Chiang Mai University, for Sudarshan Singh.

Conflicts of Interest: The authors declare no conflicts of interest.

References

1. Andersen, L.K.; Davis, M.D.P. The Epidemiology of Skin and Skin-Related Diseases: A Review of Population-Based Studies Performed by Using the Rochester Epidemiology Project. *Mayo Clin. Proc.* **2013**, *88*, 1462–1467. [CrossRef] [PubMed]
2. Nakai, K.; Tsuruta, D. What Are Reactive Oxygen Species, Free Radicals, and Oxidative Stress in Skin Diseases? *Int. J. Mol. Sci.* **2021**, *22*, 10799. [CrossRef] [PubMed]
3. Traidl, S.; Roesner, L.; Zeitvogel, J.; Werfel, T. Eczema herpeticum in atopic dermatitis. *Allergy* **2021**, *76*, 3017–3027. [CrossRef] [PubMed]
4. Wunnoo, S.; Bilhman, S.; Amnuaikit, T.; Ontong, J.C.; Singh, S.; Auepemkiate, S.; Voravuthikunchai, S.P. Rhodomyrtone as a New Natural Antibiotic Isolated from Rhodomyrtus tomentosa Leaf Extract: A Clinical Application in the Management of Acne Vulgaris. *Antibiotics* **2021**, *10*, 108. [CrossRef]
5. Patel, P.; Pal, R.; Butani, K.; Singh, S.; Prajapati, B.G. Nanomedicine-fortified cosmeceutical serums for the mitigation of psoriasis and acne. *Nanomedicine* **2023**, *18*, 1769–1793. [CrossRef]
6. Raharja, A.; Mahil, S.K.; Barker, J.N. Psoriasis: A brief overview. *Clin. Med.* **2021**, *21*, 170–173. [CrossRef]
7. Stacey, S.K.; McEleney, M. Topical Corticosteroids: Choice and Application. *Am. Fam. Physician* **2021**, *103*, 337–343.

8. Ontong, J.C.; Singh, S.; Siriyong, T.; Voravuthikunchai, S.P. Transferosomes stabilized hydrogel incorporated rhodomyrtone-rich extract from Rhodomyrtus tomentosa leaf fortified with phosphatidylcholine for the management of skin and soft-tissue infections. *Biotechnol. Lett.* **2024**, *46*, 127–142. [CrossRef]
9. Kumar, M.; Virmani, T.; Kumar, G.; Deshmukh, R.; Sharma, A.; Duarte, S.; Brandão, P.; Fonte, P. Nanocarriers in Tuberculosis Treatment: Challenges and Delivery Strategies. *Pharmaceuticals* **2023**, *16*, 1360. [CrossRef]
10. Kumar, A.; Naik, P.K.; Pradhan, D.; Ghosh, G.; Rath, G. Mucoadhesive formulations: Innovations, merits, drawbacks, and future outlook. *Pharm. Dev. Technol.* **2020**, *25*, 797–814. [CrossRef]
11. Akombaetwa, N.; Ilangala, A.B.; Thom, L.; Memvanga, P.B.; Witika, B.A.; Buya, A.B. Current Advances in Lipid Nanosystems Intended for Topical and Transdermal Drug Delivery Applications. *Pharmaceutics* **2023**, *15*, 656. [CrossRef]
12. Lyu, S.; Dong, Z.; Xu, X.; Bei, H.P.; Yuen, H.Y.; James Cheung, C.W.; Wong, M.S.; He, Y.; Zhao, X. Going below and beyond the surface: Microneedle structure, materials, drugs, fabrication, and applications for wound healing and tissue regeneration. *Bioact. Mater.* **2023**, *27*, 303–326. [CrossRef] [PubMed]
13. Lim, D.-J.; Kim, H.-J. Microneedles in Action: Microneedling and Microneedles-Assisted Transdermal Delivery. *Polymers* **2022**, *14*, 1608. [CrossRef] [PubMed]
14. Nikolić, I.; Simić, M.; Pantelić, I.; Stojanović, G.; Antić Stanković, J.; Marković, B.; Savić, S. Chemical vs. Physical Methods to Improve Dermal Drug Delivery: A Case Study with Nanoemulsions and Iontophoresis. *Pharmaceutics* **2022**, *14*, 1144. [CrossRef]
15. Yu, Y.Q.; Yang, X.; Wu, X.F.; Fan, Y.B. Enhancing Permeation of Drug Molecules Across the Skin via Delivery in Nanocarriers: Novel Strategies for Effective Transdermal Applications. *Front. Bioeng. Biotechnol.* **2021**, *9*, 646554. [CrossRef]
16. Mohite, P.; Patel, M.; Puri, A.; Pawar, A.; Singh, S.; Prajapati, B. Revisiting the advancement with painless microneedles for the diagnosis and treatment of dermal infections: A review. *Nanofabrication* **2023**, *8*. [CrossRef]
17. Amarnani, R.; Shende, P. Microneedles in diagnostic, treatment and theranostics: An advancement in minimally-invasive delivery system. *Biomed. Microdevices* **2022**, *24*, 4. [CrossRef]
18. Sharma, R.; Malviya, R.; Singh, S.; Prajapati, B. A critical review on classified excipient sodium-alginate-based hydrogels: Modification, characterization, and application in soft tissue engineering. *Gels* **2023**, *9*, 430. [CrossRef]
19. Singh, S.; Supaweera, N.; Nwabor, O.F.; Chaichompoo, W.; Suksamrarn, A.; Chittasupho, C.; Chunglok, W. Poly (vinyl alcohol)-gelatin-sericin copolymerized film fortified with vesicle-entrapped demethoxycurcumin/bisdemethoxycurcumin for improved stability, antibacterial, anti-inflammatory, and skin tissue regeneration. *Int. J. Biol. Macromol.* **2024**, *258*, 129071. [CrossRef]
20. Singh, S.; Supaweera, N.; Nwabor, O.F.; Yusakul, G.; Chaichompoo, W.; Suksamrarn, A.; Panpipat, W.; Chunglok, W. Polymeric scaffold integrated with nanovesicle-entrapped curcuminoids for enhanced therapeutic efficacy. *Nanomedicine* **2024**, *19*, 1313–1329. [CrossRef]
21. Hou, X.; Li, J.; Hong, Y.; Ruan, H.; Long, M.; Feng, N.; Zhang, Y. Advances and Prospects for Hydrogel-Forming Microneedles in Transdermal Drug Delivery. *Biomedicines* **2023**, *11*, 2119. [CrossRef] [PubMed]
22. Zhuang, J.; Rao, F.; Wu, D.; Huang, Y.; Xu, H.; Gao, W.; Zhang, J.; Sun, J. Study on the fabrication and characterization of tip-loaded dissolving microneedles for transdermal drug delivery. *Eur. J. Pharm. Biopharm.* **2020**, *157*, 66–73. [CrossRef] [PubMed]
23. Donnelly, R.F.; Singh, T.R.R.; Garland, M.J.; Migalska, K.; Majithiya, R.; McCrudden, C.M.; Kole, P.L.; Mahmood, T.M.T.; McCarthy, H.O.; Woolfson, A.D. Hydrogel-forming microneedle arrays for enhanced transdermal drug delivery. *Adv. Funct. Mater.* **2012**, *22*, 4879–4890. [CrossRef]
24. Martins, C.F.; García-Astrain, C.; Conde, J.; Liz-Marzán, L.M. Nanocomposite hydrogel microneedles: A theranostic toolbox for personalized medicine. *Drug Deliv. Transl. Res.* **2024**, *14*, 1–14. [CrossRef]
25. Omidian, H.; Dey Chowdhury, S. Swellable Microneedles in Drug Delivery and Diagnostics. *Pharmaceuticals* **2024**, *17*, 791. [CrossRef]
26. Peng, K.; Vora, L.K.; Domínguez-Robles, J.; Naser, Y.A.; Li, M.; Larrañeta, E.; Donnelly, R.F. Hydrogel-forming microneedles for rapid and efficient skin deposition of controlled release tip-implants. *Mater. Sci. Eng. C* **2021**, *127*, 112226. [CrossRef]
27. Luo, X.; Yang, L.; Cui, Y. Microneedles: Materials, fabrication, and biomedical applications. *Biomed. Microdevices* **2023**, *25*, 20. [CrossRef]
28. Sabri, A.H.B.; Anjani, Q.K.; Donnelly, R.F. Synthesis and characterization of sorbitol laced hydrogel-forming microneedles for therapeutic drug monitoring. *Int. J. Pharm.* **2021**, *607*, 121049. [CrossRef]
29. Migdadi, E.M.; Courtenay, A.J.; Tekko, I.A.; McCrudden, M.T.; Kearney, M.-C.; McAlister, E.; McCarthy, H.O.; Donnelly, R.F. Hydrogel-forming microneedles enhance transdermal delivery of metformin hydrochloride. *J. Control. Release* **2018**, *285*, 142–151. [CrossRef]
30. Feng, Y.-X.; Hu, H.; Wong, Y.-Y.; Yao, X.; He, M.-L. Microneedles: An emerging vaccine delivery tool and a prospective solution to the challenges of SARS-CoV-2 mass vaccination. *Pharmaceutics* **2023**, *15*, 1349. [CrossRef]
31. Filho, D.; Guerrero, M.; Pariguana, M.; Marican, A.; Durán-Lara, E.F. Hydrogel-Based Microneedle as a Drug Delivery System. *Pharmaceutics* **2023**, *15*, 2444. [CrossRef] [PubMed]
32. Dawud, H.; Abu Ammar, A. Rapidly dissolving microneedles for the delivery of steroid-loaded nanoparticles intended for the treatment of inflammatory skin diseases. *Pharmaceutics* **2023**, *15*, 526. [CrossRef] [PubMed]
33. Thang, N.H.; Chien, T.B.; Cuong, D.X. Polymer-based hydrogels applied in drug delivery: An overview. *Gels* **2023**, *9*, 523. [CrossRef] [PubMed]

34. Mohite, P.; Asane, G.; Rebello, N.; Munde, S.; Ade, N.; Boban, T.; Damiri, F.; Singh, S. Polymeric Hydrogel Sponges for Wound Healing Applications: A Comprehensive Review. *Regen. Eng. Transl. Med.* **2024**, *10*, 416–437. [CrossRef]
35. Israni, D.K.; Raghani, N.R.; Soni, J.; Shah, M.; Prajapati, B.G.; Chorawala, M.R.; Mangmool, S.; Singh, S.; Chittasupho, C. Harnessing Cannabis sativa Oil for Enhanced Skin Wound Healing: The Role of Reactive Oxygen Species Regulation. *Pharmaceutics* **2024**, *16*, 1277. [CrossRef]
36. Singh, S.; Nwabor, O.F.; Sukri, D.M.; Wunnoo, S.; Dumjun, K.; Lethongkam, S.; Kusolphat, P.; Hemtanon, N.; Klinprathum, K.; Sunghan, J. Poly (vinyl alcohol) copolymerized with xanthan gum/hypromellose/sodium carboxymethyl cellulose dermal dressings functionalized with biogenic nanostructured materials for antibacterial and wound healing application. *Int. J. Biol. Macromol.* **2022**, *216*, 235–250. [CrossRef]
37. Chorachoo Ontong, J.; Singh, S.; Nwabor, O.F.; Chusri, S.; Kaewnam, W.; Kanokwiroon, K.; Septama, A.W.; Panichayupakaranant, P.; Voravuthikunchai, S.P. Microwave-assisted extract of rhodomyrtone from rhodomyrtus tomentosa leaf: Anti-inflammatory, antibacterial, antioxidant, and safety assessment of topical rhodomyrtone formulation. *Sep. Sci. Technol.* **2023**, *58*, 929–943. [CrossRef]
38. Sánchez-Trasviña, C.; Coronel-Meneses, D.; Escobar-Fernández, A.M.; Mayolo-Deloisa, K. Transdermal microneedle patches as a promising drug delivery system for anti-obesogenic molecules. *Front. Bioeng. Biotechnol.* **2024**, *12*, 1380537. [CrossRef]
39. Avcil, M.; Çelik, A. Microneedles in drug delivery: Progress and challenges. *Micromachines* **2021**, *12*, 1321. [CrossRef]
40. Donnelly, R.F.; Singh, T.R.R.; Woolfson, A.D. Microneedle-based drug delivery systems: Microfabrication, drug delivery, and safety. *Drug Deliv.* **2010**, *17*, 187–207. [CrossRef]
41. Kulkarni, D.; Damiri, F.; Rojekar, S.; Zehravi, M.; Ramproshad, S.; Dhoke, D.; Musale, S.; Mulani, A.A.; Modak, P.; Paradhi, R. Recent advancements in microneedle technology for multifaceted biomedical applications. *Pharmaceutics* **2022**, *14*, 1097. [CrossRef] [PubMed]
42. Turner, J.G.; White, L.R.; Estrela, P.; Leese, H.S. Hydrogel-forming microneedles: Current advancements and future trends. *Macromol. Biosci.* **2021**, *21*, 2000307. [CrossRef] [PubMed]
43. Chen, B.Z.; He, Y.T.; Zhao, Z.Q.; Feng, Y.H.; Liang, L.; Peng, J.; Yang, C.Y.; Uyama, H.; Shahbazi, M.-A.; Guo, X.D. Strategies to develop polymeric microneedles for controlled drug release. *Adv. Drug Deliv. Rev.* **2023**, *203*, 115109. [CrossRef] [PubMed]
44. Oliveira, C.; Teixeira, J.A.; Oliveira, N.; Ferreira, S.; Botelho, C.M. Microneedles' Device: Design, Fabrication, and Applications. *Macromol.* **2024**, *4*, 320–355. [CrossRef]
45. Kulkarni, D.; Gadade, D.; Chapaitkar, N.; Shelke, S.; Pekamwar, S.; Aher, R.; Ahire, A.; Avhale, M.; Badgule, R.; Bansode, R. Polymeric microneedles: An emerging paradigm for advanced biomedical applications. *Sci. Pharm.* **2023**, *91*, 27. [CrossRef]
46. Damiri, F.; Kommineni, N.; Ebhodaghe, S.O.; Bulusu, R.; Jyothi, V.G.S.; Sayed, A.A.; Awaji, A.A.; Germoush, M.O.; Al-Malky, H.S.; Nasrullah, M.Z. Microneedle-based natural polysaccharide for drug delivery systems (DDS): Progress and challenges. *Pharmaceuticals* **2022**, *15*, 190. [CrossRef]
47. Mohite, P.; Shah, S.R.; Singh, S.; Rajput, T.; Munde, S.; Ade, N.; Prajapati, B.G.; Paliwal, H.; Mori, D.D.; Dudhrejiya, A.V. Chitosan and chito-oligosaccharide: A versatile biopolymer with endless grafting possibilities for multifarious applications. *Front. Bioeng. Biotechnol.* **2023**, *11*, 1190879. [CrossRef]
48. Mohite, P.; Rahayu, P.; Munde, S.; Ade, N.; Chidrawar, V.R.; Singh, S.; Jayeoye, T.J.; Prajapati, B.G.; Bhattacharya, S.; Patel, R.J. Chitosan-Based Hydrogel in the Management of Dermal Infections: A Review. *Gels* **2023**, *9*, 594. [CrossRef]
49. Cordeiro, A.S.; Patil-Sen, Y.; Shivkumar, M.; Patel, R.; Khedr, A.; Elsawy, M.A. Nanovaccine Delivery Approaches and Advanced Delivery Systems for the Prevention of Viral Infections: From Development to Clinical Application. *Pharmaceutics* **2021**, *13*, 2091. [CrossRef]
50. Shriky, B.; Babenko, M.; Whiteside, B.R. Dissolving and Swelling Hydrogel-Based Microneedles: An Overview of Their Materials, Fabrication, Characterization Methods, and Challenges. *Gels* **2023**, *9*, 806. [CrossRef]
51. Marinho, A.; Nunes, C.; Reis, S. Hyaluronic Acid: A Key Ingredient in the Therapy of Inflammation. *Biomolecules* **2021**, *11*, 1518. [CrossRef] [PubMed]
52. Malek-Khatabi, A.; Faraji Rad, Z.; Rad-Malekshahi, M.; Akbarijavar, H. Development of dissolvable microneedle patches by CNC machining and micromolding for drug delivery. *Mater. Lett.* **2023**, *330*, 133328. [CrossRef]
53. Chudzińska, J.; Wawrzyńczak, A.; Feliczak-Guzik, A. Microneedles Based on a Biodegradable Polymer—Hyaluronic Acid. *Polymers* **2024**, *16*, 1396. [CrossRef] [PubMed]
54. Singh, S.; Chunglok, W.; Nwabor, O.F.; Chulrik, W.; Jansakun, C.; Bhoopong, P. Porous Biodegradable Sodium Alginate Composite Fortified with *Hibiscus Sabdariffa* L. Calyx Extract for the Multifarious Biological Applications and Extension of Climacteric Fruit Shelf-Life. *J. Polym. Environ.* **2023**, *31*, 922–938. [CrossRef]
55. Liu, Y.; Vrana, N.E.; Cahill, P.A.; McGuinness, G.B. Physically crosslinked composite hydrogels of PVA with natural macromolecules: Structure, mechanical properties, and endothelial cell compatibility. *J. Biomed. Mater. Res. Part B Appl. Biomater.* **2009**, *90B*, 492–502. [CrossRef]
56. Samant, P.P.; Niedzwiecki, M.M.; Raviele, N.; Tran, V.; Mena-Lapaix, J.; Walker, D.I.; Felner, E.I.; Jones, D.P.; Miller, G.W.; Prausnitz, M.R. Sampling interstitial fluid from human skin using a microneedle patch. *Sci. Transl. Med.* **2020**, *12*, eaaw0285. [CrossRef]
57. Tang, J.; Wang, J.; Huang, K.; Ye, Y.; Su, T.; Qiao, L.; Hensley, M.T.; Caranasos, T.G.; Zhang, J.; Gu, Z.; et al. Cardiac cell-integrated microneedle patch for treating myocardial infarction. *Sci. Adv.* **2018**, *4*, eaat9365. [CrossRef]

58. Bencherif, S.A.; Srinivasan, A.; Horkay, F.; Hollinger, J.O.; Matyjaszewski, K.; Washburn, N.R. Influence of the degree of methacrylation on hyaluronic acid hydrogels properties. *Biomaterials* **2008**, *29*, 1739–1749. [CrossRef]
59. Xu, Y.; Wu, X.; Zhang, X.; Zu, Y.; Tan, Q.; Zhao, Y. Living Microneedle Patch with Adipose-Derived Stem Cells Embedding for Diabetic Ulcer Healing. *Adv. Funct. Mater.* **2023**, *33*, 2209986. [CrossRef]
60. Donnelly, R.F.; McCrudden, M.T.; Zaid Alkilani, A.; Larrañeta, E.; McAlister, E.; Courtenay, A.J.; Kearney, M.C.; Singh, T.R.; McCarthy, H.O.; Kett, V.L.; et al. Hydrogel-forming microneedles prepared from "super swelling" polymers combined with lyophilised wafers for transdermal drug delivery. *PLoS ONE* **2014**, *9*, e111547. [CrossRef]
61. Pan, X.; Li, Y.; Pang, W.; Xue, Y.; Wang, Z.; Jiang, C.; Shen, C.; Liu, Q.; Liu, L. Preparation, characterisation and comparison of glabridin-loaded hydrogel-forming microneedles by chemical and physical cross-linking. *Int. J. Pharm.* **2022**, *617*, 121612. [CrossRef] [PubMed]
62. Kolahdoozan, M.; Rahimi, T.; Taghizadeh, A.; Aghaei, H. Preparation of new hydrogels by visible light cross-linking of dextran methacrylate and poly(ethylene glycol)-maleic acid copolymer. *Int. J. Biol. Macromol.* **2023**, *227*, 1221–1233. [CrossRef] [PubMed]
63. Li, Y.; Bi, D.; Hu, Z.; Yang, Y.; Liu, Y.; Leung, W.K. Hydrogel-Forming Microneedles with Applications in Oral Diseases Management. *Mater.* **2023**, *16*, 4805. [CrossRef] [PubMed]
64. Khan, S.; Minhas, M.U.; Tekko, I.A.; Donnelly, R.F.; Thakur, R.R.S. Evaluation of microneedles-assisted in situ depot forming poloxamer gels for sustained transdermal drug delivery. *Drug Deliv. Transl. Res.* **2019**, *9*, 764–782. [CrossRef]
65. Gholami, S.; Mohebi, M.M.; Hajizadeh-Saffar, E.; Ghanian, M.H.; Zarkesh, I.; Baharvand, H. Fabrication of microporous inorganic microneedles by centrifugal casting method for transdermal extraction and delivery. *Int. J. Pharm.* **2019**, *558*, 299–310. [CrossRef]
66. Al-Abduljabbar, A.; Farooq, I. Electrospun Polymer Nanofibers: Processing, Properties, and Applications. *Polymers* **2023**, *15*, 65. [CrossRef]
67. Ali, R.; Mehta, P.; Kyriaki Monou, P.; Arshad, M.S.; Panteris, E.; Rasekh, M.; Singh, N.; Qutachi, O.; Wilson, P.; Tzetzis, D.; et al. Electrospinning/electrospraying coatings for metal microneedles: A design of experiments (DOE) and quality by design (QbD) approach. *Eur. J. Pharm. Biopharm.* **2020**, *156*, 20–39. [CrossRef]
68. Carpa, R.; Farkas, A.; Dobrota, C.; Butiuc-Keul, A. Double-Network Chitosan-Based Hydrogels with Improved Mechanical, Conductive, Antimicrobial, and Antibiofouling Properties. *Gels* **2023**, *9*, 278. [CrossRef]
69. Lutton, R.E.; Larrañeta, E.; Kearney, M.C.; Boyd, P.; Woolfson, A.D.; Donnelly, R.F. A novel scalable manufacturing process for the production of hydrogel-forming microneedle arrays. *Int. J. Pharm.* **2015**, *494*, 417–429. [CrossRef]
70. Smith, E.; Lau, W.M.; Abdelghany, T.M.; Vukajlovic, D.; Novakovic, K.; Ng, K.W. Vac-and-fill: A micromoulding technique for fabricating microneedle arrays with vacuum-activated, hands-free mould-filling. *Int. J. Pharm.* **2024**, *650*, 123706. [CrossRef]
71. Chanabodeechalermrung, B.; Chaiwarit, T.; Udomsom, S.; Rachtanapun, P.; Piboon, P.; Jantrawut, P. Determination of vat-photopolymerization parameters for microneedles fabrication and characterization of HPMC/PVP K90 dissolving microneedles utilizing 3D-printed mold. *Sci. Rep.* **2024**, *14*, 16174. [CrossRef] [PubMed]
72. Chaiwarit, T.; Chanabodeechalermrung, B.; Jantrawut, P.; Ruksiriwanich, W.; Sainakham, M. Fabrication and Characterization of Dissolving Microneedles Containing Oryza sativa L. Extract Complex for Enhancement of Transfollicular Delivery. *Polymers* **2024**, *16*, 2377. [CrossRef] [PubMed]
73. Wu, Y.; Tang, Z.; Ma, S.; Du, L. The promising application of hydrogel microneedles in medical application. *J. Pharm. Pharmacol.* **2023**, *75*, 1011–1020. [CrossRef] [PubMed]
74. Swain, S.; Pratap Singh, A.; Yadav, R.K. A review on polymer hydrogel and polymer microneedle based transdermal drug delivery system. *Mater. Today Proc.* **2022**, *61*, 1061–1066. [CrossRef]
75. Owens, G.J.; Singh, R.K.; Foroutan, F.; Alqaysi, M.; Han, C.-M.; Mahapatra, C.; Kim, H.-W.; Knowles, J.C. Sol–gel based materials for biomedical applications. *Prog. Mater. Sci.* **2016**, *77*, 1–79. [CrossRef]
76. Khan, S.; Minhas, M.U.; Singh Thakur, R.R.; Aqeel, M.T. Microneedles assisted controlled and improved transdermal delivery of high molecular drugs via in situ forming depot thermoresponsive poloxamers gels in skin microchannels. *Drug Dev. Ind. Pharm.* **2022**, *48*, 265–278. [CrossRef]
77. Aung, N.N.; Ngawhirunpat, T.; Rojanarata, T.; Patrojanasophon, P.; Pamornpathomkul, B.; Opanasopit, P. Fabrication, characterization and comparison of α-arbutin loaded dissolving and hydrogel forming microneedles. *Int. J. Pharm.* **2020**, *586*, 119508. [CrossRef]
78. Yu, K.; Yu, X.; Cao, S.; Wang, Y.; Zhai, Y.; Yang, F.; Yang, X.; Lu, Y.; Wu, C.; Xu, Y. Layered dissolving microneedles as a need-based delivery system to simultaneously alleviate skin and joint lesions in psoriatic arthritis. *Acta Pharm. Sin. B* **2021**, *11*, 505–519. [CrossRef]
79. Ding, Y.-W.; Li, Y.; Zhang, Z.-W.; Dao, J.-W.; Wei, D.-X. Hydrogel forming microneedles loaded with VEGF and Ritlecitinib/polyhydroxyalkanoates nanoparticles for mini-invasive androgenetic alopecia treatment. *Bioact. Mater.* **2024**, *38*, 95–108. [CrossRef]
80. Donnelly, R.F.; Mooney, K.; McCrudden, M.T.; Vicente-Pérez, E.M.; Belaid, L.; González-Vázquez, P.; McElnay, J.C.; Woolfson, A.D. Hydrogel-forming microneedles increase in volume during swelling in skin, but skin barrier function recovery is unaffected. *J. Pharm. Sci.* **2014**, *103*, 1478–1486. [CrossRef]
81. Leanpolchareanchai, J.; Nuchtavorn, N. Response Surface Methodology for Optimization of Hydrogel-Forming Microneedles as Rapid and Efficient Transdermal Microsampling Tools. *Gels* **2023**, *9*, 306. [CrossRef] [PubMed]

82. Chanabodeechalermrung, B.; Chaiwarit, T.; Chaichit, S.; Udomsom, S.; Baipaywad, P.; Worajittiphon, P.; Jantrawut, P. HPMC/PVP K90 Dissolving Microneedles Fabricated from 3D-Printed Master Molds: Impact on Microneedle Morphology, Mechanical Strength, and Topical Dissolving Property. *Polymers* **2024**, *16*, 452. [CrossRef] [PubMed]
83. Oh, N.G.; Hwang, S.Y.; Na, Y.H. Fabrication of a PVA-Based Hydrogel Microneedle Patch. *ACS Omega* **2022**, *7*, 25179–25185. [CrossRef] [PubMed]
84. Dawud, H.; Edelstein-Pardo, N.; Mulamukkil, K.; Amir, R.J.; Abu Ammar, A. Hydrogel Microneedles with Programmed Mesophase Transitions for Controlled Drug Delivery. *ACS Appl. Bio Mater.* **2024**, *7*, 1682–1693. [CrossRef] [PubMed]
85. Jung, J.H.; Jin, S.G. Microneedle for transdermal drug delivery: Current trends and fabrication. *J. Pharm. Investig.* **2021**, *51*, 503–517. [CrossRef]
86. Aziz, A.Y.R.; Hasir, N.A.; Imran, N.B.P.; Hamdan, M.F.; Mahfufah, U.; Wafiah, N.; Arjuna, A.; Utami, R.N.; Permana, A.D. Development of hydrogel-forming microneedles for transdermal delivery of albendazole from liquid reservoir. *J. Biomater. Sci. Polym. Ed.* **2023**, *34*, 1101–1120. [CrossRef]
87. Makvandi, P.; Shabani, M.; Rabiee, N.; Anjani, Q.K.; Maleki, A.; Zare, E.N.; Sabri, A.H.B.; De Pasquale, D.; Koskinopoulou, M.; Sharifi, E.; et al. Engineering and Development of a Tissue Model for the Evaluation of Microneedle Penetration Ability, Drug Diffusion, Photothermal Activity, and Ultrasound Imaging: A Promising Surrogate to Ex Vivo and In Vivo Tissues. *Adv. Mater.* **2023**, *35*, e2210034. [CrossRef]
88. Elim, D.; Fitri, A.M.N.; Mahfud, M.A.S.; Afika, N.; Sultan, N.A.F.; Hijrah; Asri, R.M.; Permana, A.D. Hydrogel forming microneedle-mediated transdermal delivery of sildenafil citrate from polyethylene glycol reservoir: An ex vivo proof of concept study. *Colloids Surf. B Biointerfaces* **2023**, *222*, 113018. [CrossRef]
89. Ozkaya, N.K.; Inan, Z.D.S.; Zereyak, U.; Yılmaz, S. A histopathological and clinical assessment on the effect of microneedling on the autologous platelet-rich plasma in the experimental wound healing. *Ann. Med. Res.* **2021**, *28*, 1387–1394. [CrossRef]
90. Nguyen, H.X.; Banga, A.K. Enhanced skin delivery of vismodegib by microneedle treatment. *Drug Deliv. Transl. Res.* **2015**, *5*, 407–423. [CrossRef]
91. Ripolin, A.; Volpe-Zanutto, F.; Sabri, A.H.; dos Santos, V.A.B.; Figueroba, S.R.; Bezerra, A.A.C.; Vinicius Rodrigues Louredo, B.; Agustin Vargas, P.; McGuckin, M.B.; Hutton, A.R.J.; et al. Transdermal delivery of bisphosphonates using dissolving and hydrogel-forming microarray patches: Potential for enhanced treatment of osteoporosis. *Int. J. Pharm.* **2024**, *665*, 124642. [CrossRef] [PubMed]
92. Wu, Y.; Qiu, Y.; Zhang, S.; Qin, G.; Gao, Y. Microneedle-based drug delivery: Studies on delivery parameters and biocompatibility. *Biomed. Microdevices* **2008**, *10*, 601–610. [CrossRef] [PubMed]
93. Umeyor, C.E.; Shelke, V.; Pol, A.; Kolekar, P.; Jadhav, S.; Tiwari, N.; Anure, A.; Nayak, A.; Bairagi, G.; Agale, A.; et al. Biomimetic microneedles: Exploring the recent advances on a microfabricated system for precision delivery of drugs, peptides, and proteins. *Future J. Pharm. Sci.* **2023**, *9*, 103. [CrossRef]
94. Schossleitner, K.; O'Mahony, C.; Brandstätter, S.; Haslinger, M.J.; Demuth, S.; Fechtig, D.; Petzelbauer, P. Differences in biocompatibility of microneedles from cyclic olefin polymers with human endothelial and epithelial skin cells. *J. Biomed. Mater. Res. Part A* **2019**, *107*, 505–512. [CrossRef]
95. Anju, T.R.; Parvathy, S.; Valiya Veettil, M.; Rosemary, J.; Ansalna, T.H.; Shahzabanu, M.M.; Devika, S. Green synthesis of silver nanoparticles from Aloe vera leaf extract and its antimicrobial activity. *Mater. Today Proc.* **2021**, *43*, 3956–3960. [CrossRef]
96. Jadach, B.; Nowak, A.; Długaszewska, J.; Kordyl, O.; Budnik, I.; Osmałek, T. Coated Microneedle System for Delivery of Clotrimazole in Deep-Skin Mycoses. *Gels* **2024**, *10*, 264. [CrossRef]
97. Naser, Y.A.; Tekko, I.A.; Vora, L.K.; Peng, K.; Anjani, Q.K.; Greer, B.; Elliott, C.; McCarthy, H.O.; Donnelly, R.F. Hydrogel-forming microarray patches with solid dispersion reservoirs for transdermal long-acting microdepot delivery of a hydrophobic drug. *J. Control. Release* **2023**, *356*, 416–433. [CrossRef]
98. Courtenay, A.J.; McAlister, E.; McCrudden, M.T.C.; Vora, L.; Steiner, L.; Levin, G.; Levy-Nissenbaum, E.; Shterman, N.; Kearney, M.C.; McCarthy, H.O.; et al. Hydrogel-forming microneedle arrays as a therapeutic option for transdermal esketamine delivery. *J. Control Release* **2020**, *322*, 177–186. [CrossRef]
99. Turner, J.G.; Laabei, M.; Li, S.; Estrela, P.; Leese, H.S. Antimicrobial releasing hydrogel forming microneedles. *Biomater. Adv.* **2023**, *151*, 213467. [CrossRef]
100. Abraham, A.M.; Anjani, Q.K.; Adhami, M.; Hutton, A.R.J.; Larrañeta, E.; Donnelly, R.F. Novel SmartReservoirs for hydrogel-forming microneedles to improve the transdermal delivery of rifampicin. *J. Mater. Chem. B* **2024**, *12*, 4375–4388. [CrossRef]
101. Tekko, I.A.; Chen, G.; Domínguez-Robles, J.; Thakur, R.R.S.; Hamdan, I.M.N.; Vora, L.; Larrañeta, E.; McElnay, J.C.; McCarthy, H.O.; Rooney, M.; et al. Development and characterisation of novel poly (vinyl alcohol)/poly (vinyl pyrrolidone)-based hydrogel-forming microneedle arrays for enhanced and sustained transdermal delivery of methotrexate. *Int. J. Pharm.* **2020**, *586*, 119580. [CrossRef] [PubMed]
102. Ranjan Yadav, P.; Iqbal Nasiri, M.; Vora, L.K.; Larrañeta, E.; Donnelly, R.F.; Pattanayek, S.K.; Bhusan Das, D. Super-swelling hydrogel-forming microneedle based transdermal drug delivery: Mathematical modelling, simulation and experimental validation. *Int. J. Pharm.* **2022**, *622*, 121835. [CrossRef] [PubMed]
103. Mahfufah, U.; Sultan, N.A.F.; Fitri, A.M.N.; Elim, D.; Mahfud, M.A.S.b.; Wafiah, N.; Friandini, R.A.; Chabib, L.; Permana, A.D. Application of multipolymers system in the development of hydrogel-forming microneedle integrated with polyethylene glycol reservoir for transdermal delivery of albendazole. *Eur. Polym. J.* **2023**, *183*, 111762. [CrossRef]

104. Yi, Y.; Yang, Z.; Zhou, C.; Yang, Y.; Wu, Y.; Zhang, Q. Quercetin-encapsulated GelMa hydrogel microneedle reduces oxidative stress and facilitates wound healing. *Nano TransMed* **2024**, *3*, 100030. [CrossRef]
105. Yao, W.-D.; Zhou, J.-N.; Tang, C.; Zhang, J.-L.; Chen, Z.-Y.; Li, Y.; Gong, X.-J.; Qu, M.-Y.; Zeng, Q.; Jia, Y.-L. Hydrogel Microneedle Patches Loaded with Stem Cell Mitochondria-Enriched Microvesicles Boost the Chronic Wound Healing. *ACS Nano* **2024**, *18*, 26733–26750. [CrossRef]
106. Li, Y.; Wang, Y.; Mei, R.; Lv, B.; Zhao, X.; Bi, L.; Xu, H.; Chen, L. Hydrogel-Coated SERS Microneedles for Drug Monitoring in Dermal Interstitial Fluid. *ACS Sens.* **2024**, *9*, 2567–2574. [CrossRef]
107. Razzaghi, M.; Seyfoori, A.; Pagan, E.; Askari, E.; Hassani Najafabadi, A.; Akbari, M. 3D printed hydrogel microneedle arrays for interstitial fluid biomarker extraction and colorimetric detection. *Polymers* **2023**, *15*, 1389. [CrossRef]
108. Al-Kasasbeh, R.; Brady, A.J.; Courtenay, A.J.; Larrañeta, E.; McCrudden, M.T.; O'Kane, D.; Liggett, S.; Donnelly, R.F. Evaluation of the clinical impact of repeat application of hydrogel-forming microneedle array patches. *Drug Deliv. Transl. Res.* **2020**, *10*, 690–705. [CrossRef]

gels

MDPI

Article

Marine Resources Gels as Main Ingredient for Wound Healing Biomaterials: Obtaining and Characterization

Alina Elena Coman [1], Maria Minodora Marin [2,*], Ana Maria Roșca [3,*], Madalina Georgiana Albu Kaya [1], Rodica Roxana Constantinescu [1] and Irina Titorencu [3]

1 Department of Collagen, Division of Leather and Footwear Research Institute, National Research and Development Institute for Textiles and Leather, 93 Ion Minulescu Str., 031215 Bucharest, Romania; coman.alina27@yahoo.com (A.E.C.); albu_mada@yahoo.com (M.G.A.K.); rodica.roxana@yahoo.com (R.R.C.)

2 Advanced Polymer Materials Group, University POLITEHNICA of Bucharest, 1-7 Polizu Street, 011061 Bucharest, Romania

3 Institute of Cellular Biology and Pathology "Nicolae Simionescu", 8 B. P. Hasdeu Street, District 5, 050568 Bucharest, Romania; irina.titorencu@gmail.com

* Correspondence: minodora.marin@ymail.com (M.M.M.); ana-maria.rosca@icbp.ro (A.M.R.)

Abstract: The skin, known as the largest organ of the body, is essential for maintaining physiological balance and acts as a barrier against the external environment. When skin becomes damaged and wounds appear on the skin's surface, a complex healing process, involving multiple types of cells and microenvironments, take place. Selecting a suitable dressing for a wound is crucial for accelerating healing, reducing treatment costs, and improving the patient's overall health. Starting from natural resources such as perch skin (*P. fluviatilis*), this article aims to develop biocompatible materials for regenerative medicine from collagen in the form of gels/gelatines. The extracted gels were physical/chemical and structurally analyzed. In order to obtain collagen scaffolds for wound healing, the extracted collagen gels from perch skin were further freeze-dried. The ability of these scaffolds is essential for controlling moisture levels during wound healing; therefore, it was necessary to investigate the samples' ability to absorb water. The assessed collagen-based scaffolds were microbiologically tested, and their biocompatibility was investigated by incubating human adult dermal fibroblasts. The outcomes reveal an innovative path for the production of biomaterials used in wound healing, starting from collagen derived from marine sources.

Keywords: fish wastes; marine collagen; biomaterials; wound healing

1. Introduction

In recent decades, the researchers starting to focus on new potential collagen sources due to the rising demand of high purity collagen and the limitation of porcine and bovine collagen extraction. Usually, collagen is extracted from porcine or bovine, but there are some limitations, such as the possibility of disease transmission and socio-cultural and religious concerns [1–4].

Despite mammalian collagen extraction, more efficient and sustainable sources should be exploited in order to meet the market demand [5,6]. Globally, around 20 million tons of aquaculture wastes are generated, and nearly 25% are fish wastes, an important source of high purity collagen. Fish wastes are generated in high quantities every year due to the human consumption. This includes skin, scales, viscera, bladders, ligaments and bones, representing around 75% of a fish's weight. Usually, fish wastes are burned or buried, leading to environmental, economic and health problems. A minor percentage is employed as raw materials in feed for animals [7–10].

Therefore, fish by-product valorization, as potential collagen sources, solve ecological and economic issues, leading to rentability in terms of profitability. Moreover, collagen derived from marine sources is religiously accepted by various groups [2–4].

In terms of properties, the denaturation temperature of marine collagen is lower, being in the range of 25–30 °C for most fish species (depending on the composition), in comparison with mammalian collagen, which has a denaturation temperature of 39–40 °C [4,11]. However, collagen derived from fish and invertebrate species is more bioavailable and is absorbed up to 1.5 times better than collagen from cows or pigs [12]. For example, faster blood circulation is ensured by small particle size and low molecular weight for marine collagen [13]. Also, fish collagen posed higher flexibility and a similar viscosity compared with mammalian collagen [4]. Furthermore, the amino acid content and biocompatibility of marine collagen are comparable to those of bovine and pig collagen [14].

Fish skin is a natural raw material that contains minerals, vitamins, proteins and especially collagen. Its features include improved physical/chemical properties, superior biocompatibility, easy processing, high porosity, and the capability to combine with synthetic and natural materials, which increased researchers' attention regarding fish skin. Type I collagen is known to be the most abundant protein in fish skin and in the human body.

In addition, fish skin contains omega-3 polyunsaturated fatty acids, which improves the wound healing process [3,4,15]. Thereby, wound dressing from fish wastes can be successfully used.

The largest organ of the body, the skin, plays a crucial role in preserving physiological equilibrium and providing defense against the outside world. Numerous cell types and microenvironments are involved in a complex healing process when skin is damaged and wounds appear on the skin surface. Selecting the right wound dressing is essential to promote healing, lower treatment expenses, and enhance the patient's general health. However, the variety of wound dressings on the market can be confusing. In order to avoid negative outcomes, wound care must be treated properly. Wound dressings are primarily used to create a transient physical barrier of protection, absorb wound drainage and supply the moisture required to maximize re-epithelialization. The wound's anatomical and pathophysiological features influence the dressing selection. Additional advantages of contemporary wound dressings include pain alleviation and antibacterial qualities [16–18].

The objective of this paper is represented by the development of biocompatible materials for regenerative medicine starting from collagen gels/gelatines, using natural resources such as fish skin. This research focuses on collagen extracted from perch skin (*P. fluviatilis*) in the form of a gel. To the best of our knowledge, there is no existing literature or research that addresses collagen extracted from perch skin for regenerative medicine purposes, leading to the novelty of these research studies.

The gels extracted were analyzed by proximate analysis (dry substance, protein and ash content, total nitrogen, collagen yield and pH), FT-IR spectroscopy and circular dichroism (CD).

The extracted collagen gels from perch skin were further freeze-dried in order to obtain collagen scaffolds for wound healing. Since these scaffolds are essential for controlling moisture levels during wound healing [19], the water uptake capacity of the samples obtained was investigated. The resulting collagen biomaterials were also microbiologically characterized. Fibroblasts are essential for the proper healing of wounds, having a crucial role in processes such as contracting the wound; producing new collagen and extracellular matrix structures in order to support other cells involved in successful wound healing; and decomposing the fibrin clot [20]. For this reason, the biocompatibility of the tested collagen-based scaffolds was evaluated by incubating human adult dermal fibroblasts.

The results reveal a new opportunity for the development of biomaterials employed in wound healing, starting from collagen of marine origin.

2. Results and Discussion

2.1. Characterization of Collagen Gels Extracted from Perch Skin

Collagen gels extracted from perch skin through various treatments and at different temperatures were physically/chemically and structurally analyzed.

2.1.1. Physical/Chemical Analysis

For a physical/chemical analysis of the extracted gels, a proximate analysis was performed, and the results are presented in Table 1.

Table 1. Proximate analysis of collagen gels extracted from perch skin.

Sample	Dry Substance Content, %	Ash Content, %	Total Nitrogen, %	Protein Content, %	pH, pH Units
GEL_COLL_T_{rt} *	3.41	undetectable	0.40	2.28	2.5
GEL_COLL_T_f **	1.85	undetectable	0.20	1.12	2.5
GEL_COLL_TC_{rt}	3.44	undetectable	0.40	2.25	2.5
GEL_COLL_TC_f	2.17	undetectable	0.21	1.18	2.5
GEL_COLL_A_{rt}	2.14	undetectable	0.21	1.18	2.5
GEL_COLL_A_f	2.58	undetectable	0.28	1.57	2.5

* rt = room temperature (samples kept at room temperature, at 15 °C); ** f = fridge (samples kept at refrigerator), where GEL_COLL_T represents samples treated with tartaric, GEL_COLL_TC represents samples treated with tartaric and citric acid, GEL_COLL_A represents samples treated with ascorbic acid.

Between the samples, there are some differences regarding the storage temperature during the extraction. For the samples treated with tartaric and citric acid, higher values are obtained for dry substances (represented by collagen quantity obtained after extraction, reported at 100 g, with the difference being water [21]), and for protein content (a high protein content leads to high amounts of amino acid being transformed into collagen and increased sample purity) for samples stored at room temperature, noticing the temperature influence.

The dry substance and protein content are high for all the samples, leading to adequate values for gel samples with high water content.

The pH obtained is acidic, 2.5 for all the samples, which is very good for collagen deterioration prevention and stability assurance [22].

For samples with ascorbic acid used for extraction, the results obtained for samples kept in the refrigerator are slightly higher compared with the ones kept at room temperature.

Collagen extraction is predominantly based on the treatment of fish skin in order to reduce non-collagenous components such as minerals, lipids and other impurities. The removal of non-collagenous materials occurs during the overall extraction process, starting with the pretreatment of the collagen source, and its extraction and purification process [23]. The samples' purity increased for all the samples and is demonstrated by the ash content [24], which could not be detected in any of the samples.

GEL_COLL_A_f presents the highest protein and dry substance content from samples kept in the fridge. These results will also be further confirmed by circular dichroism.

The dry substance content was used to determine the yields of collagen extraction. The dry substance is represented by the dry collagen content from the sample. Figure 1 shows the yields obtained for collagen gel extracted from perch skin. The yield is higher for all the samples kept at room temperature, compared with samples stored in the fridge.

The yields reached for collagen gel through acid extraction from *P. fluviatilis* skin are very good compared with the yields obtained in other studies. The yield of *Dasyatis zugei* skin collagen was reported to be higher when acetic acid was used for extraction (approx. 11.49%) compared with using hydrochloric acid (approx. 3.50%) [25]. Different yields were obtained for *Pangasius* sp. skin collagen extracted with 0.5 M and 0.7 M acetic acid (approx. 10.94% and 5.47%, respectively) [26]. On the contrary, *Decapterus macrosoma* collagen extracted with 0.5 M and 0.7 M acetic acid were approx. 1.01% and 1.31, respectively, which means a higher yield percentage was obtained with 0.7 M acetic acid [27].

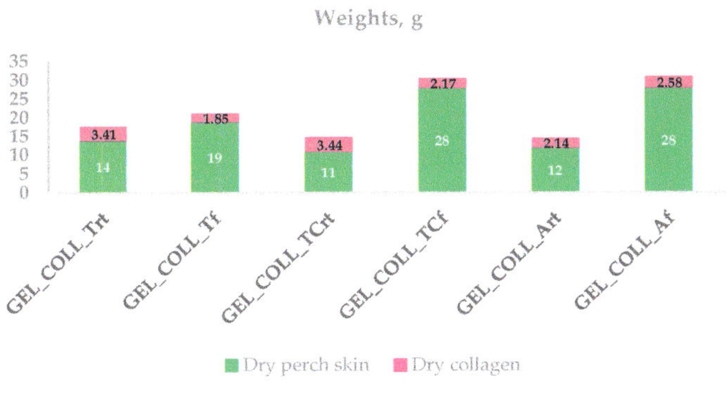

(a)

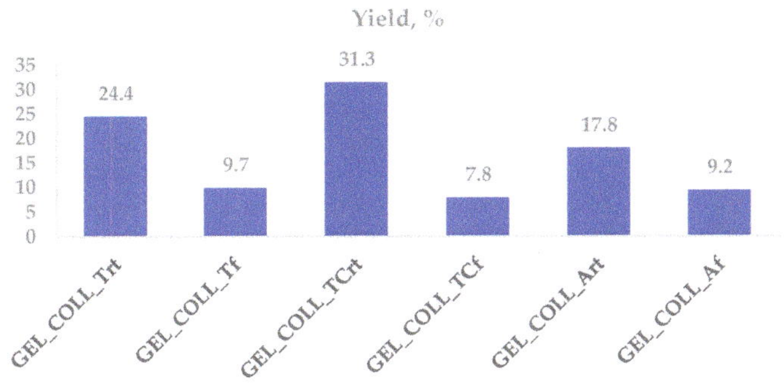

(b)

Figure 1. Yields of collagen extracted from perch skin. (**a**) Dry weights (in grams) of collagen extracted from the indicated weight of skin. (**b**) Collagen yields of the samples are calculated as (Dry collagen weight/Dry skin weight) × 100.

2.1.2. Structural Analysis

- *Circular Dichroism Spectroscopy*

Circular dichroism spectroscopy (CD) is presented in Figure 2 for all the collagen samples from perch skin. CD spectra are similar for all the samples, with a pronounced negative band around 196 to 200 nm, suggesting a random coil structure and no positive maximum around wavelength of 220 nm, specific to the triple-helix structure of collagen.

According to the literature, after complete collagen denaturation, the positive band specific to the triple-helix structure (between 220 and 230 nm) disappears and only the negative band remains around 200 nm, specific to gelatine [28–30]. Therefore, for all collagen gels extracted, were assigned a structure specific to denatured collagen, namely the gelatine structure.

Studies performed by Gopinath et al. [31] present a connection between the protein denaturation process, the maximum positive peak and minimum negative peak.

Analyzing the CD spectra profiles for all the samples, from Figure 2, and assuming the presumption that a higher ratio between the peaks, as mentioned before, we can conclude that GELL_COLL_T_{rt} is the most denatured extract from perch skin, where tartaric acid was used for extraction, and the sample was kept at room temperature (the experiments were performed during the winter, at maximum 15 °C). The less denatured sample is GELL_COLL_A_f, where ascorbic acid was used for extraction and samples were kept in the refrigerator (4 °C); therefore, the negative bands with higher values indicate a lower denaturation. Once again, the temperature influence upon conformational structure in this case is demonstrated. The prevalence of random coil structures and no bands characteristic of the triple-helix structure, which are specific to collagen, are in concordance with the FTIR spectra, presented further, demonstrating that the perch skin collagen extracts have a gelatinous structure.

Moreover, Echave et al. [32] demonstrate that the use of denatured collagen and gelatine increases cell growth, promoting the biological response of medical devices used in tissue engineering.

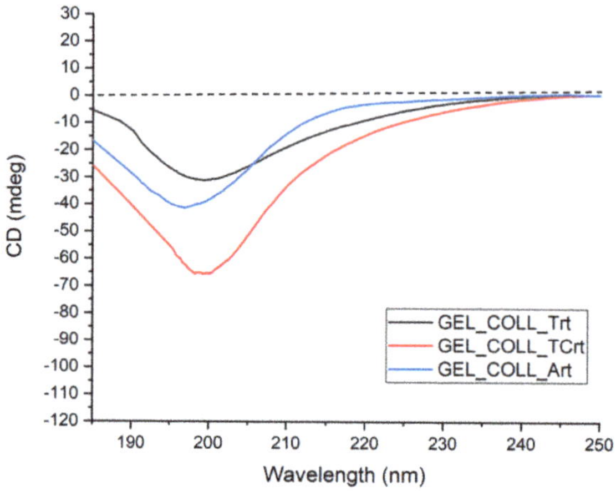

(a)

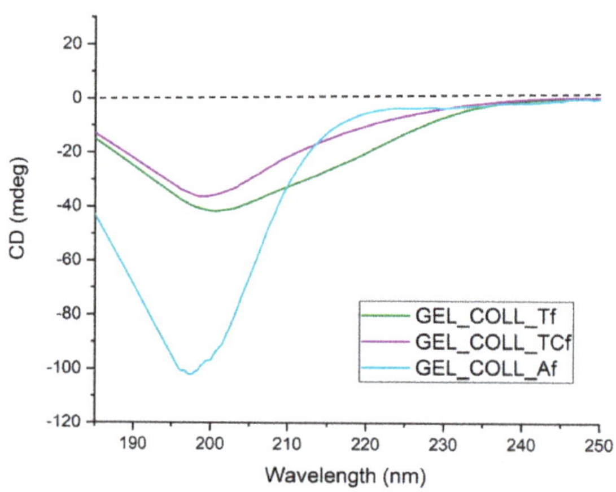

(b)

Figure 2. Circular dichroism spectra for perch gels; (**a**) samples kept at room temperature, (**b**) samples kept in the fridge.

- *Fourier transform infrared spectroscopy (FTIR)*

Gels extracted from perch skin present spectral bands characteristic of the functional groups in the collagen structure, such as amide A, B, I, II and III. In Figure 3, there are no significant differences between samples. The signal of the peaks between 3305 and 3280 cm^{-1} is represented by the amide A structure and is specific to the stretching vibrations of N-H groups coupled with hydrogen bonds from the carbonyl group in the peptide chain.

Amide B presents signals in the range of 3090–2930 cm^{-1}, with the stretching vibration of the methylene group being symmetrical and asymmetrical. The peak characteristic of amide I at approximately 1631 cm^{-1} is similar to other fish extracts [33–35].

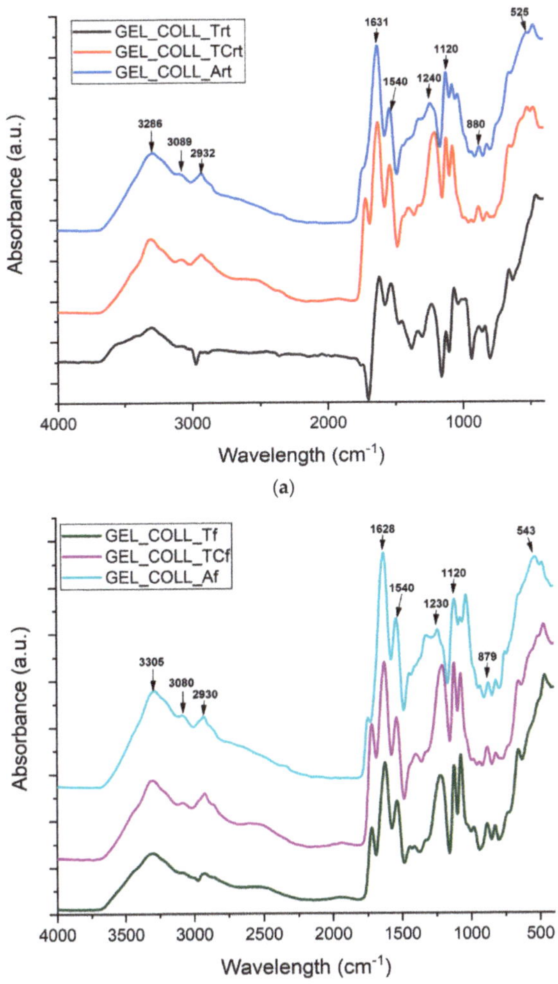

Figure 3. FTIR spectra of perch gels; (**a**) samples kept at room temperature, (**b**) samples kept at fridge.

Amide I, specific to the secondary structure of proteins, with a peak characteristic of carbonyl group stretching vibration in the peptide structure, presents an intense absorption at 1660 cm^{-1}, attributed to the collagen triple-helix structure; otherwise, the intensity decreases and the band intensification around 1630 cm^{-1} is associated with collagen denaturation, resulting gelatine [36].

The bands characteristic of amides II and III represent the bending vibrations of the N-H group (at 1540 cm^{-1}) coupled with the stretching vibrations of the C-N and C-H groups (1240–1210 cm^{-1}). In the case of collagen, the specific intensity of the amide II peak is more intense, around 1550 cm^{-1}, so the FTIR spectra clearly indicate the gelatine structure. The peaks at 1120 cm^{-1} represent the asymmetric bonds of CO-O-C glycogen and nucleic acids. The peaks appearing at wave numbers between 880 and 525 cm^{-1} represent the protein skeleton [37,38].

2.2. Characterization of Collagen Scaffolds

Following the characterization of perch gels, the best properties were obtained for samples stored in a refrigerator, despite having the lowest yield, based on physical/chemical properties and circular dichroism, which showed a lower denaturation of perch gel samples; therefore, the samples kept in a refrigerator were chosen for further analysis. The perch gels selected were poured into a glass Petri dish and freeze-dried for 48 h [35] in order to obtain collagen scaffolds (spongious forms), which were further tested to determine the water absorption, conduct a microbiological analysis and determine the biocompatibility of the synthesized collagen scaffolds.

2.2.1. Water Absorption of Collagen Scaffolds

The water uptake was estimated for three days at different intervals of time and showed that all the samples were stable, as shown in Figure 4.

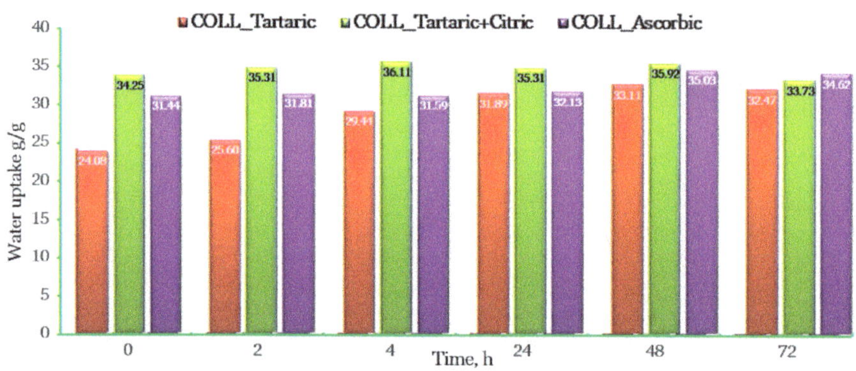

Figure 4. Water uptake of biocomposites.

The sample COLL_TC absorbed the highest amount of water, about 36 g/g water in the first 48 h. COLL_A seems to be denser, therefore absorbing a smaller amount of water, around 35 g/g water in the first 48 h. COLL_T absorbed around 33 g/g water.

All the samples present stability in the first 48 h, and then the samples start to dissolve.

Prior to selecting a wound dressing, it is critical to consider a number of criteria, including the wound dressing's cost, convenience of administration, duration of therapy and capacity to absorb exudate in an effective manner, along with other factors. Hence, water absorption is a key factor in the development of wound dressing.

2.2.2. Collagen Scaffolds Microbiological Analysis

Microbiological testing is imperative for patient health protection. Medical device manufacturers must ensure that their products meet the highest quality control standards. Microbiological testing is essential to ensure that a device is safe and effective by examining the presence of harmful pathogens that could contaminate it [39].

From Figure 5, it can be observed that all the samples presented antibacterial activity against *Escherichia coli* (*E. coli*) and *Staphylococcus aureus* (*S. aureus*), with intense activity on *E. coli*, which proves the efficiency of these collagen scaffolds for medical applications use.

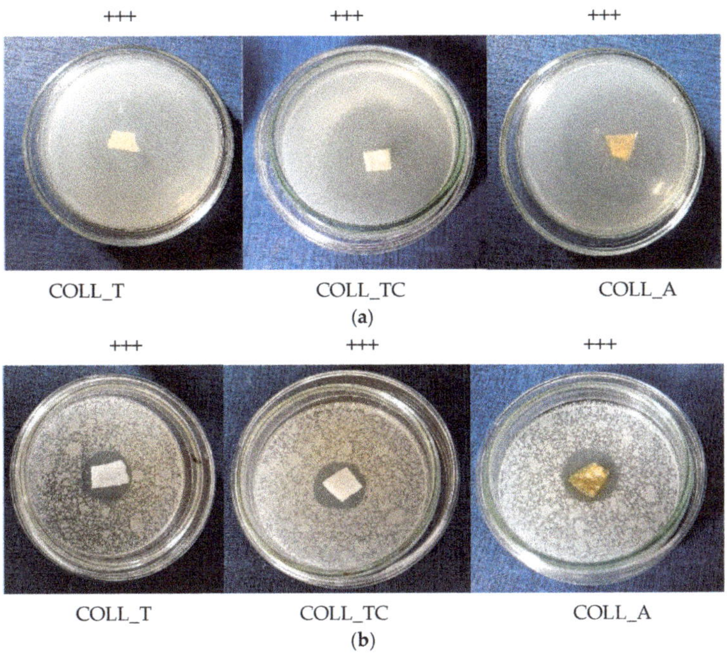

Figure 5. Antimicrobial activity of perch sponges against (**a**) *E. coli* and (**b**) *S. aureus*.

The difference between the degree of inhibition for the two types of bacteria tested may be due to the structure of the cell wall. *E. coli* is a Gram-negative bacteria unlike *S. aureus*, which is a Gram-positive bacteria with a more resistant cell wall due to the basic unit—peptidoglycan.

Depending on the diameter of the inhibition zones formed, the results are interpreted as follows:

- 0–10 mm, inactive—marked "−";
- 10–14 mm, weak activity—noted "+";
- 15–19 mm, moderate activity—marked "++";
- ≥20 mm, definite activity—marked "+++".

The scope of microbial contamination determination, in accordance with the provisions of the European Pharmacopoeia Ed. 10/20, is to identify microbial contamination of the samples (Table 2). Microbial contamination control aims to determine the total number of aerobic microorganisms or the absence of pathogenic microorganisms:

- Total number of aerobic microorganisms (TAMC);
- Total number of yeasts and filamentous fungi (TYMC).

Table 2. Determination of microbial contamination of collagen sponges.

Sample	Total Number of Aerobic Microorganisms (TAMC), CFU/g *	Total Number of Fungi and Filamentous Fungi (TYMC), CFU/g **	*E. coli* Absent	*S. aureus* Absent	*P. aeruginosa* Absent
COLL_T	5 CFU/g	3 CFU/g	absent	absent	absent
COLL_TC	6 CFU/g	2 CFU/g	absent	absent	absent
COLL_A	3 CFU/g	2 CFU/g	absent	absent	absent

* Admissibility conditions: Up to 100 CFU/g for topical products and up to 1000 CFU/g for pharmaceutical products; ** Admissibility conditions: Up to 100 CFU/g for topical products and for pharmaceutical products.

The bacteria tested on collagen scaffold were Escherichia coli (*E. coli*), Staphylococcus aureus (*S. aureus*), and Pseudomonas aeruginosa (*P. aeruginosa*).

From the obtained results, during the microbiological characterization of the tested collagen scaffolds, it can be observed that the obtained the values do not exceed the limits of admissibility provided by the European Pharmacopoeia, the currently used edition. The samples do not allow the development of aerobic germs for any of the tested bacteria [40–43].

2.2.3. Collagen Scaffolds Biocompatibility

The biocompatibility of the tested collagen-based scaffolds was assessed by incubating human adult dermal fibroblasts with extracts obtained as described in the Materials and Methods. Since the dermal fibroblasts are one of the major players in the wound healing process, we first looked at their viability in the presence of scaffold-based extracts. Moreover, given the fact that fibroblast motility is an important feature of these cells, which should be able to migrate from the areas surrounding the lesion into the injury site and colonize the scaffolds, we subsequently verified whether this ability of human dermal fibroblasts was impacted by the scaffolds.

As shown in Figure 6, no cytotoxic effect was observed for the tested scaffold extracts. Furthermore, the data indicated that, at 48 h, the COLL_T and COLL_TC scaffold sustained a slightly increased viability compared to the COLL scaffold extract; however, no statistical significance was obtained. At 72 h, the viability was similar for all extracts, except for COLL_A, which was 20% higher than the COLL extract. These data suggest that none of the tested scaffolds had any cytotoxic effect; moreover, COLL_A could have a positive impact on cell viability to some extent, possibly by promoting cell proliferation.

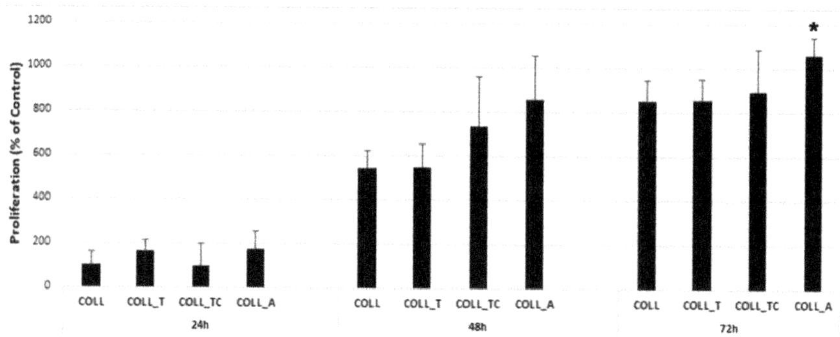

Figure 6. XTT assay showing the viability of human adult dermal fibroblasts after 24, 48 and 72 h of incubation in the presence of collagen scaffold extracts (* $p < 0.05$ versus COLL at 72 h).

As mentioned above, the migration of cells, including dermal fibroblasts, at the lesion site is an important step in the wound healing progression. Moreover, in the case of using these scaffolds for wound healing, the migration of fibroblasts in order to colonize biomaterials should not be inhibited. Therefore, we evaluated the impact of the tested scaffold extracts on this key feature. Thus, Figure 7 indicates that all extracts promoted fibroblast migration in comparison to the negative control, which was a serum-free medium (controls used in order to verify that the technique was correctly performed). No statistical significance was obtained when compared to the COLL extract, with the exception of the COLL_A extract, which induced a cell migration about 40% lower than the COLL control.

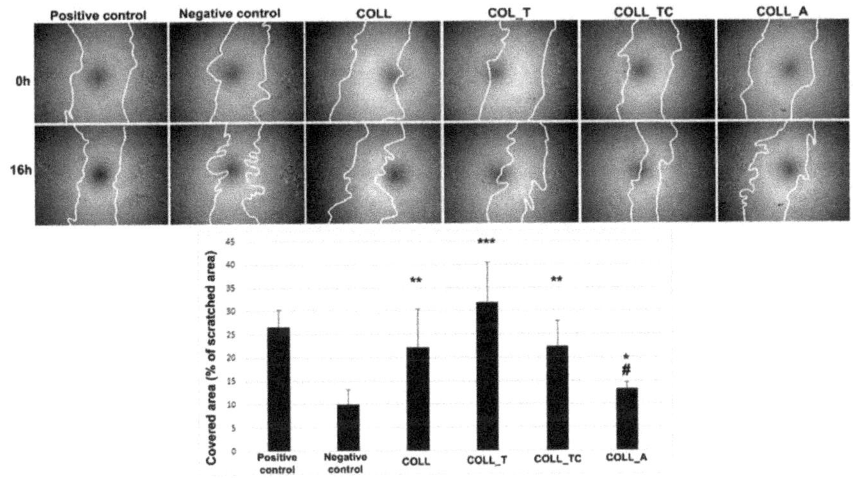

Figure 7. In vitro scratch test showing the impact of collagen scaffold extracts on the fibroblast motility: upper panel—phase-contrast microscopy showing the scratched area at 0 h and 16 h later (magnification 5×), lower panel—the quantification of covered area as percentage of the initial scratched area where positive and negative controls are serum and serum-free medium (* $p < 0.05$; ** $p < 0.005$, *** $p < 0.001$ versus negative control, # $p < 0.05$ versus COLL).

Next, the capacity of the tested scaffolds was assessed to support colonization with dermal fibroblasts. For this, cells were grown on these samples as described above and viability was evaluated. As seen in Figure 8, the viability for cells grown on the COLL_T and COLL_TC scaffolds was similar to those grown on the COLL scaffold. However, in the case of the COLL_A scaffold, the viability was 35% higher than the COLL control. This corroborates well with the previous data regarding the lack of toxicity of all extracts and the increased viability in the presence of COLL_A extract 72 h after seeding in 2D culture.

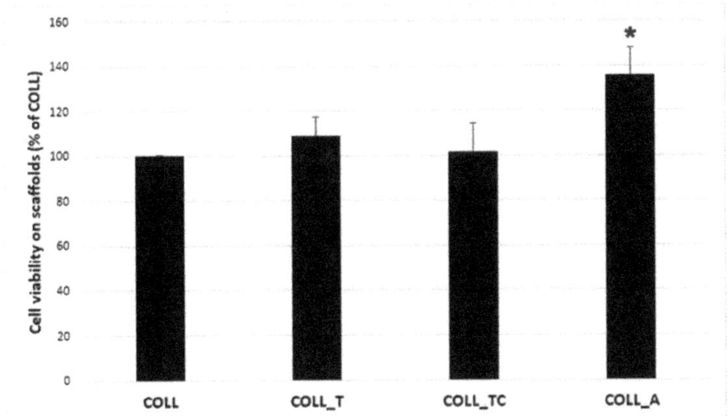

Figure 8. XTT assay showing the viability of human adult dermal fibroblasts 5 days after seeding onto collagen scaffolds (* $p < 0.05$).

The Hematoxylin and Eosin histological staining showed that all scaffolds sustained three-dimensional growth of dermal fibroblasts, both at the surface and inside the scaffolds, within the structural pores (Figure 9). In the case of COLL_T, the structure is lax, most likely due to partial degradation in the presence of cells. All the other scaffolds retained integrity in the given timeline.

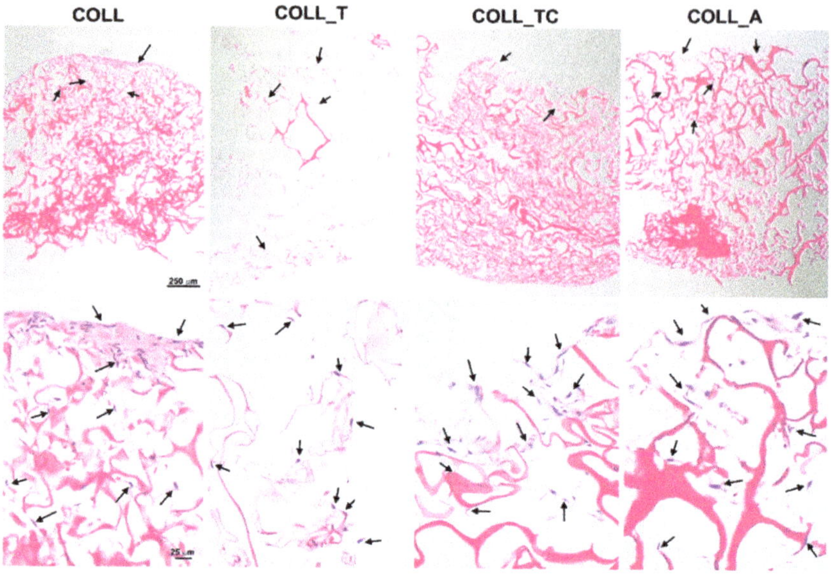

Figure 9. Hematoxylin and Eosin staining illustrating the colonization of collagen scaffolds with human dermal fibroblasts. The presence of cells attached to the collagen fibers is indicated by arrows.

Next, we checked whether the various collagen scaffolds support the ability of dermal fibroblasts to perform contraction. In Figure 10, it can be noticed that the area of the COLL-T scaffold increased after 5 days in the presence of cells. Keeping in mind that the histological analysis showed a certain degradation of collagen scaffold in the presence of fibroblasts, we assume that this increase in size and lack of contraction is due to the loss of structural integrity following the secretory activity of the cultured cells. In contrast, the other two scaffolds, COLL_TC and COLL_A, were less contracted by fibroblasts in comparison with COLL, although the difference was statistically significant only for the COLL_A scaffold. Thus, the latter showed a contraction about 25% lower than COLL.

Our data showed that all tested scaffolds were biocompatible, and COLL_A was capable of promoting a higher viability of fibroblasts in comparison with the COLL control and the other tested scaffolds, both in the case of extracts obtained by incubation in a complete culture medium and by direct contact with human dermal fibroblasts, suggesting a higher capacity to sustain colonization. Although the COLL_A extract promoted dermal fibroblast migration to a smaller extent than the COLL extract, as shown by the scratch test assay, this might not be the case in vivo, keeping in mind that the extracts were obtained in the absence of cells. Interestingly, the histological analysis showed a certain degradation of the COLL_T scaffold after 5 days in the presence of human dermal fibroblasts, suggesting that this particular biomaterial could not be appropriate for in vivo use, since the degradation of the scaffold should be synchronized with the regeneration process in order to ensure support for the migration and proliferation of cells from the surrounding tissue. All the other tested scaffolds were stable for up to 5 days in the culture and in the presence of cells. Since, throughout the wound healing process, the proliferative phase begins during the first week after injury [44,45], the scaffold should be stable in a biological environment at least for this period of time. As the fibroblasts proliferate and begin to secrete extracellular matrix, the scaffold should be able to be slowly degraded under the activity of enzymes in order to make place for the newly formed tissue. Our results indicated that, with the exception of COLL_T, all the tested scaffolds retained their structure for at least 5 days in the presence of dermal fibroblasts, suggesting they are suitable for in vivo use [44,45].

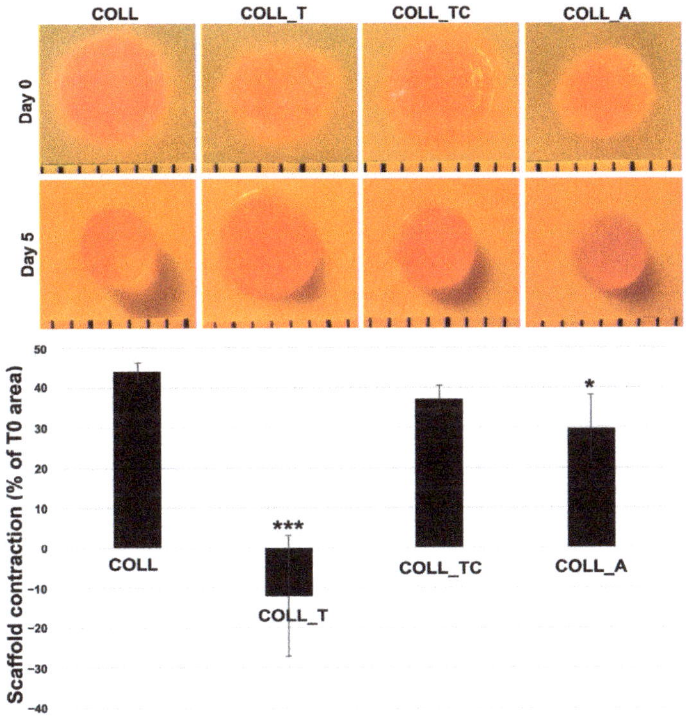

Figure 10. Quantification of collagen scaffolds contraction: upper panel—images of the scaffolds before seeding of fibroblasts and after 5 days in culture; lower panel—quantification of the contracted area (* $p < 0.05$, *** $p < 0.001$). Each image was individually calibrated.

Furthermore, we examined the capacity of the scaffolds to support dermal fibroblast contraction. It is known that although this process is normal during wound healing, having the role of pulling together the edges of the wound to minimize its size in the case of large wounds could lead to complications, such as scarring and fibrosis or even the loss of a tissue function [46]. Thus, efforts are being made to create biomaterials that inhibit or do not support a high degree of contraction to circumvent these disadvantages [47]. Data showed that, with the exception of the COLL_T scaffold, which appeared to increase in size after 5 days in culture in the presence of dermal fibroblasts most likely due to degradation, COLL_TC and COLL_A exhibited a lower contraction in comparison to the COLL scaffold, which was statistically significant for COLL_A. Thus, corroborating these data, we conclude that the COLL_A scaffold could be a valuable tool for wound healing.

3. Conclusions

This paper highlights the development of biocompatible materials for regenerative medicine starting from natural resources, such as fish skin. This research focuses on collagen extracted from perch skin (*P. fluviatilis*) in the form of a gel in order to obtain collagen scaffolds for wound healing.

The resulting collagen gel samples were analyzed by proximate analysis. The sample with ascorbic acid used for extraction and stored in the refrigerator (GEL_COLL_Af) presents the highest protein and dry substance content. The results obtained were also confirmed by circular dichroism (CD).

It can be concluded from CD spectra profiles that the most denatured sample from perch skin was GELL_COLL_Trt, with tartaric acid used for extraction and stored at room temperature (the studies were conducted during the winter, at a maximum room temperature of 15 °C). When ascorbic acid was used for extraction and the sample was kept in the refrigerator (4 °C), GELL_COLL_Af was less denatured; as a result, the negative bands with higher values indicate a lesser denaturation. At this point, it is demonstrated how temperature affects conformational structure.

The FT-IR spectra present the random coil structure preponderance and the absence of any band distinctive of the triple-helix structure specific to collagen. This indicates that the collagen extracts from perch skin have a gelatinous structure, which is in concordance with CD spectra.

The best properties of the analyzed perch gels were observed in samples stored in the refrigerator, especially for GELL_COLL_Af, despite the lowest yield; therefore, the samples kept in the refrigerator were further freeze-dried in order to obtain collagen scaffolds (spongious forms), which were further tested to determine the water absorption, conduct a microbiological analysis and analyze the biocompatibility of the synthesized collagen scaffolds. All three samples (COLL_T, COLL-TC, COLL_A) present stability in the first 48 h, and then they start to dissolve.

From the microbiological analysis, it was observed that all the samples presented antibacterial activity against *Escherichia coli* (*E. coli*) and *Staphylococcus aureus* (*S. aureus*), with intense activity on *E. coli*, which proves the efficiency of collagen scaffolds for wound dressing. The samples do not allow the development of aerobic germs for any of the tested bacteria.

The biological data demonstrated the biocompatibility of all tested scaffolds, and the COLL_A sample was able to support fibroblast viability that was higher than that of the control (COLL sample) and the other tested scaffolds, both for extracts obtained by direct contact with human dermal fibroblasts and for extracts obtained by incubation in complete culture medium, indicating a higher capacity capable to sustain colonization. Despite the fact that the scratch test assay demonstrated that the COLL_A extract facilitated dermal fibroblast migration more than the COLL sample, this may not be the case in vivo, taking into account that the extracts were produced without cells. Moreover, the capacity of the scaffolds to support dermal fibroblast contraction was examined. The contraction process is normal during wound healing. The data resulting from this analysis showed that, with the exception of the COLL_T scaffold, which appeared to increase in size after 5 days in culture in the presence of dermal fibroblasts likely due to degradation, COLL_TC and COLL_A exhibited a lower contraction in comparison with the COLL scaffold, which was statistically significant for COLL_A. Hence, it can be concluded that the COLL_A scaffold could be a valuable tool for wound healing, revealing a new opportunity for biomaterials used in regenerative medicine, starting from collagen of marine origin.

4. Materials and Methods

4.1. Process of Acidic Collagen Extraction

The fresh European perch skin was bought from a local fishing company, Tulcea, Danube Delta, Romania. In our country, perch consumption is very high, leading to large quantities of fish wastes. In this context, we tried to find a viable solution in order to valorize the by-products, which, in this case, was perch skin. The fresh skin was frozen until processing. After defrosting, the skin was washed thoroughly with bio detergent and cold distilled water in the first step. After washing, several treatments followed in order to obtain collagen gels. Figure 11 schematically shows all the treatment stages subjected to the skin, which are detailed further.

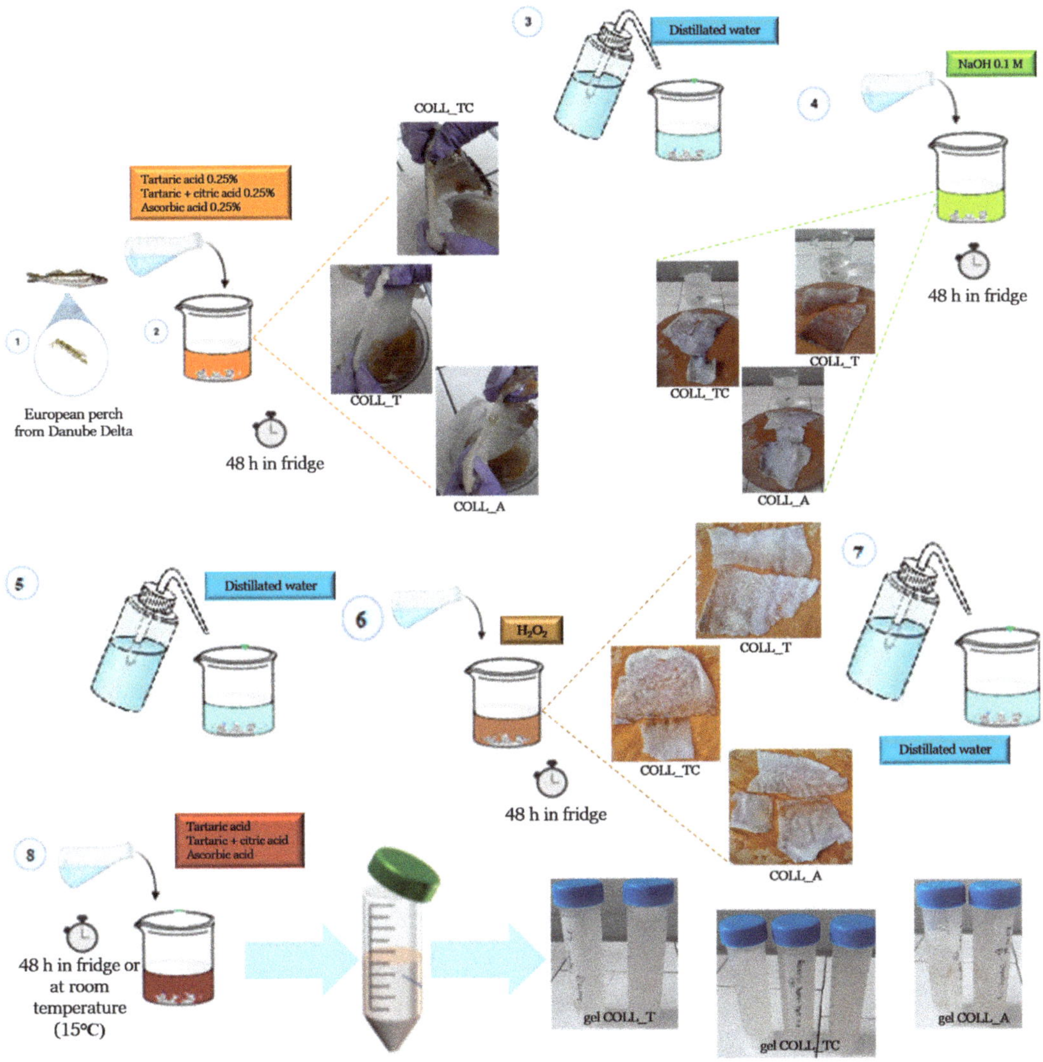

Figure 11. Schematic representation of acidic extraction of collagen gel from perch skin.

After washing, the perch skin samples were placed in three different acidic solutions with 0.25% concentration of acids and kept in the refrigerator for two days. The acids used were L (+) tartaric acid (Chimreactiv, Bucharest, Romania), L (+) tartaric and citric acid (Chimreactiv, Bucharest, Romania) in equal proportions and L (+) ascorbic acid (Scharlau, Sentmenat, Spain). After two days, it can be seen the skin is slightly swollen.

In the third stage, the samples were washed with distilled water until a neutral pH to avoid precipitation of acids remained when adding a solution of 0.1 M sodium hydroxide (Chemical Company, Iasi, Romania) in the fourth stage. In the alkaline treatment, the samples were kept in the refrigerator for 48 h. Sodium hydroxide helps to remove non-collagenous proteins, as can be seen in the pictures.

During stage five, the samples were washed with distilled water, followed by stage six, the process of pigment removal from the skin. For this, the samples were placed in a solution of 2% hydrogen peroxide (hydrogen peroxide solution 30%, Silal Trading, Bucharest, Romania) and kept 48 h in the refrigerator.

After washing the samples with distilled water, the last step for collagen gel extraction from perch skin is the addition of the acids used initially in the acidic treatment. In order to see the temperature influence on sample's properties, the treated skin was split in two: one part stayed in the refrigerator for 48 h, and the other stayed at room temperature (15 °C). The final results were collagen gels illustrated in Figure 11.

The pH of perch gels extracted was adjusted from 2.5 to 7.2–7.4 (for promoting cell growth [48]) with NaOH 0.1 M and afterward, the gels were poured into a glass Petri dish and freeze-dried for 48 h [49] to obtain collagen scaffolds (spongious forms, Figure 12).

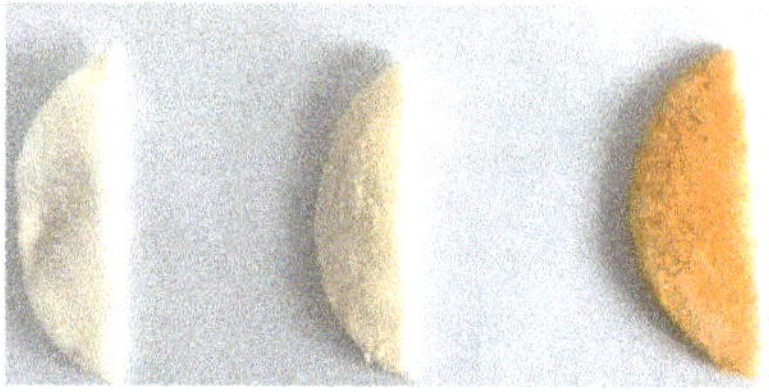

(**a**) (**b**) (**c**)

Figure 12. Collagen scaffolds, gels after freeze drying, (**a**) COLL_T, (**b**) COLL_TC and (**c**) COLL_A.

4.2. Physical/Chemical Analysis and Extracted Collagen Yields

Dry substance, ash and protein contents of extracted gels were determined according to standard methods SR EN ISO 4684:2006, SR EN ISO 4047:2002 and SR ISO 5397:1996. Total nitrogen was determined by the Kjeldahl method. The pH was determined potentiometrically according to SR EN ISO 4045:2008.

The yield of extracted collagen was calculated on basis of the weight of fresh skin:

$$\% \text{ Yield} = (\text{Dry substance content weight}/\text{Dry skin weight}) \times 100 \quad (1)$$

where *Dry substance content weight* represents dry collagen.

4.3. Water Uptake of Collagen Scaffolds

The water uptake capacity of collagen sponges was determined by weight method [16], which involves weighing the sponges before and after immersion in water. A piece of sponge of about 1 cm^3 was weighed at reference time and then placed in 3 mL water at room temperature (about 23 °C). At defined periods of time, the sponges were weighed and the capacity to retain water was calculated using the following equation (Equation (2)):

$$\text{Water uptake } (\%) = [(Wt - Wd)/Wd] \times 100 \quad (2)$$

where *Wt* represents the weight of water retained by sponges at time t and *Wd* is the weight of dry sponges. The experiment was performed in triplicate.

4.4. Structural Analysis

- *Circular Dichroism Spectroscopy*

The secondary structure of the perch collagen extracts was evaluated by circular dichroism spectroscopy (CD). Spectra acquisitions were performed on a Jasco J-1500 Spectrophotometer model, Tokyo, Japan (J-1500 Circular Dichroism Spectrophotometer) using a quartz cell with l = 10 mm.

For each reading, 500 µL of fish extracts aqueous solution of 0.05% concentration was used. The CD spectra were obtained by scanning in triplicate, using the spectral range 185–250 nm, with a scanning speed of 100 nm/min.

- *Fourier transform infrared spectroscopy (FTIR)*

Perch collagen extracts were subjected to FTIR spectral analysis using a Vertex 70 Bruker FTIR spectrometer (Bruker, Billerica, MA, USA). The following settings were used to record each FTIR spectrum in the ATR mode: resolution of 4 cm^{-1}, spectral range of 4000–600 cm^{-1} and 30 acquisitions for every sample.

4.5. Collagen Scaffolds Microbiological Analysis

The samples were tested on ATCC strains from the collection of the ICPI Biotechnology Laboratory, namely, on *E. coli* (ATCC 10536, Mediclim, Bucharest, Romania) and *S. aureus* (ATCC 6538, Mediclim, Bucharest, Romania). The working method was diffusion method. A tube containing Mueller Hinton Broth (MHB, Novachim, Bucharest, Romania) inoculated with *E. Coli* and *S. aureus* was incubated for 18 h at 37 °C. Decimal dilutions up to 10^{-5} CFU/mL were made from this tube. An amount of 200 μL of the inoculum was seeded onto the plates. Afterward, the samples thus prepared were added and kept in the incubator for 24 h at 37 °C. Antibacterial activity was determined by measuring the diameter of the zone of inhibition around every sample. For microbial contamination, Casein Soya Bean Digest Agar (Novachim, Bucharest, Romania) was employed for total aerobic microbial count (TAMC) and Sabouraud Dextrose Agar (Novachim, Bucharest, Romania) for total fungal count.

4.6. Assessment of Biocompatibility of Collagen Scaffolds

In order to have a more complete characterization of the collagen scaffolds' impact on human skin cells, the cytotoxicity of extracts obtained by incubating the samples in culture medium was tested, followed by assessment of capacity to support colonization with human dermal fibroblasts. As control, a collagen scaffold (COLL) without tartaric, tartaric plus citric and ascorbic acids addition was used.

The collagen scaffolds were incubated in complete culture medium (low glucose Dulbecco's Modified Eagle Medium from Sigma Aldrich, St. Louis, MO, USA), supplemented with 10% (*v*/*v*) fetal bovine serum from Gibco BRL, Gaithersburg, MD, USA and 100 IU/mL penicillin, 100 μg/mL streptomycin and 50 μg/mL neomycin, all from Sigma Aldrich, St. Louis, MO, USA, at a 2 mg/mL ratio for 6 h/37 °C under stirring. Subsequently, the samples were clarified by centrifugation (300 g/5 min) and sterilized by filtration (0.2 μm pore size). Next, the effect of this extract on the viability of human adult fibroblasts was assessed in addition to the impact on cell function (migration capacity). The chemotactic properties of the tested freeze-dried wafers were assessed by xCELLigence RTCA system (Acea Biosciences, Inc). The human adult fibroblasts were obtained as previously described [50] and cultured in complete culture medium, at 37 °C and 5% CO_2.

For the viability assessment, cells were seeded in complete medium on 96-well plates either in the presence of extracts (1×10^4 cells/cm^2) or on pre-cut collagen scaffolds (5×10^5 cells/well). For this, sheets of scaffolds were cropped with a 4 mm in diameter punch, sterilized in 70% ethanol overnight, followed by washing in sterile water, and maintained in DMEM without serum for at least 24 h. The viability was evaluated in triplicates by XTT assay (Thermo Fisher Scientific, Waltham, MA, USA) 24, 48 and 72 h after the addition of the extracts or 5 days after the seeding of scaffolds.

The effect of collagen scaffold extracts on the fibroblast's migration capacity was evaluated by scratch test. Thus, cells were seeded in complete medium on 96-well plates (1×10^4 cells/cm^2). Twenty-four hours before the test, cells were serum starved. A lesion was performed on the monolayer using a 200 μL pipette tip and the cells were incubated in the presence of extracts using 8 biological replicates. Pictures were taken immediately after adding the extracts (0 h) and 16 h later. The cell migration was evaluated by quantifying the area covered by the cells using the ImageJ 1.42q software (NIH, Bethesda, MD, USA). The results were presented as percentage of coverage of the scratched area.

The capacity of the tested collagen scaffolds to support colonization with dermal fibroblasts was further assessed. Thus, cells were seeded onto the cropped scaffolds as described above, and, 5 days later, the samples were fixed in 4% PFA and processed for paraffin embedding. Slices that were 5 μm thick were obtained by using a Leica microtome and subsequently subjected to hematoxylin–eosin staining. Briefly, the slices were incubated for 1 min with hematoxylin and 30 s with eosin Y, mounted in Shandon Consul-Mount (Thermo Fisher Scientific, Waltham, MA, USA) and visualized using a Zeiss Observer D1 microscope (Zeiss, Oberkochen, Germany).

The contraction of the scaffold was assessed by taking pictures of the cropped samples before seeding with cells and after 5 days in culture. The area of each sample was quantified by using the ImageJ software (NIH, Bethesda, MD, USA). Each picture was individually calibrated. The results were presented as percentage of the initial size at T0.

Author Contributions: Conceptualization, A.E.C., A.M.R., M.G.A.K. and I.T.; methodology, A.E.C. and M.G.A.K.; software, A.E.C., I.T. and M.M.M.; validation, A.E.C. and M.G.A.K.; formal analysis, A.E.C., A.M.R., R.R.C. and I.T.; investigation, A.E.C., A.M.R., I.T., M.M.M. and R.R.C.; resources, M.G.A.K., M.M.M. and I.T.; writing—original draft preparation, A.E.C., A.M.R. and M.M.M.; writing—review and editing, A.E.C., M.G.A.K. and M.M.M., visualization, A.E.C. and M.G.A.K., supervision, M.G.A.K. and I.T. All authors have read and agreed to the published version of the manuscript.

Funding: This research received no external funding.

Institutional Review Board Statement: Not applicable.

Informed Consent Statement: Not applicable.

Data Availability Statement: The original contributions presented in the study are included in the article, further inquiries can be directed to the corresponding authors.

Acknowledgments: This paper was financially supported by a grant of the Ministry of Research, Innovation and Digitalization, project number PN 23 26 01 01/2023, by an international project M-ERA NET 73/2024, and by a project PN-III-P1-1.1-TE-2021-1344.

Conflicts of Interest: The authors declare no conflicts of interest.

References

1. Susanti, E.; Lutfiana, N.; Suharti; Retnosari, R. Screening of Proteolytic Bacteria from *Tauco* Surabaya Based on Pathogenicity and Selectivity of Its Protease on Milky Fish (*Chanos chanos*) Scales for Healthy and Halal Collagen Production. *IOP Conf. Ser. Mater. Sci. Eng.* **2019**, *509*, 012044. [CrossRef]
2. Sorushanova, A.; Delgado, L.M.; Wu, Z.; Shologu, N.; Kshirsagar, A.; Raghunath, R.; Mullen, A.M.; Bayon, Y.; Pandit, A.; Raghunath, M.; et al. The Collagen Suprafamily: From Biosynthesis to Advanced Biomaterial Development. *Adv. Mater.* **2019**, *31*, 1801651. [CrossRef] [PubMed]
3. Shavandi, A.; Hou, Y.; Carne, A.; McConnell, M.; Bekhit, A.E.A. Marine Waste Utilization as a Source of Functional and Health Compounds. *Adv. Food Nutr. Res.* **2019**, *87*, 187–254. [PubMed]
4. Furtado, M.; Chen, L.; Chen, Z.; Chen, A.; Cui, W. Development of Fish Collagen in Tissue Regeneration and Drug Delivery. *Eng. Regen.* **2022**, *3*, 217–231. [CrossRef]
5. Rathod, N.K. *Extraction of Functionally Active Collagen from Fish By-Products*; Flinders University, College of Medicine and Public Health: Bedford Park, Australia, 2021.
6. Maschmeyer, T.; Luque, R.; Selva, M. Upgrading of Marine (Fish and Crustaceans) Biowaste for High Added-Value Molecules and Bio(Nano)-Materials. *Chem. Soc. Rev.* **2020**, *49*, 4527–4563. [CrossRef]
7. Shaw, C.; Knopf, K.; Kloas, W. Fish Feeds in Aquaponics and Beyond: A Novel Concept to Evaluate Protein Sources in Diets for Circular Multitrophic Food Production Systems. *Sustainability* **2022**, *14*, 4064. [CrossRef]
8. de Melo Oliveira, V.; Assis, C.R.D.; Costa, B.D.A.M.; de Araújo Neri, R.C.; Monte, F.T.D.; da Costa Vasconcelos, H.M.S.; França, R.C.P.; Santos, J.F.; de Souza Bezerra, R.; Porto, A.L.F. Physical, Biochemical, Densitometric and Spectroscopic Techniques for Characterization Collagen from Alternative Sources: A Review Based on the Sustainable Valorization of Aquatic by-Products. *J. Mol. Struct.* **2021**, *1224*, 129023. [CrossRef]
9. Rajabimashhadi, Z.; Gallo, N.; Salvatore, L.; Lionetto, F. Collagen Derived from Fish Industry Waste: Progresses and Challenges. *Polymers* **2023**, *15*, 544. [CrossRef]
10. Caruso, G.; Floris, R.; Serangeli, C.; Di Paola, L. Fishery Wastes as a Yet Undiscovered Treasure from the Sea: Biomolecules Sources, Extraction Methods and Valorization. *Mar. Drugs* **2020**, *18*, 622. [CrossRef]
11. Rodríguez, F.; Morán, L.; González, G.; Troncoso, E.; Zúñiga, R.N. Collagen Extraction from Mussel Byssus: A New Marine Collagen Source with Physicochemical Properties of Industrial Interest. *J. Food Sci. Technol.* **2017**, *54*, 1228–1238. [CrossRef]

12. Khan, S.B.; Qian, Z.-J.; Ryu, B.; Kim, S.-K. Isolation and Biochemical Characterization of Collagens from Seaweed Pipefish, Syngnathus Schlegeli. *Biotechnol. Bioprocess. Eng.* **2009**, *14*, 436–442. [CrossRef]
13. Aleman, A.; Martinez-Alvarez, O. Marine Collagen as a Source of Bioactive Molecules: A Review. *Nat. Prod. J.* **2013**, *3*, 105–114. [CrossRef]
14. Carvalho, A.M.; Marques, A.P.; Silva, T.H.; Reis, R.L. Evaluation of the Potential of Collagen from Codfish Skin as a Biomaterial for Biomedical Applications. *Mar. Drugs* **2018**, *16*, 495. [CrossRef] [PubMed]
15. Al Khawli, F.; Pateiro, M.; Domínguez, R.; Lorenzo, J.M.; Gullón, P.; Kousoulaki, K.; Ferrer, E.; Berrada, H.; Barba, F.J. Innovative Green Technologies of Intensification for Valorization of Seafood and Their By-Products. *Mar. Drugs* **2019**, *17*, 689. [CrossRef] [PubMed]
16. Albu, M.G.; Ferdes, M.; Kaya, D.A.; Ghica, M.V.; Titorencu, I.; Popa, L.; Albu, L. Collagen Wound Dressings with Anti-Inflammatory Activity. *Mol. Cryst. Liq. Cryst.* **2012**, *555*, 271–279. [CrossRef]
17. Obagi, Z.; Damiani, G.; Grada, A.; Falanga, V. Principles of Wound Dressings: A Review. *Surg. Technol. Int.* **2019**, *35*, 50–57.
18. Miguel, S.P.; Sequeira, R.S.; Moreira, A.F.; Cabral, C.S.D.; Mendonça, A.G.; Ferreira, P.; Correia, I.J. An Overview of Electrospun Membranes Loaded with Bioactive Molecules for Improving the Wound Healing Process. *Eur. J. Pharm. Biopharm.* **2019**, *139*, 1–22. [CrossRef]
19. La Monica, F.; Campora, S.; Ghersi, G. Collagen-Based Scaffolds for Chronic Skin Wound Treatment. *Gels* **2024**, *10*, 137. [CrossRef]
20. Berry, C.E.; Brenac, C.; Gonzalez, C.E.; Kendig, C.B.; Le, T.; An, N.; Griffin, M.F. Natural Compounds and Biomimetic Engineering to Influence Fibroblast Behavior in Wound Healing. *Int. J. Mol. Sci.* **2024**, *25*, 3274. [CrossRef]
21. Girsang, V.; Reveny, J.; Nainggolan, M. Isolation and Characterization Collagen of Patin Fish Skin (*Pangasius* sp.). *Asian J. Pharm. Res. Dev.* **2020**, *8*, 47–51. [CrossRef]
22. Wu, K.; Li, Y.; Chen, J. Effect of PH on the Structure, Functional Properties and Rheological Properties of Collagen from Greenfin Horse-Faced Filefish (*Thamnaconus septentrionalis*) Skin. *Mar. Drugs* **2024**, *22*, 45. [CrossRef] [PubMed]
23. Matinong, A.M.E.; Chisti, Y.; Pickering, K.L.; Haverkamp, R.G. Collagen Extraction from Animal Skin. *Biology* **2022**, *11*, 905. [CrossRef] [PubMed]
24. Agustina, M.; Patmawati, P.; Mubarok, S.; Sulmartiwi, L.; Wulandari, D.A.; Zai, K.; Siva, R.; Pujiastuti, D.Y.; Nirmala, D.; Carattri Kusuma Werdani, M.; et al. Effect of Ultrasonic Assisted Extraction with Ethanol for Removing Lipid on Catfish (*Pangasius* sp.) Skin as a Collagen Source and Its Characteristics. *J. Ilm. Perikan. Dan Kelaut.* **2023**, *16*, 274–284. [CrossRef]
25. Ong, T.Y.; Shaik, M.I.; Sarbon, N.M. Isolation and Characterization of Acid and Pepsin Soluble Collagen Extracted from Sharpnose Stingray (*Dasyatis zugei*) Skin. *Food Res.* **2021**, *5*, 214–224. [CrossRef]
26. Hadfi, N.H.; Sarbon, N.M. Physicochemical Properties of Silver Catfish (*Pangasius* sp.) Skin Collagen as Influenced by Acetic Acid Concentration. *Food Res.* **2019**, *3*, 783–790. [CrossRef]
27. Baderi, N.A. Microstructure, Extractability and Physicochemical Properties of Shortfin Scad (*Decapterus macrosoma*) Bone Collagen as Influenced by Acetic Acid Concentration. *Int. Food Res. J.* **2019**, *26*, 451–458.
28. Zhou, Y.; Li, S.; Wang, D.; Zhao, Y.; Lei, X. Estimation of Type i Collagen Structure Dissolved in Inorganical Acids from Circular Dichroism Spectra. *Biosci. J.* **2018**, *34*, 778–789. [CrossRef]
29. Drzewiecki, K.E.; Grisham, D.R.; Parmar, A.S.; Nanda, V.; Shreiber, D.I. Circular Dichroism Spectroscopy of Collagen Fibrillogenesis: A New Use for an Old Technique. *Biophys. J.* **2016**, *111*, 2377–2386. [CrossRef]
30. Perez-Puyana, V.; Ostos, F.J.; López-Cornejo, P.; Romero, A.; Guerrero, A. Assessment of the Denaturation of Collagen Protein Concentrates Using Different Techniques. *Biol. Chem.* **2019**, *400*, 1583–1591. [CrossRef]
31. Gopinath, A.; Shanmugam, G.; Madhan, B.; Rao, J.R. Differential Behavior of Native and Denatured Collagen in the Presence of Alcoholic Solvents: A Gateway to Instant Structural Analysis. *Int. J. Biol. Macromol.* **2017**, *102*, 1156–1165. [CrossRef]
32. Echave, M.C.; Hernáez-Moya, R.; Iturriaga, L.; Pedraz, J.L.; Lakshminarayanan, R.; Dolatshahi-Pirouz, A.; Taebnia, N.; Orive, G. Recent Advances in Gelatin-Based Therapeutics. *Expert. Opin. Biol. Ther.* **2019**, *19*, 773–779. [CrossRef] [PubMed]
33. Jeevithan, E.; Bao, B.; Bu, Y.; Zhou, Y.; Zhao, Q.; Wu, W. Type II Collagen and Gelatin from Silvertip Shark (*Carcharhinus albimarginatus*) Cartilage: Isolation, Purification, Physicochemical and Antioxidant Properties. *Mar. Drugs* **2014**, *12*, 3852–3873. [CrossRef] [PubMed]
34. Wang, L.; Liang, Q.; Chen, T.; Wang, Z.; Xu, J.; Ma, H. Characterization of Collagen from the Skin of Amur Sturgeon (*Acipenser schrenckii*). *Food Hydrocoll.* **2014**, *38*, 104–109. [CrossRef]
35. Wang, Y.; Wu, C.; Jia, H.; Mráz, J.; Zhao, R.; Li, S.; Dong, X.; Pan, J. Modified Structural and Functional Properties of Fish Gelatin by Glycosylation with Galacto-Oligosaccharides. *Foods* **2023**, *12*, 2828. [CrossRef]
36. Dănilă, E.; Stan, R.; Kaya, M.A.; Voicu, G.; Marin, M.M.; Moroşan, A.; Titorencu, I.; Ţuţuianu, R. Valorization of Cyprinus Carpio Skin for Biocompatible Collagen Hydrolysates with Potential Application in Foods, Cosmetics and Pharmaceuticals. *Waste Biomass Valorization* **2022**, *13*, 917–928. [CrossRef]
37. Fang, Q.; Ma, N.; Ding, K.; Zhan, S.; Lou, Q.; Huang, T. Interaction between Negatively Charged Fish Gelatin and Cyclodextrin in Aqueous Solution: Characteristics and Formation Mechanism. *Gels* **2021**, *7*, 260. [CrossRef]
38. Silva, J.C.; Barros, A.A.; Aroso, I.M.; Fassini, D.; Silva, T.H.; Reis, R.L.; Duarte, A.R.C. Extraction of Collagen/Gelatin from the Marine Demosponge *Chondrosia reniformis* (Nardo, 1847) Using Water Acidified with Carbon Dioxide—Process Optimization. *Ind. Eng. Chem. Res.* **2016**, *55*, 6922–6930. [CrossRef]

39. Tihan, G.T.; Rău, I.; Zgârian, R.G.; Ungureanu, C.; Barbaresso, R.C.; Kaya, M.G.A.; Dinu-Pîrvu, C.; Ghica, M.V. Oxytetracycline versus Doxycycline Collagen Sponges Designed as Potential Carrier Supports in Biomedical Applications. *Pharmaceutics* **2019**, *11*, 363. [CrossRef]
40. ISO-29621-2010. Available online: https://www.iso.org/standard/68310.html (accessed on 30 May 2024).
41. The European Committee on Antimicrobial Susceptibility Testing—EUCAST. Available online: https://www.eucast.org/ (accessed on 30 May 2024).
42. M02-A11: Performance Standards for Antimicrobial Disk Susceptibility Tests; Approved Standard—Eleventh Edition. Available online: https://www.researchgate.net/file.PostFileLoader.html?id=58139aa4615e27240754da03&assetKey=AS:422233756704774@1477679780485 (accessed on 31 May 2024).
43. The European Directorate for the Quality of Medicines & HealthCare (EDQM). *The European Pharmacopoeia (Ph. Eur.)*, 11th ed.; Council of Europe: London, UK; Available online: https://www.edqm.eu/en/european-pharmacopoeia-ph.-eur.-11th-edition (accessed on 1 October 2024).
44. Adib, Y.; Bensussan, A.; Michel, L. Cutaneous Wound Healing: A Review about Innate Immune Response and Current Therapeutic Applications. *Mediat. Inflamm.* **2022**, *2022*, 5344085. [CrossRef]
45. Negut, I.; Dorcioman, G.; Grumezescu, V. Scaffolds for Wound Healing Applications. *Polymers* **2020**, *12*, 2010. [CrossRef]
46. Gallant-Behm, C.L.; Hart, D.A. Genetic Analysis of Skin Wound Healing and Scarring in a Porcine Model. *Wound Repair. Regen.* **2006**, *14*, 46–54. [CrossRef] [PubMed]
47. Yannas, I.V.; Tzeranis, D.S. Mammals Fail to Regenerate Organs When Wound Contraction Drives Scar Formation. *NPJ Regen. Med.* **2021**, *6*, 39. [CrossRef] [PubMed]
48. Ibidi Cells in Focus. Available online: https://ibidi.com/img/cms/products/cells_reagents/R_5020X_CollagenI/IN_5020X_CollagenI_05mg.pdf (accessed on 1 July 2024).
49. Albu, M.G.; Ficai, A.; Lungu, A. Preparation and Characterization of Collagen Matrices Obtained at Different Freezing Temperatures. *Leather Footwear J.* **2010**, *10*, 39–50.
50. Tutuianu, R.; Rosca, A.; Albu Kaya, M.G.; Pruna, V.; Neagu, T.P.; Lascar, I.; Simionescu, M.; Titorencu, I. Mesenchymal Stromal Cell-derived Factors Promote the Colonization of Collagen 3D Scaffolds with Human Skin Cells. *J. Cell Mol. Med.* **2020**, *24*, 9692–9704. [CrossRef]

gels

MDPI

Article

3D Printed Bigel: A Novel Delivery System for Cannabidiol-Rich Hemp Extract

Anna Gościniak [1], Filip Kocaj [1], Anna Stasiłowicz-Krzemień [1], Marcin Szymański [2], Tomasz M. Karpiński [3] and Judyta Cielecka-Piontek [1,*]

1 Department of Pharmacognosy and Biomaterials, Poznan University of Medical Sciences, Rokietnicka 3, 60-806 Poznan, Poland; agosciniak@ump.edu.pl (A.G.); 83122@student.ump.edu.pl (F.K.); astasilowicz@ump.edu.pl (A.S.-K.)

2 Center for Advanced Technologies, Adam Mickiewicz University in Poznań, Uniwersytetu Poznańskiego 10, 61-614 Poznan, Poland; marcin.szymanski@amu.edu.pl

3 Department of Medical Microbiology, Medical Faculty, Poznan University of Medical Sciences, Rokietnicka 10, 60-806 Poznan, Poland; tkarpin@ump.edu.pl

* Correspondence: jpiontek@ump.edu.pl

Abstract: The therapeutic potential of *Cannabis sativa* L. extract has gained significant attention due to its diverse medical applications. Sublingual administration remains a common delivery method of cannabinoids; however, challenges often arise due to the inconvenient form of the extract and its taste. To address these issues, a novel bigel formulation was developed, combining water and oil phases to enhance stability and bioavailability. This formulation incorporates a cannabidiol-rich hemp extract, hyaluronic acid for its moisturizing properties, and a taste-masking agent to improve patient compliance and comfort. Using a standardized hemp extract rich in cannabinoids and a well-characterized terpene profile, the printability of the bigels was evaluated through 3D printing technology. A printout with known cannabidiol (CBD) and cannabidiolic acid (CBDA) content of 11.613 mg ± 0.192 of CBD and 4.732 mg ± 0.280 of CBDA in the printout was obtained. In addition, the release profile of CBD and CBDA was evaluated to determine the delivery efficiency of the active ingredient—dissolved active ingredient levels ranged from 74.84% ± 0.50 to 80.87% ± 3.20 for CBD and from 80.84 ± 1.33 to 98.31 ± 1.70 for CBDA depending on the formulation. Rheological studies were conducted to evaluate the viscosity of the bigels under varying temperature conditions, ensuring their stability and usability. Findings suggest that this 3D-printed bigel formulation could significantly enhance the delivery of cannabis extracts, offering a more convenient and effective therapeutic option for patients. This research underscores the importance of innovation in cannabinoid therapies and paves the way for further advancements in personalized medicine.

Keywords: bigels; cannabidiol; cannabidiolic acid; cannabis

1. Introduction

Bigels are innovative delivery systems that combine the structural properties of hydrophilic and hydrophobic gels, forming a biphasic network that can simultaneously encapsulate and deliver both water-soluble and fat-soluble active compounds [1]. This dual-phase system makes bigels highly versatile for a wide range of applications, particularly in pharmaceuticals and cosmetics, where controlled release and bioavailability of both types of substances are crucial [2–4]. The production process typically involves emulsifying an aqueous phase (hydrogel) with an oil phase (organogel), requiring precise control over the stability of the emulsion to achieve the desired consistency, rheological properties, and functional performance. In the study by Kurapkienė et al. [5], a bigel structured with collagen, monoglycerides, and diglycerides significantly improved the stability of curcumin, a compound known for its antioxidant and anti-inflammatory properties but that is typically unstable and poorly bioavailable. The bigel system maintained over

97% of curcumin's content during both the manufacturing process and in vitro digestion, effectively addressing curcumin's degradation and solubility issues.

The search for alternatives to traditional pharmaceuticals has intensified due to several limitations associated with conventional drug therapies. Many classic medications can cause adverse side effects, lead to tolerance, or have limited efficacy, particularly in managing chronic conditions such as pain, anxiety, and inflammatory diseases. Furthermore, issues such as drug resistance, especially in the case of antibiotics, and the environmental impact of pharmaceutical residues have driven research toward more sustainable and biocompatible options. Plant-based compounds, like cannabinoids from cannabis, offer a promising alternative as they possess therapeutic properties with generally favorable safety profiles and lower risk of severe side effects. Additionally, alternative delivery systems, such as bigels, enhance the bioavailability and targeted delivery of these compounds, potentially improving treatment outcomes while reducing systemic exposure and minimizing side effects. This push towards innovative, naturally derived treatments reflects a growing demand for safer, more effective, and patient-centric therapeutic options.

Cannabidiol (CBD)-rich cannabis extracts have garnered attention for their therapeutic potential in treating various medical conditions. These extracts are high in CBD and low in Δ9-tetrahydrocannabinol (Δ9-THC), offering non-psychoactive treatment options. They are particularly effective in managing epilepsy, cancer-related symptoms, chronic pain, and anxiety disorders [6–8]. Research also supports the use of CBD-rich extracts in veterinary medicine for pain and anxiety in animals [9]. As research progresses, the potential applications of CBD in medicine continue to expand. Mucosal and buccal delivery systems for cannabis represent an innovative approach to administering cannabinoids, offering several advantages over traditional methods [10]. These systems leverage the rich vascularization of the oral mucosa to facilitate rapid absorption of cannabinoids into the bloodstream, thereby enhancing bioavailability and providing quicker onset of effects compared to oral ingestion [11,12]. This route is particularly beneficial for patients requiring immediate relief from symptoms, such as pain or nausea, as it bypasses the gastrointestinal tract and first-pass metabolism in the liver, which can significantly reduce the effective dose of cannabinoids [13]. One of the most notable examples of a mucosal delivery system is Sativex®, an oromucosal spray that contains both THC and CBD. This formulation has been shown to provide effective symptom relief for conditions such as multiple sclerosis and cancer-related pain [11,14]. The pharmacokinetics of oromucosal delivery systems indicate that cannabinoids can achieve therapeutic plasma concentrations rapidly, making this method particularly appealing for patients who may experience acute symptoms [11].

Buccal delivery systems, such as lozenges or films, also present a viable alternative for cannabinoid administration. These formulations can be designed to dissolve slowly in the mouth, allowing for sustained release of cannabinoids and prolonged therapeutic effects. Research has demonstrated that buccal delivery can enhance the absorption of cannabinoids, leading to improved patient compliance and satisfaction due to the ease of use and discreet nature of the administration. For instance, Trokie® lozenges have been developed specifically for the buccal delivery of cannabis extracts, providing a standardized dosage form that is both effective and user-friendly [15].

An additional benefit of hemp-based bigel antibacterial properties is that it has been increasingly recognized in recent studies. For instance, hemp extract has been shown to inhibit the growth of various bacterial strains [16,17]. This adds a new dimension to the potential of application-based bigels, particularly in the field of oral care products.

Moreover, the application of 3D printing technology in the development of personalized dosage forms has become a promising area of research. Modern technologies that modify the properties of existing materials and active substances have the potential to significantly improve medical treatments [18,19]. The integration of 3D printing technology into personalized medicine represents a transformative advancement in pharmaceutical manufacturing and patient care. This technology allows for the customization of drug formulations tailored to individual patient needs, which is particularly beneficial in addressing the variability in drug response among patients. The ability to produce specific dosages, shapes, and release profiles through 3D printing enhances the precision of drug delivery systems, thereby improving therapeutic outcomes and patient compliance [20,21]. The adaptability of bigels, capable of transitioning between liquid and semi-solid states, makes them ideal candidates for extrusion-based 3D printing processes. This approach allows for precise control over drug loading, release kinetics, and dosage customization. By adjusting the composition and structure of the bigel, it is possible to tailor the release profile of active ingredients to meet individual patient needs, offering a more personalized therapeutic approach. The flexibility of 3D printing also facilitates the creation of size, making it possible to design formulations that enhance patient adherence and satisfaction with personalized doses.

The aim of the present study was to develop a novel bigel-based drug delivery system containing hemp extract, in which the oil phase consists of hemp oil and the aqueous phase incorporates hyaluronic acid, a moisturizing agent. Hyaluronic acid was included to counteract the potential drying effects of hemp extract, particularly in oral applications. Menthol was also added to enhance the formulation by improving the permeability and providing a cooling sensation [22,23]. The innovation of this approach lies in the combination of these ingredients within a bigel system, which allows for the controlled release of bioactive compounds. The system was designed as single-dose printed dosages, enabling precise control over drug loading and release. This customizable platform offers a balanced and therapeutic formulation, which can be tailored to meet individual patient needs, ensuring more effective and personalized cannabinoid delivery. By using 3D printing technology, the study also introduces a novel way to create personalized dosages, enhancing patient compliance and satisfaction while optimizing therapeutic outcomes.

2. Results and Discussion

2.1. Choosing the Strain with the Highest Content of Cannabinoids

Seven cannabis strains were extracted using supercritical carbon dioxide ($scCO_2$), and the resulting methanol-solubilized extract was analyzed through HPLC. Significant differences in total cannabinoid content were observed among the strains (Table 1). The content of cannabinoids, including CBD, CBDA, cannabigerol (CBG), cannabinol (CBN), cannabigerolic acid (CBGA), delta-9-tetrahydrocannabinol (Δ9-THC), delta-8-tetrahydrocannabinol (Δ8-THC), cannabichromene (CBC), and tetrahydrocannabinolic acid (THCA), was evaluated. The Black Widow strain exhibited the highest levels of all determined cannabinoids and was selected for further formulation studies. However, it should be noted that the extraction applied proved effective for each of the varieties analyzed. The use of $scCO_2$ extraction is one of the best methods for obtaining extracts rich in cannabinoid compounds while maintaining the principles of 'green chemistry' [24]. The variability in cannabinoid content across different cannabis strains can be attributed to several factors, including genetic variation, cultivation practices, and environmental influences [25,26]. The choice of variety has a direct effect on the cannabinoid content of the extract obtained from cannabis [27]. Depending on the desired clinical effect, varieties with different cannabinoid contents are used. The main ones are CBD and THC. In the study we conducted, all strains were high in CBD and low in THC. CBD has no psychoactive properties, and its use is not restricted by law like THC. At the same time, it can have beneficial health effects such as calming, improving sleep, antioxidant or anti-inflammatory aspects [28].

Many publications have compared cannabis strains to assess their cannabinoid content. In the study by Glivar et al. [29], 15 different hemp strains grown in Slovenia were compared, including a comparison of the two seed years. Significant differences in cannabinoid content between strains were identified for 13 analyzed cannabinoids. The uppermost inflorescences were analyzed, revealing the highest total CBD content (>5% w/w) in the bracts of Antal (9.580% ± 1.287 in 2017, 6.159% in 2018), Carmagnola (7.069% ± 3.339 in 2017, 5.726% in 2018), Helena (5.873% ± 1.816 in 2017, 8.108% in 2018), and Tiborszallasi (4.666% ± 1.931 in 2017, 4.876% in 2018).

Table 1. Cannabinoids content in different strains of *Cannabis sativa* L.

Variety	CBD * (mg/g)	CBDA (mg/g)	CBG (mg/g)	CBN (mg/g)	CBGA (mg/g)	Δ^9-THC (mg/g)	Δ^8-THC (mg/g)	CBC (mg/g)	THCA (mg/g)	Total Cannabinoids (mg/g)
Silver Haze	26.684 ± 1.067	5.616 ± 0.112	0.434 ± 0.017	0.148 ± 0.006	0.061 ± 0.002	0.641 ± 0.025	0.035 ± 0.001	0.902 ± 0.036	0.000 ± 0.000	34.520 ± 0.690
White Widow	16.435 ± 0.657	5.828 ± 0.117	0.276 ± 0.011	0.082 ± 0.003	0.085 ± 0.003	0.558 ± 0.022	0.007 ± 0.000	0.492 ± 0.020	0.000 ± 0.000	23.761 ± 0.475
Red Cherry	10.731 ± 0.429	3.811 ± 0.076	0.063 ± 0.003	0.065 ± 0.003	0.034 ± 0.001	0.318 ± 0.013	0.008 ± 0.000	0.326 ± 0.013	0.023 ± 0.001	15.379 ± 0.307
Pineapple Express	9.248 ± 0.370	3.350 ± 0.067	0.123 ± 0.005	0.054 ± 0.002	0.057 ± 0.002	0.257 ± 0.010	0.012 ± 0.000	0.346 ± 0.014	0.017 ± 0.001	13.464 ± 0.269
AK47	15.375 ± 0.615	3.860 ± 0.077	0.259 ± 0.010	0.061 ± 0.002	0.061 ± 0.002	0.393 ± 0.016	0.020 ± 0.001	0.650 ± 0.026	0.014 ± 0.001	20.694 ± 0.415
Amnesia	12.610 ± 0.504	7.399 ± 0.148	0.244 ± 0.010	0.032 ± 0.001	0.198 ± 0.008	0.522 ± 0.021	0.000 ± 0.000	0.453 ± 0.018	0.161 ± 0.003	21.618 ± 0.432
Black Widow	23.490 ± 0.940	15.355 ± 0.307	0.560 ± 0.022	0.103 ± 0.004	0.302 ± 0.012	0.931 ± 0.037	0.005 ± 0.000	0.929 ± 0.037	0.202 ± 0.004	41.877 ± 0.837

* Abbreviations used in the table: CBD: cannabidiol, CBDA: cannabidiolic acid, CBG: cannabigerol, CBN: cannabinol, CBGA: cannabigerolic acid, Δ9-THC: delta-9-tetrahydrocannabinol, Δ8-THC: delta-8-tetrahydrocannabinol, CBC: cannabichromene, THCA: tetrahydrocannabinolic acid.

Furthermore, the study by Janatova et al. [30] evaluated the performance of various strains in terms of biomass yield and cannabinoid production. This research identified strains with high yields and stable production of therapeutic cannabinoids, such as 'Nurse Jackie' and 'Jilly Bean', highlighting the importance of selecting specific strains to meet medical needs. Average Δ9-THC levels for each strain across six growing cycles ranged from 15.69 ± 2.6% to 19.31 ± 2.47% (*w*/*w*), while average CBD levels ranged from 0.45 ± 0.1% to 0.57 ± 0.08% (*w*/*w*). Another significant study, conducted by Abdollahi et al. [31], demonstrated that cannabinoid levels fluctuate during various growth stages and are influenced by regional environmental factors. This emphasizes the importance of optimal strain selection and precise timing for cultivation. CBD content across all growth stages of the strains studied in three regions ranged from 0% to 1.39%. Our results are similar to other studies that have investigated CBD-rich strains, but it should be remembered that the type of extraction used is also important.

2.2. Characteristics of the Extract Chosen for the Formulation

2.2.1. HPLC Analysis

Cannabinoids are chemical compounds found naturally in cannabis that affect the human endocannabinoid system [7]. In the cannabis plant, they are found in acidic forms, such as CBDA, THCA (tetrahydrocannabinolic acid), and CBGA (cannabigerolic acid), which are converted to active forms, such as CBD, THC, or CBG, when exposed to heat (decarboxylation process). The intra-entourage effect—referring to the synergistic interaction between cannabinoids—further increases the therapeutic potential of these compounds. Cannabinoids influence each other, which means that their combination can potentiate or diminish certain effects (the so-called synergistic or entourage effect).

For the selected extract (from the Black Widow strain), the extraction was repeated, and the winterized extract was concentrated and characterized for use in formulation development. Table 2 shows the cannabinoids' content in 1 mL of the final extract. The procedures conducted yielded an extract with CBD content suitable for creating a precise dosage formulation. The dosage regimen of CBD varies greatly depending on the expected therapeutic effect and the route of administration. For administration via oral mucosal absorption, e.g., sublingual administration, the most commonly studied doses range from 15 to 70 mg/day [32–34]. In the study by Baratta et al. [35], an oil extract was obtained with cannabinoid concentrations as follows: CBD 12.092 mg/mL, THC 6.971 mg/mL, CBDA

0.631 mg/mL, THCA 0.036 mg/mL, and CBN 0.450 mg/mL, with the note that a THC-rich cannabis strain was used. Full-spectrum cannabis extracts were also used in a study by Villate et al. [36] to obtain PLGA nanoparticles also for oral administration. In some studies, such as Taha et al. [37] where buccal film formulations were proposed, isolated CBD was used. There, CBD constituted 10% (*w*/*w*) of the film.

Table 2. Content of cannabinoids in extract assessed by HPLC method.

Cannabinoid	Content (mg/mL)
CBD	164.738 ± 10.088
CBDA	68.756 ± 5.776
CBG	3.489 ± 0.305
CBN	0.690 ± 0.038
CBGA	0.619 ± 0.026
Δ^9-THC	5.487 ± 0.443
Δ^8-THC	16.273 ± 0.921
CBC	0.733 ± 0.132
THCA	-

Abbreviations used in the table: CBD: cannabidiol, CBDA: cannabidiolic acid, CBG: cannabigerol, CBN: cannabinol, CBGA: cannabigerolic acid, Δ9-THC: delta-9-tetrahydrocannabinol, Δ8-THC: delta-8-tetrahydrocannabinol, CBC: cannabichromene, THCA: tetrahydrocannabinolic acid.

2.2.2. GC–MS Analysis

The results of the GC–MS analysis indicate the presence of various compounds in the sample (Table 3). The largest percentage (93.848%) is CBD, which is the main active compound. Other important compounds are caryophyllene (2.548%) and humulene (0.826%), terpenes known for their anti-inflammatory and analgesic properties. Rarer compounds are also present, such as cis-5,8,11,14,17-eicosapentaenoic acid (EPA) (0.324%), which is a polyunsaturated fatty acid with anti-inflammatory effects [38], which suggests that the fatty compounds were adsorbed by supercritical CO_2 extraction. The winterization process was not fully effective, resulting in some fats and waxes remaining in the final extract. The overall composition suggests a CBD-rich sample with additional terpenes and other bioactive compounds that may work together as part of an entourage effect, increasing the therapeutic potential of the sample. In addition to cannabinoids, terpenes are the key active ingredients in hemp extract. The interaction of all components, called the entourage effect, is responsible for the strain's unique effects. Among the notable terpenes identified, caryophyllene and humulene are significant due to their anti-inflammatory and analgesic properties [39–41]. Caryophyllene, a bicyclic sesquiterpene, has been documented to function as a selective agonist of the CB2 receptor, part of the endocannabinoid system [42,43]. Its activation of CB2 receptors leads to the modulation of immune responses, making it effective in reducing inflammation. Additionally, caryophyllene has been shown to provide neuroprotective benefits and assist in managing chronic pain [44]. Similarly, humulene, a monocyclic sesquiterpene, is recognized for its potential to reduce inflammation, and it may complement together with caryophyllene the effects through synergistic mechanisms [45,46]. Research indicates that humulene inhibits the production of pro-inflammatory cytokines, such as TNF-α and IL-1β, in response to inflammatory stimuli [46,47]. The sample also contains other sesquiterpenes, including α-acorenol and β-guaiene, which are less studied but exhibit promising antimicrobial properties [48–51]. Sesquiterpenes, in general, are known for their broad-spectrum biological activities, particularly in defending plants against microbial pathogens [52]. The antimicrobial potential of α-acorenol and β-guaiene suggests that these compounds may contribute to the extract's ability to combat bacterial and fungal infections, making the extract potentially useful for topical applications. The terpene profile of cannabis varies significantly depending on the strain, as confirmed by analyses using gas chromatography–mass spectrometry. A study by Ahmed et al. [53] identified six major terpenes—α-pinene, β-pinene, myrcene, limonene, β-caryophyllene, and α-humulene—in various cannabis flower samples, with concentrations differing across strains. A study by Kaur et al. [54] documented the presence of over 146 terpenes and terpenoids in cannabis, emphasizing the dominance of α-pinene and limonene in many strains. This chemical diversity and the proportions of these compounds contribute to the distinct aromas and potential therapeutic effects characteristic of individual strains.

Table 3. Content of active compounds assed by GC–MS method.

Lp.	Retention Time (min)	Percentage of Total (%)	Compound
1	5.761	0.324	cis-5.8.11.14.17-Eicosapentaenoic acid
2	13.524	2.548	Caryophyllene
3	13.624	0.191	7-epi-cis-sesquisabinene hydrate
4	13.989	0.826	Humulene
5	14.574	0.212	α-acorenol
6	15.005	0.191	ß-Guaiene
7	15.068	0.267	(4aR-trans)-decahydro-4a-methyl-1-methylene-7-(1-methylethylidene)-Naphthalene
8	15.582	0.249	(3ß.5α)-2-methylene-Cholestan-3-ol
9	16.063	0.304	8-epi-γ-eudesmol
10	16.520	0.572	α-acorenol
11	16.702	0.286	7-epi-cis-sesquisabinene hydrate
12	23.748	93.848	Cannabidiol

2.2.3. Results of the Analysis of Antimicrobial Properties

In the analysis of antimicrobial activity, the results obtained demonstrated varying antimicrobial activity of the hemp extract against pathogens associated with skin infections, oral health, and respiratory diseases (Table 4). Particularly strong effects were observed against *Streptococcus mutans*, a key contributor to dental caries. Moderate effectiveness was seen against pathogens like *Pseudomonas aeruginosa* and *Candida albicans*, which frequently cause infections in immunocompromised individuals, as well as *Porphyromonas gingivalis* and *Fusobacterium nucleatum*, both associated with periodontal diseases. The lowest activity was observed against *Staphylococcus aureus*, a bacterium responsible for skin and hospital-acquired infections, suggesting that the extract may have limited applications in treating these types of infections. These results highlight the potential of hemp extract in preventing and treating oral diseases. Given this fact, the proposed formulation has the potential not only to deliver CBD and other cannabinoids but also to provide antibacterial effects in the oral environment. Ali et al. reported that cannabis seed oil exhibited significant antibacterial effects, with inhibition zones ranging from 21 to 28 mm against *Bacillus subtilis* and *Staphylococcus aureus*, and moderate activity against *Escherichia coli* and *Pseudomonas aeruginosa* [55]. Further investigations into the specific components responsible for this activity have identified cannabinoids, terpenes, and phenolic compounds as significant contributors. For example, Malikova highlighted that cannabinoids such as THC and CBD have shown antibacterial effects, for example, against *Staphylococcus aureus* [56].

Table 4. Antimicrobial activity of the hemp extract and control octenidine.

Pathogen	Hemp Extract	Octenidine
	MIC (mg/mL)	MIC (μg/mL)
Staphylococcus aureus	73 ± 0.0	1.25 ± 0.0
Pseudomonas aeruginosa	36.5 ± 0.0	1.88 ± 0.9
Streptococcus mutansATCC 25175	4.6 ± 0.0	0.6 ± 0.0
Candida albicans	36.5 ± 0.0	2.5 ± 0.0
Porphyromonas gingivalisATCC 33277	36.5 ± 0.0	0.6 ± 0.0
Fusobacterium nucleatumATCC 25586	36.5 ± 0.0	0.6 ± 0.0

2.3. Comparison of Properties of Bigels

2.3.1. Composition and Stability Assessment of Bigels

Formulations were obtained with the compositions shown in Table 5.

Table 5. Quantitative composition of bigels.

Ingredient	Bigel 1 (%)	Bigel 2 (%)	Bigel 3 (%)	Bigel 4 (%)
Water	72.4	71.9	69.4	68.9
Oil	10	10	10	10
Lecithin	2	2	2	2
Extract	5	5	5	5
Gelatin	5	5	8	8
1.5% Hyaluronic acid salt solution	5	5	5	5
Hydroxypropyl methyl cellulose	0.5	1	0.5	1
Menthol	0.1	0.1	0.1	0.1

The preparations showed a creamy yellow color and uniform consistency. In the inverted tube test, which is used to assess the stability and gelation of the formulations, their stability was confirmed (Figure 1). This test showed that all formulations retained their integrity without any flow under gravitational conditions, indicating good stability over time. In addition, the formulations exhibited a distinct menthol aroma alongside the characteristic smell of hemp.

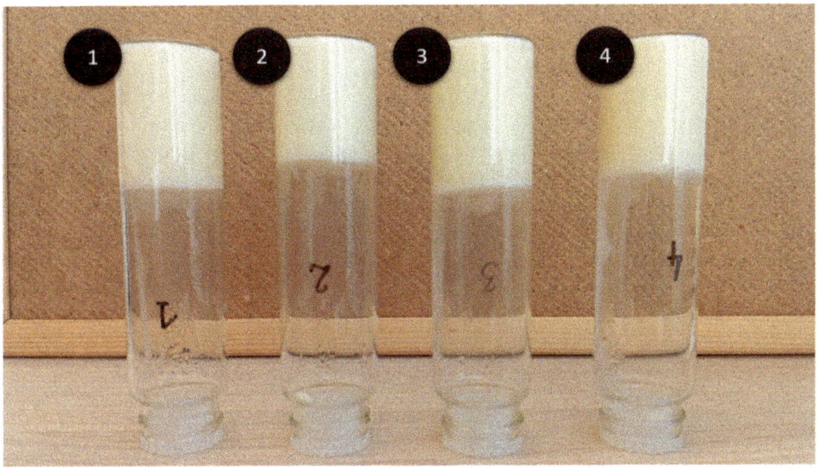

Figure 1. Results of the inverted tube test (numbers 1–4 correspond to bigels 1–4).

Similar results regarding the stability of bigel formulations containing plant extracts were reported by Sotirova et al. [57], who confirmed that a properly selected composition minimizes phase separation, enabling the creation of a uniform formulation containing St. John's Wort Extract. To date, efforts to maintain the stability of bigels containing plant extracts have been successful, including systems for delivering active compounds from Centella asiatica, as well as bigels containing 1,4-naphthoquinones [58,59]. Bigels also show potential as delivery systems, as highlighted in the review by Zampouni et al. [60] Additionally, Chen et al. [61] developed 3D-printed bigel systems based on beeswax oleogels and HPMC (hydroxypropyl methyl cellulose) hydrogels, prepared using an in situ gelation method. Their study also confirmed that bigels could be 3D printed effectively. Another important aspect is the organoleptic analysis of formulations. The cooling sensation produced by menthol can also alleviate discomfort associated with oral irritations, thereby improving the overall acceptability of buccal products [62].

2.3.2. Results of Viscosity Test

Since viscosity is influenced by the crosslinking reaction, experiments on the influence of temperature can help to develop a printing process [63,64]. In the study, the viscosity of the formulations was obtained in the temperature range of 27–35 °C. As shown in Figure 2a,b, all bigel formulations demonstrated a decrease in viscosity with increasing temperature (27 °C to 36 °C), which is characteristic of thermoresponsive materials. The viscosity profile of the four formulations indicates that the higher gelatine content (8% in formulations 3 and 4) results in a significantly higher initial viscosity compared to a formulation with lower gelatine content (5% in formulations 1 and 2). Gelatine forms a gel through the transition of its macromolecules from random coils to triple helices upon cooling, leading to the development of a compact and viscous structure, with notable increases in viscosity observed in gels 3 and 4 [65]. The higher HPMC content (1% in formulations 2 and 4) has the effect of increasing the viscosity of the formulation over the entire temperature range. Viscosity increases more rapidly above 30 °C, which is due to the presence of gelatine in the formulation. Based on the research results, it can be concluded that temperature, gelatine, and HPMC content can strongly influence the viscosity of the formulation. As the formulation is to be used as a 3D printer ink, the formulation of bigel 1 is considered to be the most suitable, as it does not show sudden viscosity changes with temperature but still can create a stable structure after cooling down. Printing parameters can remain unchanged even when the formulation cools down during the process. Figure 2c–f illustrate the influence of rotational velocity (RPM) on viscosity for all bigel formulations at different temperatures (27 °C, 30 °C, and 35 °C). The viscosity analysis of the bigels revealed a shear-thinning behavior, characteristic of non-Newtonian pseudoplastic systems. The results showed that viscosity decreased with increasing velocity (RPM), indicating structural breakdown under shear stress. Bigel 4, containing 8% gelatin and 1% HPMC, exhibited the highest viscosity values across all velocities, demonstrating enhanced structural stability and resistance to shear forces. Conversely, bigel 1, with 5% gelatin and 0.5% HPMC, showed the lowest viscosity and the steepest decrease with increasing velocity, reflecting a less cohesive gel network. The higher concentration of gelatin improved the initial viscosity, while HPMC contributed to maintaining structural integrity under shear.

Research indicates that as the concentration of gelatin increases, the viscosity of the solution also increases. For instance, Erencia et al. [66] demonstrated that gelatin solutions with higher concentrations exhibited a substantial increase in viscosity over time, particularly in the presence of a high water content and acetic acid, which is indicative of the gelation phenomenon. Temperature control is crucial in the 3D printing process of gelatine, as its viscosity changes significantly with temperature fluctuations. The addition of HPMC as an additional densifying ingredient favorably influences the rheological properties, the viscosity of the print material, and, at the same time, its mucoadhesion properties [67].

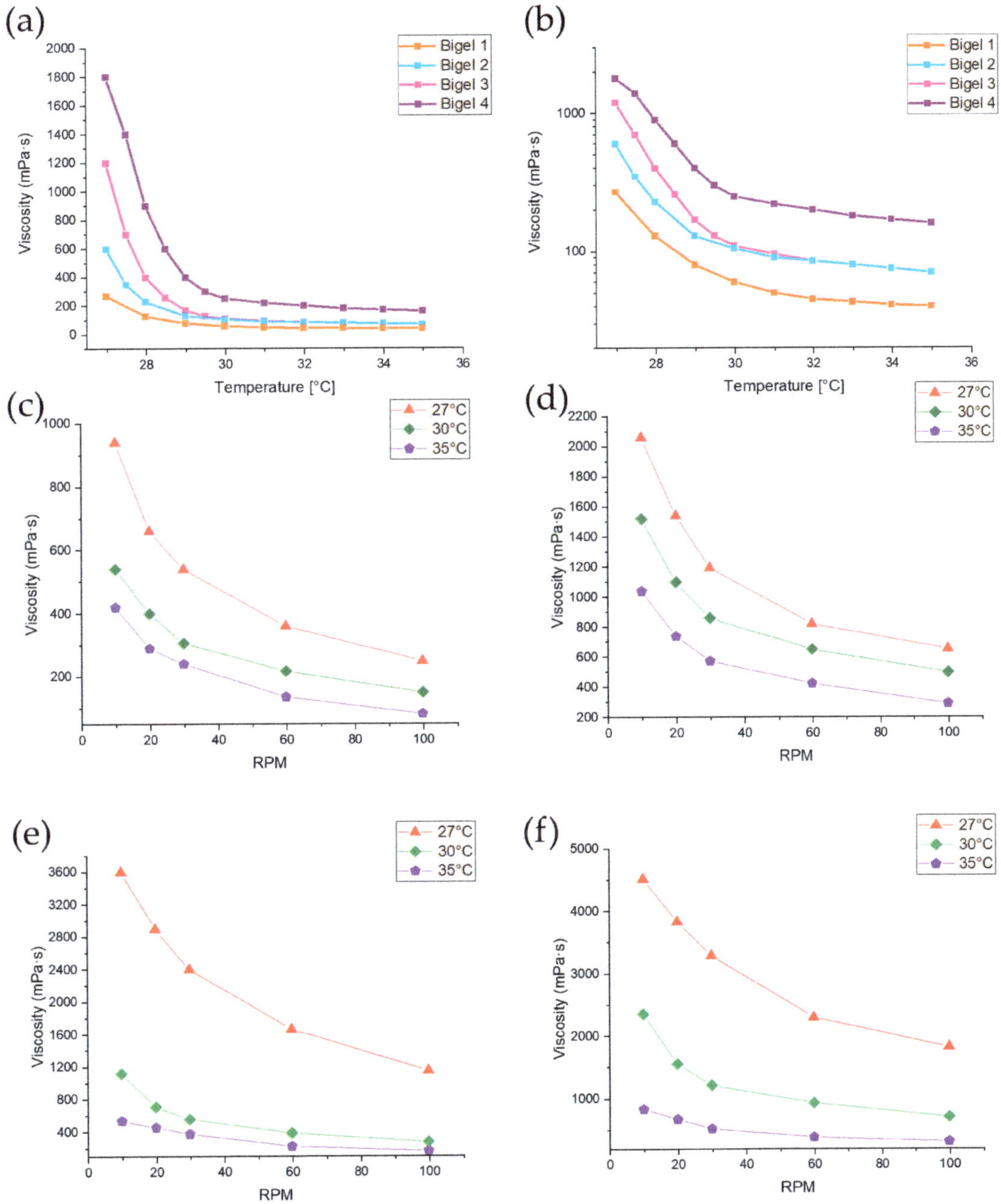

Figure 2. Viscosity of bigels as a function of temperature and velocity (RPM), temperature-dependent viscosity of bigel 1–4 (**a**,**b**), viscosity at different velocities (RPM) and temperatures (27 °C, 30 °C, 35 °C)—bigel 1 (**c**), bigel 2 (**d**), bigel 3 (**e**), bigel 4 (**f**).

2.3.3. Results of In Vitro Dissolution Study

The study was conducted for the main active compounds present in hemp extract—CBD and CBDA. From the determined curves (Figure 3), it can be concluded that each formulation allows the release of CBD and CBDA in the medium at pH 7.4, mimicking the oral cavity environment. The CBD and CBDA release curves from the four bigels formulations show that the gelatine and HPMC content significantly affects the release rate of the active substances. Bigels with a higher gelatine content (8% in bigels 3 and 4) show faster CBD release, suggesting that gelatine creates a structure that promotes diffusion. Gelatine, being a hydrophilic polymer, rapidly absorbs water, which can lead to an increase in volume and a changing of the bigel structure. Higher concentrations of gelatine may lead to a faster breakdown of the gel matrix, which may facilitate the migration of CBD and CBDA molecules. On the other hand, a higher concentration of HPMC (1% in bigels 2 and 4) slows down the release, especially for CBDA, which may be due to its ability to form a gel barrier that limits particle migration. Finding formulations that enhance the solubility of CBD and CBDA is crucial for increasing their pharmaceutical availability. Many different solutions have been proposed so far. The formation of inclusion complexes with cyclodextrins has been investigated as a method to enhance the solubility and stability of cannabinoid acids like CBDA [68]. Cyclodextrins can encapsulate these compounds, thereby improving their physicochemical properties and making them more bioavailable [68]. In the study by Abdella et al. [69], a hydroxyethyl cellulose (HEC)-based gel containing CBD-NLCs was prepared as the feedstock for pressure-assisted 3D micro-syringe printing, successfully producing buccal films with CBD. These films showed a controlled release profile, with an 84.11 ± 7.02% CBD release over six hours in vitro. Orodispersible tablets were also proposed, e.g., by Vlad et al. [70], achieving 99.3% CBD release in 30 min for pediatric epilepsy and Limpongsa's team developed directly compressible orally disintegrating tablets of cannabidiol using a liquisolid technique, achieving a dissolution efficiency of 93.5% in ethanol-based formulations [71].

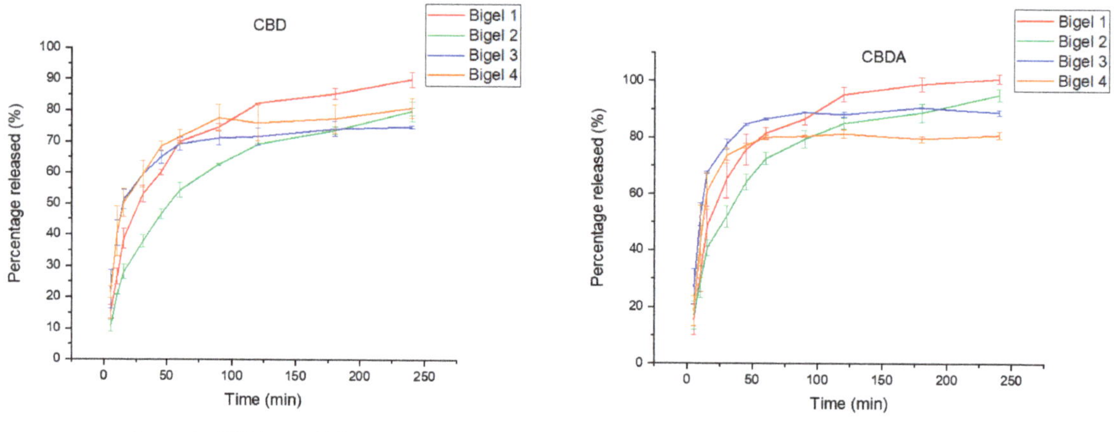

Figure 3. CBDA and CBDA release curves from bigel formulations 1–4.

The release profiles of CBD and CBDA from bigel formulations (bigel 1–4) were analyzed using five kinetic models: Zero-Order, First-Order, Higuchi, Hixson–Crowell, and Korsmeyer–Peppas [72]. Each model provided insights into the underlying release mechanisms, and the release constants (k_0, k_t, k_H, k_{HC}, k_{KP}) and diffusion exponent were calculated alongside determination coefficients (R^2) to assess the fit of the models (Tables 6 and 7). The Zero-Order model, which assumes a constant release rate independent of drug concentration, showed moderate R^2 values for most bigels, suggesting that it does not fully capture the release mechanisms. Similarly, the First-Order model, which assumes that release depends on the drug concentration remaining, provided slightly better fits for certain bigels, particularly CBDA. However, the lower R^2 values indicated that the release mechanism might not be purely concentration-dependent.

Table 6. Parameters of kinetic release models suggesting the mechanism of CBD liberation from bigel formulation.

	Zero-Order		First-Order		Higuchi		Hixson–Crowell		Korsmeyer–Peppas		
	k_0	R^2	k_1	R^2	k_H	R^2	k_{HC}	R^2	k_{KP}	n	R^2
Bigel 1	0.278	0.725	0.005	0.548	5.457	0.888	−0.009	0.864	0.435	2.315	0.921
Bigel 2	0.198	0.865	0.004	0.764	4.238	0.952	−0.006	0.932	0.37	2.404	0.974
Bigel 3	0.156	0.517	0.003	0.403	3.236	0.706	−0.004	0.598	0.264	3.04	0.804
Bigel 4	0.182	0.554	0.003	0.428	3.753	0.743	−0.005	0.649	0.294	2.959	0.827

Table 7. Parameters of kinetic release models suggesting the mechanism of CBDA liberation from bigel formulation.

	Zero-Order		First-Order		Higuchi		Hixson–Crowell		Korsmeyer–Peppas		
	k_0	R^2	k_1	R^2	k_H	R^2	k_{HC}	R^2	k_{KP}	n	R^2
Bigel 1	0.295	0.641	0.005	0.466	5.940	0.823	−0.014	0.868	0.439	2.456	0.865
Bigel 2	0.291	0.741	0.005	0.570	5.696	0.899	−0.010	0.905	0.424	2.410	0.934
Bigel 3	0.167	0.404	0.003	0.320	3.597	0.595	−0.006	0.511	0.253	3.310	0.723
Bigel 4	0.159	0.355	0.003	0.277	3.488	0.543	−0.005	0.414	0.302	2.992	0.675

The Higuchi model, which assumes Fickian diffusion as the primary release mechanism, demonstrated excellent fits for both CBD and CBDA, with $R^2 > 0.82$ in bigels 1 and 2, particularly for CBDA formulations [73]. The release constant k_H further supported diffusion-driven release from the gel matrix. The Hixson–Crowell model, which accounts for changes in surface area and particle size during release, showed moderate R^2 values for some bigels, but it was less suitable than the Higuchi and Korsmeyer–Peppas models. Notably, the k_{HC} values were low or negative in certain cases, indicating that this model might not adequately describe the release process for these formulations.

The Korsmeyer–Peppas model emerged as the most suitable model for both CBD and CBDA bigels, particularly CBDA, with R^2 values exceeding 0.95 in some cases. The release constant (k_{KP}) and the n value (diffusion exponent) consistently indicated a supercase-II transport mechanism, characterized by matrix erosion and swelling effects. This suggests that the release is predominantly driven by the erosion of the gel matrix, with diffusion playing a secondary role. For CBD formulations, n values greater than 2 confirmed supercase-II transport, highlighting the importance of matrix dynamics in controlling release. Similarly, for CBDA formulations, both Korsmeyer–Peppas and Higuchi models pointed to matrix erosion as the dominant release mechanism.

In conclusion, the analysis confirmed that the Higuchi and Korsmeyer–Peppas models best describe the release profiles of both CBD and CBDA formulations. The primary release mechanisms involve diffusion and matrix erosion, with supercase-II transport emerging as the dominant mode. While Hixson–Crowell and First-Order models provided additional insights, their lower R^2 values suggest that they are less robust in capturing the true release dynamics of these systems. These findings underscore the importance of matrix characteristics in drug release and provide a foundation for optimizing formulations to achieve desired release profiles.

2.4. 3D Printing Process

The 3D printing of the bigel yielded promising results, with the printed structures maintaining their intended shape and demonstrating high fidelity to the digital model (Figure 4). Importantly, the material's mass remained consistent across multiple prints, indicating the reproducibility of the process. The bigel exhibited stable rheological properties during printing, allowing for precise deposition and ensuring that the structural integrity was preserved throughout the fabrication process, even despite the application of no temperature control during printing. As bigel 1 showed the least rapid change in properties in viscosity tests, while retaining its structure after time, it could be used in this type of printing. These results are in line with previous studies on similar biomaterials, where bigels were also a suitable material for 3D printing [74,75]. The confirmed mass constancy (1.689 ± 0.001) indicates that 3D printing can be used to personalize the dosage of an active compound in patients who require precise dosing. The average content of CBD is 11.613 mg ± 0.192, and the average content of CBDA is 4.732 mg ± 0.280 in the printout. The proposed method can also be implemented to create delivery systems containing high-THC cannabis extract, as is needed in the treatment with this compound [76]. In the study by Andriotis et al. [77], a cannabis seed oil oleogel structured with 20% w/w glycerol monostearate was mixed with a 2% w/w xanthan gum hydrogel in various ratios (0–75% w/w hydrogel) using a syringe-to-syringe method, creating 3D-printable food inks. This process allowed a consistent mix of oleogel and hydrogel phases, incorporating air uniformly. Printability tests with a standard 3D food printer showed that higher hydrogel ratios negatively impacted print quality, while pure oleogel exhibited superior performance. However, in our study, a formulation with a high hydrogel content also performed well in 3D printing. In the study conducted by Xie et al. [78], bigels containing monoglycerides with an oleogel-to-hydrogel ratio of 7:3 exhibited mechanical properties suitable for 3D printing. This research also incorporated gelatin as a gelling agent in the aqueous phase, alongside different emulsifiers such as PGPR, monoglycerides, and lecithin. Bigels formulated with monoglycerides or lecithin successfully formed homogeneous and stable gel systems. Similarly, Qui et al. [79] identified that a bigel ink with an 80% oleogel fraction was the optimal formulation for 3D printing. Fernandes et al. [74] explored bigels with beeswax as the oleogelling agent and a combination of agar and xanthan gum as hydrogelators. Their findings indicated that bigels containing 10–20% oleogel demonstrated potential as inks for extrusion-based 3D printing. Additionally, Chen et al. [61] confirmed that O/W bigels were more suitable for printing small-area monolayer structural models. Studies carried out by other teams indicate that bigels with different oil phase contents can be successfully printed.

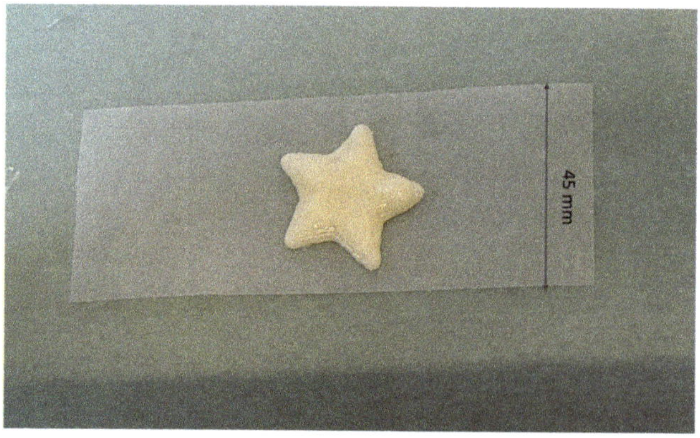

Figure 4. Star-shaped bigel after printing.

3. Conclusions

In conclusion, the successful development of a bigel-based drug delivery system incorporating hemp extract, specifically with known CBD and CBDA content of 11.613 mg ± 0.192 of CBD and 4.732 mg ± 0.280 of CBDA, hyaluronic acid, and menthol marks a significant advancement in personalized medicine. This innovative formulation not only facilitates customizable dosages but also enables controlled release of CBD and CBDA, enhancing therapeutic efficacy and patient compliance. The release profile of CBD and CBDA was evaluated to determine the delivery efficiency of the active ingredient—dissolved active ingredient levels ranged from 74.84% ± 0.50 to 80.87% ± 3.20 for CBD and from 80.84 ± 1.33 to 98.31 ± 1.70 for CBDA depending on the formulation. Bigels offer a compelling dosing option even for pediatric applications, featuring customizable textures, shapes, and flavors that improve palatability, simplify administration, and increase adherence even among younger patients. Additionally, the system demonstrated antibacterial properties against oral pathogens, further expanding its potential applications in oral health. The biphasic structure of bigels allows for the simultaneous encapsulation and delivery of diverse therapeutic agents, making them highly versatile. This platform also paves the way for the incorporation of other therapeutic extracts, broadening its potential in treating various medical conditions. Its adaptability positions the bigel-based system as a promising candidate for future personalized, multi-functional treatments tailored to individual patient needs and improving overall treatment outcomes.

4. Materials and Methods

4.1. Chemicals and Solvents

Cannabinoid standards solutions, 1 mg/mL in methanol, including CBD, CBDA, CBG, CBN, CBGA, Δ9-THC, Δ8-THC, CBC, THCA (Sigma-Aldrich, Burlington, MA, USA), hemp oil (Skolej, Kościelec, Poland), L-menthol (Sigma-Aldrich), triple hyaluronic acid 1.5% (aqueous solution with 0.5% sodium hyaluronate (0.85–1.15 MDa), 0.5% (<500 kDa), and 0.5% (<10 kDa)), gelatin 20 mesh particle size (Chempur, Karlsruhe, Germany), (Hydroxypropyl)methyl cellulose M_W = ~86 kDa, viscosity 2600–5600 cP, 2% in H_2O (20 °C) (Sigma Aldrich), phosphate buffered saline tablets (Fisher Scientific, Pittsburgh, PSA, USA), Tween 80 (Merck KGaA, Darmstadt, Germany), L-α-lecithin (EMD Millipore Corp., Darmstadt, Germany), acetonitrile for HPLC (VWR Chemicals, Radnor, PA, USA), trifluoroacetic acid (Honeywell, Albany, NY, USA); Hemp strains obtained from local markets: Silver Haze (Swiss Hemp, Biel/Bienne, Switzerland), CBD < 10%, THC < 0.2%, White Widow (Swiss Hemp), THC < 0.2%, Red Cherry (Swiss Hemp), CBD < 10%, THC < 0.2%, Pineapple Express (Swiss Hemp), CBD < 10%, THC < 0.2%, AK47 (Swiss Hemp), CBD < 10%, THC < 0.3%, Amnesia (Swiss Hemp; CBD < 10%, THC < 0.2%, Black Widow (Creathink, Nanjing, China). Mueller-Hinton broth was obtained from Graso (Poland). MTT (3-(4,5-dimethyl-2-thiazolyl)-2,5-diphenyl-2H-tetrazolium bromide) was purchased from Sigma-Aldrich.

4.2. Raw Material for Testing

In order to find the cannabis with the highest cannabinoid content, seven strains were subjected to extraction of seven strains:

1. Silver Haze
2. White Widow
3. Red Cherry
4. Pineapple Express
5. AK47
6. Amnesia
7. Black Widow

4.3. Extraction of Raw Material Using Supercritical CO_2

The extraction process with $scCO_2$ was carried out using a SFT-120 apparatus (Supercritical Fluid Technologies, Inc., Newark, DE, USA) at a pressure of 6000 PSI and a temperature of 50 °C with 250 mL of CO_2. The dried material of the above-mentioned varieties were crushed and weighed, then loaded into the 5 mL vessel of the extraction apparatus. The weight of the raw material in the dish was approximately 6.0 g and was accurately determined for each sample for further calculations. The extracts were then suspended in 5 mL of methanol and further analyzed to choose variety with the highest content of cannabinoids. The extraction of the strain selected for further study was carried out under the same conditions but repeated 5 times, each time with a fresh portion of raw material. Obtained extracts were combined and dissolved in 150 mL of ethanol (73.1 mg of pure extract/mL). The extract obtained by this technique contains many waxes, so the next step was to carry out a purification process by winterization. Winterization was carried out by placing the extract in a freezer at −18 °C for a period of 48 h. This was followed by filtration under reduced pressure, leaving the waxy impurities on the filter while the extract became clearer. The procedure was repeated twice.

4.4. Analysis of the Content of Active Compounds Using HPLC

Analysis of the cannabinoid profile of the extracts was performed by ultra-high-performance liquid chromatography using a validated method with a diode array detector (HPLC-DAD) (Shimadzu Corporation, Kyoto, Japan). The determination was performed according to the methodology [80]. The determination was carried out using a CORTECS Shield RP18, 2.7 µm; 150 mm × 4.6 mm chromatography column. 0.1% trifluoroacetic acid (41%) and acetonitrile (41:59, *v*/*v*) were used as the mobile phase. The flow rate was set at 2.0 mL/min, and the column temperature was set at 35 °C. The injection volume was 10.0 µL, the detection wavelength was 228 nm, and the analysis time was 50 min. The retention time is shown in the table below (Table 8).

Table 8. Cannabinoid retention time.

Cannabinoid	Retention Time [min]
CBD	5.84
CBDA	6.42
CBG	6.82
CBN	8.72
CBGA	9.22
Δ^9-THC	10.27
CBC	14.57
THCA	16.31

4.5. Analysis of the Content of Active Compounds Using Gas Chromatography (GC–MS)

Fifty µL of extract was taken, and 2.2 mL of absolute ethanol was added and mixed thoroughly. The whole was filtered through a 0.20 µm syringe filter and subjected to GC–MS analysis. A sample volume of 1 µL was injected into the column. The chromatograph was equipped with a VF-5ms silica column (30 m × 0.25 mm × 0.39), df = 0.25 Crawford Scientific. The electron energy was 70 eV, and the ion source was at 200 °C. Helium was used as the carrier gas at a flow rate of 1 mL/min. Identification of the compounds was based on a comparison of their retention times as well as mass spectra with standards from NIST.

4.6. Analysis of Antimicrobial Properties

The minimum inhibitory concentration (MIC) of the cannabis extract was determined using the microdilution method with 96-well plates (Nest Scientific Biotechnology, Jiangsu, China). Details are described in previous articles [81]. The activity was tested against strains of *Staphylococcus aureus*, *Pseudomonas aeruginosa*, *Candida albicans*, *Streptococcus mutans* ATCC 25175, *Porphyromonas gingivalis* ATCC 33277, *Fusobacterium nucleatum* ATCC 25586. The bacteria *S. aureus*, *P. aeruginosa*, and *S. mutans* were cultured in tryptone soy broth (Graso Biotech, Starogard Gdański, Poland), the yeast *C. albicans* was cultured in Sabouraud broth (Graso Biotech, Starogard Gdański, Poland), and the anaerobes *P. gingivalis* and *F. nucleatum* were cultured in Schaedler broth (Graso Biotech, Starogard Gdański, Poland). Serial dilutions of each antiseptic were prepared, starting from a concentration of 73 mg/mL. The plates were incubated at 36 °C for 24–48 h. Additionally, octenidine dihydrochloride

(Schülke & Mayr, Norderstedt, Germany) was used as a control substance, starting at a concentration of 10 µg/mL.

4.7. Bigel Preparation

To prepare bigels with the desired properties, ingredients were carefully selected in various proportions to achieve the desired effects. The substances used in each formulation tested include the following:

- Purified water—aqueous phase
- Hemp oil—oil phase (carrier for hemp extract)
- Gelatine—hydrogelator
- Lecithin—oleogelator
- Hydroxypropyl methyl cellulose (HPMC)—adhesion enhancer
- 1.5% Hyaluronic acid salt solution—moisturizer
- Menthol—taste enhancer

Formulations were obtained with the compositions shown in Table 5 in Section 2.3. For each formulation, the execution followed the same process. In a glass beaker, hemp oil was heated to 80 °C, and then lecithin and menthol were added and mixed with a dipstick. Water in the beaker was then heated to 80 °C, gelatine and HPMC were added and mixed until dissolved, then hyaluronic acid was added and mixed again. The 5-fold concentrated hemp extract was added to the cooled oil phase and mixed. The two phases were combined and mixed on a magnetic stirrer at low speed for one minute. Homogenization of the bigel was carried out for one minute at 1500 rpm. The formulations are shown in Table 5. Formulations were put into glass containers and cooled to room temperature (RT, 25 °C) for 24 h forming bigels. The formation of bigels was confirmed by the inverted tube method [4].

4.8. Viscosity Test

Analysis was performed using a Rotating Disc Viscometer DV2T-RV Extra5 (Ametek Brookfield, Middleboro, MA, USA) equipped with a temperature probe and an RV05 spindle system. The substance was initially heated and then cooled over time, with simultaneous testing performed as the temperature decreased in 1 °C increments. The analysis was conducted in the same beaker with a diameter of 8.25 cm. This measurement corresponds to apparent viscosity, as it reflects the flow behavior of the substance under the applied conditions.

4.9. In Vitro Dissolution Study

A release study was conducted in simulated saliva to select the formulation with the highest pharmaceutical availability among the four proposed formulations. Approximately 1.5 g of each formulation was placed in a saliva-simulating fluid, which was phosphate buffer pH 7.4 with 1% Tween 80 as surfactant. The test was carried out using a 708-DS Dissolution Apparatus (Agilent Technologies) with a basket rotation speed of 50 RPM. Dissolution samples were taken at appropriate time points and were filtered through 0.22 µm nylon membrane syringe filters.

To determine the release mechanisms of CBD and CBDA from bigel formulations, the release data were fitted to five mathematical kinetic models: Zero-Order, First-Order, Higuchi, Hixson–Crowell, and Korsmeyer–Peppas [72]. These models were selected based on their ability to describe various drug release mechanisms, including diffusion, erosion, and their combinations. Linear regression was applied to each dataset for all models. The release constants were obtained from the slopes or intercepts of the fitted lines, depending on the model. The fit of each model was evaluated using the correlation coefficient (R^2), with the highest R^2 value indicating the best-fitting model and the most probable release mechanism. The models are represented by the following equations:

$$F_t = k_0 \times t \quad (1)$$

$$F_t = 1 - e^{-k_1 t} \tag{2}$$

$$F_t = k_H \sqrt{t} \tag{3}$$

$$\sqrt[3]{F_0} - \sqrt[3]{F_t} = k_{HC}{}^t \tag{4}$$

$$F_t = kt^n \tag{5}$$

F_t—the fraction of CBD/CBDA released in time
$k_0, k_1, k_H, k_{HC}, k_{KP}$—release constants of particular kinetic models
n—the diffusion exponent

For the Korsmeyer–Peppas model, the n value was calculated to classify the release mechanism [82]:

- $n \leq 0.45$: Fickian diffusion
- $0.45 < n < 0.89$: Anomalous transport
- $n = 0.89$: Erosion-controlled (Case II transport)
- $n > 0.89$: Supercase-II transport

4.10. 3D Printing

The printing process was carried out using a 3D printer, model Moore 2 Pro (Shenzen Tronxy Technology, Shenzhen, Guangdong, China) using a 1.4 mm nozzle. Using computer software (Audodesk's Tinkecad, online access: https://www.tinkercad.com/ accessed on 1 October 2024), a design of the formula shape was created and then transferred to the printer system (Ultimaker Cura 4.13.1). The design is a single-layer star shape with dimensions of 30 mm × 35 mm × 2 mm. The print speed was set to 10 mm/s, and the nozzle height to 4 mm. The bigel was heated to 35 °C before printing and allowed to cool and crosslink for 24 h after printing. The average CBD and CBDA content of the printed products was determined by dissolving them in methanol, sonification, and determination by the HPLC method.

Author Contributions: Conceptualization, A.G. and J.C.-P.; methodology, A.G., A.S.-K., T.M.K. and M.S.; software, A.G.; validation, A.G., A.S.-K. and T.M.K., formal analysis, A.G.; investigation, A.G., F.K., T.M.K. and M.S.; resources, J.C.-P., T.M.K. and A.S.-K.; data curation, A.G. writing—original draft preparation, A.G.; writing—review and editing, J.C.-P., A.S.-K., T.M.K. and M.S.; visualization, A.G. supervision, J.C.-P., project administration, J.C.-P., funding acquisition, J.C.-P. and A.S.-K. All authors have read and agreed to the published version of the manuscript.

Funding: This research was funded in whole by the National Science Centre, Poland, the grant Preludium nr UMO-2021/41/N/NZ7/01125. For the purpose of Open Access, the author has applied a CC-BY public copyright license to any Author Accepted Manuscript (AAM) version arising from this submission.

Institutional Review Board Statement: Not applicable.

Informed Consent Statement: Not applicable.

Data Availability Statement: The data presented in this study will be openly available in the Ze-nodo repository.

Conflicts of Interest: The authors declare no conflicts of interest.

References

1. Chao, E.; Li, J.; Duan, Z.; Fan, L. Bigels as Emerging Biphasic Systems: Properties, Applications, and Prospects in the Food Industry. *Food Hydrocoll.* **2024**, *154*, 110089. [CrossRef]
2. Hashemi, B.; Assadpour, E.; Jafari, S.M. Bigels as Novel Carriers of Bioactive Compounds: Applications and Research Trends. *Food Hydrocoll.* **2024**, *147*, 109427. [CrossRef]
3. Francavilla, A.; Corradini, M.G.; Joye, I.J. Bigels as Delivery Systems: Potential Uses and Applicability in Food. *Gels* **2023**, *9*, 648. [CrossRef] [PubMed]
4. Martín-Illana, A.; Notario-Pérez, F.; Cazorla-Luna, R.; Ruiz-Caro, R.; Bonferoni, M.C.; Tamayo, A.; Veiga, M.D. Bigels as Drug Delivery Systems: From Their Components to Their Applications. *Drug Discov. Today* **2022**, *27*, 1008–1026. [CrossRef] [PubMed]

5. Kurapkienė, A.; Vinauskienė, R.; Jasutienė, I.; Keršienė, M.; Damulevičienė, G.; Knašienė, J.; Lesauskaitė, V.; Sulmont-Rossé, C.; Eisinaitė, V.; Leskauskaitė, D. Bigel as a Curcumin Delivery System and Its Application in 3D-Printed in-between-Meal Foods to Boost the Immune System of Elderly People. *Food Biosci.* **2024**, *61*, 104789. [CrossRef]
6. Leinen, Z.J.; Mohan, R.; Premadasa, L.S.; Acharya, A.; Mohan, M.; Byrareddy, S.N. Therapeutic Potential of Cannabis: A Comprehensive Review of Current and Future Applications. *Biomedicines* **2023**, *11*, 2630. [CrossRef]
7. Stasiłowicz, A.; Tomala, A.; Podolak, I.; Cielecka-Piontek, J. *Cannabis sativa* L. as a Natural Drug Meeting the Criteria of a Multitarget Approach to Treatment. *Int. J. Mol. Sci.* **2021**, *22*, 778. [CrossRef]
8. Voicu, V.; Brehar, F.-M.; Toader, C.; Covache-Busuioc, R.-A.; Corlatescu, A.D.; Bordeianu, A.; Costin, H.P.; Bratu, B.-G.; Glavan, L.-A.; Ciurea, A.V. Cannabinoids in Medicine: A Multifaceted Exploration of Types, Therapeutic Applications, and Emerging Opportunities in Neurodegenerative Diseases and Cancer Therapy. *Biomolecules* **2023**, *13*, 1388. [CrossRef]
9. Landa, L.; Trojan, V.; Demlova, R.; Jurica, J.; Hrib, R. Cannabidiol and the Possibilities of Its Use in Veterinary Medicine of Dogs and Horses: A Brief Review. *Vet. Med.* **2022**, *67*, 455. [CrossRef]
10. Tabboon, P.; Pongjanyakul, T.; Limpongsa, E.; Jaipakdee, N. Mucosal Delivery of Cannabidiol: Influence of Vehicles and Enhancers. *Pharmaceutics* **2022**, *14*, 1687. [CrossRef]
11. Karschner, E.L.; Darwin, W.D.; Goodwin, R.S.; Wright, S.; Huestis, M.A. Plasma Cannabinoid Pharmacokinetics Following Controlled Oral Δ9-Tetrahydrocannabinol and Oromucosal Cannabis Extract Administration. *Clin. Chem.* **2011**, *57*, 66–75. [CrossRef] [PubMed]
12. O'Sullivan, S.E.; Jensen, S.S.; Kolli, A.R.; Nikolajsen, G.N.; Bruun, H.Z.; Hoeng, J. Strategies to Improve Cannabidiol Bioavailability and Drug Delivery. *Pharmaceuticals* **2024**, *17*, 244. [CrossRef] [PubMed]
13. Oberoi, S.; Protudjer, J.L.P.; Rapoport, A.; Rassekh, S.R.; Crooks, B.; Siden, H.; Decker, K.; Ananth, P.; Chapman, S.; Balneaves, L.G.; et al. Perspectives of Pediatric Oncologists and Palliative Care Physicians on the Therapeutic Use of Cannabis in Children with Cancer. *Cancer Rep.* **2022**, *5*, e1551. [CrossRef] [PubMed]
14. Stella, B.; Baratta, F.; Della Pepa, C.; Arpicco, S.; Gastaldi, D.; Dosio, F. Cannabinoid Formulations and Delivery Systems: Current and Future Options to Treat Pain. *Drugs* **2021**, *81*, 1513–1557. [CrossRef] [PubMed]
15. Crowley, K.; de Vries, S.T.; Moreno-Sanz, G. Self-Reported Effectiveness and Safety of Trokie® Lozenges: A Standardized Formulation for the Buccal Delivery of Cannabis Extracts. *Front. Neurosci.* **2018**, *12*, 564. [CrossRef] [PubMed]
16. Ribeiro, A.; Alsayyed, R.; Oliveira, D.; Loureiro, R.; Cabral-Marques, H. Cannabinoids from *C. sativa* L.: Systematic Review on Potential Pharmacological Effects against Infectious Diseases Downstream and Multidrug-Resistant Pathogens. *Future Pharmacol.* **2024**, *4*, 590–625. [CrossRef]
17. Blaskovich, M.A.T.; Kavanagh, A.M.; Elliott, A.G.; Zhang, B.; Ramu, S.; Amado, M.; Lowe, G.J.; Hinton, A.O.; Pham, D.M.T.; Zuegg, J.; et al. The Antimicrobial Potential of Cannabidiol. *Commun. Biol.* **2021**, *4*, 7. [CrossRef]
18. Fellah, M.; Hezil, N.; Bouras, D.; Habeeb, M.A.; Hamadi, F.; Bouchareb, N.; Laouini, S.E.; Perez Larios, A.; Aleksei, O.; El-Hiti, G.A. Microstructural and Photocatalytic Properties of Nanostructured Near-β Ti-Nb-Zr Alloy for Total Hip Prosthesis Use. *Kuwait J. Sci.* **2024**, *51*, 100276. [CrossRef]
19. Gu, S.; Luo, Q.; Wen, C.; Zhang, Y.; Liu, L.; Liu, L.; Liu, S.; Chen, C.; Lei, Q.; Zeng, S. Application of Advanced Technologies—Nanotechnology, Genomics Technology, and 3D Printing Technology—In Precision Anesthesia: A Comprehensive Narrative Review. *Pharmaceutics* **2023**, *15*, 2289. [CrossRef]
20. Wang, S.; Chen, X.; Han, X.; Hong, X.; Li, X.; Zhang, H.; Li, M.; Wang, Z.; Zheng, A. A Review of 3D Printing Technology in Pharmaceutics: Technology and Applications, Now and Future. *Pharmaceutics* **2023**, *15*, 416. [CrossRef]
21. Alghahtani, M.S. Assessment of Pharmacist's Knowledge and Perception toward 3D Printing Technology as a Dispensing Method for Personalized Medicine and the Readiness for Implementation. *Pharmacy* **2021**, *9*, 68. [CrossRef] [PubMed]
22. Chen, L.; Ma, L.; Yang, S.; Wu, X.; Dai, X.; Wang, S.; Shi, X. A Multiscale Study of the Penetration-Enhancing Mechanism of Menthol. *J. Tradit. Chin. Med. Sci.* **2019**, *6*, 347–354. [CrossRef]
23. Eleftheriadis, G.K.; Monou, P.K.; Bouropoulos, N.; Boetker, J.; Rantanen, J.; Jacobsen, J.; Vizirianakis, I.S.; Fatouros, D.G. Fabrication of Mucoadhesive Buccal Films for Local Administration of Ketoprofen and Lidocaine Hydrochloride by Combining Fused Deposition Modeling and Inkjet Printing. *J. Pharm. Sci.* **2020**, *109*, 2757–2766. [CrossRef] [PubMed]
24. Arumugham, T.; Rambabu, K.; Hasan, S.W.; Show, P.L.; Rinklebe, J.; Banat, F. Supercritical Carbon Dioxide Extraction of Plant Phytochemicals for Biological and Environmental Applications—A Review. *Chemosphere* **2021**, *271*, 129525. [CrossRef] [PubMed]
25. Zandkarimi, F.; Decatur, J.; Casali, J.; Gordon, T.; Skibola, C.; Nuckolls, C. Comparison of the Cannabinoid and Terpene Profiles in Commercial Cannabis from Natural and Artificial Cultivation. *Molecules* **2023**, *28*, 833. [CrossRef]
26. Lynch, R.C.; Vergara, D.; Tittes, S.; White, K.; Schwartz, C.J.; Gibbs, M.J.; Ruthenburg, T.C.; deCesare, K.; Land, D.P.; Kane, N.C. Genomic and Chemical Diversity in Cannabis. *Crit. Rev. Plant Sci.* **2016**, *35*, 349–363. [CrossRef]
27. Karğılı, U.; Aytaç, E. Evaluation of Cannabinoid (CBD and THC) Content of Four Different Strains of Cannabis Grown in Four Different Regions. *Eur. Food Res. Technol.* **2022**, *248*, 1351–1364. [CrossRef]
28. Jîtcă, G.; Ősz, B.E.; Vari, C.E.; Rusz, C.-M.; Tero-Vescan, A.; Pușcaș, A. Cannabidiol: Bridge between Antioxidant Effect, Cellular Protection, and Cognitive and Physical Performance. *Antioxidants* **2023**, *12*, 485. [CrossRef]
29. Glivar, T.; Eržen, J.; Kreft, S.; Zagožen, M.; Čerenak, A.; Čeh, B.; Tavčar Benković, E. Cannabinoid Content in Industrial Hemp (*Cannabis sativa* L.) Varieties Grown in Slovenia. *Ind. Crops Prod.* **2020**, *145*, 112082. [CrossRef]

30. Janatová, A.; Fraňková, A.; Tlustoš, P.; Hamouz, K.; Božik, M.; Klouček, P. Yield and Cannabinoids Contents in Different Cannabis (*Cannabis sativa* L.) Genotypes for Medical Use. *Ind. Crops Prod.* **2018**, *112*, 363–367. [CrossRef]
31. Abdollahi, M.; Sefidkon, F.; Peirovi, A.; Calagari, M.; Mousavi, A. Assessment of the Cannabinoid Content from Different Varieties of *Cannabis sativa* L. during the Growth Stages in Three Regions. *Chem. Biodivers.* **2021**, *18*, e2100247. [CrossRef] [PubMed]
32. Johnson, D.A.; Funnell, M.P.; Heaney, L.M.; Cable, T.G.; Wheeler, P.C.; Bailey, S.J.; Clifford, T.; James, L.J. Cannabidiol Oil Ingested as Sublingual Drops or Within Gelatin Capsules Shows Similar Pharmacokinetic Profiles in Healthy Males. *Cannabis Cannabinoid Res.* **2024**, *9*, e1423–e1432. [CrossRef] [PubMed]
33. Hosseini, A.; McLachlan, A.J.; Lickliter, J.D. A Phase I Trial of the Safety, Tolerability and Pharmacokinetics of Cannabidiol Administered as Single-Dose Oil Solution and Single and Multiple Doses of a Sublingual Wafer in Healthy Volunteers. *Br. J. Clin. Pharmacol.* **2021**, *87*, 2070–2077. [CrossRef] [PubMed]
34. Notcutt, W.; Price, M.; Miller, R.; Newport, S.; Phillips, C.; Simmons, S.; Sansom, C. Initial Experiences with Medicinal Extracts of Cannabis for Chronic Pain: Results from 34 'N of 1' Studies. *Anaesthesia* **2004**, *59*, 440–452. [CrossRef] [PubMed]
35. Baratta, F.; Simiele, M.; Pignata, I.; Ravetto Enri, L.; D'Avolio, A.; Torta, R.; De Luca, A.; Collino, M.; Brusa, P. Cannabis-Based Oral Formulations for Medical Purposes: Preparation, Quality and Stability. *Pharmaceuticals* **2021**, *14*, 171. [CrossRef]
36. Villate, A.; Barreto, G.P.; Nicolás, M.S.; Aizpurua-Olaizola, O.; Olivares, M.; Usobiaga, A. Development, Characterization and In Vitro Gastrointestinal Release of PLGA Nanoparticles Loaded with Full-Spectrum Cannabis Extracts. *AAPS PharmSciTech* **2024**, *25*, 120. [CrossRef]
37. Taha, I.E.; ElSohly, M.A.; Radwan, M.M.; Omari, S.; Repka, M.A.; Ashour, E.A. Development and in Vitro Evaluation of Cannabidiol Mucoadhesive Buccal Film Formulations Using Hot-Melt Extrusion Technology. *Med. Cannabis Cannabinoids* **2024**, *7*, 171–182. [CrossRef]
38. Crupi, R.; Cuzzocrea, S. Role of EPA in Inflammation: Mechanisms, Effects, and Clinical Relevance. *Biomolecules* **2022**, *12*, 242. [CrossRef]
39. Fernandes, E.S.; Passos, G.; Medeiros, R.; Da Cunha, F.; Ferreira, J.; Campos, M.; Pianowski, L.; Calixto, J. Anti-Inflammatory Effects of Compounds Alpha-Humulene and (−)-Trans-Caryophyllene Isolated from the Essential Oil of Cordia Verbenacea. *Eur. J. Pharmacol.* **2007**, *569*, 228–236. [CrossRef]
40. Moghrovyan, A.; Parseghyan, L.; Sevoyan, G.; Darbinyan, A.; Sahakyan, N.; Gaboyan, M.; Karabekian, Z.; Voskanyan, A. Antinociceptive, Anti-Inflammatory, and Cytotoxic Properties of Origanum Vulgare Essential Oil, Rich with β-Caryophyllene and β-Caryophyllene Oxide. *Korean J. Pain* **2022**, *35*, 140–151. [CrossRef]
41. Becker, L.; Holtmann, D. Anti-Inflammatory Effects of α-Humulene on the Release of pro-Inflammatory Cytokines in Lipopolysaccharide-Induced THP-1 Cells. *Cell Biochem. Biophys.* **2024**, *82*, 839–847. [CrossRef] [PubMed]
42. Hashiesh, H.M.; Sharma, C.; Goyal, S.N.; Sadek, B.; Jha, N.K.; Kaabi, J.A.; Ojha, S. A Focused Review on CB2 Receptor-Selective Pharmacological Properties and Therapeutic Potential of β-Caryophyllene, a Dietary Cannabinoid. *Biomed. Pharmacother.* **2021**, *140*, 111639. [CrossRef] [PubMed]
43. Ricardi, C.; Barachini, S.; Consoli, G.; Marazziti, D.; Polini, B.; Chiellini, G. Beta-Caryophyllene, a Cannabinoid Receptor Type 2 Selective Agonist, in Emotional and Cognitive Disorders. *Int. J. Mol. Sci.* **2024**, *25*, 3203. [CrossRef] [PubMed]
44. Viveros-Paredes, J.M.; González-Castañeda, R.E.; Gertsch, J.; Chaparro-Huerta, V.; López-Roa, R.I.; Vázquez-Valls, E.; Beas-Zarate, C.; Camins-Espuny, A.; Flores-Soto, M.E. Neuroprotective Effects of β-Caryophyllene against Dopaminergic Neuron Injury in a Murine Model of Parkinson's Disease Induced by MPTP. *Pharmaceuticals* **2017**, *10*, 60. [CrossRef] [PubMed]
45. Legault, J.; Pichette, A. Potentiating Effect of Beta-Caryophyllene on Anticancer Activity of Alpha-Humulene, Isocaryophyllene and Paclitaxel. *J. Pharm. Pharmacol.* **2007**, *59*, 1643–1647. [CrossRef]
46. Viveiros, M.M.H.; Silva, M.G.; da Costa, J.G.M.; de Oliveira, A.G.; Rubio, C.; Padovani, C.R.; Rainho, C.A.; Schellini, S.A. Anti-Inflammatory Effects of α-Humulene and β-Caryophyllene on Pterygium Fibroblasts. *Int. J. Ophthalmol.* **2022**, *15*, 1903. [CrossRef]
47. Medeiros, R.; Passos, G.F.; Vitor, C.E.; Koepp, J.; Mazzuco, T.L.; Pianowski, L.F.; Campos, M.M.; Calixto, J.B. Effect of Two Active Compounds Obtained from the Essential Oil of Cordia Verbenacea on the Acute Inflammatory Responses Elicited by LPS in the Rat Paw. *Br. J. Pharmacol.* **2007**, *151*, 618–627. [CrossRef]
48. Jalil, V.; Khan, M.; Haider, S.Z.; Shamim, S. Investigation of the Antibacterial, Anti-Biofilm, and Antioxidative Effect of Piper Betle Leaf Extract against Bacillus Gaemokensis MW067143 Isolated from Dental Caries, an In Vitro-In Silico Approach. *Microorganisms* **2022**, *10*, 2485. [CrossRef]
49. Riyadi, S.A.; Naini, A.A.; Supratman, U. Sesquiterpenoids from Meliaceae Family and Their Biological Activities. *Molecules* **2023**, *28*, 4874. [CrossRef]
50. Sharifi-Rad, J.; Hoseini-Alfatemi, S.M.; Sharifi-Rad, M.; Sharifi-Rad, M.; Iriti, M.; Sharifi-Rad, M.; Sharifi-Rad, R.; Raeisi, S. Phytochemical Compositions and Biological Activities of Essential Oil from *Xanthium strumarium* L. *Molecules* **2015**, *20*, 7034–7047. [CrossRef]
51. Walasek-Janusz, M.; Grzegorczyk, A.; Malm, A.; Nurzyńska-Wierdak, R.; Zalewski, D. Chemical Composition, and Antioxidant and Antimicrobial Activity of Oregano Essential Oil. *Molecules* **2024**, *29*, 435. [CrossRef] [PubMed]
52. Sharifi-Rad, J.; Sureda, A.; Tenore, G.C.; Daglia, M.; Sharifi-Rad, M.; Valussi, M.; Tundis, R.; Sharifi-Rad, M.; Loizzo, M.R.; Ademiluyi, A.O.; et al. Biological Activities of Essential Oils: From Plant Chemoecology to Traditional Healing Systems. *Mol. A J. Synth. Chem. Nat. Prod. Chem.* **2017**, *22*, 70. [CrossRef] [PubMed]

53. Ahmed, A.Q.; Park, R.Y.; Noshad, D.; Li, P.C.H. Fast GC–MS Method for Identification and Quantification of Terpenes from Cannabis Species. *Chromatographia* 2024. [CrossRef]
54. Kaur, J.; Sun, N.; Hill, J.E. Comprehensive Profiling of Terpenes and Terpenoids in Different Cannabis Strains Using GC × GC-TOFMS. *Separations* **2023**, *10*, 500. [CrossRef]
55. Ali, E.M.M.; Almagboul, A.Z.I.; Khogali, S.M.E.; Gergeir, U.M.A. Antimicrobial Activity of *Cannabis sativa* L. *Chin. Med.* **2012**, *3*, 61–64. [CrossRef]
56. Malikova, L.; Malik, M.; Pavlik, J.; Ulman, M.; Pechouckova, E.; Skrivan, M.; Kokoska, L.; Tlustos, P. Anti-Staphylococcal Activity of Soilless Cultivated Cannabis across the Whole Vegetation Cycle under Various Nutritional Treatments in Relation to Cannabinoid Content. *Sci. Rep.* **2024**, *14*, 4343. [CrossRef]
57. Sotirova, Y.; Gugleva, V.; Stoeva, S.; Kolev, I.; Nikolova, R.; Marudova, M.; Nikolova, K.; Kiselova-Kaneva, Y.; Hristova, M.; Andonova, V. Bigel Formulations of Nanoencapsulated St. John's Wort Extract—An Approach for Enhanced Wound Healing. *Gels* **2023**, *9*, 360. [CrossRef]
58. Khelifi, I.; Saada, M.; Hayouni, E.A.; Tourette, A.; Bouajila, J.; Ksouri, R. Development and Characterization of Novel Bigel-Based 1,4-Naphthoquinones for Topical Application with Antioxidant Potential. *Arab. J. Sci. Eng.* **2020**, *45*, 53–61. [CrossRef]
59. Kulawik-Pióro, A.; Osak, E.; Mendrycka, M.; Trześniewska-Ofiara, Z. Bigels as Novel Systems for the Delivery Active Compounds from Centella Asiatica. *Soft Mater.* **2023**, *21*, 316–338. [CrossRef]
60. Zampouni, K.; Dimakopoulou-Papazoglou, D.; Katsanidis, E. Food-Grade Bigel Systems: Formulation, Characterization, and Applications for Novel Food Product Development. *Gels* **2024**, *10*, 712. [CrossRef]
61. Chen, Z.; Bian, F.; Cao, X.; Shi, Z.; Meng, Z. Novel Bigels Constructed from Oleogels and Hydrogels with Contrary Thermal Characteristics: Phase Inversion and 3D Printing Applications. *Food Hydrocoll.* **2023**, *134*, 108063. [CrossRef]
62. Barwood, M.; Corbett, J.; Thomas, K.; Twentyman, P. Relieving Thermal Discomfort: Effects of Sprayed L-Menthol on Perception, Performance, and Time Trial Cycling in the Heat: Menthol, Perception, Pacing, and TT Performance. *Scand. J. Med. Sci. Sports* **2015**, *25* (Suppl. S1), 211–218. [CrossRef] [PubMed]
63. Kalkandelen, C.; Ozbek, B.; Ergul, N.M.; Akyol, S.; Moukbil, Y.; Oktar, F.N.; Ekren, N.; Kılıc, O.; Kılıc, B.; Gunduz, O. Effect of Temperature, Viscosity and Surface Tension on Gelatine Structures Produced by Modified 3D Printer. *IOP Conf. Ser. Mater. Sci. Eng.* **2017**, *293*, 012001. [CrossRef]
64. Xu, X.; Zhou, J.; Jiang, Y.; Zhang, Q.; Shi, H.; Liu, D. 3D Printing Process of Oxidized Nanocellulose and Gelatin Scaffold. *J. Biomater. Sci. Polym. Ed.* **2018**, *29*, 1498–1513. [CrossRef] [PubMed]
65. Ilyin, S.O. Structural Rheology in the Development and Study of Complex Polymer Materials. *Polymers* **2024**, *16*, 2458. [CrossRef]
66. Erencia, M.; Cano, F.; Tornero, J.A.; Fernandes, M.M.; Tzanov, T.; Macanás, J.; Carrillo, F. Electrospinning of Gelatin Fibers Using Solutions with Low Acetic Acid Concentration: Effect of Solvent Composition on Both Diameter of Electrospun Fibers and Cytotoxicity. *J. Appl. Polym. Sci.* **2015**, *132*, 42115. [CrossRef]
67. Zhang, Q.; Li, X.; Jasti, B.R. Role of Physicochemical Properties of Some Grades of Hydroxypropyl Methylcellulose on in Vitro Mucoadhesion. *Int. J. Pharm.* **2021**, *609*, 121218. [CrossRef]
68. Park, C.; Zuo, J.; Gil, M.-C.; Löbenberg, R.; Lee, B.-J. Investigation of Cannabinoid Acid/Cyclodextrin Inclusion Complex for Improving Physicochemical and Biological Performance. *Pharmaceutics* **2023**, *15*, 2533. [CrossRef]
69. Abdella, S.; Kim, S.; Afinjuomo, F.; Song, Y.; Upton, R.; Garg, S. Combining the Potential of 3D Printed Buccal Films and Nanostructured Lipid Carriers for Personalised Cannabidiol Delivery. *Drug Deliv. Transl. Res.* **2024**, *14*, 984–1004. [CrossRef]
70. Vlad, R.-A.; Antonoaea, P.; Todoran, N.; Rédai, E.-M.; Bîrsan, M.; Muntean, D.-L.; Imre, S.; Hancu, G.; Farczádi, L.; Ciurba, A. Development and Evaluation of Cannabidiol Orodispersible Tablets Using a 23-Factorial Design. *Pharmaceutics* **2022**, *14*, 1467. [CrossRef]
71. Limpongsa, E.; Tabboon, P.; Pongjanyakul, T.; Jaipakdee, N. Preparation and Evaluation of Directly Compressible Orally Disintegrating Tablets of Cannabidiol Formulated Using Liquisolid Technique. *Pharmaceutics* **2022**, *14*, 2407. [CrossRef] [PubMed]
72. Dash, S.; Murthy, P.N.; Nath, L.; Chowdhury, P. Kinetic Modeling on Drug Release from Controlled Drug Delivery Systems. *Acta Pol. Pharm.* **2010**, *67*, 217–223. [PubMed]
73. Paul, D.R. Elaborations on the Higuchi Model for Drug Delivery. *Int. J. Pharm.* **2011**, *418*, 13–17. [CrossRef] [PubMed]
74. Fernandes, A.S.; Neves, B.V.; Mazzo, T.M.; Longo, E.; Jacob-Lopez, E.; Zepka, L.Q.; de Rosso, V.V. Bigels as Potential Inks for Extrusion-Based 3d Food Printing: Effect of Oleogel Fraction on Physical Characterization and Printability. *Food Hydrocoll.* **2023**, *144*, 108986. [CrossRef]
75. De Salvo, M.I.; Palla, C.A.; Cotabarren, I.M. Development of Beetroot Powder-Enriched Inks for 3D Food Printing Based on Hydrogel/Oleogel Bigels. *Food Biosci.* **2024**, *62*, 105278. [CrossRef]
76. Schlag, A.K.; Hindocha, C.; Zafar, R.; Nutt, D.J.; Curran, H.V. Cannabis Based Medicines and Cannabis Dependence: A Critical Review of Issues and Evidence. *J. Psychopharmacol.* **2021**, *35*, 773–785. [CrossRef]
77. Andriotis, E.G.; Paraskevopoulou, A.; Fatouros, D.G.; Zhang, H.; Ritzoulis, C. Design of Aerated Oleogel–Hydrogel Mixtures for 3D Printing of Personalized Cannabis Edibles. *Gels* **2024**, *10*, 654. [CrossRef]
78. Xie, D.; Hu, H.; Huang, Q.; Lu, X. Development and Characterization of Food-Grade Bigel System for 3D Printing Applications: Role of Oleogel/Hydrogel Ratios and Emulsifiers. *Food Hydrocoll.* **2023**, *139*, 108565. [CrossRef]
79. Qiu, R.; Wang, K.; Tian, H.; Liu, X.; Liu, G.; Hu, Z.; Zhao, L. Analysis on the Printability and Rheological Characteristics of Bigel Inks: Potential in 3D Food Printing. *Food Hydrocoll.* **2022**, *129*, 107675. [CrossRef]

80. Stasiłowicz-Krzemień, A.; Sip, S.; Szulc, P.; Cielecka-Piontek, J. Determining Antioxidant Activity of Cannabis Leaves Extracts from Different Varieties—Unveiling Nature's Treasure Trove. *Antioxidants* **2023**, *12*, 1390. [CrossRef]
81. Karpiński, T.M.; Ożarowski, M. Plant Organic Acids as Natural Inhibitors of Foodborne Pathogens. *Appl. Sci.* **2024**, *14*, 6340. [CrossRef]
82. Ahmed, L.; Atif, R.; Eldeen, T.; Yahya, I.; Omara, A.; Eltayeb, M. Study the Using of Nanoparticles as Drug Delivery System Based on Mathematical Models for Controlled Release. *Int. J. Latest Technol. Eng. Manag. Appl. Sci. IJLTEMAS* **2019**, *8*, 52–56.

gels

MDPI

Article

Investigation of a Thermoresponsive In Situ Hydrogel Loaded with Nanotriphala: Implications for Antioxidant, Anti-Inflammatory, and Antimicrobial Therapy in Nasal Disorders

Rungsinee Phongpradist [1], Chuda Chittasupho [1], Sudarshan Singh [2,3], Julalak Chorachoo Ontong [4], Sarin Tadtong [5], Puriputt Akachaipaibul [6], Charatda Punvittayagul [7], Kriangkrai Thongkorn [8], Pornngarm Dejkriengkraikul [9,10,11], Jutamas Jiaranaikulwanitch [1], Sunee Chansakaow [1] and Darunee Hongwiset [1,*]

1 Department of Pharmaceutical Sciences, Faculty of Pharmacy, Chiang Mai University, Muang, Chiang Mai 50200, Thailand; rungsinee.p@cmu.ac.th (R.P.); chuda.c@cmu.ac.th (C.C.); jutamas.jia@cmu.ac.th (J.J.); sunee.c@cmu.ac.th (S.C.)
2 Faculty of Pharmacy, Chiang Mai University, Muang, Chiang Mai 50200, Thailand; sudarshan.s@cmu.ac.th
3 Office of Research Administration, Chiang Mai University, Muang, Chiang Mai 50200, Thailand
4 Cosmetic Technology and Dietary Supplement Products Program, Faculty of Agro and Bio Industry, Thaksin University, Ban Pa Phayom, Phatthalung 93210, Thailand; julalak.o@tsu.ac.th
5 Department of Pharmacognosy, Faculty of Pharmacy, Srinakharinwirot University, Ongkharak, Nakhon Nayok 26120, Thailand; sarin@g.swu.ac.th
6 Faculty of Pharmacy, Srinakharinwirot University, Ongkharak, Nakhon Nayok 26120, Thailand; puriputt.akachaipaibul@g.swu.ac.th
7 Center of Veterinary Medical Diagnostic and Animal Health Innovation, Faculty of Veterinary Medicine, Chiang Mai University, Muang, Chiang Mai 50100, Thailand; charatda.pun@cmu.ac.th
8 Faculty of Veterinary Medicine, Chiang Mai University, Muang, Chiang Mai 50100, Thailand; kriangkrai.th@cmu.ac.th
9 Department of Biochemistry, Faculty of Medicine, Chiang Mai University, Muang, Chiang Mai 50200, Thailand; pornngarm.d@cmu.ac.th
10 Center for Research and Development of Natural Products for Health, Chiang Mai University, Muang, Chiang Mai 50200, Thailand
11 Anticarcinogenesis and Apoptosis Research Cluster, Faculty of Medicine, Chiang Mai University, Muang, Chiang Mai 50200, Thailand
* Correspondence: darunee.h@cmu.ac.th

Abstract: Oxidative stress plays a crucial role in chronic nasal disorders, contributing to inflammation, tissue damage, and impaired mucosal function, highlighting the need for targeted therapies. Recent advancements in nasal drug delivery systems have expanded their applications for treating respiratory and inflammatory conditions. Among these, hydrogel-based systems offer prolonged release of active pharmaceutical ingredients (APIs), enhancing therapeutic efficacy and reducing dosing frequency. This study initially evaluates the antioxidant, anti-inflammatory, antimicrobial, and cytotoxic properties of Nanotriphala, followed by its incorporation into a thermoresponsive in situ hydrogel system, which was subsequently developed and characterized as a novel formulation. Nanotriphala exhibited >90% cell viability and significantly reduced nitric oxide (NO) levels by 40.55 μg/mL at 250 μg/mL. The hydrogel was characterized by key parameters, including viscosity, gelling time, pH, gelling temperature, texture analysis, and ex vivo spreadability. Stability was assessed under various conditions, and mutagenicity and antimutagenicity were evaluated using the Ames test. Results showed that the hydrogel gelled at 34 °C, exhibited good spreadability (10.25 ± 0.28 cm), a viscosity of 227 ± 22 cP, and maintained a pH of 5.75 ± 0.01, with optimal hardness and adhesiveness suitable for nasal application. It demonstrated antimicrobial activity against *E. coli*, *P. aeruginosa*, *S. aureus*, and *S.*

epidermidis at minimal bactericidal concentrations (MBCs) of 32, 2, 4, and 8 μg/mL, respectively, with low mutagenicity (mutagenic index < 2) and strong antimutagenic activity (>60%). The gallic acid content was 0.5796 ± 0.0218 μg/100 mL. Stability studies confirmed optimal storage at 4 °C. These findings suggest that in situ hydrogel loaded with Nanotriphala is a promising nasal drug delivery system for managing oxidative stress and related inflammatory conditions.

Keywords: in situ hydrogel; triphala; nasal delivery pathway; antioxidant; antiinflammation; antimicrobial; nanoparticles; nasal disorder

1. Introduction

Nasal disorders, such as allergic rhinitis, chronic sinusitis, and rhinosinusitis, have a significant burden on individual health and healthcare systems. These conditions are characterized by chronic inflammation, tissue damage, and impaired mucociliary clearance, which are often exacerbated by oxidative stress [1,2]. Oxidative stress occurs due to an imbalance between the production of reactive oxygen species (ROS) and the antioxidant defenses, playing a pivotal role in the pathogenesis and progression of these disorders [3]. Chronic inflammation and oxidative damage contribute to the ongoing nature of nasal disorders, underscoring the need for innovative treatments that address these core issues. Current nasal therapies, including corticosteroids and antihistamines, effectively alleviate symptoms and reduce oxidative stress. When used together, these treatments amplify their effects, leading to a notable reduction in total oxidative stress and offering a more targeted approach to managing these conditions [4,5]. However, systemic treatments may cause undesired side effects, emphasizing the importance of localized therapies that deliver relief directly to the nasal cavity. In this light, recent advancements in drug delivery systems designed for sustained and localized release of medications, have drawn considerable attention [6,7].

Triphala is a polyherbal formulation composed of three plants: *Emblica officinalis*, *Terminalia chebula*, and *Terminalia bellerica*. It is traditionally prepared with equal parts of *E. officinalis*, *T. chebula*, and *T. bellerica*. However, a modified formulation with varying ratios of *T. chebula*, *T. bellerica*, and *E. officinalis* has been reported to optimize the therapeutic effects of Triphala, enabling targeted benefits tailored to specific health concerns [8,9]. This herbal combination is rich in bioactive compounds, including polyphenols (gallic acid, ellagic acid, chebulinic acid, chebulagic acid, and emblicanin A and B), flavonoids (quercetin and kaempferol), and tannins, which provide strong antioxidant, anti-inflammatory, and antimicrobial effects [10–13]. Chemical analysis of Triphala reveals numerous biologically active constituents, including chebulinic acid, gallic acid, rutin, quercetin, tannins, flavonoids, pectin, and vitamin C, which collectively contribute to its potent antioxidant and health-promoting effects [10]. The amount of each phytochemical is influenced by the extraction techniques utilized, the type of solvents applied, and the specific geographic location where the parent plant is grown [13]. Pharmacological studies have demonstrated that Triphala extract possesses potent antioxidant activity, helping to reduce damage caused by oxidative stress [9]. This has led to its growing recognition as a potential remedy for oxidative stress-related disorders. Despite its therapeutic potential, the clinical use of Triphala is often hindered by challenges related to the poor solubility, stability, and bioavailability of its active components [14]. To overcome these limitations, advancements in nanotechnology and modern drug delivery systems offer a promising approach to enhance its efficacy and application.

Nanocarrier systems have been shown to enhance the solubility, stability, and bioavailability of herbal extracts, leading to improved therapeutic outcomes [15]. Among these, thermoresponsive in situ hydrogels have emerged as innovative solutions for nasal drug delivery [16]. These hydrogels exhibit a sol-to-gel transition when exposed to physiological temperatures, enabling convenient administration in liquid form followed by gelation within the nasal cavity [17]. This transition not only ensures prolonged retention and controlled release of encapsulated therapeutic agents but also enhances local efficacy while reducing systemic exposure [18]. Advancements in nanotechnology-based delivery systems have shown notable success in improving the bioavailability and therapeutic effectiveness of herbal extracts [19]. Similarly, nanoformulations of other herbal products have demonstrated enhanced penetration through biological barriers, leading to better therapeutic results in preclinical studies. These developments highlight the potential of integrating nanotechnology with traditional herbal therapies to overcome limitations and optimize clinical outcomes [20,21].

The development of a thermoresponsive in situ hydrogel loaded with Nanotriphala (In situ Tri) represents a novel approach to leverage the therapeutic potential of this traditional formulation for treating nasal disorders. By merging the benefits of nanotechnology with the unique properties of in situ gelling systems, this approach aims to overcome the limitations associated with conventional formulations of herbal extracts. A thorough evaluation of the hydrogel's physicochemical properties, antioxidant capacity, anti-inflammatory effects, cytotoxicity profile, and antimicrobial effectiveness against clinically relevant pathogens will be critical to validate its potential. Furthermore, safety assessment remains a cornerstone of pharmaceutical development. The Salmonella/human S9 mutagenicity test, a well-established method for assessing the genotoxicity of compounds, provides vital information about the safety profile of the developed formulation [22]. This comprehensive framework for characterization and safety evaluation not only ensures alignment with regulatory standards but also underscores adherence to best practices in modern pharmaceutical development.

Merging traditional herbal medicine with advanced drug delivery technologies offers valuable insights into enhancing the efficacy and safety of herbal formulations, bridging traditional knowledge with modern pharmaceutical advancements. Thus, incorporating Triphala extract into a nanoformulation and combining it with an in situ hydrogel could be a promising strategy to overcome the limitations of traditional Triphala formulations for nasal application. The nanoformulation will enhance the solubility, stability, and bioavailability of Triphala's active components [23], addressing challenges such as poor absorption and rapid degradation, as mentioned earlier. Integrating this nanoformulation into a thermoresponsive in situ hydrogel could amplify its benefits by enabling sustained and localized drug release within the nasal cavity [24]. This dual approach not only improves the therapeutic efficacy of Triphala but also reduces systemic exposure, thereby minimizing potential side effects. Consequently, the combined system may promote the potential to maximize the antioxidant, anti-inflammatory, and antimicrobial activities of Triphala, making it a highly effective treatment option for oxidative stress-related nasal disorders.

This study explores the development of a thermoresponsive in situ hydrogel incorporating Nanotriphala, with the goal of evaluating its biological and pharmacological properties. The research focuses on the antioxidant activity, anti-inflammatory effects, cytotoxicity, and antimicrobial efficacy of Nanotriphala. The antioxidant activity was assessed using established assays, such as DPPH, ABTS, and FRAP. The anti-inflammatory effect was quantified through nitric oxide assays, while cytotoxicity was evaluated using MTT assays to analyze the compound's impact on cell viability. The antimicrobial potential was tested against key pathogens, including *Escherichia coli, Pseudomonas aeruginosa, Staphylococcus aureus*, and *Staphylococcus epidermidis*. Subsequently, Nanotriphala was integrated into a thermoresponsive in situ hydrogel, which undergoes detailed characterization of its physicochemical properties, including gelation behavior, viscosity, and thermal stability. The stability of the hydrogel formulation was also evaluated under various storage conditions. To ensure safety, the genotoxic potential of in situ hydrogel loaded with Nanotriphala was analyzed using the Salmonella/human S9 mutagenicity test.

This research aims to uncover the therapeutic potential and safety of this innovative hydrogel system for managing oxidative stress-related nasal disorders. The outcomes may contribute to the development of novel treatment options that bridge traditional knowledge and modern pharmaceutical science.

2. Results and Discussion

2.1. Antioxidant Activities of Triphala Extract and Nanotirphala

The assessment of antioxidant activity for gallic acid, Triphala extract (Tri ext), and Nanotriphala (Tri Np) using DPPH, ABTS, and FRAP assays provides crucial insights into the potential therapeutic benefits of these compounds in combating oxidative stress. For the DPPH assay (Figure 1A), gallic acid, a standard antioxidant compound, exhibited an IC_{50} value of 1.863 ± 0.191 μg/mL. In contrast, Triphala extract demonstrated higher IC_{50} values of 17.07 ± 2.02 μg/mL, indicating relatively lower antioxidant efficiency compared to gallic acid. However, Nanotriphala displayed lower IC_{50} values of 0.004 ± 0.111 μg/mL, demonstrating a significant increase in free radical-scavenging capacity for the nanoformulation. This significant improvement in antioxidant activity can be attributed to nanoformulation, which enhances the solubility of the active compounds in Triphala. This observation aligns with findings from our previous study, which demonstrated that nanoformulation improves the solubility of Triphala extract [23]. The reduced particle size in Nanotriphala likely facilitates better interaction with DPPH radicals, resulting in improved radical-scavenging efficiency. This observation aligns with a previous report, which highlighted that the nanoscale dimensions of nanoparticles play a critical role in amplifying their surface area [25]. The increased surface area facilitates enhanced interactions with free radicals, thereby significantly bolstering their scavenging capabilities. These amplified antioxidant properties are crucial for combating oxidative stress, which plays a significant role in the development of various conditions, including neurodegenerative diseases, cardiovascular disorders, and cancer [26,27].

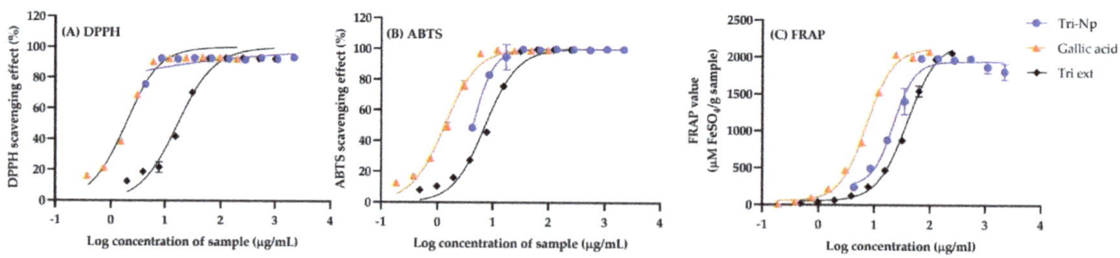

Figure 1. The antioxidant activity of gallic acid, Triphala extract, and Nanotriphala as determined by (**A**) DPPH free radical-scavenging assay, (**B**) ABTS free radical-scavenging assay, and (**C**) ferric reducing antioxidant power (FRAP) assay. Data are presented as mean ± SD (n = 3).

Furthermore, the ABTS assay (Figure 1B) showed IC_{50} values of 1.383 ± 0.117 μg/mL for gallic acid, 7.343 ± 0.707 μg/mL for Triphala extract, and 4.533 ± 0.211 μg/mL for Nanotriphala. The remarkably low IC_{50} for Nanotriphala confirms its superior ability to scavenge ABTS radicals, which could be attributed to the synergistic action of the diverse phytochemicals in Triphala. This synergy aligns with evidence suggesting that combinations of phytochemicals often outperform individual compounds in antioxidant efficacy, as they target a broader spectrum of oxidative pathways [28,29].

The ferric-reducing antioxidant power (FRAP) of gallic acid, Triphala extract, and Nanotriphala is summarized in Figure 1C. A calibration curve for ferrous sulfate (Fe^{2+}) was constructed, demonstrating excellent linearity within the concentration range of 12.5 to 200 μM, with a correlation coefficient (R^2) of 0.9957. The FRAP values were expressed in terms of Fe^{2+} equivalents. The data indicated a concentration-dependent increase in the FRAP values for gallic acid, Triphala extract, and Nanotriphala. Specifically, the FRAP values for gallic acid ranged from 11.58 ± 6.42 to 2084.22 ± 24.09 μM, from 19.38 ± 2.44 to 2062.00 ± 48.00 μM for Triphala extract, and from 241.75 ± 3.94 to 1812.37 ± 108.15 μM for Nanotriphala. The ferric-reducing antioxidant power (FRAP) results for Triphala extract and Nanotriphala demonstrate a concentration-dependent increase in antioxidant activity. The concentration range for Triphala extract is 0.49–250 μg/mL, while for Nanotriphala, it is 4.43–2272 μg/mL, which is equivalent to the weight of Triphala extract per milliliter. In the case of Triphala extract, the FRAP values ranged from 19.38 ± 2.44 μM to 2062.00 ± 48.00 μM, showing an increase in antioxidant activity as the concentration increased. For Nanotriphala, with concentrations between 4.43 and 2272 μg/mL, the FRAP values ranged from 241.75 ± 3.94 μM to 1812.37 ± 108.15 μM. Despite the wider concentration range of Nanotriphala, its FRAP values were generally higher at lower concentrations than those of Triphala extract, indicating that Nanotriphala provides more efficient or potent antioxidant activity per unit concentration. This enhanced reducing capability emphasizes the formulation's role in maintaining the stability of antioxidant compounds, critical for their efficacy in biological systems where environmental factors often lead to the breakdown of these compounds, worsening the effects of oxidative stress [30,31].

The notable increase in antioxidant activity observed with the Nanotriphala formulation underscores the potential of nanoparticulate systems to enhance the therapeutic effectiveness of herbal extracts. When compared to Triphala extract, Nanotriphala stands out as a promising innovation for improving the antioxidant benefits of natural compounds. Future research should focus on elucidating the specific mechanisms driving these improvements and exploring the clinical applications of Nanotriphala in treating oxidative stress-related disorders.

2.2. *Antimicrobial Activities of Triphala Extract and Nanotriphala*

The antimicrobial activity results (see Table 1) for Triphala extract (Tri ext), Nanotriphala (Tri Np), and standard antibiotic treatments demonstrate significant differences in efficacy against various bacterial strains associated with oxidative stress-related nasal diseases. These results indicate that while Triphala extract demonstrates moderate antibacterial properties, particularly against *E. coli* and *S. aureus*, its efficacy is limited, as evidenced by high MBC values. The high MIC and MBC for *P. aeruginosa*, a pathogen known for its resistance, suggest that Triphala extract may require multiple doses of treatment for infections caused by this bacterium. In comparison, Nanotriphala exhibited slightly reduced antimicrobial activity compared to the Triphala extract at equivalent concentrations, likely due to the slower release of the active ingredients from the nanoparticle matrix, which may enable prolonged interaction with bacterial cells [11]. However, Nanotriphala demonstrated activity against *P. aeruginosa*, achieving MIC and MBC values of 12,500 μg/mL and 25,000 μg/mL, respectively; this suggests potential utility for Nanotriphala in treating resistant bacterial infections. While the MIC and MBC values for both Tri ext and Tri Np were higher than those of standard antibiotics, this indicates limited efficacy compared to established treatments. Standard antibiotics (Gentamicin and Vancomycin) served as controls, displaying low MIC and MBC values (0.5 μg/mL for Gentamicin against *S. aureus* and varying for Vancomycin). The results confirm the effectiveness of these antibiotics. However, the enhanced activity of Nanotriphala suggests that it may serve as a complementary or alternative approach, especially in cases of antibiotic resistance [32]. The findings indicate that Nanotriphala not only enhances the antimicrobial properties of Triphala extract but also provides a promising strategy for addressing oxidative stress-related nasal diseases. This enhanced efficacy could be attributed to the encapsulation of bioactive compounds within nanoparticles or a gel matrix, which may protect them from degradation and facilitate sustained release, thus improving their interaction with bacterial cells [33]. However, further optimization of the formulation, including release kinetics and concentration adjustments, is necessary to enhance its antimicrobial efficacy to levels comparable with standard antibiotics. Previous studies have demonstrated the potential of Triphala as an antimicrobial agent due to its rich polyphenolic content [34,35]. Additionally, the therapeutic potential of Triphala's as a delivery system for improving the therapeutic index of herbal extracts has been highlighted by Peterson et al., in their review, suggesting that nanoencapsulation may prolong the efficacy, improve bioavailability, and protect bioactive compounds from premature degradation [36]. Thus, iterations of this study could compare activity against multidrug-resistant strains, as seen in other nanoparticle-based antimicrobial formulations. In conclusion, Nanotriphala presents significant potential as an innovative therapeutic strategy for bacterial infections related to oxidative stress in nasal conditions.

Table 1. MIC and MBC of Triphala extract and Nanotriphala for different microorganism strains.

Sample	MIC:MBC (μg/mL)			
	E. coli	*P. aeruginosa*	*S. aureus*	*S. epidermidis*
Tri ext	128:1024	>1024:>1024	1024:>1024	1024:>1024
Tri Np	390:1562	12,500:25,000	1562:12,500	1562:6250
Antibiotics	0.5:0.5 [Gen]	0.5:1 [Gen]	0.5: 0.5 [VA]	0.5:1 [VA]

Gen: Gentamicin; VA: Vancomycin. The data represent the mean of three independent experiments (n = 3).

2.3. Cytotoxicity of Triphala Extract and Nanotriphala

Due to the importance of ensuring cell viability, the primary purpose of assessing the cytotoxicity of gallic acid, Triphala extract, and Nanotriphala against RAW264.7 cells (used as an anti-inflammatory model) was to establish the maximum non-toxic concentration suitable for the nitric oxide (NO) assay, which serves as a critical evaluation of their anti-inflammatory potential. The results, depicted in Figure 2, show the cell viability percentage, with the control group set at 100%. At 500 μg/mL, gallic acid significantly reduced cell viability, while Triphala extract and Nanotriphala, at concentrations ranging from 3.91 to 500 μg/mL, maintained cell viability above 80%, indicating minimal toxicity [37]. In general, all formulations exhibited favorable cytotoxicity profiles at lower concentrations, with Nanotriphala and Triphala extract maintaining viability above 90% at most doses. Notably, Nanotriphala consistently preserved cell viability at above 94%, even at higher doses, demonstrating excellent biocompatibility. These findings align with previous studies assessing the cytotoxicity of nanoparticles, further supporting the safety and potential of Nanotriphala for biomedical applications [38]. A slight reduction in viability was noted at 500 μg/mL, indicating a threshold beyond which toxicity might occur. While gallic acid showed high cell viability at lower doses, it caused a significant decrease (51.43%) at 500 μg/mL, reflecting dose-dependent cytotoxicity, as noted in previous studies [39]. Blank nanoparticles maintained stable viability at all concentrations, confirming the non-toxic nature of the nanoparticle excipient and its ability to support cell health effectively. Based on these findings, concentrations of 250 μg/mL or lower for gallic acid, Triphala extract, and Nanotriphala were selected for the nitric oxide (NO) assay to ensure cell viability and reliable assessment of their anti-inflammatory potential.

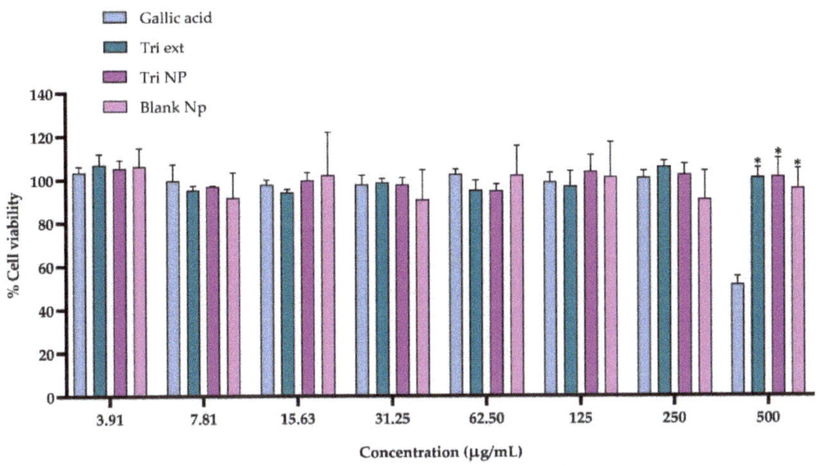

Figure 2. Cell viability (MTT assay) in RAW 267.4 cells cultured on callic acid, Triphala extract (Tri ext), Nanotriphala (Tri Np), and blank nanoparticles (Blank Np). The data represent the mean ± standard deviation (SD) of three independent experiments (n = 3). * indicates a significant difference ($p < 0.05$) when compared to gallic acid at the same concentration.

2.4. Anti-Inflammatory Activity of Nanotriphala

The results from the nitric oxide (NO) assay (Figure 3) demonstrate the anti-inflammatory potential of gallic acid, Triphala extract (Tri ext), and Nanotriphala (Tri Np) at various concentrations. Nitric oxide, produced by nitric oxide synthase (NOS), plays a crucial role in inflammation, and its inhibition can indicate anti-inflammatory effects [40]. At lower concentrations (1.953 μg/mL to 31.25 μg/mL), gallic acid caused only a slight reduction in NO levels, which remained close to 80 μg/mL. However, as the concentration increased beyond 62.5 μg/mL, there was a notable decline in NO production. At 250 μg/mL, the NO level was reduced significantly to 9.99 μg/mL. Gallic acid demonstrated the strongest anti-inflammatory effects at higher concentrations, in agreement with its known ability to inhibit pro-inflammatory mediators [41]. This steep decline suggests that gallic acid possesses potent anti-inflammatory activity at higher concentrations, possibly through the inhibition of NOS activity and the reduction in NO production, as shown in previous studies [42,43]. Triphala extract (Tri ext) showed a more gradual decrease in NO production compared to gallic acid. At lower concentrations of Triphala extract (1.953 μg/mL to 31.25 μg/mL), the NO level was still high and ranged from 98 to 104 μg/mL. Contrastingly, a drastic decline in NO levels was seen as the doses reached 125 μg/mL and 250 μg/mL, with NO levels of 22.73 μg/mL and 14.29 μg/mL, respectively. This implies that higher doses of Triphala extract may, therefore, be required to achieve a similar level of NO inhibition as with gallic acid. However, Triphala extract can also have an anti-inflammatory effect. These findings also confirm an earlier study that identified Triphala's bioactive compounds (such as tannins, flavonoids, and polyphenols) with anti-inflammatory and antioxidant activity [44,45]. The Nanotriphala (Tri Np) formulation demonstrated a unique profile of NO inhibition. At lower concentrations (1.953 μg/mL to 31.25 μg/mL), the NO levels produced by Tri Np were comparable to the control group, demonstrating limited anti-inflammatory activity at these doses. However, NO production began to decrease at concentrations of 62.5 μg/mL and above, with NO levels at 250 μg/mL measuring 40.55 μg/mL. This suggests that Tri Np still exhibited anti-inflammatory properties at higher doses, but the reduction in NO levels was not as significant as that of gallic acid. When comparing the concentration range of 62.5–250 μg/mL between Nanotriphala and Triphala extract, the initial results indicated that Triphala extract significantly reduced NO levels compared to Nanotriphala at the same concentrations. However, when calculating the equivalent concentration of Triphala extract in Nanotriphala, it was found that 62.5, 125, and 250 μg/mL of Nanotriphala correspond to approximately 2.84, 5.68, and 11.36 μg/mL of Triphala extract, respectively. At 2.84 and 5.68 μg/mL, the reduction in NO levels by Nanotriphala was not significantly different from the reductions observed at the nearest higher concentrations of Triphala extract (3.91 and 7.81 μg/mL, respectively). Interestingly, at 250 μg/mL of Nanotriphala, which is equivalent to 11.36 μg/mL of Triphala extract, the NO level reduction was significantly greater when compared to 15.63 μg/mL of Triphala extract. Hence, we demonstrate the anti-inflammatory properties of Nanotriphala by considering the significant reduction in NO generation in inflammatory RAW267.4 macrophage cells. These delivery systems are known to improve the solubility, stability, and therapeutic effectiveness of bioactive components of food, thus increasing their ability to modulate negative inflammatory responses [46].

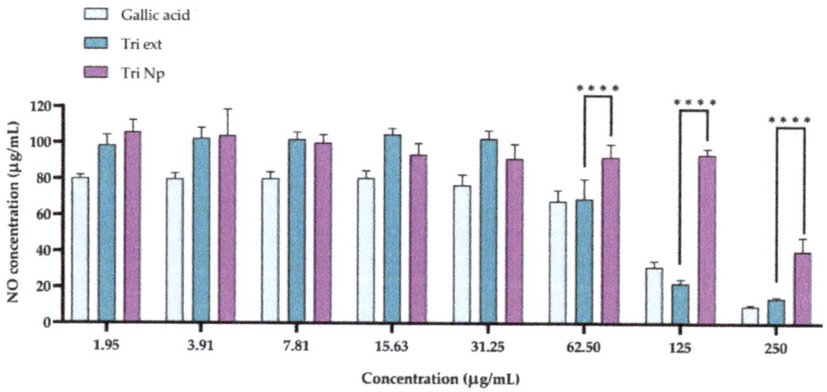

Figure 3. Inhibition of nitric oxide production by gallic acid, Triphala extract, and Nano-Triphala in lipopolysaccharide (LPS)-induced RAW 264.7 macrophages. The data represent the mean ± standard deviation (SD) of three independent experiments (n = 3). **** indicates $p < 0.0001$ when compared with Triphala extract at the same concentration.

The results from the nitric oxide assay demonstrate that the anti-inflammatory effect of Tri ext and Tri Np were concentration-dependent. Hence, according to this study, gallic acid and Triphala extract, as well as Nanotriphala, exhibited nitric oxide synthesis inhibition in a concentration-dependent manner, thereby indicating their anti-inflammatory potential. These results highlight the potential application of Nanotriphala as a biocompatible and effective delivery system for anti-inflammatory therapy, especially for diseases associated with oxidative stress.

2.5. Physicochemical Properties of In Situ Gel Loaded with Nanotriphala

After incorporating Nanotriphala, with a size of 137.6 ± 1.9 nm, a PDI of 0.13 ± 0.01, and a zeta potential of −22.73 ± 0.23 mV, into an in situ hydrogel system, the resulting formulation was characterized for its physicochemical properties. Numerous important inferences related to the properties of the in situ gel comprising nanoparticles with Triphala extract that are useful in treating oxidative stress-mediated nasal disorders are drawn from the characterization results (Table 2). The obtained pH value of 5.75 falls within the physiological values of nasal secretions, which are generally between 5.5 and 6.5 [47,48]. This slightly acidic pH is essential for several reasons. First, it reduces the potential for nasal irritation, a concern specific to topical preparations. Research shows that products with pH above or below the physiological range can cause irritation and even damage to the nasal mucosa [49]. The gelling time of 26.27 ± 1.16 s falls within the suitable range reported in previous studies, indicating that the formulation is well suited for nasal application [50–52]. The short gelation time will ensure a prolonged residence time in the nasal cavity, effectively counteracting mucociliary inflammation [53]. A rapid-to-gel phase transition upon administration can effectively prevent draining from the nasal cavity and allow sustained contact with the mucosal surface. This property is consistent with previous results from Ivano et al. [54], who reported that the bioavailability of thermosensitive gels was significantly greater than that of conventional delivery in the case of gels (32–34 °C) with the same gelling temperatures. Moreover, the gelation temperature (34.0 °C) is also well in the range of the human body temperature, which enables the fluid to be smoothly administered and gel quickly upon contact with nasal mucosa [55]. In our previous investigation, gallic acid, chebulagic acid, and chebulinic acid were found to be the major components of the Nanotriphala preparation. Nevertheless, to reflect the actual studies, for this study, gallic acid was chosen as the predominant active compound for its well-known therapeutic effects. The retention time of gallic acid was about 3.960 min (Figure 4A), and the quantification analysis presented a linear response from 3.001 to 9.004 μg/mL with an R^2 value over 0.99, supporting the precision and reliability of the analytical method. This was coupled with a tailing factor of 1.755 ± 0.040, theoretical plate count of 18,018 ± 377, resolution of 4.092 ± 0.084, and a signal-to-noise ratio of 50.12 ± 38.00, collectively demonstrating excellent system suitability for chromatographic analysis. Gallic acid in In situ Tri (Figure 4B) recorded a retention time of 3.961 ± 0.002 min. The chromatogram of the blank in situ hydrogel (Figure 4D) reveals a major peak around 27 min, likely representing components or impurities inherent to the hydrogel formulation that elute at this retention time. Importantly, this peak does not overlap with the retention time of gallic acid (3.960 min), confirming the method's selectivity and suitability for the accurate quantification of the gallic acid without interference from the hydrogel matrix. For In situ Tri, temperature control was crucial throughout the sample preparation process. The sample temperature was kept below 30 °C to avoid premature gelation and the column temperature was set at 17 °C to provide optimal separation and accurate determination of the chromatographic analysis. The final concentration of gallic acid in the In situ Tri formulation was determined as 0.5796 ± 0.0218 μg/100 mL, indicating that while the amount of gallic acid achieved in the preparation was not very high, it is nevertheless therapeutically important for the action of intra-nasal therapy. Gallic acid is well known for being a potent antioxidant, anti-inflammatory, and antimicrobial agent, which makes it a promising agent for the treatment of nasal disorders like allergic rhinitis, sinusitis, and other diseases related to oxidative stress, inflammation, and microbial infection [56]. The viscosity of the formulation at 227 cP is likely to lie within the range of optimal nasal gels (200–1000 cP). Such intermediate viscosity is suitable for easy administration but offers sufficient resistance to the mucociliary clearance processes to prolong the contact between the drug and the nasal epithelium [57]. Viscosity and mucoadhesion must be well balanced to guarantee drug absorption and therapeutic effectiveness. A relatively high spreadability value of 10.25 cm was reported as one of the delivery properties of the developed formulations, which guarantees good and even nasal mucus coverage [58]. This value suggests that all the tested formulations have good spreadability and are therefore appropriate to be used nasally, which is in line with the results obtained from previous studies [58]. Adequate viscosity is essential to prolong nasal residence time, ensuring sustained contact with the mucosa for effective drug delivery [58]. Low viscosity allows easy packing, handling, and hassle-free administration of the formulation, while a higher viscosity may accompany a prolonged retention time in the nasal cavity, which also limits the permeation rate. Thus, it is important to achieve optimal viscosity. The viscosity of Nanotriphala in this study was observed to be between 100 and 200 cP, which falls in the range of viscosity that is reported to be optimal for nasal administration [59,60].

Table 2. Characterization of in situ gel.

Sample	pH	Gelation Time (s)	Gelation Temperature (°C)	Viscosity (cP)	Spreadability (cm)	Gallic Acid Content (μg/100 mL)
In situ Tri	5.75 ±0.01	26.27 ± 1.16	34.0 ± 0.0	227 ± 22	10.25 ± 0.28	0.5796 ± 0.0218

Values are mean ± SD. The data represent the mean of three independent experiments (n = 3).

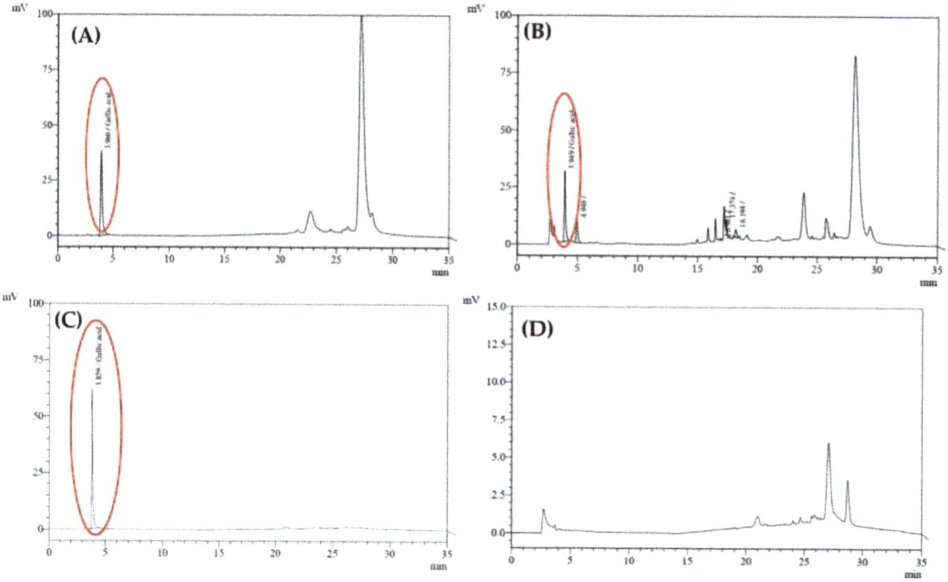

Figure 4. HPLC chromatogram of (**A**) standard gallic acid in blank hydrogel sample, (**B**) gallic acid in in situ hydrogel Nanotriphala, (**C**) gallic acid standard solution, and (**D**) blank in situ hydrogel.

Overall, the In situ Tri formulation demonstrates favorable physicochemical properties, such as an appropriate pH, rapid gelling, optimal viscosity, and good spreadability, all of which are crucial for effective nasal drug delivery. These characteristics suggest potential for improved drug retention and absorption in the nasal cavity, which could translate to enhanced therapeutic outcomes.

2.6. Texture Profile Analysis

The desirable attributes of mucoadhesive formulation gels include ease of removal from the primary packaging, ease of application, and the ability to retain the product at the application site without disintegration [61]. These properties are crucial for ensuring effective delivery, prolonged contact with the mucosal surface, and enhanced therapeutic outcomes [61,62]. The texture analysis of the in situ hydrogel loaded with Nanotriphala (Table 3) reveals critical insights into its mechanical and adhesive properties, which directly relate to its mucoadhesive potential for nasal drug delivery [63]. The hardness of the hydrogel, measured at 14.05 ± 0.35 g, indicates its structural stability and ability to withstand external forces during application and retention within the nasal cavity [61]. This value aligns with the findings of Basu et al., who reported that a hardness of less than 28 g is considered optimal for trans-nasal formulations, ensuring both ease of administration and effective retention [64]. This moderate hardness is ideal for nasal formulations, as it ensures the gel is not too rigid to cause discomfort nor too soft to compromise its mechanical integrity during administration. These properties suggest that the formulation can be easily administered in vivo, ensuring smooth and efficient application during use [65].

Table 3. Texture profile of in situ hydrogel loaded with Nanotriphala.

	Hardness (g)	Adhesiveness (g·s)
In situ Tri	14.05 ± 0.35	−13.84 ± 1.48

Values are mean ± SD. The data represent the mean of three independent experiments (n = 3).

The recorded adhesiveness was −13.84 ± 1.48 g·s. Our findings show that the adhesive results fall within the range corresponding to those of previous studies [62,66]. In more detail, adhesiveness is related to bioadhesion and is a measure of the force required to overcome the attractive forces between the surfaces of the sample and the probe [67,68]. This property is crucial for ensuring that the formulation can effectively adhere to the mucosal surfaces, allowing for prolonged retention and enhanced therapeutic effects at the application site [67]. The relationship between texture analysis and mucoadhesion is crucial in designing nasal formulations. Mucoadhesion relies on the ability of the hydrogel to adhere to the mucosal surface, which is influenced by its mechanical and adhesive properties [69]. A hydrogel with suitable hardness ensures ease of application without collapsing, while optimal adhesiveness enhances retention within the dynamic environment of the nasal cavity, making it a promising candidate for nasal drug delivery.

2.7. Physical Stability of In Situ Hydrogel Loaded with Nanotriphala

In situ hydrogels for nasal drug delivery must be stable during storage to effectively deliver drugs, and temperature and pH are important factors. This study evaluated a thermoresponsive In situ Tri at three storage temperatures (4 °C, 30 °C, and 40 °C) during a six-month stability study. Hydrogel pH was 5.75 ± 0.01 at baseline, an ideal value for nasal mucosa as previously described. However, this showed significant changes over time, where the pH was most stable at 4 °C, with only slight decreases to 5.29 by month 5, and returning to 5.75 by month 6. At 30 °C, the pH value significantly decreased to 5.24 after 6 months of storage compared to the initial value at 0 months. Moreover, the pH level at 40 °C decreased more extensively, with pH decreasing to 3.96 ± 0.01 by month 6 at 40 °C (Figure 5A), indicating accelerated degradation and potential risks for nasal irritation [49]. Gelling time measurements (Figure 5B) revealed similar temperature-dependent behaviors. The initial gelling time of 26.26 ± 1.16 s remained consistent across all temperatures at baseline, which is suitable for nasal delivery. However, at 4 °C, gelling time progressively increased over time, reaching 55.64 ± 0.46 s by month 6, indicating slower gelation. At 30 °C, gelling time remained stable, suggesting it is an optimal storage condition. At 40 °C, premature gelation was observed after incubation, indicating that the formulation at this temperature lacks long-term storage stability. Therefore, data for this temperature could not be presented in Figure 5B. The temperature-sensitive property of the hydrogel was also confirmed by viscosity analysis (Figure 5C). The baseline viscosity of 131 ± 10 cP underwent notable transformations. The viscosity at 4 °C decreased relatively slowly until it was 67 ± 14 cP, whilst that at 30 °C was unstable. At 40 °C the most substantial changes were observed, with the viscosity rocketing up to 388 ± 568 cP by month 3, indicating a degree of nanoparticle aggregation and gelation of the polymer. All these changes can influence mucoadhesion, drug release, and general performance. The viscosity at 4 °C was within an acceptable range for proper nasal application, but at 40 °C, the hydrogel showed high viscosity and impaired effectiveness.

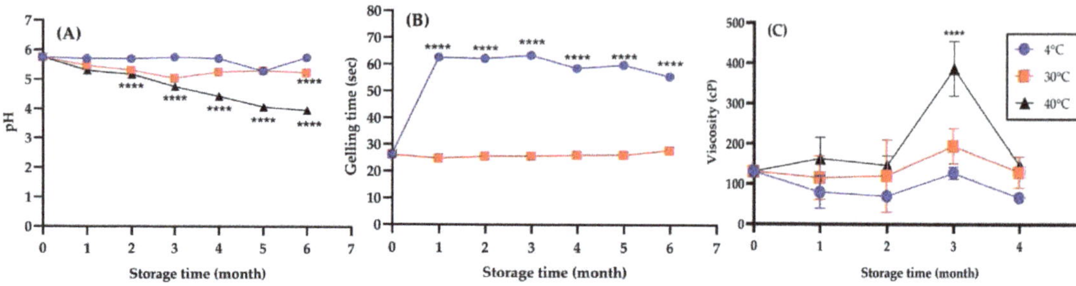

Figure 5. pH stability (**A**), gelling time (**B**), and viscosity (**C**) of In situ Tri at different storage temperatures (4 °C, 30 °C, and 40 °C) over a specified period. The data represent the mean ± standard deviation (SD) of three independent experiments (n = 3). **** indicates a significant difference ($p < 0.0001$) compared to the initial storage period.

Based on the thorough analysis described above, 4 °C is the most appropriate storage temperature for In situ Tri. This is the condition that best maintains the pH stability, gelling properties, and viscosity of the formulation. For short-term storage, 30 °C seems acceptable, while 40 °C should be avoided because of substantial degradation of critical hydrogel properties. These conclusions highlight the importance of temperature when maintaining the integrity of systems for advanced drug delivery. The temperature sensitivity showcases the fragile aspects of In situ Tri and indicates that appropriate storage conditions must be strictly adhered to in order to maintain optimal therapeutic performance. It is also a significant consideration for storage in the nasal drug delivery system.

2.8. Antimicrobial Activities of In Situ Hydrogel Loaded with Nanotriphala

The results of antimicrobial activity for In situ Tri are essential knowledge about their potential activity against bacterial pathogens that are relevant to oxidative stress-related nasal diseases. As shown in Table 4, the minimum inhibitory concentration (MIC), minimum bactericidal concentration (MBC), and MBC/MIC ratios for different microorganisms demonstrate that all the tested strains were susceptible to the formulation's antimicrobial action. The MBC/MIC ratios of all microorganisms, being less than 4, demonstrate that the concentrations necessary to kill the bacteria (MBC) are near those needed to stop their growth (MIC), thus confirming the bactericidal properties of the formulation [70]. These results align with similar studies where nanostructured formulations demonstrated enhanced antimicrobial efficacy [71]. Overall, In situ Tri has shown excellent broad-spectrum antimicrobial activities against Gram-negative (*E. coli*, *P. aeruginosa*) and Gram-positive (*S. aureus*, *S. epidermidis*) bacteria, indicating that it can provide a new potential antibiotic for oxidative stress-related nasal diseases. The present study also showcased the low minimum inhibitory concentration (MIC) and minimum bactericidal concentration (MBC) values of the examined formulation against *P. aeruginosa*, which indicates the potential of this formulation to target pathogens that have developed resistance to common antibiotic treatment, which is of particular interest as the phenomenon of resistance needs to be investigated more and more in clinical settings. This also reinforces the notion stated here that natural extracts such as Triphala could offer a viable alternative or adjunct to traditional antibiotics [11,72]. The efficacy of the formulation can be attributed to the synergistic actions of bioactive compounds in Triphala, which are further augmented by the nanocarrier system offered by in situ hydrogel, wherein comparable optimization of activity has been reported in other studies utilizing nanoformulations [11]. Furthermore, the enhanced bioavailability and site-specific release of active compounds that can be provided at the nanoscale are important advantages, which were emphasized in recent reviews regarding the involvement of nanomedicine in the treatment of pathogenic microorganisms [73,74]. Additional studies are warranted to explore the specific mechanisms of action, optimal dosing regimens, and therapeutic potential of this formulation for the management of oxidative stress-related bacterial infections in nasal diseases. This highlights the increasing potential of natural product-derived nanotherapeutics as a safe and potent alternative to conventional antibiotic agents against antimicrobial resistance.

Table 4. MIC and MBC of in situ hydrogel loaded with Nanotriphala for different microorganism strains.

Microorganism	μg/mL			
	MIC	**MBC**	**MBC/MIC**	**Activity**
E. coli	128	32	<4	Bactericidal
P. aeruginosa	4	2	<4	Bactericidal
S. aureus	32	4	<4	Bactericidal
S. epidermidis	32	8	<4	Bactericidal

The data represent the mean of three independent experiments (n = 3).

2.9. Mutagenicity of In Situ Hydrogel Loaded with Nanotriphala

The results of the revertant colony assay for TA98 and TA100 strains with and without S9 activation reveal the mutagenic potential of various treatments (Table 5). The DMSO control, used as a solvent, showed consistent baseline revertant colonies, with values of 31.56 ± 0.56 for TA98 and 28.89 ± 0.48 for TA100 without S9 activation, and 136.89 ± 2.23 and 144.67 ± 1.92 with S9 activation, respectively. For 2AA, a known mutagen, a significant increase in revertant colonies was observed, especially with S9 activation, where the colony count reached 703.11 ± 13.18 for TA98 and 778.67 ± 4.81 for TA100. AF-2, at a concentration of 0.1 μg/plate, showed a moderate mutagenic response, with 349.00 ± 2.22 revertant colonies in TA98 without S9 activation and 786.67 ± 14.05 for TA100 with S9 activation. The blank hydrogel, used as a formulation vehicle, exhibited minimal mutagenic activity, with revertant colonies of 29.78 ± 0.95 for TA98 and 28.22 ± 0.44 for TA100 without S9 activation, and 169.89 ± 1.22 and 179.33 ± 2.85 with S9 activation, respectively. In situ Tri, a formulation containing Nanotriphala, demonstrated no significant mutagenic activity across different concentrations. At 40 μg/plate, the revertant colony count for TA98 was 27.22 ± 0.95 (without S9) and 28.78 ± 1.18 (with S9), and for TA100, it was 134.33 ± 7.43 (without S9) and 145.11 ± 5.10 (with S9). As the concentration increased to 200 μg/plate and 1000 μg/plate, revertant colonies for both strains remained within the range of the control, with no signs of mutagenic effects, indicating that In situ Tri is not mutagenic at these concentrations. At the highest concentration tested, 5000 μg/plate, In situ Tri still showed no significant increase in revertant colonies, with values of 42.22 ± 0.40 for TA98 and 41.56 ± 0.97 for TA100 without S9, and 188.56 ± 2.23 and 202.67 ± 2.36 with S9, respectively. These results suggest that, under the conditions tested, In situ Tri does not exhibit mutagenic potential and could be considered safe in terms of genetic toxicity.

The mutagenicity index, as shown in Figure 6, reveals that for all concentrations of In situ Tri, the mutagenic index is consistently below 2. A mutagenic index equal to or greater than 2 is considered the threshold for classifying a substance as a mutagenic agent [75,76]. These results are in agreement with several mutagenicity studies performed with plant-derived compounds, where nonmutagenicity was also attributed to dose effects [77]. The absence of mutagenic effects in both the presence and absence of the S9-activating enzyme further supports the nonmutagenic nature of In situ Tri, as similar results have been observed in other studies of Triphala extract [78].

Table 5. Mutagenicity of in situ hydrogel loaded with Nanotriphala (In situ Tri).

Treatment	Concentration (µg/Plate)	Average of Revertant Colonies			
		TA 98		TA 100	
		−S9	+S9	−S9	+S9
DMSO	50 (µL/plate)	31.56 ± 0.56	28.89 ± 0.48	136.89 ± 2.23	144.67 ± 1.92
2AA	0.5	N/A	703.11 ± 13.18	N/A	778.67 ± 4.81
AF-2	0.1	349.00 ± 2.22	N/A	786.67 ± 14.05	N/A
Blank hydrogel	5000	29.78 ± 0.95	28.22 ± 0.44	169.89 ± 1.22	179.33 ± 2.85
In situ Tri	40	27.22 ± 0.95	28.78 ± 1.18	134.33 ± 7.43	145.11 ± 5.10
	200	36.44 ± 0.97	32.89 ± 0.99	143.00 ± 8.19	160.56 ± 1.25
	1000	38.11 ± 0.56	36.67 ± 1.07	161.22 ± 9.88	182.22 ± 1.46
	5000	42.22 ± 0.40	41.56 ± 0.97	188.56 ± 2.23	202.67 ± 2.36

Values are mean ± SD. AF-2: 2-(2-furyl)-3-(5-nitro-2-furyl)-acrylamide, 2-AA: 2-amino anthracine, NA: Not analyzed. The data represent the mean of three independent experiments (n = 3).

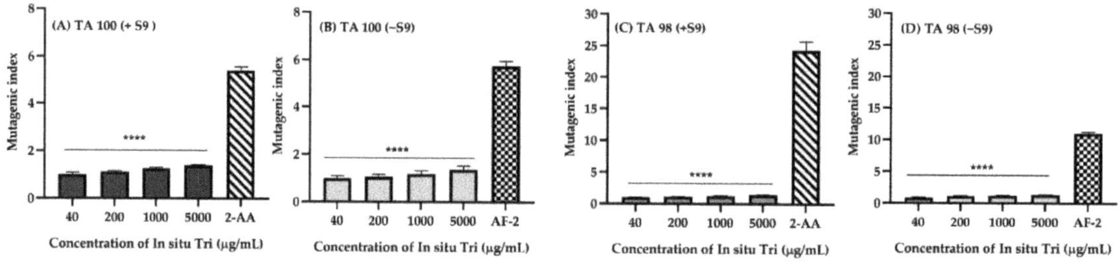

Figure 6. Mutagenic activity expressed by the mean of revertant/plate index of mutagenicity (IM) induced by different concentrations of in situ Tri in the TA98 and TA100 strains of *S. typhimurium* in the presence (+S9) and absence (−S9) of metabolic activation. The data represent the mean ± standard deviation (SD) of three independent experiments (n = 3). **** indicates a significant difference ($p < 0.0001$) when compared to the standard mutant for each condition.

For instance, as shown in the following results of the Salmonella/human S9 mutagenicity test, all of the In situ Tri concentrations 40, 200, 1000, and 5000 µg/mL did not affect either viability or metabolic activity of the bacteria/yeast/liver, with readings close to 1.0 indicating that In situ Tri in either non-treated or treated forms is not mutagenic, as mentioned above. Though a slight increase in values with increasing concentrations might indicate a possible growth-stimulating effect, these values still fell within an expected range for nonmutagenicity. Mutagen control AF-2 displayed much higher numbers of revertant colonies, especially in the TA 98 strains, confirming its status as a highly mutagenic constituent of the plant. The increased sensitivity of TA 98 strains, in comparison to the TA 100 strain responsive to base-pair substitutions, to frame-shift mutations is consistent with the specificity of AF-2's mutagenic effects [79].

Based on the mutagenicity test results, In situ Tri does not exhibit any detectable mutagenic activity. These findings support a positive safety profile for the In situ Tri formulation, particularly for therapeutic use in addressing oxidative stress-related nasal disorders. Additionally, there is evidence suggesting that Triphala-based products are nonmutagenic, which is consistent with the results of this mutagenicity test [78]. This further reinforces the safety and suitability of In situ Tri for potential clinical applications.

2.10. Antimutagenic Activity of In Situ Hydrogel Loaded with Nanotriphala

The antimutagenic activity was assessed by comparing the number of revertant colonies of the test substances with those of the mutagen alone, as shown in Figure 7A–D. The inhibition percentage (% inhibition) of mutagenicity was calculated with the Ames test, indicating a moderate antimutagenic effect when the inhibitory effect is between 25 and 40% and a strong effect when it exceeds 45%. Inhibitory effects of less than 25% are considered weak [80]. The antimutagenic activity of In situ *Tri* was assessed by evaluating its inhibitory effects against various mutagens, including the indirect mutagen Aflatoxin B1 (AFB1) in the TA98 strain, MeIQ in the TA100 strain, and the direct mutagens AF-2 in the TA98 strain and sodium azide (NaN3) in the TA100 strain. At a concentration of 40 μg/mL, In situ *Tri* exhibited weak inhibition across the tested mutagens. The inhibition against AFB1 was 5.91 ± 3.01%, while AF-2 showed a negative inhibition of −8.81 ± 1.59%, suggesting a potential enhancing effect rather than inhibition. MeIQ showed a modest 9.91 ± 5.59% inhibition, and NaN_3 inhibition was negative at −12.87 ± 4.74%, indicating little to no antimutagenic activity at this low concentration. At 200 μg/mL, moderate inhibition was observed for most mutagens. AFB1 exhibited 26.6 ± 1.65% inhibition, AF-2 showed 10.20 ± 1.06%, MeIQ had 26.83 ± 11.81%, and NaN_3 exhibited 22.64 ± 3.95% inhibition. These results suggest a moderate antimutagenic effect, particularly for AFB1 and MeIQ. At 1000 μg/mL, In situ *Tri* demonstrated stronger inhibition, with AFB1 showing 48.47 ± 3.91%, AF-2 showing 37.46 ± 1.14%, MeIQ showing 43.46 ± 6.12%, and NaN_3 showing 35.73 ± 3.10%. These results indicate moderate to strong antimutagenic activity across the mutagens tested. At the highest concentration of 5000 μg/mL, In situ Tri demonstrated strong inhibitory effects across all mutagens, with AFB1 showing 62.95 ± 0.96%, AF-2 at 53.34 ± 9.79%, MeIQ at 80.41 ± 5.77%, and NaN_3 at 76.12 ± 1.74%. Our findings align with the previous study by Kaur et al., which reported significant antimutagenic activity of Triphala in the TA98 and TA100 bacterial strains [78]. In more detail, gallic acid, a major component of Triphala, has been suggested in previous reports to exhibit antimutagenic activity through several mechanisms, one of which could involve gallic acid acting as a nucleophile to scavenge electrophilic mutagens [81]. These results indicate that In situ Tri exhibits potent antimutagenic activity, particularly against MeIQ and NaN_3, at higher concentrations, providing strong evidence of its potential as an effective antimutagenic agent.

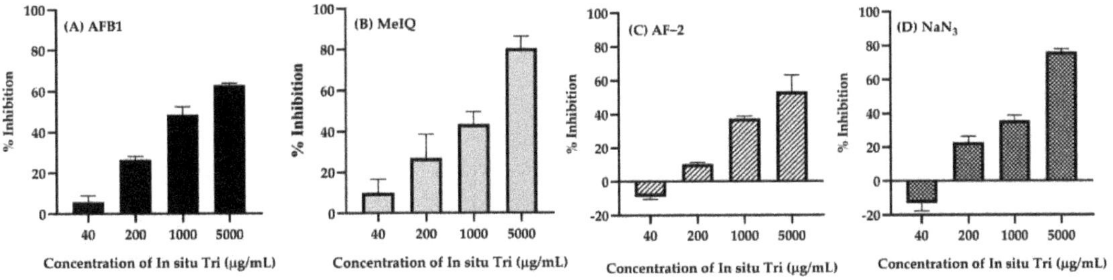

Figure 7. Antimutagenicity of various concentrations of in situ *Tri* against the mutagenicity of indirect mutagens, (**A**) AFB1 in TA98 and (**B**) MeIQ in TA100, as well as direct mutagens: (**C**) AF−2 in TA98 and (**D**) NaN_3 in TA100. Values are expressed as mean ± SD (n = 3).

3. Conclusions

Overall, this wide-ranging investigation of the thermoresponsive in situ hydrogel loaded with Nanotriphala sheds light on its role as an innovative and potential nasal drug delivery system in the treatment of oxidative stress-induced nasal disorders. The Nanotriphala formulation exhibited excellent antioxidant activity in more than one assay and its radical-scavenging potential was severalfold greater than that of the existing Triphala extract. The nanoencapsulation method employed in this study significantly enhanced the biological efficacy of active components, as evidenced by a marked reduction in IC_{50} values in DPPH, ABTS, and FRAP assays compared to Triphala extract, effectively demonstrating its superior ability to alleviate oxidative stress. Antimicrobial studies showed broad-spectrum activity against several Gram-positive and Gram-negative strains of bacteria, with improved efficacy against difficult pathogens such as *Pseudomonas aeruginosa*. The formulation's improved antimicrobial properties suggest its potential therapeutic benefit in complicated nasal infections of oxidative stress origin. The anti-inflammatory property of the Nanotriphala was assessed by the nitric oxide inhibition assays, which showed concentration-dependent effects, highlighting its potential therapeutic applications in managing oxidative stress-related inflammatory diseases. After incorporating Nanotriphala into an in situ hydrogel system, the resulting formulation exhibited excellent physicochemical characteristics, positioning it as a promising therapeutic strategy. With a physiological pH of 5.75 ± 0.01, a gelling temperature of 34.0 °C, and a rapid gelation time of 26.27 ± 1.16 s, the hydrogel demonstrated optimal properties for nasal application. It also displayed good spreadability (10.25 ± 0.28 cm) and suitable hardness and adhesiveness, ensuring enhanced nasal drug delivery performance. These features promote prolonged contact with the mucosa, minimize clearance, and enable engineered drug-release profiles, addressing significant challenges faced by nasal therapies in clinical practice. The biocompatibility and safety profile of Nanotriphala hydrogel at different concentrations were confirmed by high cell viability and its reverse mutagenic potential in Salmonella typhimurium strains. Stability studies strongly recommended achieving ideal physicochemical properties of the formulation at a storage temperature of 4 °C. The temperature sensitivity demonstrates the delicate nature of in situ hydrogel loaded with Nanotriphala, highlighting the importance of exact storage conditions to preserve therapeutic efficacy.

In summary, the thermoresponsive in situ hydrogel loaded with Nanotriphala has demonstrated significant potential as a novel nasal delivery system for managing nasal disorders. Our findings highlight its optimal properties for nasal application, including an excellent safety profile, along with remarkable anti-inflammatory, antibacterial, antioxidant, and antimutagenic activities. This research provides strong preliminary evidence supporting the use of Nanotriphala-loaded in situ hydrogel as an effective therapeutic approach for addressing complex nasal disorders.

4. Materials and Methods

Poloxamer 407 was sourced from Chanjao Longevity Co., Ltd. (Bangkok, Thailand), and polyethylene glycol 400 was obtained from Dow Corporate Headquarters (Midland, MI, USA). *Staphylococcus aureus* DMST 8013, *Pseudomonas aeruginosa* DMST 15501 and *Candida albicans* DMST 5815 were purchased from Department of Medical Sciences, Ministry of Public Health, Thailand (DMST). *Aspergillus niger* ATCC 10578 was purchased from American Type Culture Collection, Manassas, VA, USA. The cetrimide agar base was from Himedia, Mumbai, Maharashtra, India. Glycerol was purchased from SL quality supply, Bangkok, Thailand. Standard gallic acid with 99.6% purity was purchased from Sigma-Aldrich, USA. HPLC grades of acetonitrile and methanol were obtained from J.T. Baker, Phillipsburg, NJ, USA. HPLC water was purchased from RCI lab-scan, Bangkok Thailand. Potassium dihydrogen phosphate, AR grade, was obtained from Merck, Darmstadt, Hesse, Germany.

4.1. Preparation of Nanotriphala

Triphala nanoparticles were formulated based on our previous method [23]. Briefly, 500 mg of Triphala ethanolic extract was dissolved in 1 mL of acetone and added dropwise at 1 mL per hour to a solution containing 8 mL deionized water, 1 mL of 1% (*w*/*v*) poloxamer 407, and 1 mL of PEG 400, under continuous magnetic stirring at 600 rpm. The mixture was stirred overnight to allow complete evaporation of the organic solvent. For the blank control, the organic solvent was added to the surfactant and stabilizer solution without Triphala extract, leading to micelle formation when the PEO-PPO block copolymer concentration reached its critical micellization concentration (CMC). The nanoparticle size, polydispersity index (PDI), and zeta potential of the Nanotriphala (5 mg/mL) were analyzed using dynamic light scattering (DLS) at a 173° scattering angle and 25 °C with a Zetasizer Nanoseries (Malvern Instruments, Malvern, UK).

4.2. Antioxidant Activities of Nanotriphala

4.2.1. DPPH Free Radical-Scavenging Activity Assay

The free radical-scavenging capacity of both Triphala extract (Tri ext) and Nanotriphala (Tri Np) was evaluated using the DPPH assay, following the method described by Chittasupho et al. [82]. Gallic acid was used as the positive control, prepared in concentrations ranging from 0.4 to 200 µg/mL. Aliquots of Triphala extract (1.95 to 1000 µg/mL) and Nanotriphala (0.1 to 50 mg/mL) were prepared. The concentrations of Nanotriphala (Tri Np) used in the DPPH, ABTS, and FRAP experiments were based on the weight of the Nanotriphala formulation (0.1–50 mg/mL). This weight corresponds to an equivalent weight of Triphala extract (Tri ext) ranging from 4.43 to 2000 µg/mL, aligning with the concentrations used for Triphala extract in the same assays. For the assay, 100 µL of each sample was added to a 96-well plate. Following this, 100 µL of a 500 µM DPPH solution was added to each well. The mixture was incubated in the dark for 30 min, after which absorbance was measured at 517 nm. The percentage of inhibition for both the standard and the extract was calculated at each concentration, and data were plotted as % inhibition versus log concentration. The IC_{50} values, representing the concentration needed to reduce DPPH absorbance by 50% compared to the control, were determined for each sample.

$$\text{DPPH Free radical scavenging (\%)} = [(\text{A} - \text{B})/\text{A}] \times 100$$

where A is the absorbance of the reaction with solvent control, and B is the absorbance of the DPPH with the extract or Nanotriphala.

4.2.2. ABTS Free Radical-Scavenging Activity Assay

The ABTS radical-scavenging assay was conducted to further evaluate the free radical-scavenging activity of Tri ext and Tri Np, following the method described by Chittasupho et al. [82]. The ABTS radical stock solution was prepared by mixing 7 mM ABTS solution with 2.45 mM potassium persulfate in a 1:1 ratio and allowing the mixture to react in the dark at room temperature for 12 h. For the assay, 20 µL of gallic acid (0.4 to 200 µg/mL), Triphala extract (1.95 to 1000 µg/mL), and Nanotriphala (0.1 to 50 mg/mL) were added to a 96-well plate, followed by the addition of 180 µL of the ABTS solution. The plates were incubated in the dark for 30 min, after which the absorbance was measured at 734 nm. The percentage of inhibition was calculated for both the standard and the extract, and the IC_{50} values were determined from the resulting graph.

$$\text{ABTS Free radical scavenging (\%)} = [(\text{A} - \text{B})/\text{A}] \times 100$$

where A is the absorbance of the reaction with solvent control, and B is the absorbance of the reaction with the extract.

4.2.3. Ferric-Reducing Antioxidant Power (FRAP) Assay

The FRAP assay was conducted following the method described by Chittasupho et al. [82]. The FRAP reagent was prepared by combining 300 mM acetate buffer (pH 3.6), 10 mM 2,4,6-tripyridyl-s-triazine (TPTZ) solution in 40 mM HCl, and 20 mM $FeCl_3{\cdot}6H_2O$ solution in a 10:1:1 ratio. Gallic acid (0.4 to 200 μg/mL) served as the standard, while solutions of Triphala extract (1.95 to 1000 μg/mL) and Nanotriphala (0.1 to 50 mg/mL) were also prepared. Samples (20 μL) were incubated with 180 μL of FRAP solution in 96-well plates at 37 °C for 30 min in the dark. The absorbance of the ferrous tripyridyltriazine complex was measured at 595 nm. The FRAP content of the extract was expressed as μM Fe (II) equivalent, calculated using a standard curve constructed with ferrous sulfate solution (9.8–5000 μM).

4.3. Antimicrobial Activity of Triphala Extract and Nanotriphala

The antimicrobial activities of Triphala extract and Nanotriphala were evaluated using the broth dilution technique. Minimum inhibitory concentrations (MICs) and minimum bactericidal concentrations (MBCs) against *Escherichia coli* (ATCC 25922), *Pseudomonas aeruginosa* (DMST15501), *Staphylococcus aureus* (DMST8013), and *Staphylococcus epidermidis* (DMST15055) were determined by the broth microdilution method [83]. Triphala extract was tested at concentrations of 32–1024 μg/mL, and Nanotriphala at 390–25,000 μg/mL. The MIC was defined as the lowest concentration that completely inhibited bacterial growth. MBC values were determined by the drop plate technique and recorded as the lowest concentration, showing no bacterial growth on TSA plates.

4.4. Cell Culture

The RAW264.7 (ATCC TIB-71) cell line was obtained from Dr. Natthachai Duangnin (Regional Medical Science Center 1, Chiang Mai, Thailand). Cells were cultured in Dulbecco's Modified Eagle's Medium (DMEM) with high glucose, supplemented with 10% fetal bovine serum (FBS) and 1% penicillin–streptomycin, and incubated at 37 °C in 5% CO_2. Subculturing was performed every three days using 0.25% trypsin-EDTA.

4.5. Cytotoxicity Assay of Triphala Extract and Nanotriphala Against RAW264.7 Cells

The cytotoxicity of gallic acid, Triphala extract, and Nanotriphala against RAW264.7 cells was evaluated to determine the maximum concentration suitable for use in the NO assay, an anti-inflammatory test. Cell viability was assessed at various concentrations of gallic acid, Triphala extract, and Nanotriphala using the MTT assay, following the method described by Chittasupho et al. [84]. RAW264.7 cells were seeded in 96-well plates at a density of 8×10^3 cells/well in culture medium and incubated at 37 °C with 5% CO_2. After a 24 h adhesion period, Triphala extracts and Nanotriphala were applied to the cells, followed by incubation at 37 °C in 5% CO_2 for 24 h. At 24 h post-treatment, an MTT solution (0.5 mg/mL in culture medium) was added to each well, and the cells were incubated for an additional 2 h at 37 °C. Formazan crystals formed by metabolically active cells were dissolved in 100 μL DMSO per well, and absorbance was measured at 550 nm. IC_{50} values were calculated using GraphPad Prism v.7.0 (La Jolla, CA, USA).

4.6. Anti-Inflammation Activity Assay of Triphala Extract and Nanotriphala

The nitric oxide (NO) assay was employed to assess the anti-inflammatory activity of the Triphala extract and Nanotriphala by measuring nitrite, the final stable product of nitric oxide in the culture medium. Nitric oxide secretion was evaluated in RAW

264.7 macrophages following the method described by Chittasupho et al. [85]. RAW 264.7 macrophage cells were seeded at a density of 1×10^5 cells per well in 96-well plates and incubated for 24 h. Following this, the cells were pretreated with Triphala extract (15.6–2000 μg/mL), Nanotriphala (62.5–8000 μg/mL), or gallic acid standard (1.95–250 μg/mL) for 1 h. After pretreatment, cells were exposed to LPS (50 ng/mL) to induce an inflammatory response. After 18 h of incubation, nitric oxide levels in the supernatant were measured using the Griess reagent following the previous report [85]. The supernatant from each well was collected to assess nitrite levels, with absorbance measured at 540 nm. Nitrite concentrations were quantified based on a standard nitrite calibration curve. Results were expressed as the percentage (%) of nitrite secreted by treated cells relative to the control (LPS-treated cells).

4.7. Preparation of In Situ Hydrogel Loaded with Nanotriphala

The in situ hydrogel containing Nanotriphala (In situ Tri) was prepared by dissolving Nanotriphala (1 g), 0.25% *w*/*v* benzalkonium chloride (4 g), and sodium chloride (0.76 g) in deionized water (77.8 g). The above excipients were stirred thoroughly using an overhead stirrer set to 600 rpm until a homogenous solution was achieved. Next, poloxamer 188 was slowly added to the solution by sprinkling it gradually while maintaining continuous stirring until fully dissolved. Then, poloxamer 407 and introduced into the solution and stirred continuously for another 2 h. The clear solution was stored at 4 °C for 24 h and was transferred into a spray bottle for subsequent application.

4.8. Characterization of In Situ Hydrogel Loaded with Nanotriphala

4.8.1. Gelation Temperature

The gelation temperature is defined as the temperature at which the drug solution transforms into a gel. This was determined using the test tube inversion method [86]. A 10 mL amount of In situ Tri was placed in a test tube within a water bath. The solution was then heated. A thermometer was immersed in the solution to monitor temperature continuously. The gelation temperature was recorded as the point at which the solution ceased movement due to gel formation. This experiment was performed in triplicate.

4.8.2. Gelation Time

The gelling time of the In situ Tri formulation was assessed using the test tube inversion method described by Sherafudeen et al. [86]. Specifically, 10 mL of the formulation was added to a glass test tube. The test tube was then placed in a temperature-controlled water bath set at 34 °C. Periodically, the test tube was inverted at a 90° angle, and the time required for the liquid to gel was recorded in seconds as the gelation time.

4.8.3. pH

The pH of the developed In situ Tri formulation was measured using a calibrated digital pH meter (Mettler Toledo, OH, USA). Prior to measurement, the pH meter was calibrated with standard buffer solutions. The pH was determined by immersing the electrode fully into the formulation at room temperature. Measurements were conducted in triplicate, and the results are reported as the average value.

4.8.4. Rheology and Viscosity

The amount of gel that can be introduced into the nasal cavity is limited due to its small volume. Therefore, the rheology and viscosity of the In situ Tri must be low at the time of application to facilitate easy delivery but should increase afterward to ensure the drug remains at the disease site for a sufficient duration. The viscosity of In situ Tri formulations was measured using Haake Modular Advance Rheometer System MARS

40 Rheometer (Thermo Fisher Scientific Inc., MA, USA). The rheology and viscosity of formulation were evaluated at 25 °C.

4.8.5. Ex Vivo Spreadability

The spreadability was evaluated based on the method described by Sherafudeen et al. with slight modifications [86]. A 10 × 4 cm rectangular glass slide was used to assess spreadability. The porcine nasal mucosa, with the serosal side facing outward, was secured onto the slide using a thread. The slide was then placed in a hot air oven at 37 °C. A single drop of In situ Tri was applied to the mucosa at a 120° angle. Spreadability was determined by measuring the distance traveled by the In situ Tri drop before it gelled. The average of three measurements was recorded. The protocol for the use of cadavers was approved by the Animal Care and Use Committee, Faculty of Veterinary Medicine, Chiang Mai University, Thailand (FVM-CMU-ICUC Ref. No. 2567/BR-0001. C2).

4.8.6. Quantification of Gallic Acid in In Situ Hydrogel Loaded with Nanotriphala Formulation by High-Performance Liquid Chromatography (HPLC)

Chromatographic separation was performed using a Shimadzu LC-10ATvp high-performance liquid chromatography (HPLC) system equipped with a UV detector (Shimadzu, Kyoto, Japan). Separation was carried out on a Mightysil C18 column (250 mm × 4.6 mm, 5.0 µm particle size; Kanto Chemical Co., Inc., Tokyo, Japan) at a column temperature of 17 °C. A 20 µL aliquot of the sample was injected, and detection was conducted at 270 nm. The flow rate was set to 1.0 mL/min. Gradient elution was employed using a mobile phase consisting of solvent A (acetonitrile) and solvent B (20 mM potassium dihydrogen phosphate buffer), with the following gradient: 1:90 (A) at 0 min, 1:90 at 5 min, 70:30 at 20 min, 10:90 at 25 min, and 10:90 at 35 min. For calibration, a standard curve was generated using gallic acid standard solutions at five concentrations ranging from 3.001 to 9.004 µg/mL. The calibration curve was constructed by plotting peak areas against the corresponding concentrations, with triplicate analysis of the gallic acid standard.

Sample preparation involved dissolving 500 mg of the In situ Tri formulation in 0.5 mL methanol, followed by shaking at 2500 rpm and sonication for 10 min at temperatures below 30 °C. The mixture was then centrifuged at 10,900 rpm for 10 min and filtered through a 0.2 µm PTFE syringe filter. Prior to analysis, 450 µL of the supernatant was mixed with 50 µL of 20 mM potassium dihydrogen phosphate buffer, shaken, and transferred to an injection vial for HPLC analysis

4.9. Texture Profile Analysis of In Situ Hydrogel Loaded with Nanotriphala

Texture profile analysis was conducted following the method described by Xu et al., with slight modifications [87]. The texture parameters, including hardness, stickiness, and adhesiveness, were measured using a TA-XT Plus texture analyzer (Stable Micro System, Surrey, UK) in a simple compression mode. For the experiment, 10 g of the sample was transferred into a 15 mL glass vial to achieve a sample height of 25 mm. The beaker was kept in a thermostatic water bath at a temperature of 34 ± 1 °C. A spherical analytical probe (Type P/0.5HS) was used, which was lowered at a speed of 2 mm/s to a depth of 10 mm before being retracted at a faster rate of 10 mm/s until it fully detached from the gel surface. The resulting force–distance curve was analyzed using Texture Exponent 32 software to determine hardness, stickiness, and adhesiveness. All tests were performed in triplicate.

4.10. Physical Stability of In Situ Hydrogel Loaded with Nanotriphala

To assess the stability of the In situ Tri formulation, samples were stored at 4 °C, 30 °C, and 40 °C for three months, with gelation time, gelation temperature, pH, rheological properties, and viscosity measured at baseline (0 months), 1 month, 2 months, and 3 months. Aliquots were placed in individual containers and monitored at each time point to observe potential changes due to temperature. The physical characteristics of samples were determined according to the above methods.

4.11. Antimicrobial and Microbiological Stability of In Situ Hydrogel Loaded with Nanotriphala

The microbial limitation assay was assessed by measuring total aerobic microbial counts (TAMCs) and total yeast and mold counts (TYMCs). This was performed using $3M^{TM}$ $Petrifilm^{TM}$ aerobic count plates and $3M^{TM}$ $Petrifilm^{TM}$ yeast and mold count plates. Positive controls for TAMC included *S. aureus* (DMST 8013) and *P. aeruginosa* (DMST 15501), while positive controls for TYMC were *Candida albicans* (DMST 5815) and *Aspergillus niger* (ATCC 10578). The $3M^{TM}$ $Petrifilm^{TM}$ Staph Express plate and Cetrimide agar plate were used to examine the contamination of specified microorganisms, *S. aureus* and *P. aeruginosa*, respectively. The positive control for the presence of *S. aureus* on $3M^{TM}$ $Petrifilm^{TM}$ Staph Express plate was *S. aureus*, and the positive control for the presence of *P. aeruginosa* on the Cetrmide agar plate was *P. aeruginosa*. In situ Tri contamination was identified according to standards set by the U.S. Pharmacopoeia (USP) 41, British Pharmacopoeia (BP) 2024, and Thai Herbal Pharmacopoeia 2022.

4.12. Mutagenicity Determination of In Situ Hydrogel Loaded with Nanotriphala

The mutagenicity of Triphala extract and In situ Tri was assessed using the Ames test, following the method described by Punvittayagul et al. [88]. The assay utilized *Salmonella typhimurium* strains TA98 and TA100, with and without an exogenous metabolic activation system (S9 mix). Distilled water or DMSO served as the negative control, and the standard mutagens 2-AA and AF-2 were used as positive controls in the presence of metabolic activation and the presence of metabolic activation, respectively.

The number of mutant bacterial colonies was counted after incubating the test substance (or standard mutagen) with the bacteria and liver enzyme (or buffer in the absence of enzyme activation) for 48 h on nutrient agar. The mutagenic index was then calculated (number of revertant colonies of the test substance divided by the number of revertant colonies in the negative control). If the mutagenic index was greater than 2, the test sample was considered to have potential mutagenic effects.

4.13. Antimutagenicity Test of In Situ Hydrogel Loaded with Nanotriphala

For the antimutagenicity test, the assay steps were conducted following the same procedure as the mutagenicity test, as described in the method of Punvittayagul et al. [88]. In the study of the antimutagenic effects of the test substance, the mutagens used to induce bacterial mutation were divided into two groups. The first group consists of indirect mutagens, which require the activity of enzymes to alter their structure. The mutagens used in this study included Aflatoxin B1 (AFB1), which was tested in TA98, and 3-methyl-3, 4-dimethyl-3H-imidazo[4,5-f]quinolin-2-amine (MeIQ), which was tested in TA100. The second group is direct mutagens, which do not require enzyme activation. The direct mutagens used in this study were 2-(2-furyl)-3-(5-nitro-2-furyl)-acrylamide (AF-2), tested in the TA98 strain, and sodium azide (NaN_3), tested in the TA100 strain. The number of histidine-independent revertant colonies was counted after incubation and compared with the positive control. Antimutagenicity was expressed as the percentage of inhibition of mutagenicity using the following formula:

$$\% \text{ Inhibition} = \{[(A - B) - (C - B)]/(A - B)\} \times 100$$

where A represents the number of revertants in standard mutagen plates, B denotes the number of spontaneous revertants, and C corresponds to the number of revertants observed in the test plates.

4.14. Statical Analysis

All experiments were performed in triplicate. All data are presented as mean ± standard deviation (mean ± S.D.) values. Prism version 8.0 software was used for statistical analysis using an independent *t*-test, one-way ANOVA, and two-way ANOVA. Statistical significance was determined at * $p < 0.05$ and **** $p < 0.0001$.

Author Contributions: Formal analysis, R.P., C.C., J.J., S.C., S.S., J.C.O., S.T., P.A., C.P., K.T. and D.H.; investigation, R.P., C.C., J.J., S.C., S.S., J.C.O., S.T., P.A., C.P. and K.T.; resources, P.D.; data curation, R.P., C.C., J.J., S.C., S.S., J.C.O., S.T., P.A., C.P., K.T. and D.H.; writing—original draft preparation, R.P., C.C.; writing—review and editing, R.P., C.C. and D.H. funding acquisition, D.H. All authors have read and agreed to the published version of the manuscript.

Funding: This research project was supported by Fundamental Fund 2024, Chiang Mai University (FF002/2567) and also Thailand Science Research and Innovation (TSRI) [grant numbers FRB670083/0162].

Institutional Review Board Statement: The animal study protocol for the use of cadavers was approved by the Animal Care and Use Committee, Faculty of Veterinary Medicine, Chiang Mai University, Thailand (FVM-CMU-ICUC Ref. No. 2567/BR-0001. C2).

Informed Consent Statement: Not applicable.

Data Availability Statement: The data that support the findings of this study are available from the corresponding author upon reasonable request.

Acknowledgments: We are thankful to the Faculty of Pharmacy at Chiang Mai University for providing facilities and equipment. We also extend our heartfelt appreciation to the staff of the Pharmacy Service Center (PSC), Faculty of Pharmacy, Chiang Mai University, especially Saowarunee Sangsrijan, Siriluk Sangsrijan, Kunthawat Siangwong, Akharapon Saiboukham, and Supaporn Bourjai from the Central Equipment Laboratory, for their invaluable analytical support and assistance.

Conflicts of Interest: The authors have indicated that they have no other conflicts of interest regarding the content of this article.

References

1. Sies, H.; Berndt, C.; Jones, D.P. Oxidative stress. *Annu. Rev. Biochem.* **2017**, *86*, 715–748. [CrossRef] [PubMed]
2. Tai, J.; Shin, J.-M.; Park, J.; Han, M.; Kim, T.H. Oxidative stress and antioxidants in chronic rhinosinusitis with nasal polyps. *Antioxidants* **2023**, *12*, 195. [CrossRef]
3. Holguin, F. Oxidative stress in airway diseases. *Ann. Am. Thorac. Soc.* **2013**, *10*, S150–S157. [CrossRef] [PubMed]
4. Kahveci, O.K.; Kuzu, S.; Altıntaş, M.; Vurmaz, A.; Çelik, S. The effect of nasal steroid and antihistamine use on total oxidative stress and antioxidant status in the treatment of allergic rhinitis. *Am. J. Rhinol. Allergy* **2021**, *35*, 52–58. [CrossRef] [PubMed]
5. Arnaudova Danevska, I.; Jakjovska, T.; Atanasovska, E.; Petrushevska, M.; Dzekova Vidimliski, P.; Krstevska Balkanov, S.; Balkanov, T.; Zendelovska, D. Effect of nasal corticosteriods on oxidative stress parameters in children with allergic rhinitis. *J. Morphol. Sci.* **2023**, *6*, 1–7.
6. Tai, J.; Lee, K.; Kim, T.H. Current perspective on nasal delivery systems for chronic rhinosinusitis. *Pharmaceutics* **2021**, *13*, 246. [CrossRef]
7. Djupesland, P.G. Nasal drug delivery devices: Characteristics and performance in a clinical perspective—A review. *Drug Deliv. Transl. Res.* **2013**, *3*, 42–62. [CrossRef]

8. Charoenchai, L.; Pathompak, P.; Madaka, F.; Settharaksa, S.; Saingam, W. HPLC-MS profiles and quantitative analysis of triphala formulation. *Interprof. J. Health Sci.* **2016**, *14*, 57–67.
9. Nariya, M.; Shukla, V.; Jain, S.; Ravishankar, B. Comparison of enteroprotective efficacy of triphala formulations (Indian Herbal Drug) on methotrexate-induced small intestinal damage in rats. *Phytother. Res. Int. J. Devoted Pharmacol. Toxicol. Eval. Nat. Prod. Deriv.* **2009**, *23*, 1092–1098. [CrossRef]
10. Prasad, S.; Srivastava, S.K. Oxidative stress and cancer: Chemopreventive and therapeutic role of triphala. *Antioxidants* **2020**, *9*, 72. [CrossRef]
11. Omran, Z.; Bader, A.; Porta, A.; Vandamme, T.; Anton, N.; Alehaideb, Z.; El-Said, H.; Faidah, H.; Essa, A.; Vassallo, A.; et al. Evaluation of antimicrobial activity of Triphala constituents and nanoformulation. *Evid.-Based Complement. Altern. Med.* **2020**, *2020*, 6976973. [CrossRef]
12. Kalaiselvan, S.; Rasool, M.K. Triphala herbal extract suppresses inflammatory responses in LPS-stimulated RAW 264.7 macrophages and adjuvant-induced arthritic rats via inhibition of NF-κB pathway. *J. Immunotoxicol.* **2016**, *13*, 509–525. [CrossRef] [PubMed]
13. Jantrapirom, S.; Hirunsatitpron, P.; Potikanond, S.; Nimlamool, W.; Hanprasertpong, N. Pharmacological benefits of Triphala: A perspective for allergic rhinitis. *Front. Pharmacol.* **2021**, *12*, 628198. [CrossRef] [PubMed]
14. Huang, H.-Z.; Zhao, S.-Y.; Ke, X.-M.; Lin, J.-Z.; Huang, S.-S.; Xu, R.-C.; Ma, H.-Y.; Zhang, Y.; Han, L.; Zhang, D.-K. Study on the stability control strategy of Triphala solution based on the balance of physical stability and chemical stabilities. *J. Pharm. Biomed. Anal.* **2018**, *158*, 247–256. [CrossRef] [PubMed]
15. Huang, L.; Huang, X.-H.; Yang, X.; Hu, J.-Q.; Zhu, Y.-Z.; Yan, P.-Y.; Xie, Y. Novel nano-drug delivery system for natural products and their application. *Pharmacol. Res.* **2024**, *201*, 107100. [CrossRef] [PubMed]
16. Wang, X.; Liu, G.; Ma, J.; Guo, S.; Gao, L.; Jia, Y.; Li, X.; Zhang, Q. In situ gel-forming system: An attractive alternative for nasal drug delivery. *Crit. Rev. Ther. Drug Carr. Syst.* **2013**, *30*, 411–434. [CrossRef] [PubMed]
17. Nazar, H.; Fatouros, D.; van der Merwe, S.; Bouropoulos, N.; Avgouropoulos, G.; Tsibouklis, J.; Roldo, M. Thermosensitive hydrogels for nasal drug delivery: The formulation and characterisation of systems based on N-trimethyl chitosan chloride. *Eur. J. Pharm. Biopharm.* **2011**, *77*, 225–232. [CrossRef] [PubMed]
18. Karnaki, A.; Siamidi, A.; Karalis, V.; Lagopati, N.; Pippa, N.; Vlachou, M. Thermoresponsive Hydrogels: Current Status and Future Perspectives. In *Bioinspired Technology and Biomechanics*; IntechOpen: Rijeka, Croatia, 2024.
19. Kumar, R. Nanotechnology in herbal medicine: Challenges and future perspectives. In *Nanotechnology in Herbal Medicine*; Elsevier: Amsterdam, The Netherlands, 2023; pp. 515–548.
20. Moradi, S.Z.; Momtaz, S.; Bayrami, Z.; Farzaei, M.H.; Abdollahi, M. Nanoformulations of herbal extracts in treatment of neurodegenerative disorders. *Front. Bioeng. Biotechnol.* **2020**, *8*, 238. [CrossRef]
21. Namuga, C.; Ocan, M.; Kinengyere, A.A.; Richard, S.; Namisango, E.; Muwonge, H.; Kirabira, J.B.; Lawrence, M.; Obuku, E.A. Efficacy of nano encapsulated herbal extracts in the treatment of induced wounds in animal models: A systematic review protocol. *Syst. Rev.* **2023**, *12*, 215. [CrossRef] [PubMed]
22. Horn, R.C.; Vargas, V.M.F. Antimutagenic activity of extracts of natural substances in the Salmonella/microsome assay. *Mutagenesis* **2003**, *18*, 113–118. [CrossRef]
23. Chittasupho, C.; Umsumarng, S.; Srisawad, K.; Arjsri, P.; Phongpradist, R.; Samee, W.; Tingya, W.; Ampasavate, C.; Dejkriengkraikul, P. Inhibition of SARS-CoV-2-Induced NLRP3 Inflammasome-Mediated Lung Cell Inflammation by Triphala-Loaded Nanoparticle Targeting Spike Glycoprotein S1. *Pharmaceutics* **2024**, *16*, 751. [CrossRef] [PubMed]
24. Lofts, A.; Campea, M.A.; Winterhelt, E.; Rigg, N.; Rivera, N.P.; Macdonald, C.; Frey, B.N.; Mishra, R.K.; Hoare, T. In situ-gelling hydrophobized starch nanoparticle-based nanoparticle network hydrogels for the effective delivery of intranasal olanzapine to treat brain disorders. *Int. J. Biol. Macromol.* **2024**, *277*, 134385. [CrossRef] [PubMed]
25. Abdullah, J.A.A.; Perdomo, C.A.A.; Núnez, L.A.H.; Rivera-Flores, O.; Sánchez-Barahona, M.; Guerrero, A.; Romero, A. Lychee peel extract-based magnetic iron oxide nanoparticles: Sustainable synthesis, multifaceted antioxidant system, and prowess in eco-friendly food preservation. *Food Bioprod. Process.* **2024**, *145*, 148–157. [CrossRef]
26. Niedzielska, E.; Smaga, I.; Gawlik, M.; Moniczewski, A.; Stankowicz, P.; Pera, J.; Filip, M. Oxidative stress in neurodegenerative diseases. *Mol. Neurobiol.* **2016**, *53*, 4094–4125. [CrossRef] [PubMed]
27. Muscolo, A.; Mariateresa, O.; Giulio, T.; Mariateresa, R. Oxidative stress: The role of antioxidant phytochemicals in the prevention and treatment of diseases. *Int. J. Mol. Sci.* **2024**, *25*, 3264. [CrossRef]
28. Fisher, D.R.; Zheng, T.; Bielinski, D.F.; Kelly, M.E.; Cahoon, D.S.; Shukitt-Hale, B. Phytochemical combination is more effective than individual components in reducing stress signaling in rat hippocampal neurons and microglia in vitro. *Int. J. Mol. Sci.* **2022**, *23*, 12651. [CrossRef] [PubMed]
29. Zhang, L.; Virgous, C.; Si, H. Synergistic anti-inflammatory effects and mechanisms of combined phytochemicals. *J. Nutr. Biochem.* **2019**, *69*, 19–30. [CrossRef] [PubMed]

30. Ling, J.K.U.; Sam, J.H.; Jeevanandam, J.; Chan, Y.S.; Nandong, J. Thermal degradation of antioxidant compounds: Effects of parameters, thermal degradation kinetics, and formulation strategies. *Food Bioprocess Technol.* **2022**, *15*, 1919–1935. [CrossRef]
31. Zargoosh, Z.; Ghavam, M.; Bacchetta, G.; Tavili, A. Effects of ecological factors on the antioxidant potential and total phenol content of Scrophularia striata Boiss. *Sci. Rep.* **2019**, *9*, 16021. [CrossRef]
32. Muteeb, G. Nanotechnology—A light of hope for combating antibiotic resistance. *Microorganisms* **2023**, *11*, 1489. [CrossRef]
33. Culas, M.; Popovich, D.; Rashidinejad, A. Recent advances in encapsulation techniques for cinnamon bioactive compounds: A review on stability, effectiveness, and potential applications. *Food Biosci.* **2023**, *57*, 103470. [CrossRef]
34. Bhattacharya, A.; Ghosal, S.; Bhattacharya, S. Antioxidant activity of tannoid principles of *Emblica officinalis* (amla) in chronic stress induced changes in rat brain. *Indian J. Exp. Biol.* **2000**, *38*, 877–880. [PubMed]
35. Mishra, S.; Anuradha, J.; Tripathi, S.; Kumar, S. In vitro antioxidant and antimicrobial efficacy of Triphala constituents: *Emblica officinalis*, *Terminalia belerica* and *Terminalia chebula*. *J. Pharmacogn. Phytochem.* **2016**, *5*, 273–277.
36. Peterson, C.T.; Denniston, K.; Chopra, D. Therapeutic uses of triphala in ayurvedic medicine. *J. Altern. Complement. Med.* **2017**, *23*, 607–614. [CrossRef] [PubMed]
37. López-García, J.; Lehocký, M.; Humpolíček, P.; Sáha, P. HaCaT keratinocytes response on antimicrobial atelocollagen substrates: Extent of cytotoxicity, cell viability and proliferation. *J. Funct. Biomater.* **2014**, *5*, 43–57. [CrossRef] [PubMed]
38. Wu, P.-C.; Su, C.-H.; Cheng, F.-Y.; Weng, J.-C.; Chen, J.-H.; Tsai, T.-L.; Yeh, C.-S.; Su, W.-C.; Hwu, J.R.; Tzeng, Y.; et al. Modularly assembled magnetite nanoparticles enhance in vivo targeting for magnetic resonance cancer imaging. *Bioconjug. Chem.* **2008**, *19*, 1972–1979. [CrossRef] [PubMed]
39. Aborehab, N.M.; Osama, N. Effect of Gallic acid in potentiating chemotherapeutic effect of Paclitaxel in HeLa cervical cancer cells. *Cancer Cell Int.* **2019**, *19*, 154. [CrossRef]
40. Sharma, J.; Al-Omran, A.; Parvathy, S. Role of nitric oxide in inflammatory diseases. *Inflammopharmacology* **2007**, *15*, 252–259. [CrossRef] [PubMed]
41. Kim, S.-H.; Jun, C.-D.; Suk, K.; Choi, B.-J.; Lim, H.; Park, S.; Lee, S.H.; Shin, H.-Y.; Kim, D.-K.; Shin, T.-Y. Gallic acid inhibits histamine release and pro-inflammatory cytokine production in mast cells. *Toxicol. Sci.* **2006**, *91*, 123–131. [CrossRef] [PubMed]
42. Oyawaluja, B.; Oyawaluja, A.; Babasanmi, J.; Soneye, O. Phytochemistry and antioxidant assays of *Entandrophragma angolense* (Welw) C. DC.(meliaceae) using DPPH and nitric oxide free radical scavenging methods. *Niger. J. Pharm. Res.* **2019**, *15*, 229–235. [CrossRef]
43. Afsar, T.; Razak, S.; Shabbir, M.; Khan, M.R. Antioxidant activity of polyphenolic compounds isolated from ethyl-acetate fraction of *Acacia hydaspica* R. Parker. *Chem. Cent. J.* **2018**, *12*, 5. [CrossRef] [PubMed]
44. Kalaiselvan, S.; Rasool, M.K. The anti-inflammatory effect of triphala in arthritic-induced rats. *Pharm. Biol.* **2015**, *53*, 51–60. [CrossRef] [PubMed]
45. Parveen, R.; Shamsi, T.N.; Singh, G.; Athar, T.; Fatima, S. Phytochemical analysis and in-vitro biochemical characterization of aqueous and methanolic extract of Triphala, a conventional herbal remedy. *Biotechnol. Rep.* **2018**, *17*, 126–136. [CrossRef]
46. Conte, R.; Marturano, V.; Peluso, G.; Calarco, A.; Cerruti, P. Recent advances in nanoparticle-mediated delivery of anti-inflammatory phytocompounds. *Int. J. Mol. Sci.* **2017**, *18*, 709. [CrossRef]
47. Kapoor, M.; Cloyd, J.C.; Siegel, R.A. A review of intranasal formulations for the treatment of seizure emergencies. *J. Control. Release* **2016**, *237*, 147–159. [CrossRef]
48. Hinchcliffe, M. The Novel Application of Chitosan for the Intranasal Delivery of Insulin. Doctoral Dissertation, University of Nottingham, Nottingham, UK, 1996.
49. Behl, C.; Pimplaskar, H.; Sileno, A.; Demeireles, J.; Romeo, V. Effects of physicochemical properties and other factors on systemic nasal drug delivery. *Adv. Drug Deliv. Rev.* **1998**, *29*, 89–116. [CrossRef]
50. Salatin, S.; Alami-Milani, M.; Daneshgar, R.; Jelvehgari, M. Box–Behnken experimental design for preparation and optimization of the intranasal gels of selegiline hydrochloride. *Drug Dev. Ind. Pharm.* **2018**, *44*, 1613–1621. [CrossRef]
51. Chen, X.; Zhi, F.; Jia, X.; Zhang, X.; Ambardekar, R.; Meng, Z.; Paradkar, A.R.; Hu, Y.; Yang, Y. Enhanced brain targeting of curcumin by intranasal administration of a thermosensitive poloxamer hydrogel. *J. Pharm. Pharmacol.* **2013**, *65*, 807–816. [CrossRef]
52. Wang, M.; Ma, X.; Zong, S.; Su, Y.; Su, R.; Zhang, H.; Liu, Y.; Wang, C.; Li, Y. The prescription design and key properties of nasal gel for CNS drug delivery: A review. *Eur. J. Pharm. Sci.* **2024**, *192*, 106623. [CrossRef] [PubMed]
53. González, N.N.; Rassu, G.; Cossu, M.; Catenacci, L.; Sorrenti, M.L.; Cama, E.S.; Serri, C.; Giunchedi, P.; Gavini, E. A thermosensitive chitosan hydrogel: An attempt for the nasal delivery of dimethyl fumarate. *Int. J. Biol. Macromol.* **2024**, *278*, 134908. [CrossRef]
54. Ivanova, N.; Ermenlieva, N.; Simeonova, L.; Vilhelmova-Ilieva, N.; Bratoeva, K.; Stoyanov, G.; Andonova, V. In Situ Gelling Behavior and Biopharmaceutical Characterization of Nano-Silver-Loaded Poloxamer Matrices Designed for Nasal Drug Delivery. *Gels* **2024**, *10*, 385. [CrossRef]

55. Majithiya, R.J.; Ghosh, P.K.; Umrethia, M.L.; Murthy, R.S. Thermoreversible-mucoadhesive gel for nasal delivery of sumatriptan. *AAPS Pharmscitech* **2006**, *7*, E80–E86. [CrossRef] [PubMed]
56. Hadidi, M.; Liñán-Atero, R.; Tarahi, M.; Christodoulou, M.C.; Aghababaei, F. The potential health benefits of gallic acid: Therapeutic and food applications. *Antioxidants* **2024**, *13*, 1001. [CrossRef] [PubMed]
57. Marttin, E.; Schipper, N.G.; Verhoef, J.C.; Merkus, F.W. Nasal mucociliary clearance as a factor in nasal drug delivery. *Adv. Drug Deliv. Rev.* **1998**, *29*, 13–38. [CrossRef]
58. Nair, A.B.; Chaudhary, S.; Shah, H.; Jacob, S.; Mewada, V.; Shinu, P.; Aldhubiab, B.; Sreeharsha, N.; Venugopala, K.N.; Attimarad, M.; et al. Intranasal delivery of darunavir-loaded mucoadhesive in situ gel: Experimental design, in vitro evaluation, and pharmacokinetic studies. *Gels* **2022**, *8*, 342. [CrossRef]
59. Lin, H.; Gebhardt, M.; Bian, S.; Kwon, K.A.; Shim, C.-K.; Chung, S.-J.; Kim, D.D. Enhancing effect of surfactants on fexofenadineĚHCl transport across the human nasal epithelial cell monolayer. *Int. J. Pharm.* **2007**, *330*, 23–31. [CrossRef] [PubMed]
60. Phongpradist, R.; Thongchai, W.; Thongkorn, K.; Lekawanvijit, S.; Chittasupho, C. Surface modification of curcumin microemulsions by coupling of KLVFF peptide: A prototype for targeted bifunctional microemulsions. *Polymers* **2022**, *14*, 443. [CrossRef]
61. Phongpradist, R.; Jiaranaikulwanitch, J.; Thongkorn, K.; Lekawanvijit, S.; Sirilun, S.; Chittasupho, C.; Poomanee, W. KLVFF Conjugated Curcumin Microemulsion-Based Hydrogel for Transnasal Route: Formulation Development, Optimization, Physicochemical Characterization, and Ex Vivo Evaluation. *Gels* **2023**, *9*, 610. [CrossRef] [PubMed]
62. Cevher, E.; Taha, M.; Orlu, M.; Araman, A. Evaluation of mechanical and mucoadhesive properties of clomiphene citrate gel formulations containing carbomers and their thiolated derivatives. *Drug Deliv.* **2008**, *15*, 57–67. [CrossRef] [PubMed]
63. Basu, S.; Maity, S. Preparation and characterisation of mucoadhesive nasal gel of venlafaxine hydrochloride for treatment of anxiety disorders. *Indian J. Pharm. Sci.* **2012**, *74*, 428. [CrossRef]
64. Basu, S.; Bandyopadhyay, A.K. Characterization of mucoadhesive nasal gels containing midazolam hydrochloride prepared from *Linum usitatissimum* L. mucilage. *Braz. J. Pharm. Sci.* **2011**, *47*, 817–823. [CrossRef]
65. Saudagar, R.B.; Deore, S.B. In-Situ Nasal Gel Drug Delivery: An Overview. *Res. J. Pharm. Dos. Forms Technol.* **2016**, *8*, 9–14. [CrossRef]
66. Dawre, S.; Waghela, S.; Saraogi, G. Statistically designed vitamin D3 Encapsulated PLGA microspheres dispersed in thermoresponsive in-situ gel for nasal delivery. *J. Drug Deliv. Sci. Technol.* **2022**, *75*, 103688. [CrossRef]
67. Tichota, D.M.; Silva, A.C.; Sousa Lobo, J.M.; Amaral, M.H. Design, characterization, and clinical evaluation of argan oil nanostructured lipid carriers to improve skin hydration. *Int. J. Nanomed.* **2014**, *9*, 3855–3864.
68. Çelik, Y.S.; Örenli, B.; Al-Mohaya, M.; Mesut, B.; Özsoy, Y. Nasal in situ gels as a drug delivery system: An overview of literature and clinical studies. *J. Res. Pharm.* **2023**, *27*, 1875.
69. Hanafy, N.A.; Leporatti, S.; El-Kemary, M.A. Mucoadhesive hydrogel nanoparticles as smart biomedical drug delivery system. *Appl. Sci.* **2019**, *9*, 825. [CrossRef]
70. Makade, C.S.; Shenoi, P.R.; Bhongade, B.A.; Shingane, S.A.; Ambulkar, P.C.; Shewale, A.M. Estimation of MBC: MIC Ratio of Herbal Extracts against Common Endodontic Pathogens. *J. Pharm. Bioallied Sci.* **2024**, *16* (Suppl. 2), S1414–S1416. [CrossRef]
71. Ahluwalia, V.; Elumalai, S.; Kumar, V.; Kumar, S.; Sangwan, R.S. Nano silver particle synthesis using *Swertia paniculata* herbal extract and its antimicrobial activity. *Microb. Pathog.* **2018**, *114*, 402–408. [CrossRef] [PubMed]
72. Biradar, Y.S.; Jagatap, S.; Khandelwal, K.; Singhania, S.S. Exploring of antimicrobial activity of Triphala Mashi—An ayurvedic formulation. *Evid.-Based Complement. Altern. Med.* **2008**, *5*, 107–113. [CrossRef]
73. Osman, N.; Devnarain, N.; Omolo, C.A.; Fasiku, V.; Jaglal, Y.; Govender, T. Surface modification of nano-drug delivery systems for enhancing antibiotic delivery and activity. *Wiley Interdiscip. Rev. Nanomed. Nanobiotechnol.* **2022**, *14*, e1758. [CrossRef] [PubMed]
74. Raza, A.; Sime, F.B.; Cabot, P.J.; Maqbool, F.; Roberts, J.A.; Falconer, J.R. Solid nanoparticles for oral antimicrobial drug delivery: A review. *Drug Discov. Today* **2019**, *24*, 858–866. [CrossRef] [PubMed]
75. Gontijo, V.S.; Espuri, P.F.; Alves, R.B.; de Camargos, L.F.; dos Santos, F.V.; de Souza Judice, W.A.; Marques, M.J.; Freitas, R.P. Leishmanicidal, antiproteolytic, and mutagenic evaluation of alkyltriazoles and alkylphosphocholines. *Eur. J. Med. Chem.* **2015**, *101*, 24–33. [CrossRef]
76. Silva, V.A.; Gonçalves, G.F.; Pereira, M.S.; Gomes, I.F.; Freitas, A.F.; Diniz, M.F.; Pessôa, H.L. Assessment of mutagenic, antimutagenic and genotoxicity effects of Mimosa tenuiflora. *Rev. Bras. Farmacogn.* **2013**, *23*, 329–334. [CrossRef]
77. Borges, F.F.V.; Silva, C.R.; Véras, J.H.; Cardoso, C.G.; da Cruz, A.D.; Chen, L.C. Antimutagenic, antigenotoxic, and anticytotoxic activities of *Silybum marianum* [L.] Gaertn assessed by the *Salmonella* mutagenicity assay (Ames test) and the micronucleus test in mice bone marrow. *Nutr. Cancer* **2016**, *68*, 848–855. [CrossRef] [PubMed]
78. Kaur, S.; Arora, S.; Kaur, K.; Kumar, S. The in vitro antimutagenic activity of Triphala—An Indian herbal drug. *Food Chem. Toxicol.* **2002**, *40*, 527–534. [CrossRef] [PubMed]

79. Buschini, A.; Ferrarini, L.; Franzoni, S.; Galati, S.; Lazzaretti, M.; Mussi, F.; Northfleet de Albuquerque, C.; Maria Araújo Domingues Zucchi, T.; Poli, P. Genotoxicity revaluation of three commercial nitroheterocyclic drugs: Nifurtimox, benznidazole, and metronidazole. *J. Parasitol. Res.* **2009**, *2009*, 463575. [CrossRef] [PubMed]
80. Makhafola, T.J.; Elgorashi, E.E.; McGaw, L.J.; Verschaeve, L.; Eloff, J.N. The correlation between antimutagenic activity and total phenolic content of extracts of 31 plant species with high antioxidant activity. *BMC Complement. Altern. Med.* **2016**, *16*, 490. [CrossRef]
81. Hour, T.-C.; Liang, Y.-C.; Chu, I.-S.; Lin, J.-K. Inhibition of eleven mutagens by various tea extracts, (−) epigallocatechin-3-gallate, gallic acid and caffeine. *Food Chem. Toxicol.* **1999**, *37*, 569–579. [CrossRef]
82. Chittasupho, C.; Athikomkulchai, S.; Samee, W.; Na Takuathung, M.; Yooin, W.; Sawangrat, K.; Saenjum, C. Phenylethanoid Glycoside-Enriched Extract Prepared from *Clerodendrum chinense* Leaf Inhibits A549 Lung Cancer Cell Migration and Apoptosis Induction through Enhancing ROS Production. *Antioxidants* **2023**, *12*, 461. [CrossRef] [PubMed]
83. Singh, S.; Chidrawar, V.R.; Hermawan, D.; Nwabor, O.F.; Olatunde, O.O.; Jayeoye, T.J.; Samee, W.; Ontong, J.C.; Chittasupho, C. Solvent-assisted dechlorophyllization of *Psidium guajava* leaf extract: Effects on the polyphenol content, cytocompatibility, antibacterial, anti-inflammatory, and anticancer activities. *S. Afr. J. Bot.* **2023**, *158*, 166–179. [CrossRef]
84. Chittasupho, C.; Kengtrong, K.; Chalermnithiwong, S.; Sarisuta, N. Anti-angiogenesis by dual action of R5K peptide conjugated itraconazole nanoparticles. *AAPS PharmSciTech* **2020**, *21*, 74. [CrossRef]
85. Angsusing, J.; Singh, S.; Samee, W.; Tadtong, S.; Stokes, L.; O'connell, M.; Bielecka, H.; Toolmal, N.; Mangmool, S.; Chittasupho, C. Anti-inflammatory activities of Yataprasen Thai traditional formulary and its active compounds, beta-amyrin and stigmasterol, in RAW264. 7 and THP-1 cells. *Pharmaceuticals* **2024**, *17*, 1018. [CrossRef] [PubMed]
86. Sherafudeen, S.P.; Vasantha, P.V. Development and evaluation of in situ nasal gel formulations of loratadine. *Res. Pharm. Sci.* **2015**, *10*, 466–476. [PubMed]
87. Xu, X.; Shen, Y.; Wang, W.; Sun, C.; Li, C.; Xiong, Y.; Tu, J. Preparation and in vitro characterization of thermosensitive and mucoadhesive hydrogels for nasal delivery of phenylephrine hydrochloride. *Eur. J. Pharm. Biopharm.* **2014**, *88*, 998–1004. [CrossRef] [PubMed]
88. Punvittayagul, C.; Sringarm, K.; Chaiyasut, C.; Wongpoomchai, R. Mutagenicity and antimutagenicity of hydrophilic and lipophilic extracts of Thai northern purple rice. *Asian Pac. J. Cancer Prev.* **2014**, *15*, 9517–9522. [CrossRef] [PubMed]

gels

MDPI

Review

Polydopamine Nanocomposite Hydrogel for Drug Slow-Release in Bone Defect Repair: A Review of Research Advances

Xiaoman Li [1,2,3], Jianhua Tang [4], Weiwei Guo [1,2,3], Xuan Dong [1,2,3], Kaisen Cao [1,2,3] and Fushan Tang [1,2,3,*]

1 Department of Clinical Pharmacy, Key Laboratory of Basic Pharmacology of Guizhou Province and School of Pharmacy, Zunyi Medical University, Zunyi 563006, China; manmanoooo@126.com (X.L.); gww4567@outlook.com (W.G.); dongxuan07202000@163.com (X.D.); kscao20250227@163.com (K.C.)

2 Key Laboratory of Basic Pharmacology of Ministry of Education and Joint International Research Laboratory of Ethnomedicine of Ministry of Education, Zunyi Medical University, Zunyi 563006, China

3 Key Laboratory of Clinical Pharmacy of Zunyi City, Zunyi Medical University, Zunyi 563006, China

4 Cancer Research UK Manchester Institute, The University of Manchester, Cheshire SK10 4TG, UK; jianhua.tang@manchester.ac.uk

* Correspondence: fstang@zmu.edu.cn or fstang@vip.163.com; Tel.: +86-851-2864-2337; Fax: +86-851-2864-2334

Abstract: In recent years, hydrogels have emerged as promising candidates for bone defect repair due to their excellent biocompatibility, high porosity, and water-retentive properties. However, conventional hydrogels face significant challenges in clinical translation, including brittleness, low mechanical strength, and poorly controlled drug degradation rates. To address these limitations, as a multifunctional polymer, polydopamine (PDA) has shown great potential in both bone regeneration and drug delivery systems. Its robust adhesive properties, biocompatibility, and responsiveness to photothermal stimulation make it an ideal candidate for enhancing hydrogel performance. Integrating PDA into conventional hydrogels not only improves their mechanical properties but also creates an environment conducive to cell adhesion, proliferation, and differentiation, thereby promoting bone defect repair. Moreover, PDA facilitates controlled drug release, offering a promising approach to optimizing treatment outcomes. This paper first explores the mechanisms through which PDA promotes bone regeneration, laying the foundation for its clinical translation. Additionally, it discusses the application of PDA-based nanocomposite hydrogels as advanced drug delivery systems for bone defect repair, providing valuable insights for both research and clinical translation.

Keywords: polydopamine; nanocomposite hydrogel; bone defect repair; drug delivery system

1. Introduction

Bone defects due to trauma, infection or osteoporosis pose a substantial challenge to the global healthcare system, affecting over 20 million patients annually [1–3]. Currently, autologous and allogeneic bone grafts remain the gold standard for the treatment of bone defect repair, but other repair strategies are necessary due to high donor site morbidity, limited availability, and immune refractory reactions [4,5]. In addition, effective bone repair requires sustained pharmacological activity to promote osteoblast proliferation and bone regeneration, a requirement that synthetic implants and systemic drug therapies often fail to meet due to issues of malintegration, off-target toxicity, and inadequate control over osteogenic factor delivery [6–8]. As a result, there is an urgent need to develop a drug delivery system with excellent slow-release properties to enhance bone repair and overcome the limitations of existing treatment options. Combining osteogenic drugs with biocompatible and biodegradable carrier materials can create a system that ensures effective

https://doi.org/10.3390/gels11030190

loading and controlled release of drugs, thereby sustaining therapeutic action at the defect site and enhancing efficiency while minimizing systemic side effects [9].

Hydrogel shows unique advantages in bone tissue engineering due to its three-dimensional hydration network and extracellular matrix (ECM)-like microenvironment [10–12]. It not only has good biocompatibility but also effectively promotes bone regeneration by supporting cellular infiltration, facilitating nutrient diffusion, and enabling local drug delivery [13–15]. However, conventional hydrogels often lack the mechanical elasticity and dynamic responsiveness required for load-bearing applications or controlled therapeutic release [16–18]. These challenges have led researchers to work on the development of enhanced hydrogels to optimize their mechanical elasticity and dynamic responsiveness to meet the clinical needs of bone regeneration.

Inspired by the adhesive properties of marine mussels, polydopamine (PDA)—a dopamine-based polymer—has emerged as a promising material in the development of advanced hydrogels and bone tissue engineering [19,20]. PDA is formed through the spontaneous polymerization of dopamine monomers under alkaline conditions. Its formation mechanism involves multiple pathways, including both noncovalent self-assembly and covalent polymerization [21] (Figure 1). Initially, dopamine is oxidized to dopamine quinone (DQ), which undergoes cyclization and rearrangement to produce intermediates such as 5,6-dihydroxyindole (DHI) and indole quinone. These intermediates are further polymerized to form oligomers, ultimately producing PDA [21,22]. The resulting polymer is rich in catechol groups, which confer several functional properties, as follows: (i) strong interfacial adhesion, allowing stable binding to both organic (e.g., hydrogels, peptide copolymers) and inorganic (e.g., metal and silicon-based) substrates, facilitating composite material design [23–25]; (ii) photo-thermal responsiveness, as the conjugated single-double bonds in its structure enable significant near-infrared (NIR) absorption and efficient photothermal conversion, enabling remote drug release and antimicrobial effects [26–29]; and (iii) multifunctional modification potential, with abundant amine, imine, and aromatic ring structures that facilitate efficient drug loading and targeted delivery via chemical reactions or π-π stacking [30–33]. Additionally, PDA's antioxidant and immunomodulatory properties, such as promoting macrophage M2 polarization, contribute to a pro-regenerative microenvironment for bone repair, enhancing osteogenesis and angiogenesis [34,35]. The diverse nanostructural forms of PDA—such as nanosheets [36], nanoparticles [37], nanocapsules [38], and mesoporous PDAs [39]—offer high modification flexibility, optimizing drug delivery and bone repair effectiveness. Figure 2 illustrates how different PDA structures integrated with hydrogels enable controlled drug release in bone defect repair, regulate inflammation, and promote bone and vascular remodeling. These attributes make PDA a key component in enhancing the mechanical properties and bioactivity of hydrogels, providing a novel approach for developing a smart, responsive platform for bone repair.

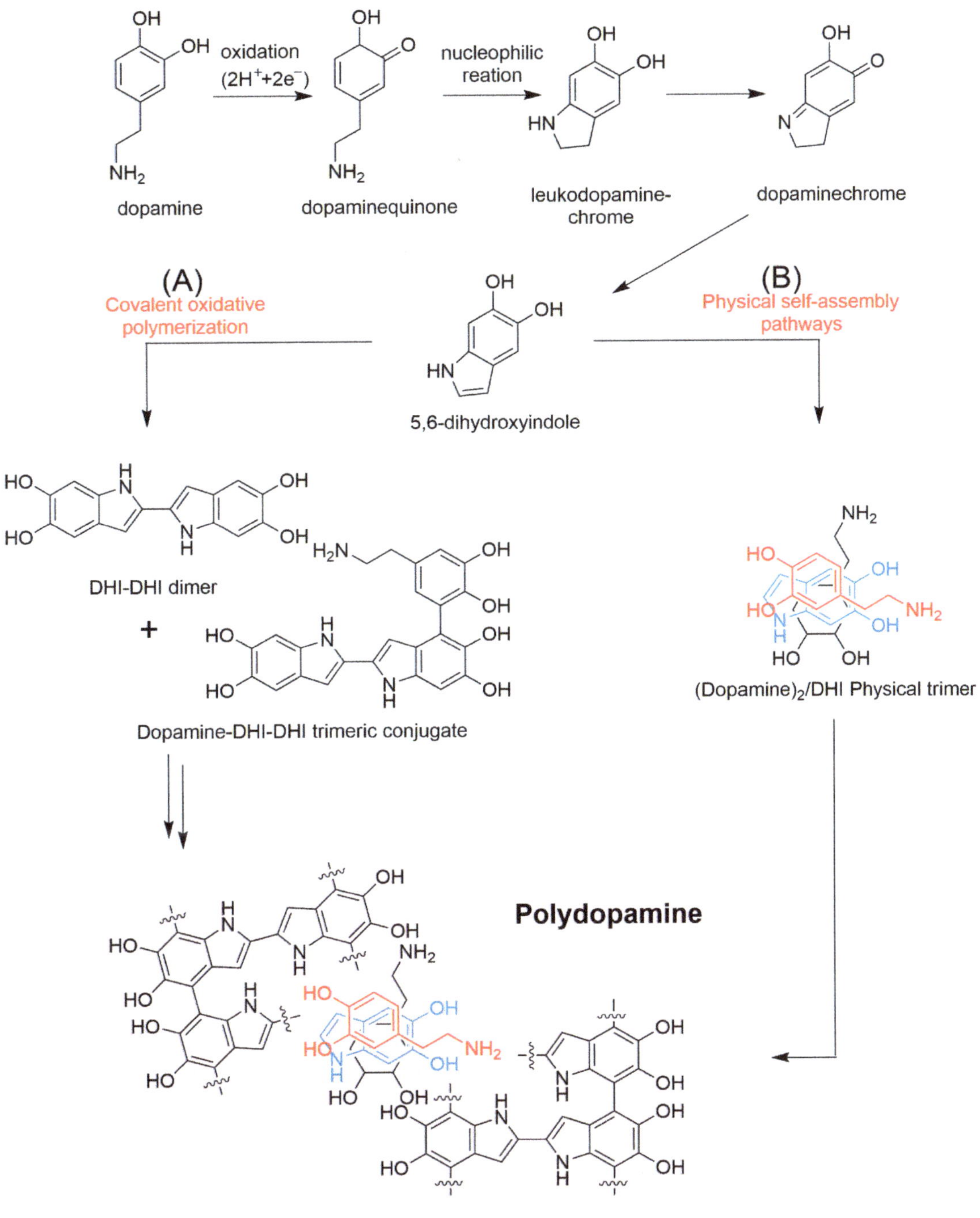

Figure 1. Two synthetic pathways of polydopamine: (A) Covalent polymerization pathway, (B) Non-covalent self-assembly pathway [21].

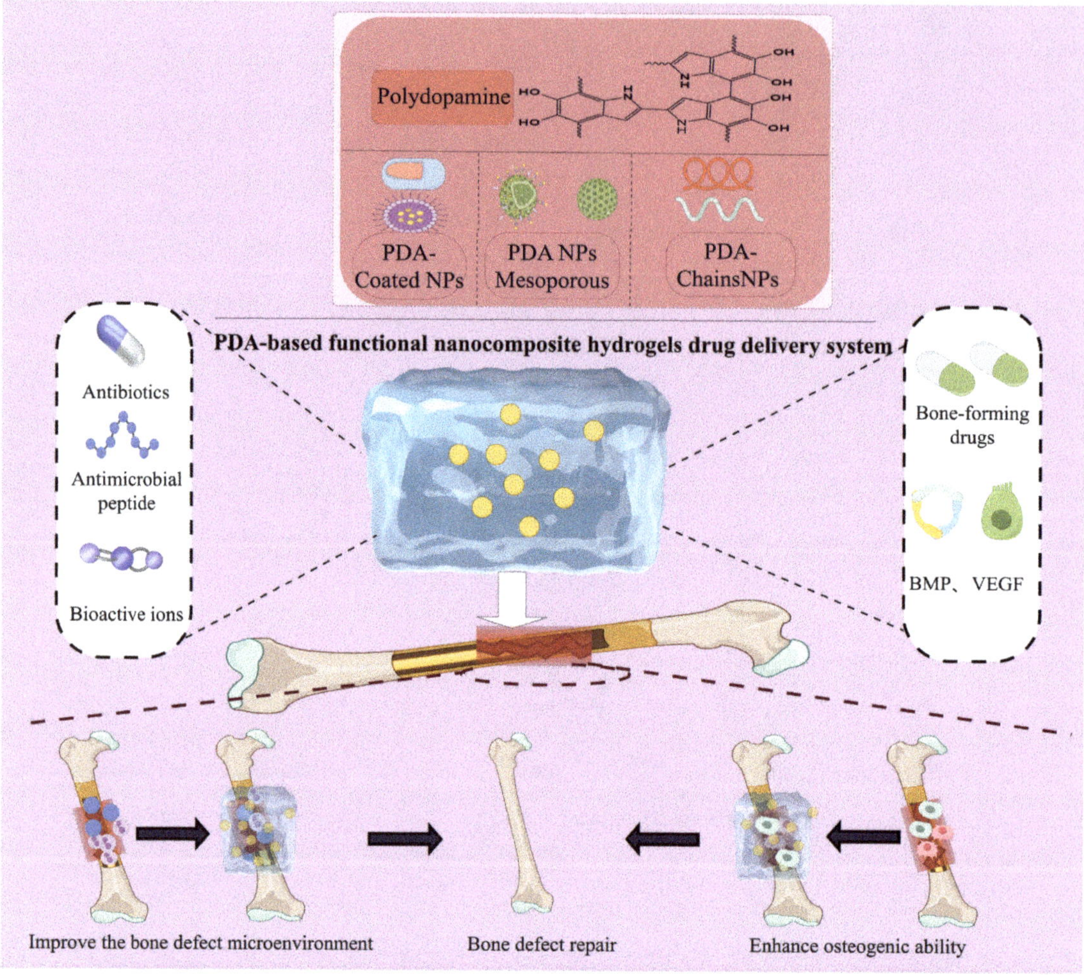

Figure 2. Schematic representation of PDA nanocomposite hydrogel applied to bone defect repair.

Despite significant research on PDA-based nanocomposite hydrogels, current reviews often focus on the physicochemical properties of PDA, with less emphasis on its role in bone repair mechanisms or a systematic classification of PDA hydrogel composites. This paper aims to bridge this gap by delineating the molecular and cellular mechanisms through which PDA promotes bone regeneration, including macrophage polarization, angiogenesis, and Runx2-mediated osteogenesis. It provides a comprehensive classification of PDA-based nanocomposite hydrogels, highlighting design principles, drug loading strategies, and preclinical outcomes. The paper also identifies challenges in clinical translation, such as polymerization variability and long-term biocompatibility, and suggests directions for materials optimization. By integrating materials science with orthopedic application, this study seeks to expedite the development of PDA hydrogels as a versatile platform for bone defect repair. With this comprehensive review, we hope to pave the way for future research and clinical applications of PDA nanocomposite hydrogels in bone defect repair.

2. Application and Function of PDA in Bone Defect Repair

A variety of organic and inorganic nanodrug delivery systems have been developed for the treatment of bone diseases, such as silica nanoparticles, gold nanoparticles, calcium phosphate nanoparticles, chitosan nanoparticles, liposome nanoparticles, and polymer nanoparticles [40,41]. However, these systems still face some important limitations, including low drug loading, limited physiological compatibility, poor degradability, and too fast drug release rates [42,43]. To address these drawbacks, PDA has gradually attracted widespread attention as an adjunctive drug delivery system in recent years. PDA not only significantly enhances drug loading capacity, but also improves drug delivery by increasing cell capture efficiency. In addition, PDA itself has a photothermal effect, which can respond to the stimulation of an external light source and thus regulate drug release. In addition, PDA can promote cell adhesion and regulate cell differentiation, which makes it a material with wide application potential in the treatment of orthopedic diseases. Studies have gradually revealed [44–46] the multifaceted functions and mechanisms of PDA in bone regeneration, and that it can provide favorable conditions for bone tissue repair by altering the microenvironment, regulating the immune response, and promoting the proliferation and differentiation of osteoblasts.

In this section, we will focus on the different functions of PDA in promoting bone regeneration, especially how it can be further developed in bone defect repair through photothermal effects, cell adhesion enhancement, and regulation of differentiation.

2.1. Anti-Inflammation

The inflammatory response plays a crucial role in physiological processes such as tissue injury and bone defect repair. On the one hand, angiogenesis triggered by immune inflammation contributes to the promotion of bone regeneration. Therefore, excessive suppression of early inflammation may interfere with angiogenesis, thereby affecting the healing process of bone defects [47,48]. On the other hand, excessive immune inflammatory response may lead to localized granulomas and fibrous encapsulation, which in turn prevents stable fixation of the implant [49,50]. For this reason, balancing the intensity and duration of the inflammatory response during bone defect repair is crucial for promoting bone healing. The aromatic ring structure and hydrophilic catechol groups on the surface of PDA have antioxidant properties, which can scavenge free radicals in the body and alleviate oxidative stress, thus reducing the inflammatory response triggered by oxidative stress. Through this antioxidant mechanism, PDA helps to improve the local immune environment during bone repair and promotes the osteogenesis process [51–53]. In addition, in the local inflammatory region, PDA can reduce the activity of inflammatory cells and the release of inflammatory factors, such as tumor necrosis factor (TNF)-α, interleukin (IL)-1β, and IL-6, through its unique photothermal effect, thus controlling the inflammatory response and preventing the adverse effects of excessive inflammation on bone tissue repair [54]. At the same time, PDA can also promote macrophage M2 type polarization, thereby creating an immune microenvironment conducive to bone repair [48]. Li et al. [55] showed that PDA could inhibit NF-κB expression by increasing i -κB expression in macrophages, thereby reducing the inflammatory response induced by implants.

2.2. Promoting Cell Adhesion and Proliferation

PDA can promote cell adhesion through several mechanisms. First, the amine and catechol groups in PDA can strongly chelate with calcium ions (Ca^{2+}). This chelation promotes the interaction of blood Ca_{2+} with phosphate ions ($PO_4{}^{3-}$), which in turn precipitates and forms a mineralized coating on the PDA surface [52,56]. This mineralization process not only enhances the bioactivity of the material but also provides an ideal surface for osteoblasts and promotes cell attachment and proliferation. Meanwhile, a calcium phosphate crystal is deposited on the surface of PDA, which usually shows a coral like or amorphous nanohemispherical structure [57,58]. This amorphous calcium phosphate is a precursor for the formation of biogenic bone-like apatite (i.e., the inorganic component of bone), which plays an important role in bone repair [59,60]. Studies have shown that, on PDA surfaces containing calcium phosphate, osteoblasts are able to form larger cell clusters. In contrast, on smooth, pure PDA surfaces, osteoblasts show a tendency to diffuse and have difficulty aggregating. This shows that the rough structure of the mineralized coating on the surface of PDA and the formation of the mineralized layer have a facilitating effect on the adhesion and aggregation behavior of osteoblasts [61].

Secondly, PDA, through its surface hydrophilicity and chemical reactivity, can promote the production of a large number of extracellular matrix (ECM) proteins, such as collagen, fibronectin, and vitronectin, by cells. Binding of integrin receptors on cells to these extracellular matrices can activate intracellular signaling pathways (e.g., FAK signaling pathway) to further regulate cellular value addition and differentiation [62–64]. In addition to exhibiting changes in cell adhesion capacity, it was found that cells cultured on the PDA surface showed a significant increase in the number of cells in the S phase and a decrease in the number of cells in the sub-G1 phase. This suggests that the PDA-coated material has a promotional effect on cell proliferation [65]. In summary, PDA not only promotes cell adhesion, but also promotes the mineralization process by regulating cell proliferation, promoting osteogenic differentiation, and through interaction with minerals such as calcium phosphate. This provides an ideal support platform for bone defect repair.

2.3. Promoting Osteogenesis and Angiogenesis

It has been found that bone tissue is rich in dopaminergic neurons and expresses various DA receptors [34,44]. These receptors, categorized into five types (D1 to D5) [66–68], play critical roles in cellular signaling and regulating numerous physiological processes. PDA materials feature dopamine-related reactive groups on their surfaces, enabling interactions with dopamine receptors on cell surfaces, thereby influencing cellular behavior and responses. In bone tissue, the regulation of the extracellular signal regulated kinase (ERK) signaling pathway significantly affects osteoblast behavior. Wang et al. [69] identified D1 as a specific target through which dopamine promotes osteogenic expression by enhancing ERK phosphorylation. This phosphorylation increases the transcriptional activity of RUNX2, a key osteogenic transcription factor that directly drives osteogenic differentiation. The activity of this pathway may also vary depending on the cell type involved. Furthermore, the dopamine D1 receptor (D1R) regulates osteogenic signaling and promotes bone regeneration by activating signaling pathways such as the cyclic adenosine monophosphate (cAMP)/protein kinase A (PKA)/cAMP responsive element binding protein (CREB) pathway [34,70,71]. The coordinated activity of osteoblasts and osteoclasts is crucial during the later stages of bone repair, maintaining the balance necessary for bone tissue health and reconstruction. Osteoblasts facilitate the formation of new bone, while osteoclasts mediate bone resorption, with their interaction ensuring proper bone metabolism. Excessive bone resorption, however, may lead to osteoporosis, potentially compromising bone repair effectiveness. While findings on PDA's regulation of osteoblast activity remain inconsistent, some studies suggest it may be closely linked to the local degradation concentration of PDA, a relationship that requires clarifying through further investigation [72].

3. Advances in the Application of PDA-Hydrogel Based Drug Slow Release System in the Repair of Bone Defects

PDA-based nanocomposite hydrogels, particularly in controlled drug delivery, have driven significant advancements in bone defect repair. These hydrogels are composed of both synthetic and natural polymers. Common synthetic polymers include polyacrylic acid and its derivatives, poly(vinyl alcohol), poly(vinyl oxide), poly(acrylamide), and self-assembling peptides. Natural polymers typically used are collagen, gelatin, hyaluronic acid, alginate, and chitosan. The fabrication of PDA-based hydrogels involves diverse and complex methods, such as hydrogels with dopamine (DA) side-chain branches [73–75], hydrogels loaded with PDA nanoparticles (NPs) [76–78], and hydrogels incorporating PDA-modified nanomaterials [79–82]. These hydrogels, including chitosan, gelatin, PEG, and peptides, are often functionalized with PDA to enhance their adhesion properties and bioactivity, offering novel solutions for bone defect repair and laying the groundwork for clinical application (Figure 3). This review explores the unique properties of PDA and examines its integration with various hydrogel types, highlighting several representative composite hydrogels from recent studies (Table 1).

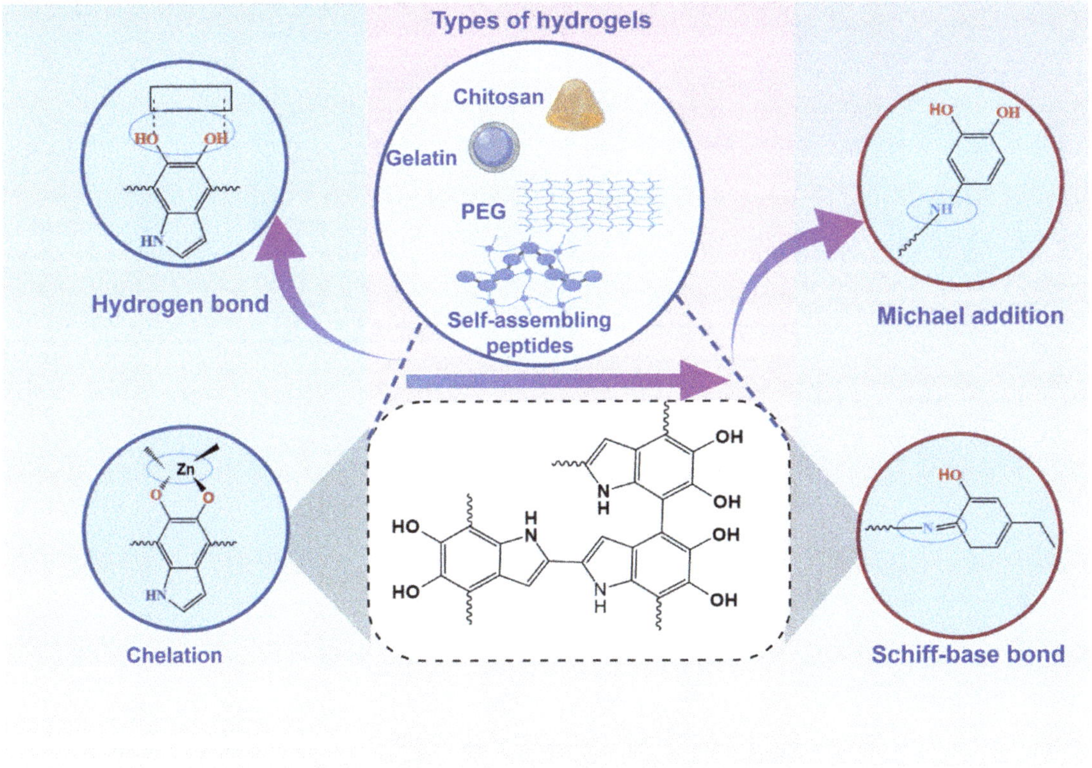

Figure 3. The mechanism of polydopamine-based modified hydrogels.

Table 1. Recent advances in PDA-based hydrogel delivery system for bone defect repair.

Type of Composite Hydrogel	Types of Cells/Bacteria	Type of Animal Model	Drugs/Growth Factors/Others	Advantages	Disadvantages	Reference
PDA/Hydroxybutyl chitosan hydrogel	hBMMSCs	SD rats	Aspirin	Dual responsive properties	Complex processing	Wan et al. [82]
PDA/alginate hydrogel	BMSCs	/	Silver Nanoparticles	Antibacterial/anti-infective properties	Insufficient mechanical strength	Zhang et al. [83]
PDA/Alginate-allylated double-cross-linked hydrogels	MG63 rBMSCs	/	DOX	Fast kinetic response/High UV cross-linking conversion efficiency/Excellent mechanical properties	Insufficient stability of drug release	Chen et al. [84]
GelMA-PDA/HA hydrogel	BMSCs	New Zealand white rabbits	BMP-2 TGF-β3	Excellent osteochondral repair	Reducing degradation speed	Gan et al. [85]
GelMA/PMMA/PDA hydrogel	BMSCs	BALB/c rats	/	Good biocompatibility/degradation properties	Local overheating	Wu et al. [86]
PLGA-PDA-/Alginate-RGD hydrogel	BMSCs HUVECs HELA MC3T3-E1	Fischer 344 rats SD rats	BMP-2 VEGF BP Doxorubicin Hydrochloride	Precise and timely drug release	Complex processing	Dashtimoghaamet al. [87]
Polyvinyl alcohol (PVA)/PDA@HAP hydrogel	BMSCs	SD rats	Silver Nanoparticles HAP	Long-lasting antimicrobial effect	Induction of cytotoxicity by silver nanoparticles	Li et al. [88]
PDA/Hyaluronic acid methacrylate hydrogel MPs	BMSCs	SD rats Rabbits	Barium titanate nanoparticles Stem cell recruitment peptides	Precise electrical stimulation	Poor stability	Han et al. [89]
PDA hydrogel	hBMSCs	SD rats	CNT PLA	High mechanical strength	Large manufacturing scale	Sun et al. [90]
PDA@E2/HA/GelMA/Gel hydrogel	BMSCs	/	Employing estradiol BMSCs	Adaptation of complex defects	Degradation rate/trigger conditions need to be optimized	Chen et al. [91]
MSN@pDA/Chitosan (CS) hydrogel	SMSCs	SD rats Rabbits	TGF-β3 IGF-I PDGF-BB	Activation of endogenous cartilage repair	Insufficient stability	Li et al. [92]
PDA/Gelatin methacrylate/sodium alginate methacrylate (GA) hybrid hydrogel	HUVECs MC3T3-E1	SD rats	DFO PO_4^{3-}	Improving the microenvironment of bone regeneration	Insufficient biocompatibility/photothermal efficiency	Wu et al. [93]

Table 1. *Cont.*

Type of Composite Hydrogel	Types of Cells/Bacteria	Type of Animal Model	Drugs/Growth Factors/Others	Advantages	Disadvantages	Reference
PDA/Hydroxypropyl chitosan/Gelatin (HG) hydrogel	HUVECs MC3T3-E1	BALB/c rats	aFGF Ti3C2Tx Mxene nanosheets	Accelerating critical bone defect healing	Inadequate biosecurity/limited demand for light control devices	Wu et al. [94]
KGN@PDA/UPy hydrogel	BMSCs	Rabbits	KGN miRNA@CaP NPs	Stable mechanical properties/strong self-healing ability	Complex forming process/insufficient transfection efficiency	Kang et al. [95]
PDA/ PEEK/Gelatin hydrogel	hMSCs	/	BMP-2	Enhanced osteogenic differentiation./Improved bio-inertness of the material	Limited drug loading	Zhang et al. [96]
PDA/Fpolyacrylamide/ Silk fibroin hydrogel	BMSCs HUVECs	SD rats	BMP-2DFO	Excellent interfacial adhesion/structural toughness/mechanical stiffness.	Need for multiple photothermal interventions, large implants to trigger foreign body reactions	Li et al. [97]
BML@β-TCP/PDA carboxymethyl chitosan hydrogel	MC3T3-E1	SD rats	BML-284	Multipurpose bone repair	High preparation costs	Wu et al. [98]
GPEGD/PDA hydrogel	MC3T3-E1	SD rats	BMP-2 Heparin	Excellent mechanical properties/biocompatibility	Limited cell infiltration/Insufficient stability of ROS scavengers	Wu et al. [99]
PDA@zeolitic imidazolate framework-8/Soft matrix hydrogel	MC3T3-E1 RAW264.7 HUVECs	SD rats	Zn^{2+}	Good structural stability/mechanical support	The complex diabetic microenvironment impairs the therapeutic effect	Wu et al. [100]
PDA/Al/GP/Fibrin hydrogels	EMSCs	SD rats	Al GP	Dual functions of osteoinduction and immunomodulation	Alendronate affects the balance of bone remodeling	Shi et al. [101]
Methacrylated silk fibroin (SFMA)/ PDA hydrogel	HUVECs BMSCs	SD rats	MAP	Exhibits good biocompatibility/physicochemical properties	Uneven distribution of photothermal agent/local overheating	Ma et al. [102]
Alginate methacrylate/Alginate/ PDA hydrogel	MC3T3-E1	SD rats	Ti_3C_2 MXene nanosheets	Good biocompatibility/osteogenic activity/immune-regulatory functions	Phototherapy produces free radicals that damage cells	Wu et al. [103]
PDA/Polysaccharide chitin hydrogel	MC3T3-E1 BMSCs	Wistar male rats	Cu^{2+} Nano HAP	High biocompatibility/Significant osteogenic activity.	Insufficient interfacial bonding strength	Huang et al. [104]

Table 1. *Cont.*

Type of Composite Hydrogel	Types of Cells/Bacteria	Type of Animal Model	Drugs/Growth Factors/Others	Advantages	Disadvantages	Reference
PDA/Polyethylene hydrogel (PEG)	MC3T3-E1	SD rats	AgNPs	Mineralization/anti-infection dual function	Reducing the elasticity of hydrogel	Xu et al. [105]
PDA/Chitosan/Gelatin hydrogel	HUVECs MC3T3-E1 RAW 264.7	SD rats	Hydroxyapatite $BaTiO_3$ NPs	Excellent immunomodulation/angiogenesis/osteogenesis/suitable for combat wound repair	Complex material processing	Wu et al. [106]
PDACS/PCL/Hydrogel	HUVECs WJMSCs	/	HUVECs WJMSCs	Synergized to promote osteogenesis/vascularization	Calcium silicate degradation products affect pH/limited microstructure control	Chen et al. [107]
Oxidized sodium alginate (OSA)/Gelatin (Gel)/PDA-nHA hydrogel	BMSCs	Japanese big-ear white rabbits	nHA	Injectable/easy to operate	Long-term stability of nano-hydroxyapatite (nHA) in vivo is insufficient	Liu et al. [108]
CGH/PDA@HAP hydrogel	BMSCs	SD rats	Gallic acid Hydroxyapatite	Enhanced antibacterial and osteogenic synergy	Generation of acidic degradation products	Pang et al. [109]
Characterization of the fucoidan/PDA hydrogel	PDLSCs	/	/	Enhanced osteogenic potential	Quality control of fucoidan sulfate was low	Kwack et al. [110]
Polyacrylamide/PDA hydrogel	MG-63	/	/	Matrix stiffness targets osteosarcoma cell apoptosis	Stiffness parameters need to be highly precise/difficult to adjust in clinical application	Deng et al. [111]
Xanthan gum-PDA hydrogel	BMSCs	SD rats	SDF-1α Mg^{2+}	Excellent injectability/mechanical properties	High SDF-1α inactivation	Li et al. [28]
OSA-GelDA@ACP/DA/Ag hydrogel	/	/	ACP DA Ag^+	Composite hydrogel combines tissue adhesion and anti-infection functions	The hydrogel flexibility/bond strength decreased	Zhong et al. [112]
PDA/Chondroitin sulfate hydrogel	rBMSCs	New Zealand rabbits	SDF-1α	Sustained-release SDF-1α	Lack of control over release kinetics	Wu et al. [113]
ALG/GelAGE-PDA@DOX hydrogels	rBMSCs MG 63	/	Sr^{2+} DOX	Synergistic effect of chemotherapy and photothermal therapy (PTT)	Degree of cross-linking affects the stability of drug release	Chen et al. [84]
PDA/GMS/Osteogenic hydrogel	*P. gingivalis*	SD rats	Amino antibacterial nanoparticle Magnetic nanoparticles	Precision antimicrobial therapy	Magnetic field conditioning devices limit clinical applications	Zhou et al. [114]

Table 1. *Cont.*

Type of Composite Hydrogel	Types of Cells/Bacteria	Type of Animal Model	Drugs/Growth Factors/Others	Advantages	Disadvantages	Reference
PDA/Nano-hydroxyapatite (nHAP) hydrogel	MC3T3-E1	/	PEEK Aspirin	Good biocompatibility/compressive strength/modulus	Poor cell adhesion to the inert surface of PEEK	Li et al. [115]
CS/PDA hydrogel	HUVECs	/	DFO	Enhanced bond strength/angiogenic effect	Short half-life of deferoxamine/frequent injections required	Liu et al. [116]
BNP-PEDOT-PSF-AG hydrogel	PDLSCs	SD rats	Bovine serum albumin nanoparticles Hydrogen sulfide	Promoting alveolar bone regeneration/reversing inflammatory microenvironment under diabetic conditions	Difficulty in controlling the release of H_2S gas	Fang et al. [117]
Alginate/TOCNF/PDA hydrogel	MC3T3-E1	/	TOCNFs PDANPs	High osteogenic activity	Low structural fidelity after printing	Im et al. [118]
GO-PHA-CPs hydrogel	MC3T3-E1	SD rats	CPs	Exhibits excellent injectability/adhesion/antioxidant activity/osteoinductive properties	Limited self-repair capacity/degradation rate mismatch with bone formation rate	Ma et al. [119]
DA-nano-hydroxyapatite hydrogel	4T1 BMSCs	BALB/c mice	DDP	Synergistic photothermal anti-tumor/bone regeneration capabilities	Photothermal agents are potentially toxic	Luo et al. [120]
MCG-HG-PLGA-PD-B hydrogel	ATDC5 MC3T3-E1	/	BMP-7	Promoting Structural Bionicity in Cartilage Regeneration	Insufficient scaffold porosity connectivity	Jung et al. [121]
Gellan gum/PDA hydrogel	MC3T3-E1	/	ALP	Polydopamine enhances the efficiency of mineralization	Increased material brittleness/complex preparation process	Douglas et al. [122]
PF-127/HAMA/M@S (PH/M@S) hydrogel	rBMSCs HUVEC RAW264.7	Mice	M@S NPs	Cost-effective/easy to synthesize/possesses multiple therapeutic capabilities	Nanoparticles prone to leakage	Liu et al. [123]
PDA/LC hydrogel	BMSCs E. coli S. aureus	SD rats	/	Excellent osteogenic activity/angiogenic capacity/antimicrobial effects	Chitosan causes allergic reactions/complex preparation	Li et al. [124]

Table 1. *Cont.*

Type of Composite Hydrogel	Types of Cells/Bacteria	Type of Animal Model	Drugs/Growth Factors/Others	Advantages	Disadvantages	Reference
Gel-PHA hydrogel	MC3T3-E1	SD rats	nHA	Enhanced mechanical and osteogenic properties of gelatin hydrogels	Reduced hydrogel elasticity	Ma et al. [125]
T/DOP-IL 4/CG-RGD hydrogel	BMSCs	/	IL-4 RGD peptide	IL-4 and RGD synergistically regulate the osteoimmune microenvironment	IL-4 short half-life/RGD overexpression	Li et al. [126]
PDA/Gel-PAA hydrogel	BMSCs	New Zealand rabbits	TGF-β3	Enhances the toughness and cell affinity of PAA hydrogels	Catechol oxidative cross-linking is irreversible/affects controllability of degradation	Yan et al. [127]
AD/CS/RSF/EXO hydrogel	BMSCs	SD rats	Exosomes	Excellent mechanical properties/ biodegradability/biocompatibility/ the ability	Low efficiency in exosome extraction and loading	Zhang et al. [128]
CTP-SA/TiO2@PDA hydrogel	HUVEC BMSCs Staphylococcus aureus Escherichia coli Streptococcus mutans	SD rats	Cu_2O TiO_2 NPs	Enhanced antimicrobial activity	Insufficient mechanical properties	Xu et al. [129]
PDA@SiO2-PRF hydrogel	BMSCs	SD rats	PRF	Multi-level regulation of microenvironment	Proteins are prone to degradation/short shelf life	Ren et al. [130]
Chitosan/ Polydopamine/NO-PVA hydrogel	MRSA MC3T3-E1	SD rats	Ti-RP/PCP/RSNO NO	With combined photother-mal/immunotherapy	Photothermal effect damages surrounding healthy tissue	Li et al. [131]
PnP-iPRF hydrogel	BMSCs RAW 264.7	Rats	i-PRF	Multiple pathways regulate the microenvironment	Immunogenic risk has not been completely ruled out	Li et al. [132]
SP@MX/GelMA hydrogel	MG-63 MC3T3-E1	Kunming mice	Tobramycin	Significantly enhances the initial adhesion and proliferation of cells	MXene nanosheets trigger inflammation	Yin et al. [133]
Gelatin-Silkfibroin-Oxidized dextran/PLLA-PLGA-PCL/PDA hydrogel	BMSCs	SD rats	Kartogenin P24 peptides	Excellent cell compatibility/Dual-layer scaffolds synergistically repair osteochondral defects	Weak interfacial bonding strength between the two layers	Zheng et al. [134]

Table 1. *Cont.*

Type of Composite Hydrogel	Types of Cells/Bacteria	Type of Animal Model	Drugs/Growth Factors/Others	Advantages	Disadvantages	Reference
SFO-TA-BGNF-PDA hydrogel	MG-63	/	Bioactive glass	Integrated antimicrobial activity/antiosteosarcoma properties/osteoinduction of multiple functions	Aerogel has low mechanical strength and is not suitable for load-bearing applications	Abie et al. [135]

Abbreviations: hBM(M)SCs, human bone marrow mesenchymal stem cells; MG63, human osteosarcoma cells; rBMSCs, rat bone mesenchymal stem cells; BMSCs, bone marrow mesenchymal stem cells; HUVECs, human umbilical vein endothelial cells; HELA, human cervical cancer cell; MC3T3-E1, mouse embryo osteoblast precursor cells; hMSCs, human mesenchymal stem cells; RAW264.7, murine monocyte-macrophage leukemia cells; EMSCs, ecto-mesenchymal stem cells; WJMSCs, human Wharton's jelly mesenchymal stem cells; PDLSCs, periodontal ligament stem cells; *P. gingivalis*, *Porphyromonas gingivalis*; 4T1, mouse breast cancer cells; ATDC5, mouse chondrocyte; E. coli, Escherichia coli; S. aureus, Staphylococcus aureus; MRSA, Methicillin-resistant staphylococcus aureus; BMP-2, bone morphogenetic protein-2; DOX, doxorubicin; TGF-β3, transforming growth factor-β3; VEGF, vascular endothelial growth factor; BP, black phosphorus; HAP, hydroxyapatite; CNT, carbon nanotube; PLA, polylactic acid; IGF-I, insulin-like growth factors; PDGF-BB, platelet-derived growth factor-BB; PO_4^{3-}, phosphate; aFGF, acid fibro-blast growth factor; KGN, kartogenin; miRNA@CaP NPs, microRNA@calcium phosphate nanoparticles; DFO, deferoxamine; BML-284, wnt agonist 1; Zn^{2+}, zinc ion; Al, aluminum; GP, genipin; MAP, magnesium ascorbyl phosphate; Ti_3C_2 MXene nanosheets, titanium carbide MXene nanosheets; Cu^{2+}, cupric ion; Nano HAP, nano-hydroxyapatite; AgNPs, silver nanoparticles; BaTiO3 NPs, barium titanate nanoparticles; nHA, nanohydroxyapatite; SDF-1α, stromal cell-derived factor-1α; Mg^{2+}, magnesium ion; ACP, amorphous calcium phosphate; DA, dopamine; Ag^+, silver ion; Sr^{2+}, strontium ions; PEEK, polyetheretherketone; TOCNFs, tempo-oxidized cellulose nanofibrils; PDANPs, polydopamine nanoparticles; CPs, bioactive cod peptides; DDP, cisplatin; BMP-7, bone morphogenetic protein-7; ALP; alkaline phosphatase; M@SNPs, spermidine-modified mesoporous polydopamine nano-particles; IL-4, interleukin-4; Cu_2O, cuprous oxide; TiO_2NPs, titanium dioxide nanoparticles; PRF, platelet-rich fibrin; Ti-RP/PCP/RSNO, titanium implant; NO, nitric oxide; i-PRF, injectable platelet-rich fibrin.

3.1. Composite Nanohydrogels of Natural Materials with Polydopamine Nanostructures

Natural polymers are highly favored in bone defect repair due to their superior biocompatibility and biodegradability. However, their hydrogels often lack adequate mechanical properties, limiting clinical applications. Incorporating polydopamine (PDA) into these hydrogels can significantly improve their mechanical attributes and functional capabilities, making them excellent candidates for drug delivery in bone defect repair.

3.1.1. Chitosan-Based PDA Hydrogel

Chitosan, a natural polysaccharide, is widely recognized as an ideal biomaterial for hydrogel preparation due to its excellent biocompatibility, cell adhesion properties, and versatile applications in drug delivery and tissue engineering [134,135]. However, it has limitations, such as poor mechanical strength and instability in high-humidity or acidic environments [136,137]. Incorporating polydopamine (PDA) significantly enhances the functionality of chitosan hydrogels, expanding their potential in biomedical and smart material applications [138–140]. These interactions improve the mechanical properties of the hydrogel, increasing stiffness and toughness while reducing swelling and overcoming the mechanical degradation and adhesion loss typically observed in chitosan hydrogels due to their high hygroscopicity [141–143]. Additionally, while conventional chitosan hydrogels are often prepared under acidic conditions, their pH stability is limited, and acidic environments can harm bioactive components [144]. Cross-linking with PDA creates a stable network on the chitosan surface, improving water stability and allowing the hydrogel to maintain integrity under acidic or humid conditions, while also enhancing thermal stability [145]. Moreover, PDA-modified chitosan hydrogels offer improved drug delivery capacity by forming a dense network structure that prolongs drug release and enables controlled, slow-release effects [146,147]. The combination of PDA and chitosan not only addresses the limitations of traditional chitosan hydrogels but also advances the development of smart-responsive biomaterials [148]. To further enhance the osteogenic potential, bioactive molecules, mineral particles, or nanomaterials such as hydroxyapatite, silica gel, or calcium–phosphorus complexes can be incorporated.

Rahnama et al. [149] developed an injectable hydrogel combining chitosan, dopamine, and inositol aldehyde for drug delivery. The hydrogel rapidly gels under physiological conditions and exhibits sustained indomethacin release across various pH environments. Its cytocompatibility with L-929 fibroblasts underscores its potential for controlled drug delivery.

Wan et al. [82] used PDA-modified hydroxybutyl chitosan hydrogels for bone repair. The hydrogels, with NIR light responsive microspheres, facilitated a sequential release of aspirin and BMP-2, aligning with the bone healing process (Figure 4). This approach offers a novel therapeutic strategy for bone-related conditions.

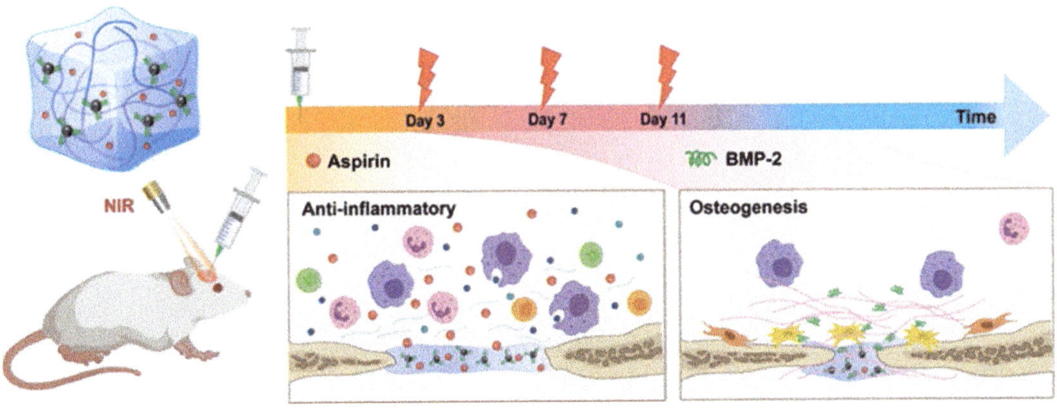

Figure 4. Synthesis of PDA-coated magnesium calcium carbonate microspheres and thermally responsive hydroxybutyl chitosan (HBC) dual responsive hydrogel used for near infrared (NIR) triggered continuous delivery of aspirin (Asp) and BMP-2 to promote in situ calvaria bone regeneration. Adapted with permission from Ref. [82]. Copyright 2022 Carbohydrate polymers.

3.1.2. Alginate-Based PDA Hydrogel

Alginate (Alg), a hydrophilic polysaccharide derived from brown algae, is valued for its excellent biocompatibility and degradability, making it ideal for applications in wound healing, microencapsulation, drug delivery, and 3D scaffolds for bone and soft tissue engineering [150,151]. However, alginate hydrogels often suffer from low mechanical strength and slow degradation rates [152–155]. Recent studies indicate that incorporating PDA significantly enhances the biocompatibility, mechanical strength, and adhesion of alginate hydrogels, particularly in underwater environments [83,156]. PDA modification improves the mechanical and adhesive properties of the hydrogels through catechol interactions, balancing stiffness and flexibility. This enhancement not only broadens the applicability of alginate hydrogels in tissue engineering but also boosts their diffusion capabilities at contact surfaces [157]. Additionally, PDA-modified alginate hydrogels demonstrate improved cohesion, stability, drug loading capacity, and sustained release properties, offering superior drug delivery performance compared to unmodified alginate hydrogels [158,159]. In summary, alginate–PDA hydrogels provide better control over bioviscosity and osteogenic induction compared to pure alginate hydrogels.

Zhang et al. [83] modified alginate with PDA, resulting in hydrogels that promoted MSC cell survival, proliferation, and osteogenic differentiation (Figure 5). Additionally, PDA's adhesive properties enabled the coating of silver nanoparticles on the alginate PDA gel surface, thereby conferring significant antimicrobial properties to the gel (Figure 6). This hydrogel could be a good tool to promote cell encapsulation and bone regeneration, especially for contaminated bone defects.

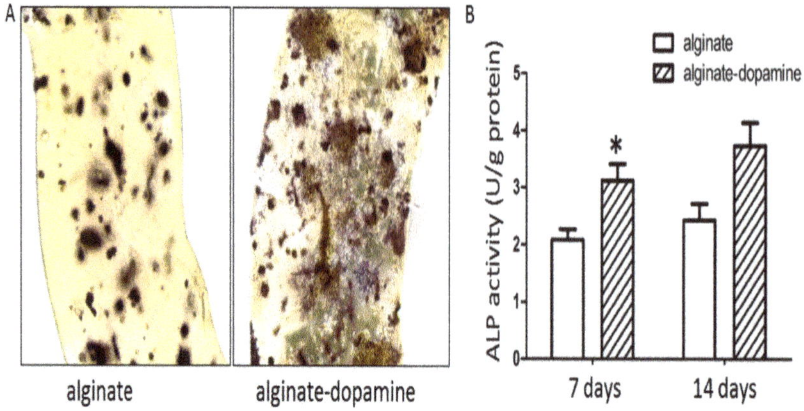

Figure 5. Osteogenic differentiation analysis: (**A**) Alkaline phosphatase (ALP) staining showed the distribution and activity of BMSC in alginate and alginate DA fibrous matrices after 14 days of osteogenic induction. (**B**) ALP activity of BMSC cultured in alginate and alginate dopamine fiber matrices on days 7 and 14 of osteoinduction; data shown as mean ± SD (n = 3), "*" indicates significant difference with $p < 0.05$. Adapted with permission from Ref. [83]. Copyright 2016 Materials Science and Engineering: C.

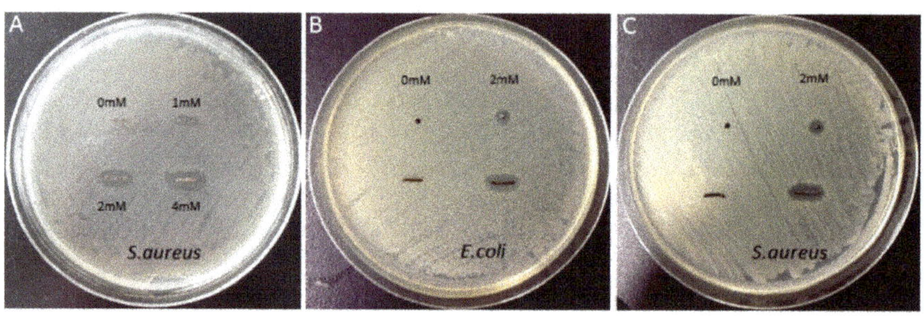

Figure 6. Antibacterial activity analysis: No inhibition zone against * Salmonella * was observed for nanosilver that was not modified with dopamine (**A**). However, alginate dopamine beads and fibers coated with nanosilver exhibited significant inhibition zones against both Gram-positive and Gram-negative bacteria (**B**,**C**). Adapted with permission from Ref. [83]. Copyright 2016 Materials Science and Engineering: C.

3.1.3. Gelatin-Based PDA Hydrogel

Gelatin, derived from the hydrolysis of collagen, is widely used in tissue engineering and drug delivery due to its biocompatibility, degradability, and cell adhesion properties [160,161]. However, gelatin hydrogels face challenges such as weak mechanical strength, poor thermal stability, and limited osteoinductivity, which hinder their effectiveness as bone repair materials [162–164]. Similar to chitosan and alginate, the incorporation of PDA enhances gelatin hydrogels by improving their mechanical strength, thermal stability, and cell affinity. These improvements result from noncovalent interactions, particularly those involving the catechol groups of PDA [165,166].

Chen et al. [84] prepared a bifunctional alginate (ALG)/allylated gelatin (GelAGE) hydrogel with UV and Sr^{2+} cross-linking, incorporating PDA particles. This hydrogel showed enhanced mechanical strength compared to other injectable hydrogels. Additionally, the inclusion of PDA@DOX particles increased porosity, facilitating cell penetration. Experimental results revealed that the ALG/GelAGE-PDA@DOX hydrogel achieved a high in vitro killing rate of MG63 cells and exhibited promising bone-like mineralization properties, indicating its potential for bone tissue regeneration.

Gan et al. [85] developed a mussel inspired bilayer hydrogel for cartilage defect repair (Figure 7). The upper layer comprises a methacrylamide polydopamine (Gel-MA-PDA) hydrogel loaded with transforming growth factor β3 (TGF-β3) to support cartilage regeneration, while the lower layer is a methacrylamide polydopamine/hydroxyapatite gelatin (GelMA-PDA/HA) hydrogel containing bone morphogenetic protein 2 (BMP-2) to aid subchondral bone repair. PDA in the lower layer facilitates hydroxyapatite mineralization, mimicking subchondral bone structure and enhancing mechanical strength. This bilayer hydrogel supports cell proliferation and differentiation, effectively delivering BMP-2 and TGF-β3 for targeted cartilage and subchondral bone regeneration.

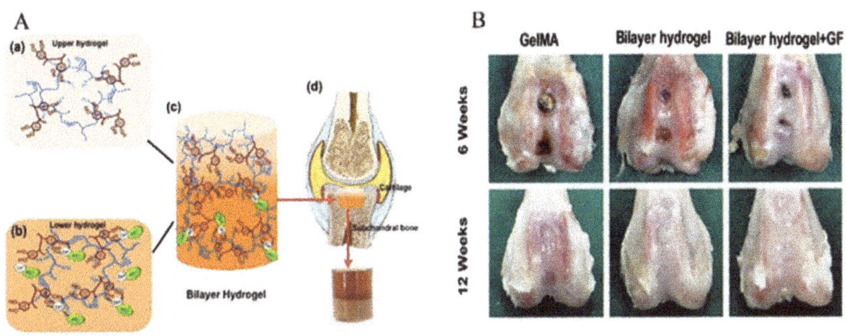

Figure 7. (**A**) Preparation of bilayer hydrogel for cartilage defect repair. (**a**) Gelatin methacryloyl (GelMA) was mixed with polydopamine (PDA) to prepare the upper layer hydrogel for cartilage defect repair. (**b**) Ca^{2+} GelMA was mixed with PO_4^{3-} GelMA to mineralize hydroxyapatite (HA) in situ, to prepare the lower layer hydrogel for subchondral bone repair. (**c**) Polymerization to generate bilayer hydrogels. (**d**) Schematic of osteochondral defect repair. (**B**) Gross morphological examination of osteochondral defects in the knee joint of rabbits at 6 and 12 weeks after operation was performed. Adapted with permission from Ref. [85]. Copyright 2022 Advanced Healthcare Materials.

3.2. *Composite Nanohydrogels of Synthetic Materials with Polydopamine Nanostructures*

3.2.1. Nanohydrogels Based on Frequently Studied Synthetic Materials

Compared to natural materials, traditional synthetic materials, such as polyethylene glycol (PEG), polyvinyl alcohol (PVA), and poly (methyl methacrylate) (PMMA), are frequently employed to construct strong hydrogels due to their cost effectiveness and robust mechanical attributes [167,168]. Despite these advantages, they typically lack the necessary biocompatibility that facilitates cell adhesion, proliferation, and differentiation. Furthermore, the degradation of polyester compounds like PLGA, PGA, and PLA within the body can result in acidic byproducts that may provoke inflammatory responses, potentially hindering bone healing [169]. The integration of (PDA) into these materials has shown promise in overcoming these limitations, thereby enhancing their utility for bone repair purposes [170,171].

Wu et al. [86] have developed a gelatin methacryloyl/poly (methyl methacrylate)/polydopamine (GelMA/PMMA/PDA) photohydrothermal gel aimed at addressing bone defects. This hydrogel underwent rigorous testing through in vitro cell culture experiments and in vivo animal studies to evaluate its biocompatibility and bone repair efficacy. The data revealed its potent osteogenic potential, marking it as a viable treatment for bone defects.

Dashtimoghadam et al. [87] utilized PLGA to create monodisperse microcarriers encapsulating VEGF, which were then functionalized with a biomimetic PDA coating to bind

BMP-2. These microcarriers were integrated with an injectable alginate RGD hydrogel to facilitate the controlled release of VEGF and BMP-2 (Figure 8). The findings indicated that the PDA functionalized microcarriers not only improved the immobilization and bioavailability of BMP-2, but also enhanced the attachment and proliferation of mesenchymal stem cells (MSCs), suggesting a promising approach for stem cell therapy in bone defect treatment.

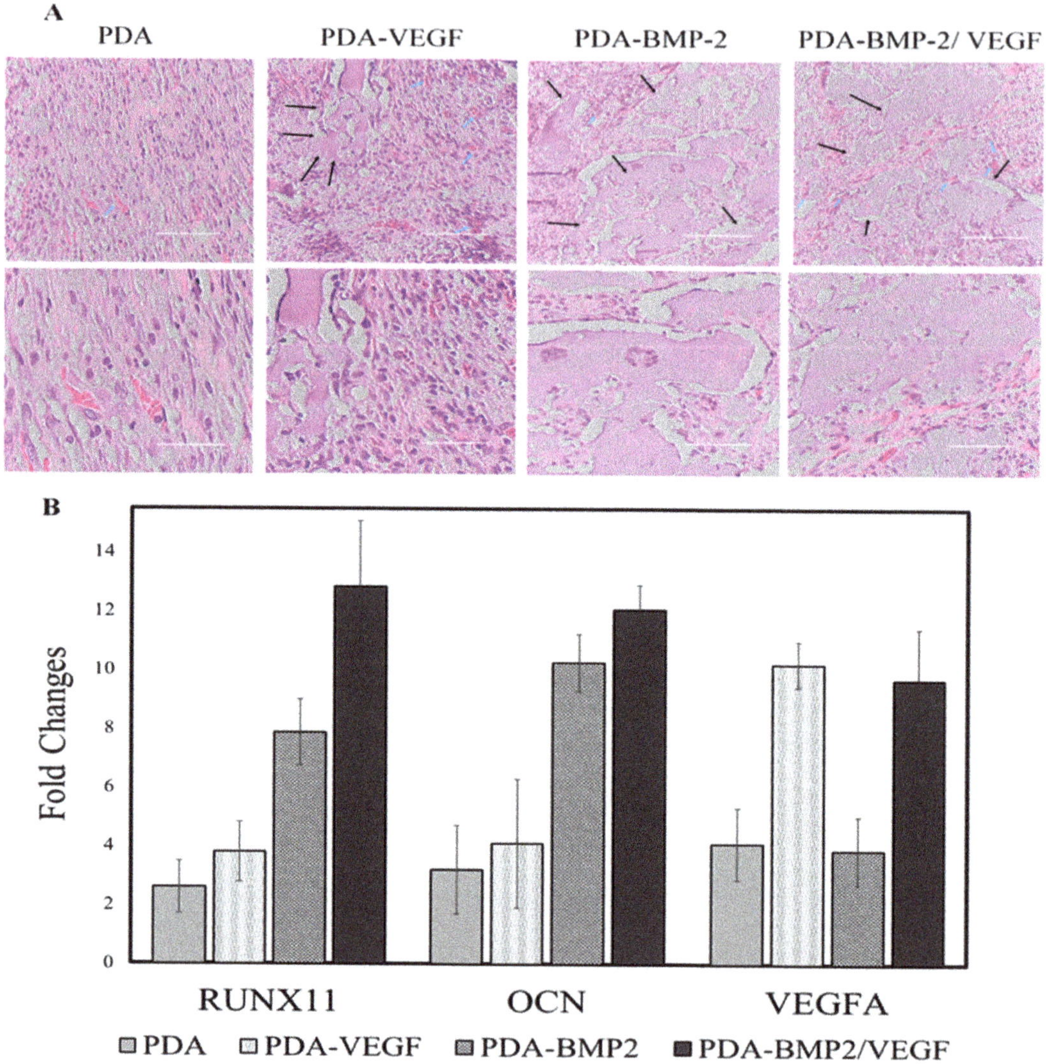

Figure 8. (**A**) H&E staining of decalcified gel matrix sections with cell laden microcarriers: PDA treated (control), VEGF encapsulated, BMP-2 conjugated, and VEGF encapsulated microcarriers with BMP-2 after 6 weeks of subcutaneous implantation. (**B**) Real-time PCR analysis of RUNX2, OCN, and ALP expression after 6 weeks of subcutaneous implantation. Data are presented as means ± standard deviations. Modified from Dashtimoghadam et al. [87]. (2020) under the terms of the Creative Commons Attribution International License (CCBY4.0).

In another study, Xu et al. [105] synthesized a silver nanoparticles/PDA/PEG hydrogel, providing both antimicrobial capabilities and promoting bone mineralization. This utilized PDA mineralization on polyethylene (PEG) hydrogels, and then improved the hydrogel's adhesion to bone tissue and biocompatibility. Experimental results demonstrated that this hydrogel promotes the proliferation and differentiation of osteoblasts, while inducing bone mineralization and offering antimicrobial protection against infections (Figures 9 and 10). A recent study [27] also describes the preparation of a multifunctional gelatin methacrylate/dopamine gelatin methacrylate adhesive hydrogel coating that includes two-dimensional black phosphorus (BP) nanoparticles coated with dopamine. This multifunctional hydrogel coating, in combination with BP, facilitates photothermal mediated drug delivery and bacterial eradication through photodynamic therapy, aiding in bone healing.

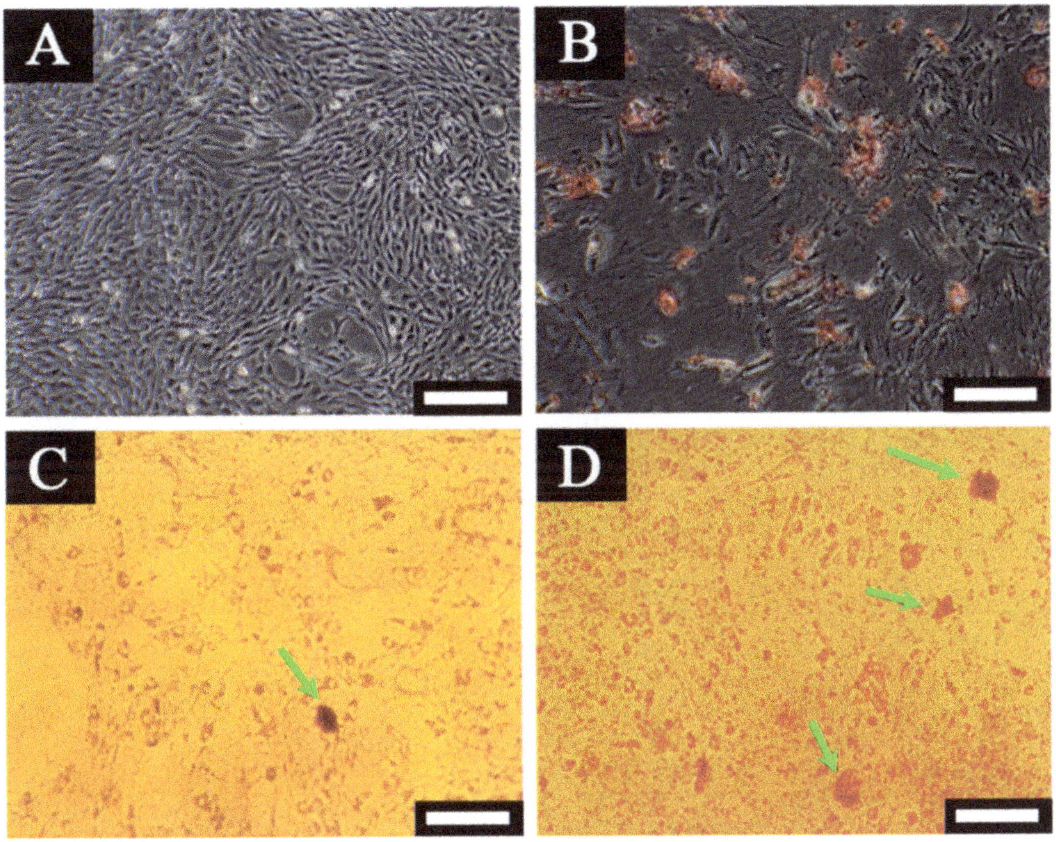

Figure 9. The osteoblastic ability of the AgNPs/PDA gel detected by Alizarin red staining: Alizarin red staining shows osteoblastic activity of AgNPs/PDA gel. (**A**) Cells on a 2D plate. (**B**) Cells on a 2D plate with osteogenic inducer. (**C**) Cells on the gel. (**D**) Cells on the gel with osteogenic inducer. Green arrows indicate calcium nodes. Scale bar: 250 μm. Adapted with permission from Ref. [105]. Copyright 2018 Materials Science and Engineering: C.

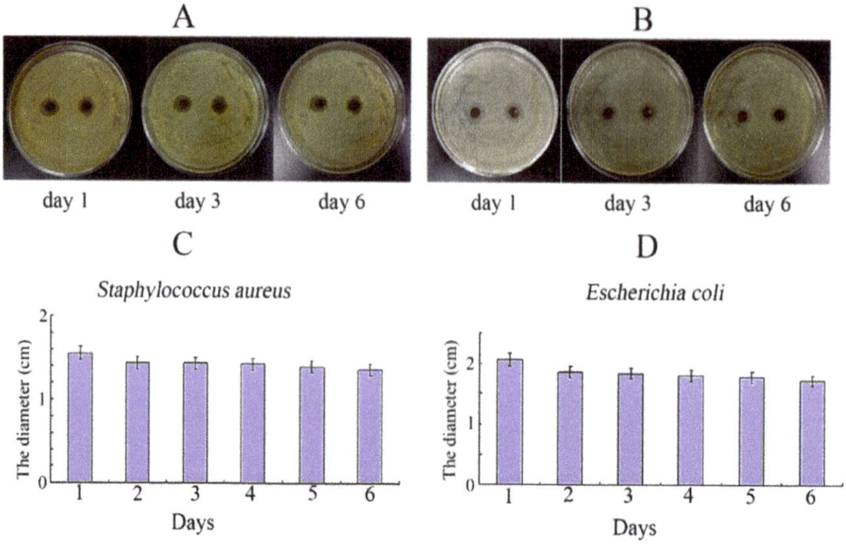

Figure 10. Antibacterial activity of AgNPs/PDA gel: (**A**,**C**) S. aureus groups. (**B**,**D**) *E. coli* groups. (**C**,**D**) Statistical analysis of antibacterial ring diameter. Data are presented as mean ± standard deviation (SD). Adapted with permission from Ref. [105]. Copyright 2018 Materials Science and Engineering: C.

3.2.2. Nanohydrogels Based on Self-Assembling Peptides

Beyond the traditional hydrogels of synthetic materials, peptide-based self-assembling hydrogels have garnered significant attention in materials science and biomedical applications in recent years [172,173]. These peptide-based supramolecular gel scaffolds are extensively utilized in cell culture, tissue engineering, drug delivery, and wound healing, thanks to their straightforward preparation, biocompatibility, and degradability. Previous studies have demonstrated that self-assembling peptide hydrogels are effective in facilitating the repair of bone and cartilage, as well as promoting wound healing [174].

Despite their utility, peptide-based hydrogels often exhibit insufficient functionality and mechanical strength [175,176]. To overcome this limitation, researchers have started to incorporate various inorganic nanomaterials and polymers into these hydrogels, creating hybrid heteropeptide hydrogels that enhance their properties. Studies have demonstrated [177–179] that incorporating appropriate amounts of inorganic nanoparticles can significantly improve the mechanical strength and endow new functionalities to the gels. However, achieving compatibility between certain inorganic nanomaterials and the gel matrix can be challenging. The introduction of polymers like (PNIPAAm) can enhance compatibility, but their synthesis is often complex and typically requires organic solvents, which may introduce residues that can adversely affect the biomedical properties of the gels. Therefore, developing novel hydrogel systems that are multifunctionalized and stable in physiological environments is crucial for advancing hydrogel applications in biomedicine.

In light of the mechanical and functional limitations of hydrogels, researchers have started to incorporate polydopamine into peptide hydrogels. This integration not only reduces the critical gel concentration but also significantly enhances their mechanical properties. For example, Fichman et al. [180] showed that self-polymerized dopamine can react with lysine residues in peptides, effectively tuning the viscoelastic properties of the gels (Figure 11). Their findings indicated that incorporating dopamine during gelation significantly increases the storage modulus of the peptide gel while maintaining their shear thinning recovery behavior.

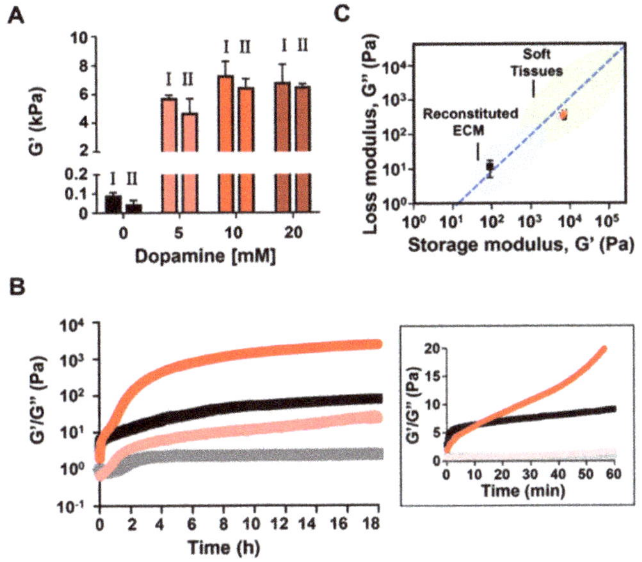

Figure 11. Rheological studies of the 0.5 wt.% MAX1 dopamine gel system. (**A**) Rheological analysis of 0.5 wt.% MAX1 gel 3 days post gelation with varying dopamine concentrations. Left bar (I) shows the initial G′ value before shear thinning (1000% strain, 30 s), and right bar (II) shows the recovered G′ value 10 min after shear thinning. Data are presented as means ± standard deviations. (**B**) Time sweep measurements of 0.5 wt.% MAX1 gel without dopamine (black) and with 5 mM dopamine (red), tracking G and G″ (dark and light, respectively) over time at 37 °C, pH 7.4. (**C**) Presheared G and G values of preformed 0.5 wt.% MAX1 gel. Modified from Fichman et al. [180]. (2021) under the terms of the Creative Commons Attribution International License (CCBY4.0).

Additionally, the remarkable photothermal properties of PDA have been utilized to facilitate the loading of drug carrying agents through π-π bonding, leading to the development of a therapeutic platform that integrates photothermal therapy with controlled drug release, thus achieving multifunctionality in hydrogels. For instance, Falcone et al. [181] encapsulated polydopamine nanoparticles (PDNPs) loaded with the hydrophobic drug rifampicin within a C14-FF hydrogel and used laser heating to trigger drug release (Figure 12). By adjusting the laser power and duration, precise control over the drug release rate was achieved. When the laser irradiates the polydopamine layer in the nanocomposite hydrogel, the PDA absorbs the laser energy and converts it into thermal energy, raising the temperature within the hydrogel and altering its structure to facilitate drug release. The results indicate that the C14-FF hydrogel containing PDNPs can sustain the delivery of high concentrations of rifampin after laser induction, effectively preventing bacterial growth (Figure 13). Overall, initiating peptide-based gels in the presence of dopamine offers a simple yet effective method for modulating their viscoelastic mechanical properties, with promising applications in medical wound dressings and controlled drug delivery.

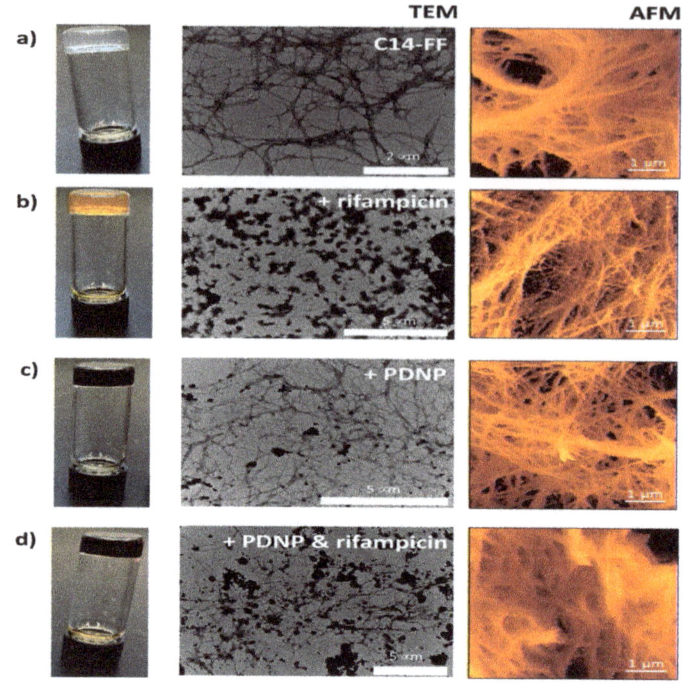

Figure 12. Morphological characterization map of nanocomposite hydrogels: TEM, and AFM images of (**a**) C14-FF gels alone, (**b**) C14-FF + rifampicin, (**c**) C14-FF + PDNP, and (**d**) C14-FF + PDNP + rifampicin. Modified from Falcone et al. [181]. (2021) under the terms of the Creative Commons Attribution International License (CC BY 4.0).

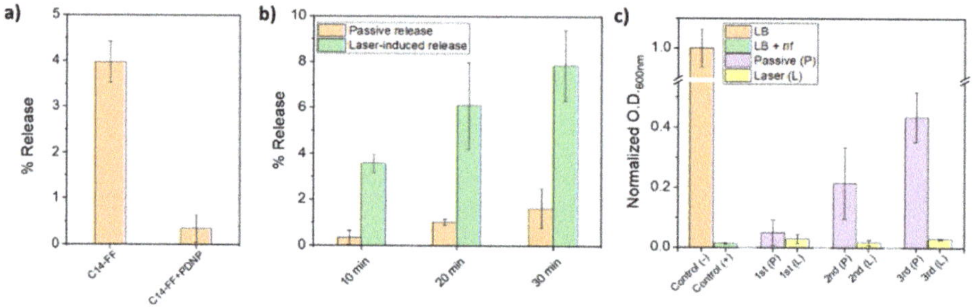

Figure 13. Passive release of rifampicin from the C14-FF hydrogel alone versus the nanocomposite hydrogel with PDNP, and the growth of *Escherichia coli* after laser induced release (**a**–**c**). Data are presented as means ± standard deviations. Modified from Falcone et al. [181]. (2021) under the terms of the Creative Commons Attribution International License (CC BY 4.0).

While the use of dopamine self-polymerization as a technique for enhancing peptide-based gels has been proposed, there is a scarcity of detailed reports on its specific applications and effects. Moreover, research into the mechanisms of action and optimization conditions for dopamine in peptide-based gels is limited, particularly in terms of evaluating and comparing effects across different peptide systems and application scenarios. Therefore, despite its potential, the application prospects and advantages of dopamine self-polymerization in peptide-based gels require further validation through more in-depth experimental studies.

4. Conclusions and Outlook

Polydopamine (PDA)-based nanocomposite hydrogels represent a promising advancement in drug delivery, offering significant improvements over conventional hydrogels in terms of biocompatibility, drug loading capacity, mechanical strength, and controlled release capabilities. These hydrogels have diverse applications in medicine, including tissue adhesion, sealing, and hemostasis during surgical procedures. By leveraging the unique properties of PDA alongside the advantages of hydrogels, these systems can be engineered to deliver drugs in a controlled manner, often through the integration of nanoparticles or drug carriers. This approach can enhance drug stability, bioactivity, and concentration at target sites, potentially benefiting bone tissue regeneration and addressing bone defect-related conditions.

However, PDA-based hydrogels remain in the research and development stage and have not yet reached widespread commercialization. In contrast, other biomaterials such as chitosan, PEG hydrogel, and fibrin have achieved industrial-scale production, driven by advancements in synthesis, clinical trials, and regulatory approval. For PDA-based hydrogels to follow a similar path, further optimization of the synthesis process and biodegradation properties is essential to ensure consistent polymerization and batch stability, meeting the stringent regulatory standards for medical devices.

Despite their potential, PDA-based hydrogels face three main challenges: (1) limited understanding of PDA polymerization mechanisms, (2) risk of drug leakage during nanoparticle coating, and (3) dependence on cytotoxic cross-linking agents in fabrication. Thus, developing a simplified, one-step method to prepare PDA-based hydrogels without cross-linkers or oxidizers under mild conditions remains a key challenge.

Future research will focus on refining the design and synthesis of PDA-based nanocomposite hydrogels to improve drug-loading efficiency, controlled release, and long-term stability. Collaboration with medical device companies will be crucial to expedite the registration and commercialization of PDA-based products, ultimately advancing these hydrogels into more effective and practical clinical drug delivery tools.

Author Contributions: Conceptualization, F.T.; writing—original draft preparation, X.L., J.T., W.G., X.D. and K.C.; writing—review and editing, F.T. and X.L. All authors have read and agreed to the published version of the manuscript.

Funding: This work was supported by the Project of Guizhou Provincial Science and Technology Program (Key 055 of Qiankehe-ZK [2023]); the Science and Technology Fund of Guizhou Provincial Health Commission (gzwkj2023-235); the Project of Special Funds for Science and Technology Cooperation in Guizhou Province and Zunyi City (Shengshikehe [2015] 53) and the National Natural Science Foundation of China (No. 32160225, 31460246).

Institutional Review Board Statement: Not applicable.

Informed Consent Statement: Informed consent was obtained from all subjects involved in the study.

Data Availability Statement: Not applicable.

Acknowledgments: The authors sincerely appreciate the financial support provided by the aforementioned funding sources. We would like to extend our gratitude to Qiang Huang for his meticulous work in creating Figure 1. Additionally, we thank Figdraw (www.figdraw.com) for assistance with the creation of Figures 2 and 3.

Conflicts of Interest: The authors report no conflicts of interest. The authors alone are responsible for the content and writing of this article.

References

1. Fan, S.; Sun, X.; Su, C.; Xue, Y.; Song, X.; Deng, R. Macrophages—Bone marrow mesenchymal stem cells crosstalk in bone healing. *Front. Cell Dev. Biol.* **2023**, *11*, 1193765. [CrossRef] [PubMed]
2. Goodman, S.B.; Lin, T. Modifying MSC Phenotype to Facilitate Bone Healing: Biological Approaches. *Front. Bioeng. Biotechnol.* **2020**, *8*, 641. [CrossRef] [PubMed]
3. Habibovic, P. Strategic Directions in Osteoinduction and Biomimetics. *Tissue Eng. Part A* **2017**, *23*, 1295–1296. [CrossRef]
4. Amini, A.R.; Laurencin, C.T.; Nukavarapu, S.P. Bone Tissue Engineering: Recent Advances and Challenges. *Crit. Rev. Biomed. Eng.* **2012**, *40*, 363–408. [CrossRef] [PubMed]
5. Kawecki, F.; Clafshenkel, W.P.; Fortin, M.; Auger, F.A.; Fradette, J. Biomimetic Tissue-Engineered Bone Substitutes for Maxillofacial and Craniofacial Repair: The Potential of Cell Sheet Technologies. *Adv. Healthc. Mater.* **2018**, *7*, e1700919. [CrossRef]
6. Subbiah, R.; Lin, E.Y.; Athirasala, A.; Romanowicz, G.E.; Lin, A.S.P.; Califano, J.V.; Guldberg, R.E.; Bertassoni, L.E. Engineering of an osteoinductive and growth factor-free injectable bone-like microgel for bone regeneration. *Adv. Healthc. Mater.* **2023**, *12*, e2200976. [CrossRef]
7. Zeng, Y.; Hoque, J.; Varghese, S. Biomaterial-assisted local and systemic delivery of bioactive agents for bone repair. *Acta Biomater.* **2019**, *93*, 152–168. [CrossRef]
8. Chen, J.; Ashames, A.; Buabeid, M.A.; Fahelelbom, K.M.; Ijaz, M.; Murtaza, G. Nanocomposites drug delivery systems for the healing of bone fractures. *Int. J. Pharm.* **2020**, *585*, 119477. [CrossRef]
9. Wang, Y.; Newman, M.R.; Benoit, D.S. Development of controlled drug delivery systems for bone fracture-targeted therapeutic delivery: A review. *Eur. J. Pharm. Biopharm.* **2018**, *127*, 223–236. [CrossRef]
10. Bai, X.; Gao, M.; Syed, S.; Zhuang, J.; Xu, X.; Zhang, X.-Q. Bioactive hydrogels for bone regeneration. *Bioact. Mater.* **2018**, *3*, 401–417. [CrossRef]
11. Shi, W.; Jiang, Y.; Wu, T.; Zhang, Y.; Li, T. Advancements in drug-loaded hydrogel systems for bone defect repair. *Regen. Ther.* **2023**, *25*, 174–185. [CrossRef] [PubMed]
12. Zhang, H.; Wu, S.; Chen, W.; Hu, Y.; Geng, Z.; Su, J. Bone/cartilage targeted hydrogel: Strategies and applications. *Bioact. Mater.* **2022**, *23*, 156–169. [CrossRef] [PubMed]
13. Wei, W.; Tang, J.; Hu, L.; Feng, Y.; Li, H.; Yin, C.; Tang, F. Experimental anti-tumor effect of emodin in suspension—In situ hydrogels formed with self-assembling peptide. *Drug Deliv.* **2021**, *28*, 1810–1821. [CrossRef] [PubMed]
14. Raeisi, A.; Farjadian, F. Commercial hydrogel product for drug delivery based on route of administration. *Front. Chem.* **2024**, *12*, 1336717. [CrossRef]
15. Farjadian, F.; Mirkiani, S.; Ghasemiyeh, P.; Kafshboran, H.R.; Mehdi-Alamdarlou, S.; Raeisi, A.; Esfandiarinejad, R.; Soleymani, S.; Goshtasbi, G.; Firouzabadi, N.; et al. Smart nanogels as promising platform for delivery of drug, gene, and vaccine; therapeutic applications and active targeting mechanism. *Eur. Polym. J.* **2024**, *219*, 113400. [CrossRef]
16. Dhand, A.P.; Galarraga, J.H.; Burdick, J.A. Enhancing Biopolymer Hydrogel Functionality through Interpenetrating Networks. *Trends Biotechnol.* **2021**, *39*, 519–538. [CrossRef]
17. Zheng, F.; Yang, X.; Li, J.; Tian, Z.; Xiao, B.; Yi, S.; Duan, L. Coordination with zirconium: A facile approach to improve the mechanical properties and thermostability of gelatin hydrogel. *Int. J. Biol. Macromol.* **2022**, *205*, 595–603. [CrossRef]
18. Chen, M.; Le, D.Q.; Baatrup, A.; Nygaard, J.V.; Hein, S.; Bjerre, L.; Kassem, M.; Zou, X.; Bünger, C. Self-assembled composite matrix in a hierarchical 3-D scaffold for bone tissue engineering. *Acta Biomater.* **2011**, *7*, 2244–2255. [CrossRef]
19. Wu, L.; Chen, G.; Li, Z. Layered Rare-Earth Hydroxide/Polyacrylamide Nanocomposite Hydrogels with Highly Tunable Photoluminescence. *Small* **2017**, *13*, 1604070. [CrossRef]
20. Bedhiafi, T.; Idoudi, S.; Alhams, A.A.; Fernandes, Q.; Iqbal, H.; Basineni, R.; Uddin, S.; Dermime, S.; Merhi, M.; Billa, N. Applications of polydopaminic nanomaterials in mucosal drug delivery. *J. Control. Release* **2023**, *353*, 842–849. [CrossRef]
21. Hong, S.; Na, Y.S.; Choi, S.; Song, I.T.; Kim, W.Y.; Lee, H. Non-Covalent Self-Assembly and Covalent Polymerization Co-Contribute to Polydopamine Formation. *Adv. Funct. Mater.* **2012**, *22*, 4711–4717. [CrossRef]
22. Sarkari, S.; Khajehmohammadi, M.; Davari, N.; Li, D.; Yu, B. The effects of process parameters on polydopamine coatings employed in tissue engineering applications. *Front. Bioeng. Biotechnol.* **2022**, *10*, 1005413. [CrossRef]
23. Hong, D.; Lee, H.; Kim, B.J.; Park, T.; Choi, J.Y.; Park, M.; Lee, J.; Cho, H.; Hong, S.-P.; Yang, S.H.; et al. A degradable polydopamine coating based on disulfide-exchange reaction. *Nanoscale* **2015**, *7*, 20149–20154. [CrossRef] [PubMed]
24. Wang, Z.; Li, C.; Xu, J.; Wang, K.; Lu, X.; Zhang, H.; Qu, S.; Zhen, G.; Ren, F. Bioadhesive Microporous Architectures by Self-Assembling Polydopamine Microcapsules for Biomedical Applications. *Chem. Mater.* **2015**, *27*, 848–856. [CrossRef]
25. Ku, S.H.; Ryu, J.; Hong, S.K.; Lee, H.; Park, C.B. General functionalization route for cell adhesion on non-wetting surfaces. *Biomaterials* **2010**, *31*, 2535–2541. [CrossRef] [PubMed]
26. Su, T.; Zhang, M.; Zeng, Q.; Pan, W.; Huang, Y.; Qian, Y.; Dong, W.; Qi, X.; Shen, J. Mussel-inspired agarose hydrogel scaffolds for skin tissue engineering. *Bioact. Mater.* **2021**, *6*, 579–588. [CrossRef]

27. Li, Y.; Liu, C.; Cheng, X.; Wang, J.; Pan, Y.; Zhang, S.; Jian, X. PDA-BPs integrated mussel-inspired multifunctional hydrogel coating on PPENK implants for anti-tumor therapy, antibacterial infection and bone regeneration. *Bioact. Mater.* **2023**, *27*, 546–559. [CrossRef]
28. Li, Z.; Lin, H.; Shi, S.; Su, K.; Zheng, G.; Gao, S.; Zeng, X.; Ning, H.; Yu, M.; Li, X.; et al. Controlled and Sequential Delivery of Stromal Derived Factor-1 α (SDF-1α) and Magnesium Ions from Bifunctional Hydrogel for Bone Regeneration. *Polymers* **2022**, *14*, 2872. [CrossRef]
29. Hathout, R.M.; Metwally, A.A.; El-Ahmady, S.H.; Metwally, E.S.; Ghonim, N.A.; Bayoumy, S.A.; Erfan, T.; Ashraf, R.; Fadel, M.; El-Kholy, A.I.; et al. Dual stimuli-responsive polypyrrole nanoparticles for anticancer therapy. *J. Drug Deliv. Sci. Technol.* **2018**, *47*, 176–180. [CrossRef]
30. Ni, X.; Gao, Y.; Zhang, X.; Lei, Y.; Sun, G.; You, B. An eco-friendly smart self-healing coating with NIR and pH dual-responsive superhydrophobic properties based on biomimetic stimuli-responsive mesoporous polydopamine microspheres. *Chem. Eng. J.* **2021**, *406*, 126725. [CrossRef]
31. Zhong, Z.; Fang, C.; He, S.; Zhang, T.; Liu, S.; Zhang, Y.; Wang, Q.; Ding, X.; Zhou, W.; Wang, X. Sequential Release Platform of Heparin and Urokinase with Dual Physical (NIR-II and Bubbles) Assistance for Deep Venous Thrombosis. *ACS Biomater. Sci. Eng.* **2020**, *6*, 6790–6799. [CrossRef]
32. Li, H.; Li, Y.; Wang, X.; Hou, Y.; Hong, X.; Gong, T.; Zhang, Z.; Sun, X. Rational design of Polymeric Hybrid Micelles to Overcome Lymphatic and Intracellular Delivery Barriers in Cancer Immunotherapy. *Theranostics* **2017**, *7*, 4383–4398. [CrossRef]
33. Xie, Y.; Zheng, Y.; Fan, J.; Wang, Y.; Yue, L.; Zhang, N. Novel Electronic–Ionic Hybrid Conductive Composites for Multifunctional Flexible Bioelectrode Based on in Situ Synthesis of Poly(dopamine) on Bacterial Cellulose. *ACS Appl. Mater. Interfaces* **2018**, *10*, 22692–22702. [CrossRef]
34. Wang, L.; Han, L.; Xue, P.; Hu, X.; Wong, S.-W.; Deng, M.; Tseng, H.C.; Huang, B.-W.; Ko, C.-C. Dopamine suppresses osteoclast differentiation via cAMP/PKA/CREB pathway. *Cell. Signal.* **2021**, *78*, 109847. [CrossRef] [PubMed]
35. Yuan, Z.; Tao, B.; He, Y.; Mu, C.; Liu, G.; Zhang, J.; Liao, Q.; Liu, P.; Cai, K. Remote eradication of biofilm on titanium implant via near-infrared light triggered photothermal/photodynamic therapy strategy. *Biomaterials* **2019**, *223*, 119479. [CrossRef] [PubMed]
36. Sheng, W.; Li, W.; Yu, B.; Li, B.; Jordan, R.; Jia, X.; Zhou, F. Mussel-Inspired Two-Dimensional Freestanding Alkyl-Polydopamine Janus Nanosheets. *Angew. Chem. Int. Ed. Engl.* **2019**, *58*, 12018–12022. [CrossRef] [PubMed]
37. Park, J.; Brust, T.F.; Lee, H.J.; Lee, S.C.; Watts, V.J.; Yeo, Y. Polydopamine-Based Simple and Versatile Surface Modification of Polymeric Nano Drug Carriers. *ACS Nano* **2014**, *8*, 3347–3356. [CrossRef]
38. Zhu, M.; Shi, Y.; Shan, Y.; Guo, J.; Song, X.; Wu, Y.; Wu, M.; Lu, Y.; Chen, W.; Xu, X.; et al. Recent developments in mesoporous polydopamine-derived nanoplatforms for cancer theranostics. *J. Nanobiotechnol.* **2021**, *19*, 387. [CrossRef]
39. Jing, X.; Mi, H.-Y.; Lin, Y.-J.; Enriquez, E.; Peng, X.-F.; Turng, L.-S. Highly Stretchable and Biocompatible Strain Sensors Based on Mussel-Inspired Super-Adhesive Self-Healing Hydrogels for Human Motion Monitoring. *ACS Appl. Mater. Interfaces* **2018**, *10*, 20897–20909. [CrossRef]
40. Rossi, F.; Kurashina, Y.; Onoe, H. Can nanoparticles enhance drug-delivery performance of hydrogels? *Nanomedicine* **2023**, *18*, 653–657. [CrossRef]
41. Mohammadpour, R.; Dobrovolskaia, M.A.; Cheney, D.L.; Greish, K.F.; Ghandehari, H. Subchronic and chronic toxicity evaluation of inorganic nanoparticles for delivery applications. *Adv. Drug Deliv. Rev.* **2019**, *144*, 112–132. [CrossRef] [PubMed]
42. Paris, J.L.; Baeza, A.; Vallet-Regí, M. Overcoming the stability, toxicity, and biodegradation challenges of tumor stimuli-responsive inorganic nanoparticles for delivery of cancer therapeutics. *Expert Opin. Drug Deliv.* **2019**, *16*, 1095–1112. [CrossRef] [PubMed]
43. Wang, X.; Yu, X.; Wang, X.; Qi, M.; Pan, J.; Wang, Q. One-Step Nanosurface Self-Assembly of d-Peptides Renders Bubble-Free Ultrasound Theranostics. *Nano Lett.* **2019**, *19*, 2251–2258. [CrossRef]
44. Zhu, J.; Feng, C.; Zhang, W.; Zhong, M.; Tang, W.; Wang, Z.; Shi, H.; Yin, Z.; Shi, J.; Huang, Y.; et al. Activation of dopamine receptor D1 promotes osteogenic differentiation and reduces glucocorticoid-induced bone loss by upregulating the ERK1/2 signaling pathway. *Mol. Med.* **2022**, *28*, 23. [CrossRef] [PubMed]
45. Zhu, Y.; Liu, D.; Wang, X.; He, Y.; Luan, W.; Qi, F.; Ding, J. Polydopamine-mediated covalent functionalization of collagen on a titanium alloy to promote biocompatibility with soft tissues. *J. Mater. Chem. B* **2019**, *7*, 2019–2031. [CrossRef]
46. Kim, H.; Lee, Y.H.; Kim, N.K.; Kang, I.K. Immobilization of Collagen on the Surface of a PEEK Implant with Monolayer Nanopores. *Polymers* **2022**, *14*, 1633. [CrossRef]
47. Xue, X.; Hu, Y.; Wang, S.; Chen, X.; Jiang, Y.; Su, J. Fabrication of physical and chemical crosslinked hydrogels for bone tissue engineering. *Bioact. Mater.* **2021**, *12*, 327–339. [CrossRef]
48. Lu, G.; Xu, Y.; Liu, Q.; Chen, M.; Sun, H.; Wang, P.; Wang, Y.; Li, X.; Hui, X.; Luo, E.; et al. An instantly fixable and self-adaptive scaffold for skull regeneration by autologous stem cell recruitment and angiogenesis. *Nat. Commun.* **2022**, *13*, 2499. [CrossRef]
49. Wang, Y.; Qi, H.; Miron, R.J.; Zhang, Y. Modulating macrophage polarization on titanium implant surface by poly(dopamine)-assisted immobilization of IL4. *Clin. Implant. Dent. Relat. Res.* **2019**, *21*, 977–986. [CrossRef]

50. Su, J.; Du, Z.; Xiao, L.; Wei, F.; Yang, Y.; Li, M.; Qiu, Y.; Liu, J.; Chen, J.; Xiao, Y. Graphene oxide coated Titanium Surfaces with Osteoimmunomodulatory Role to Enhance Osteogenesis. *Mater. Sci. Eng. C* **2020**, *113*, 110983. [CrossRef]
51. Zhang, D.; Zheng, H.; Geng, K.; Shen, J.; Feng, X.; Xu, P.; Duan, Y.; Li, Y.; Wu, R.; Gou, Z.; et al. Large fuzzy biodegradable polyester microspheres with dopamine deposition enhance cell adhesion and bone regeneration in vivo. *Biomaterials* **2021**, *272*, 120783. [CrossRef] [PubMed]
52. Agilan, P.; Saranya, K.; Rajendran, N. Bio-inspired polydopamine incorporated titania nanotube arrays for biomedical applications. *Colloids Surf. A Physicochem. Eng. Asp.* **2021**, *629*, 127489. [CrossRef]
53. Qiaoxia, L.; Yujie, Z.; Meng, Y.; Yizhu, C.; Yan, W.; Yinchun, H.; Xiaojie, L.; Weiyi, C.; Di, H. Hydroxyapatite/tannic acid composite coating formation based on Ti modified by TiO_2 nanotubes. *Colloids Surf. B Biointerfaces* **2020**, *196*, 111304. [CrossRef] [PubMed]
54. Yang, H.; Xu, Y.; Zhu, M.; Gu, Y.; Zhang, W.; Shao, H.; Wang, Y.; Ping, Z.; Hu, X.; Wang, L.; et al. Inhibition of titanium-particle-induced inflammatory osteolysis after local administration of dopamine and suppression of osteoclastogenesis via D2-like receptor signaling pathway. *Biomaterials* **2016**, *80*, 1–10. [CrossRef]
55. Li, Y.; Yang, C.; Yin, X.; Sun, Y.; Weng, J.; Zhou, J.; Feng, B. Inflammatory responses to micro/nano-structured titanium surfaces with silver nanoparticles in vitro. *J. Mater. Chem. B* **2019**, *7*, 3546–3559. [CrossRef]
56. Feng, P.; Liu, M.; Peng, S.; Bin, S.; Zhao, Z.; Shuai, C. Polydopamine modified polycaprolactone powder for fabrication bone scaffold owing intrinsic bioactivity. *J. Mater. Res. Technol.* **2021**, *15*, 3375–3385. [CrossRef]
57. Cheng, J.; Liu, H.; Zhao, B.; Shen, R.; Liu, D.; Hong, J.; Wei, H.; Xi, P.; Chen, F.; Bai, D. MC3T3-E1 preosteoblast cell-mediated mineralization of hydroxyapatite by poly-dopamine-functionalized graphene oxide. *J. Bioact. Compat. Polym.* **2015**, *30*, 289–301. [CrossRef]
58. Chen, J.; Mei, M.L.; Li, Q.-L.; Chu, C.-H. Mussel-inspired silver-nanoparticle coating on porous titanium surfaces to promote mineralization. *RSC Adv.* **2016**, *6*, 104025–104035. [CrossRef]
59. Wu, M.; Wang, T.; Wang, Y.; Wang, H. Ultrafast bone-like apatite formation on bioactive tricalcium silicate cement using mussel-inspired polydopamine. *Ceram. Int.* **2019**, *45*, 3033–3043. [CrossRef]
60. Lin, H.; Fu, Y.; Gao, Y.; Mo, A. Integrated design of a mussel-inspired hydrogel biofilm composite structure to guide bone regeneration. *Macromol. Mater. Eng.* **2020**, *305*, 2000064. [CrossRef]
61. Chien, C.; Liu, T.; Kuo, W.; Wang, M.; Tsai, W. Dopamine-assisted immobilization of hydroxyapatite nanoparticles and RGD peptides to improve the osteoconductivity of titanium. *J. Biomed. Mater. Res. Part A* **2013**, *101*, 740–747. [CrossRef] [PubMed]
62. Bachir, A.I.; Zareno, J.; Moissoglu, K.; Plow, E.F.; Gratton, E.; Horwitz, A.R. Integrin-associated complexes form hierarchically with variable stoichiometry in nascent adhesions. *Curr. Biol.* **2014**, *24*, 1845–1853. [CrossRef]
63. Yuan, Z.; Huang, S.; Lan, S.; Xiong, H.; Tao, B.; Ding, Y.; Liu, Y.; Liu, P.; Cai, K. Surface engineering of titanium implants with enzyme-triggered antibacterial properties and enhanced osseointegration in vivo. *J. Mater. Chem. B* **2018**, *6*, 8090–8104. [CrossRef] [PubMed]
64. Yin, H.-M.; Mao, C.; Liu, W.; Liu, Y.-H.; Ren, Y.; Xu, L.; Xu, J.-Z.; Zhao, B.; Gul, R.M.; Li, Z.-M. Nanotopographical polymeric surface with mussel-inspired decoration to enhance osteoblast differentiation. *Appl. Surf. Sci.* **2019**, *481*, 987–993. [CrossRef]
65. Yang, Y.; Xu, T.; Bei, H.P.; Zhao, Y.; Zhao, X. Sculpting bio-inspired surface textures: An adhesive janus periosteum. *Adv. Funct. Mater.* **2021**, *31*, 2104636. [CrossRef]
66. Hanami, K.; Nakano, K.; Saito, K.; Okada, Y.; Yamaoka, K.; Kubo, S.; Kondo, M.; Tanaka, Y. Dopamine D2-like receptor signaling suppresses human osteoclastogenesis. *Bone* **2013**, *56*, 1–8. [CrossRef]
67. Chiang, T.-I.; Lane, H.-Y.; Lin, C.-H. D2 dopamine receptor gene (DRD2) Taq1A (rs1800497) affects bone density. *Sci. Rep.* **2020**, *10*, 13236. [CrossRef]
68. Liu, Y.; Chen, Q.; Jeong, H.-W.; Han, D.; Fabian, J.; Drexler, H.C.; Stehling, M.; Schöler, H.R.; Adams, R.H. Dopamine signaling regulates hematopoietic stem and progenitor cell function. *Blood* **2021**, *138*, 2051–2065. [CrossRef]
69. Wang, C.-X.; Ge, X.-Y.; Wang, M.-Y.; Ma, T.; Zhang, Y.; Lin, Y. Dopamine D1 receptor-mediated activation of the ERK signaling pathway is involved in the osteogenic differentiation of bone mesenchymal stem cells. *Stem Cell Res. Ther.* **2020**, *11*, 12. [CrossRef]
70. Taylor, E.L.; Weaver, S.R.; Lorang, I.M.; Arnold, K.M.; Bradley, E.W.; de Velasco, E.M.F.; Wickman, K.; Westendorf, J.J. GIRK3 deletion facilitates kappa opioid signaling in chondrocytes, delays vascularization and promotes bone lengthening in mice. *Bone* **2022**, *159*, 116391. [CrossRef]
71. Wang, J.; Cui, Y.; Zhang, B.; Sun, S.; Xu, H.; Yao, M.; Wu, D.; Wang, Y. Polydopamine-Modified functional materials promote bone regeneration. *Mater. Des.* **2024**, *238*, 112655. [CrossRef]
72. Gao, B.; Chen, L.; Zhao, Y.; Yan, X.; Wang, X.; Zhou, C.; Shi, Y.; Xue, W. Methods to prepare dopamine/polydopamine modified alginate hydrogels and their special improved properties for drug delivery. *Eur. Polym. J.* **2019**, *110*, 192–201. [CrossRef]
73. Jing, X.; Mi, H.-Y.; Napiwocki, B.N.; Peng, X.-F.; Turng, L.-S. Mussel-inspired electroactive chitosan/graphene oxide composite hydrogel with rapid self-healing and recovery behavior for tissue engineering. *Carbon* **2017**, *125*, 557–570. [CrossRef]

74. Di, X.; Hang, C.; Xu, Y.; Ma, Q.; Li, F.; Sun, P.; Wu, G. Bioinspired tough, conductive hydrogels with thermally reversible adhesiveness based on nanoclay confined NIPAM polymerization and a dopamine modified polypeptide. *Mater. Chem. Front.* **2020**, *4*, 189–196. [CrossRef]
75. Wang, X.; Wang, C.; Wang, X.; Wang, Y.; Zhang, Q.; Cheng, Y. A Polydopamine Nanoparticle-Knotted Poly(ethylene glycol) Hydrogel for On-Demand Drug Delivery and Chemo-photothermal Therapy. *Chem. Mater.* **2017**, *29*, 1370–1376. [CrossRef]
76. Han, L.; Li, P.; Tang, P.; Wang, X.; Zhou, T.; Wang, K.; Ren, F.; Guo, T.; Lu, X. Mussel-inspired cryogels for promoting wound regeneration through photobiostimulation, modulating inflammatory responses and suppressing bacterial invasion. *Nanoscale* **2019**, *11*, 15846–15861. [CrossRef]
77. Liu, Y.; Xi, Y.; Zhao, J.; Zhao, J.; Li, J.; Huang, G.; Li, J.; Fang, F.; Gu, L.; Wang, S. Preparation of therapeutic-laden konjac hydrogel for tumor combination therapy. *Chem. Eng. J.* **2019**, *375*, 122048. [CrossRef]
78. Zeng, J.; Shi, D.; Gu, Y.; Kaneko, T.; Zhang, L.; Zhang, H.; Kaneko, D.; Chen, M. Injectable and Near-Infrared-Responsive Hydrogels Encapsulating Dopamine-Stabilized Gold Nanorods with Long Photothermal Activity Controlled for Tumor Therapy. *Biomacromolecules* **2019**, *20*, 3375–3384. [CrossRef]
79. Wu, Y.; Wang, H.; Gao, F.; Xu, Z.; Dai, F.; Liu, W. An Injectable Supramolecular Polymer Nanocomposite Hydrogel for Prevention of Breast Cancer Recurrence with Theranostic and Mammoplastic Functions. *Adv. Funct. Mater.* **2018**, *28*, 1801000. [CrossRef]
80. Song, J.; Hu, H.; Jian, C.; Wu, K.; Chen, X. New Generation of Gold Nanoshell-Coated Esophageal Stent: Preparation and Biomedical Applications. *ACS Appl. Mater. Interfaces* **2016**, *8*, 27523–27529. [CrossRef]
81. Han, L.; Liu, K.; Wang, M.; Wang, K.; Fang, L.; Chen, H.; Zhou, J.; Lu, X. Mussel-Inspired Adhesive and Conductive Hydrogel with Long-Lasting Moisture and Extreme Temperature Tolerance. *Adv. Funct. Mater.* **2018**, *28*, 1704195. [CrossRef]
82. Wan, Z.; Dong, Q.; Guo, X.; Bai, X.; Zhang, X.; Zhang, P.; Liu, Y.; Lv, L.; Zhou, Y. A dual-responsive polydopamine-modified hydroxybutyl chitosan hydrogel for sequential regulation of bone regeneration. *Carbohydr. Polym.* **2022**, *297*, 120027. [CrossRef]
83. Zhang, S.; Xu, K.; Darabi, M.A.; Yuan, Q.; Xing, M. Mussel-inspired alginate gel promoting the osteogenic differentiation of mesenchymal stem cells and anti-infection. *Mater. Sci. Eng. C* **2016**, *69*, 496–504. [CrossRef]
84. Chen, S.; Wang, Y.; Zhang, X.; Ma, J.; Wang, M. Double-crosslinked bifunctional hydrogels with encapsulated anti-cancer drug for bone tumor cell ablation and bone tissue regeneration. *Colloids Surf. B Biointerfaces* **2022**, *213*, 112364. [CrossRef]
85. Gan, D.; Wang, Z.; Xie, C.; Wang, X.; Xing, W.; Ge, X.; Yuan, H.; Wang, K.; Tan, H.; Lu, X. Mussel-Inspired Tough Hydrogel with In Situ Nanohydroxyapatite Mineralization for Osteochondral Defect Repair. *Adv. Healthc. Mater.* **2019**, *12*, e2203040. [CrossRef] [PubMed]
86. Wu, Y.; Zhang, X.; Tan, B.; Shan, Y.; Zhao, X.; Liao, J. Near-infrared light control of GelMA/PMMA/PDA hydrogel with mild photothermal therapy for skull regeneration. *Mater. Sci. Eng. C Mater. Biol. Appl.* **2022**, *133*, 112641. [CrossRef] [PubMed]
87. Dashtimoghadam, E.; Fahimipour, F.; Tongas, N.; Tayebi, L. Microfluidic fabrication of microcarriers with sequential delivery of VEGF and BMP-2 for bone regeneration. *Sci. Rep.* **2020**, *10*, 11764. [CrossRef]
88. Li, X.; Pang, Y.; Guan, L.; Li, L.; Zhu, Y.; Whittaker, A.K.; Yang, B.; Zhu, S.; Lin, Q. Mussel-inspired antimicrobial hydrogel with cellulose nanocrystals/tannic acid modified silver nanoparticles for enhanced calvarial bone regeneration. *Int. J. Biol. Macromol.* **2024**, *270 Pt 2*, 132419. [CrossRef]
89. Han, Z.; Wang, F.; Xiong, W.; Meng, C.; Yao, Y.; Cui, W.; Zhang, M. Precise Cell Type Electrical Stimulation Therapy Via Force-electric Hydrogel Microspheres for Cartilage Healing. *Adv. Mater.* **2024**, *37*, e2414555. [CrossRef]
90. Sun, H.; Shang, Y.; Guo, J.; Maihemuti, A.; Shen, S.; Shi, Y.; Liu, H.; Che, J.; Jiang, Q. Artificial Periosteum with Oriented Surface Nanotopography and High Tissue Adherent Property. *ACS Appl. Mater. Interfaces* **2023**, *15*, 45549–45560. [CrossRef]
91. Chen, S.; Tan, S.; Zheng, L.; Wang, M. Multilayered Shape-Morphing Scaffolds with a Hierarchical Structure for Uterine Tissue Regeneration. *ACS Appl. Mater. Interfaces* **2024**, *16*, 6772–6788. [CrossRef]
92. Li, H.; Zhao, T.; Yuan, Z.; Gao, T.; Yang, Y.; Li, R.; Tian, Q.; Tang, P.; Guo, Q.; Zhang, L. Cartilage lacuna-biomimetic hydrogel microspheres endowed with integrated biological signal boost endogenous articular cartilage regeneration. *Bioact. Mater.* **2024**, *41*, 61–82. [CrossRef]
93. Wu, M.; Liu, H.; Li, D.; Zhu, Y.; Wu, P.; Chen, Z.; Chen, F.; Chen, Y.; Deng, Z.; Cai, L. Smart-Responsive Multifunctional Therapeutic System for Improved Regenerative Microenvironment and Accelerated Bone Regeneration via Mild Photothermal Therapy. *Adv. Sci.* **2024**, *11*, e2304641. [CrossRef] [PubMed]
94. Wu, M.; Zhang, Y.; Zhao, Y.; Chu, L.; Meng, X.; Ye, L.; Li, X.; Wang, Z.; Wu, P. Photoactivated Hydrogel Therapeutic System with MXene-Based Nanoarchitectonics Potentiates Endogenous Bone Repair Through Reshaping the Osteo-Vascularization Network. *Small* **2024**, *20*, e2403003. [CrossRef] [PubMed]
95. Kang, J.; Li, Y.; Qin, Y.; Huang, Z.; Wu, Y.; Sun, L.; Wang, C.; Wang, W.; Feng, G.; Qi, Y. In Situ Deposition of Drug and Gene Nanoparticles on a Patterned Supramolecular Hydrogel to Construct a Directionally Osteochondral Plug. *Nano-Micro Lett.* **2023**, *16*, 18. [CrossRef] [PubMed]

96. Zhang, R.; Jo, J.-I.; Kanda, R.; Nishiura, A.; Hashimoto, Y.; Matsumoto, N. Bioactive Polyetheretherketone with Gelatin Hydrogel Leads to Sustained Release of Bone Morphogenetic Protein-2 and Promotes Osteogenic Differentiation. *Int. J. Mol. Sci.* **2023**, *24*, 12741. [CrossRef]
97. Li, M.; Wu, H.; Gao, K.; Wang, Y.; Hu, J.; Guo, Z.; Hu, R.; Zhang, M.; Pang, X.; Guo, M.; et al. Smart Implantable Hydrogel for Large Segmental Bone Regeneration. *Adv. Healthc. Mater.* **2024**, *13*, e2402916. [CrossRef]
98. Wu, M.; Chen, F.; Liu, H.; Wu, P.; Yang, Z.; Zhang, Z.; Su, J.; Cai, L.; Zhang, Y. Bioinspired sandwich-like hybrid surface functionalized scaffold capable of regulating osteogenesis, angiogenesis, and osteoclastogenesis for robust bone regeneration. *Mater. Today Bio* **2022**, *17*, 100458. [CrossRef]
99. Wu, Y.; Li, X.; Sun, Y.; Tan, X.; Wang, C.; Wang, Z.; Ye, L. Multiscale design of stiffening and ROS scavenging hydrogels for the augmentation of mandibular bone regeneration. *Bioact. Mater.* **2022**, *20*, 111–125. [CrossRef]
100. Wu, M.; Liu, H.; Zhu, Y.; Wu, P.; Chen, Y.; Deng, Z.; Zhu, X.; Cai, L. Bioinspired soft-hard combined system with mild photothermal therapeutic activity promotes diabetic bone defect healing via synergetic effects of immune activation and angiogenesis. *Theranostics* **2024**, *14*, 4014–4057. [CrossRef]
101. Shi, W.; Gao, Y.; Wu, Y.; Sun, J.; Xu, B.; Lu, X.; Wang, Q. A multifunctional polydopamine/genipin/alendronate nanoparticle licences fibrin hydrogels osteoinductive and immunomodulatory potencies for repairing bone defects. *Int. J. Biol. Macromol.* **2023**, *249*, 126072. [CrossRef] [PubMed]
102. Ma, K.; Yang, L.; Li, W.; Chen, K.; Shang, L.; Bai, Y.; Zhao, Y. Mussel-inspired multi-bioactive microsphere scaffolds for bone defect photothermal therapy. *Mater. Today Bio* **2024**, *29*, 101363. [CrossRef]
103. Wu, M.; Liu, H.; Zhu, Y.; Chen, F.; Chen, Z.; Guo, L.; Wu, P.; Li, G.; Zhang, C.; Wei, R.; et al. Mild Photothermal-Stimulation Based on Injectable and Photocurable Hydrogels Orchestrates Immunomodulation and Osteogenesis for High-Performance Bone Regeneration. *Small* **2023**, *19*, e2300111. [CrossRef]
104. Huang, L.; Wu, T.; Sun, J.; Lin, X.; Peng, Y.; Zhang, R.; Gao, Y.; Xu, S.; Sun, Y.; Zhou, Y.; et al. Biocompatible chitin-based Janus hydrogel membranes for periodontal repair. *Acta Biomater.* **2024**, *190*, 219–232. [CrossRef] [PubMed]
105. Xu, H.; Zhang, G.; Xu, K.; Wang, L.; Yu, L.; Xing, M.M.; Qiu, X. Mussel-inspired dual-functional PEG hydrogel inducing mineralization and inhibiting infection in maxillary bone reconstruction. *Mater. Sci. Eng. C* **2018**, *90*, 379–386. [CrossRef] [PubMed]
106. Wu, P.; Shen, L.; Liu, H.-F.; Zou, X.-H.; Zhao, J.; Huang, Y.; Zhu, Y.-F.; Li, Z.-Y.; Xu, C.; Luo, L.-H.; et al. The marriage of immunomodulatory, angiogenic, and osteogenic capabilities in a piezoelectric hydrogel tissue engineering scaffold for military medicine. *Mil. Med. Res.* **2023**, *10*, 35. [CrossRef]
107. Chen, Y.-W.; Shen, Y.-F.; Ho, C.-C.; Yu, J.; Wu, Y.-H.A.; Wang, K.; Shih, C.-T.; Shie, M.-Y. Osteogenic and angiogenic potentials of the cell-laden hydrogel/mussel-inspired calcium silicate complex hierarchical porous scaffold fabricated by 3D bioprinting. *Mater. Sci. Eng. C* **2018**, *91*, 679–687. [CrossRef]
108. Liu, C.; Wu, J.; Gan, D.; Li, Z.; Shen, J.; Tang, P.; Luo, S.; Li, P.; Lu, X.; Zheng, W. The characteristics of mussel-inspired nHA/OSA injectable hydrogel and repaired bone defect in rabbit. *J. Biomed. Mater. Res. Part B Appl. Biomater.* **2020**, *108*, 1814–1825. [CrossRef]
109. Pang, Y.; Guan, L.; Zhu, Y.; Niu, R.; Zhu, S.; Lin, Q. Gallic acid-grafted chitosan antibacterial hydrogel incorporated with polydopamine-modified hydroxyapatite for enhancing bone healing. *Front. Bioeng. Biotechnol.* **2023**, *11*, 1162202. [CrossRef]
110. Kwack, K.H.; Ji, J.Y.; Park, B.; Heo, J.S. Fucoidan (*Undaria pinnatifida*)/Polydopamine Composite-Modified Surface Promotes Osteogenic Potential of Periodontal Ligament Stem Cells. *Mar. Drugs* **2022**, *20*, 181. [CrossRef]
111. Deng, H.; Shu, X.; Wang, Y.; Zhang, J.; Yin, Y.; Wu, F.; He, J. Matrix Stiffness Regulated Endoplasmic Reticulum Stress-mediated Apoptosis of Osteosarcoma Cell through Ras Signal Cascades. *Cell Biochem. Biophys.* **2023**, *81*, 839–850. [CrossRef] [PubMed]
112. Zhong, W.; Xiong, Y.; Wang, X.; Yu, T.; Zhou, C. Synthesis and characterization of multifunctional organic-inorganic composite hydrogel formed with tissue-adhesive property and inhibiting infection. *Mater. Sci. Eng. C* **2021**, *118*, 111532. [CrossRef] [PubMed]
113. Wu, Y.; Lyu, Z.; Hu, F.; Yang, L.; Yang, K.; Chen, M.; Wang, Y. A chondroitin sulphate hydrogel with sustained release of SDF-1α for extensive cartilage defect repair through induction of cell homing and promotion of chondrogenesis. *J. Mater. Chem. B* **2024**, *12*, 8672–8687. [CrossRef]
114. Zhou, Q.; Liu, J.; Yan, J.; Guo, Z.; Zhang, F. Magnetic microspheres mimicking certain functions of macrophages: Towards precise antibacterial potency for bone defect healing. *Mater. Today Bio* **2023**, *20*, 100651. [CrossRef]
115. Li, S.; Jia, C.; Han, H.; Yang, Y.; Xiaowen, Y.; Chen, Z. Characterization and biocompatibility of a bilayer PEEK-based scaffold for guiding bone regeneration. *BMC Oral Health* **2024**, *24*, 1138. [CrossRef]
116. Liu, H.; Li, K.; Yi, D.; Ding, Y.; Gao, Y.; Zheng, X. Deferoxamine-Loaded Chitosan-Based Hydrogel on Bone Implants Showing Enhanced Bond Strength and Pro-Angiogenic Effects. *J. Funct. Biomater.* **2024**, *15*, 112. [CrossRef] [PubMed]
117. Fang, X.; Wang, J.; Ye, C.; Lin, J.; Ran, J.; Jia, Z.; Gong, J.; Zhang, Y.; Xiang, J.; Lu, X.; et al. Polyphenol-mediated redox-active hydrogel with H2S gaseous-bioelectric coupling for periodontal bone healing in diabetes. *Nat. Commun.* **2024**, *15*, 9071. [CrossRef]

118. Im, S.; Choe, G.; Seok, J.M.; Yeo, S.J.; Lee, J.H.; Kim, W.D.; Lee, J.Y.; Park, S.A. An osteogenic bioink composed of alginate, cellulose nanofibrils, and polydopamine nanoparticles for 3D bioprinting and bone tissue engineering. *Int. J. Biol. Macromol.* **2022**, *205*, 520–529. [CrossRef]
119. Ma, W.; Yang, M.; Wu, C.; Wang, S.; Du, M. Bioinspired self-healing injectable nanocomposite hydrogels based on oxidized dextran and gelatin for growth-factor-free bone regeneration. *Int. J. Biol. Macromol.* **2023**, *251*, 126145. [CrossRef]
120. Luo, S.; Wu, J.; Jia, Z.; Tang, P.; Sheng, J.; Xie, C.; Liu, C.; Gan, D.; Hu, D.; Zheng, W.; et al. An Injectable, Bifunctional Hydrogel with Photothermal Effects for Tumor Therapy and Bone Regeneration. *Macromol. Biosci.* **2019**, *19*, e1900047. [CrossRef]
121. Jung, A.; Makkar, P.; Amirian, J.; Lee, B.-T. A novel hybrid multichannel biphasic calcium phosphate granule-based composite scaffold for cartilage tissue regeneration. *J. Biomater. Appl.* **2018**, *32*, 775–787. [CrossRef] [PubMed]
122. Douglas, T.; Wlodarczyk, M.; Pamula, E.; Declercq, H.; de Mulder, E.; Bucko, M.; Balcaen, L.; Vanhaecke, F.; Cornelissen, R.; Dubruel, P.; et al. Enzymatic mineralization of gellan gum hydrogel for bone tissue-engineering applications and its enhancement by polydopamine. *J. Tissue Eng. Regen. Med.* **2014**, *8*, 906–918. [CrossRef]
123. Liu, Y.; Wei, X.; Yang, T.; Wang, X.; Li, T.; Sun, M.; Jiao, K.; Jia, W.; Yang, Y.; Yan, Y.; et al. Hyaluronic acid methacrylate/Pluronic F127 hydrogel enhanced with spermidine-modified mesoporous polydopamine nanoparticles for efficient synergistic periodontitis treatment. *Int. J. Biol. Macromol.* **2024**, *281 Pt 1*, 136085. [CrossRef] [PubMed]
124. Li, Y.; Tang, S.; Luo, Z.; Liu, K.; Luo, Y.; Wen, W.; Ding, S.; Li, L.; Liu, M.; Zhou, C.; et al. Chitin whisker/chitosan liquid crystal hydrogel assisted scaffolds with bone-like ECM microenvironment for bone regeneration. *Carbohydr. Polym.* **2024**, *332*, 121927. [CrossRef] [PubMed]
125. Ma, W.; Chen, H.; Cheng, S.; Wu, C.; Wang, L.; Du, M. Gelatin hydrogel reinforced with mussel-inspired polydopamine-functionalized nanohydroxyapatite for bone regeneration. *Int. J. Biol. Macromol.* **2023**, *240*, 124287. [CrossRef]
126. Li, M.; Wei, F.; Yin, X.; Xiao, L.; Yang, L.; Su, J.; Weng, J.; Feng, B.; Xiao, Y.; Zhou, Y. Synergistic regulation of osteoimmune microenvironment by IL-4 and RGD to accelerate osteogenesis. *Mater. Sci. Eng. C* **2020**, *109*, 110508. [CrossRef]
127. Yan, L.; Zhou, T.; Ni, R.; Jia, Z.; Jiang, Y.; Guo, T.; Wang, K.; Chen, X.; Han, L.; Lu, X. Adhesive Gelatin-Catechol Complex Reinforced Poly(Acrylic Acid) Hydrogel with Enhanced Toughness and Cell Affinity for Cartilage Regeneration. *ACS Appl. Bio Mater.* **2020**, *5*, 4366–4377. [CrossRef]
128. Zhang, F.-X.; Liu, P.; Ding, W.; Meng, Q.-B.; Su, D.-H.; Zhang, Q.-C.; Lian, R.-X.; Yu, B.-Q.; Zhao, M.-D.; Dong, J.; et al. Injectable Mussel-Inspired highly adhesive hydrogel with exosomes for endogenous cell recruitment and cartilage defect regeneration. *Biomaterials* **2021**, *278*, 121169. [CrossRef]
129. Xu, Y.; Zhao, S.; Weng, Z.; Zhang, W.; Wan, X.; Cui, T.; Ye, J.; Liao, L.; Wang, X. Jelly-Inspired Injectable Guided Tissue Regeneration Strategy with Shape Auto-Matched and Dual-Light-Defined Antibacterial/Osteogenic Pattern Switch Properties. *ACS Appl. Mater. Interfaces* **2020**, *12*, 54497–54506. [CrossRef]
130. Ren, S.; Tang, X.; Liu, L.; Meng, F.; Yang, X.; Li, N.; Zhang, Z.; Aimaijiang, M.; Liu, M.; Liu, X.; et al. Reinforced Blood-Derived Protein Hydrogels Enable Dual-Level Regulation of Bio-Physiochemical Microenvironments for Personalized Bone Regeneration with Remarkable Enhanced Efficacy. *Nano Lett.* **2022**, *22*, 3904–3913. [CrossRef]
131. Li, Y.; Liu, X.; Li, B.; Zheng, Y.; Han, Y.; Chen, D.-F.; Yeung, K.W.K.; Cui, Z.; Liang, Y.; Li, Z.; et al. Near-Infrared Light Triggered Phototherapy and Immunotherapy for Elimination of Methicillin-Resistant *Staphylococcus aureus* Biofilm Infection on Bone Implant. *ACS Nano* **2020**, *14*, 8157–8170. [CrossRef] [PubMed]
132. Li, N.; Liu, L.; Wei, C.; Ren, S.; Liu, X.; Wang, X.; Song, J.; Li, Y.; Wang, Z.; Qiao, S.; et al. Immunomodulatory Blood-Derived Hybrid Hydrogels as Multichannel Microenvironment Modulators for Augmented Bone Regeneration. *ACS Appl. Mater. Interfaces* **2022**, *14*, 53523–53534. [CrossRef]
133. Yin, J.; Han, Q.; Zhang, J.; Liu, Y.; Gan, X.; Xie, K.; Xie, L.; Deng, Y. MXene-Based Hydrogels Endow Polyetheretherketone with Effective Osteogenicity and Combined Treatment of Osteosarcoma and Bacterial Infection. *ACS Appl. Mater. Interfaces* **2020**, *12*, 45891–45903. [CrossRef]
134. Zheng, L.; Li, D.; Wang, W.; Zhang, Q.; Zhou, X.; Liu, D.; Zhang, J.; You, Z.; Zhang, J.; He, C. Bilayered Scaffold Prepared from a Kartogenin-Loaded Hydrogel and BMP-2-Derived Peptide-Loaded Porous Nanofibrous Scaffold for Osteochondral Defect Repair. *ACS Biomater. Sci. Eng.* **2019**, *5*, 4564–4573. [CrossRef]
135. Abie, N.; Ünlü, C.; Pinho, A.R.; Gomes, M.C.; Remmler, T.; Herb, M.; Grumme, D.; Tabesh, E.; Shahbazi, M.-A.; Mathur, S.; et al. Designing of a Multifunctional 3D-Printed Biomimetic Theragenerative Aerogel Scaffold via Mussel-Inspired Chemistry: Bioactive Glass Nanofiber-Incorporated Self-Assembled Silk Fibroin with Antibacterial, Antiosteosarcoma, and Osteoinductive Properties. *ACS Appl. Mater. Interfaces* **2024**, *16*, 22809–22827. [CrossRef]
136. Zhao, J.; Qiu, P.; Wang, Y.; Wang, Y.; Zhou, J.; Zhang, B.; Zhang, L.; Gou, D. Chitosan-based hydrogel wound dressing: From mechanism to applications, a review. *Int. J. Biol. Macromol.* **2023**, *244*, 125250. [CrossRef]
137. Sarmah, D.; Rather, M.A.; Sarkar, A.; Mandal, M.; Sankaranarayanan, K.; Karak, N. Self-cross-linked starch/chitosan hydrogel as a biocompatible vehicle for controlled release of drug. *Int. J. Biol. Macromol.* **2023**, *237*, 124206. [CrossRef] [PubMed]

138. Hu, Z.; Liu, D.; Wang, M.; Yu, C.; Han, Z.; Xu, M.; Yue, W.; Nie, G. β-Alanine enhancing the crosslink of chitosan/poly-(γ-glutamic acid) hydrogel for a potential alkaline-adapted wound dressing. *Int. J. Biol. Macromol.* **2023**, *231*, 123157. [CrossRef] [PubMed]
139. Mu, M.; Li, X.; Tong, A.; Guo, G. Multi-functional chitosan-based smart hydrogels mediated biomedical application. *Expert Opin. Drug Deliv.* **2019**, *16*, 239–250. [CrossRef]
140. Gou, D.; Qiu, P.; Hong, F.; Wang, Y.; Ren, P.; Cheng, X.; Wang, L.; Liu, T.; Liu, J.; Zhao, J. Polydopamine modified multifunctional carboxymethyl chitosan/pectin hydrogel loaded with recombinant human epidermal growth factor for diabetic wound healing. *Int. J. Biol. Macromol.* **2024**, *274*, 132917. [CrossRef]
141. Oh, D.X.; Hwang, D.S. A biomimetic chitosan composite with improved mechanical properties in wet conditions. *Biotechnol. Prog.* **2013**, *29*, 505–512. [CrossRef] [PubMed]
142. Zhang, X.; Hassanzadeh, P.; Miyake, T.; Jin, J.; Rolandi, M. Squid beak inspired water processable chitosan composites with tunable mechanical properties. *J. Mater. Chem. B* **2016**, *4*, 2273–2279. [CrossRef]
143. Ryu, J.H.; Jo, S.; Koh, M.; Lee, H. Bio-Inspired, Water-Soluble to Insoluble Self-Conversion for Flexible, Biocompatible, Transparent, Catecholamine Polysaccharide Thin Films. *Adv. Funct. Mater.* **2014**, *24*, 7709–7716. [CrossRef]
144. Edson, J.A.; Ingato, D.; Wu, S.; Lee, B.; Kwon, Y.J. Aqueous-Soluble, Acid-Transforming Chitosan for Efficient and Stimuli-Responsive Gene Silencing. *Biomacromolecules* **2018**, *19*, 1508–1516. [CrossRef] [PubMed]
145. Kim, K.; Ryu, J.H.; Lee, D.Y.; Lee, H. Bio-inspired catechol conjugation converts water-insoluble chitosan into a highly water-soluble, adhesive chitosan derivative for hydrogels and LbL assembly. *Biomater. Sci.* **2013**, *1*, 783–790. [CrossRef]
146. Qiao, H.; Sun, M.; Su, Z.; Xie, Y.; Chen, M.; Zong, L.; Gao, Y.; Li, H.; Qi, J.; Zhao, Q.; et al. Kidney-specific drug delivery system for renal fibrosis based on coordination-driven assembly of catechol-derived chitosan. *Biomaterials* **2014**, *35*, 7157–7171. [CrossRef]
147. Sakono, N.; Nakamura, K.; Ohshima, T.; Hayakawa, R.; Sakono, M. Tyrosinase-mediated Peptide Conjugation with Chitosan-coated Gold Nanoparticles. *Anal. Sci.* **2018**, *35*, 79–83. [CrossRef]
148. Samyn, P. A platform for functionalization of cellulose, chitin/chitosan, alginate with polydopamine: A review on fundamentals and technical applications. *Int. J. Biol. Macromol.* **2021**, *178*, 71–93. [CrossRef]
149. Rahnama, H.; Khorasani, S.N.; Aminoroaya, A.; Molavian, M.R.; Allafchian, A.; Khalili, S. Facile preparation of chitosan-dopamine-inulin aldehyde hydrogel for drug delivery application. *Int. J. Biol. Macromol.* **2021**, *185*, 716–724. [CrossRef]
150. Zhang, M.; Zhao, X. Alginate hydrogel dressings for advanced wound management. *Int. J. Biol. Macromol.* **2020**, *162*, 1414–1428. [CrossRef]
151. Rastogi, P.; Kandasubramanian, B. Review of alginate-based hydrogel bioprinting for application in tissue engineering. *Biofabrication* **2019**, *11*, 042001. [CrossRef]
152. Nagakura, T.; Hirata, H.; Tsujii, M.; Sugimoto, T.; Miyamoto, K.; Horiuchi, T.; Nagao, M.; Nakashima, T.; Uchida, A. Effect of viscous injectable pure alginate sol on cultured fibroblasts. *Plast. Reconstr. Surg.* **2005**, *116*, 831–838. [CrossRef] [PubMed]
153. Schulz, A.; Gepp, M.M.; Stracke, F.; von Briesen, H.; Neubauer, J.C.; Zimmermann, H. Tyramine-conjugated alginate hydrogels as a platform for bioactive scaffolds. *J. Biomed. Mater. Res. Part A* **2019**, *107*, 114–121. [CrossRef] [PubMed]
154. Yuan, N.; Shao, K.; Huang, S.; Chen, C. Chitosan, alginate, hyaluronic acid and other novel multifunctional hydrogel dressings for wound healing: A review. *Int. J. Biol. Macromol.* **2023**, *240*, 124321. [CrossRef]
155. Raus, R.A.; Nawawi, W.M.F.W.; Nasaruddin, R.R. Alginate and alginate composites for biomedical applications. *Asian J. Pharm. Sci.* **2021**, *16*, 280–306. [CrossRef]
156. Lan, L.; Ping, J.; Li, H.; Wang, C.; Li, G.; Song, J.; Ying, Y. Skin-Inspired All-Natural Biogel for Bioadhesive Interface. *Adv. Mater.* **2024**, *36*, e2401151. [CrossRef]
157. Ye, Z.; Mao, Z. Research Progress on the Regulation of Structure and Antioxidant Properties of Polydopamine-Based Nanomaterials and Their Biomedical Applications. *Mater. China* **2022**, *41*, 679–688. [CrossRef]
158. Kashi, M.; Nazarpak, M.H.; Nourmohammadi, J.; Moztarzadeh, F. Study the effect of different concentrations of polydopamine as a secure and bioactive crosslinker on dual crosslinking of oxidized alginate and gelatin wound dressings. *Int. J. Biol. Macromol.* **2024**, *277 Pt 3*, 134199. [CrossRef]
159. Rezk, A.I.; Obiweluozor, F.O.; Choukrani, G.; Park, C.H.; Kim, C.S. Drug release and kinetic models of anticancer drug (BTZ) from a pH-responsive alginate polydopamine hydrogel: Towards cancer chemotherapy. *Int. J. Biol. Macromol.* **2019**, *141*, 388–400. [CrossRef]
160. Liang, M.; He, C.; Dai, J.; Ren, P.; Fu, Y.; Wang, F.; Ge, X.; Zhang, T.; Lu, Z. A high-strength double network polydopamine nanocomposite hydrogel for adhesion under seawater. *J. Mater. Chem. B* **2020**, *8*, 8232–8241. [CrossRef]
161. Xu, J.; Wang, G.; Wu, Y.; Ren, X.; Gao, G. Ultrastretchable Wearable Strain and Pressure Sensors Based on Adhesive, Tough, and Self-healing Hydrogels for Human Motion Monitoring. *ACS Appl. Mater. Interfaces* **2019**, *11*, 25613–25623. [CrossRef] [PubMed]
162. Montazerian, H.; Baidya, A.; Haghniaz, R.; Davoodi, E.; Ahadian, S.; Annabi, N.; Khademhosseini, A.; Weiss, P.S. Stretchable and Bioadhesive Gelatin Methacryloyl-Based Hydrogels Enabled by in Situ Dopamine Polymerization. *ACS Appl. Mater. Interfaces* **2021**, *13*, 40290–40301. [CrossRef] [PubMed]

163. Wu, E.; Huang, L.; Shen, Y.; Wei, Z.; Li, Y.; Wang, J.; Chen, Z. Application of gelatin-based composites in bone tissue engineering. *Heliyon* **2024**, *10*, e36258. [CrossRef]
164. Afewerki, S.; Sheikhi, A.; Kannan, S.; Ahadian, S.; Khademhosseini, A. Gelatin-polysaccharide composite scaffolds for 3D cell culture and tissue engineering: Towards natural therapeutics. *Bioeng. Transl. Med.* **2018**, *4*, 96–115. [CrossRef]
165. Pei, X.; Zhang, H.; Zhou, Y.; Zhou, L.; Fu, J. Stretchable, self-healing and tissue-adhesive zwitterionic hydrogels as strain sensors for wireless monitoring of organ motions. *Mater. Horizons* **2020**, *7*, 1872–1882. [CrossRef]
166. Lee, H.A.; Park, E.; Lee, H. Polydopamine and Its Derivative Surface Chemistry in Material Science: A Focused Review for Studies at KAIST. *Adv. Mater.* **2020**, *32*, e1907505. [CrossRef] [PubMed]
167. Chen, Y.; Song, J.; Wang, S.; Liu, W. PVA-Based Hydrogels: Promising Candidates for Articular Cartilage Repair. *Macromol. Biosci.* **2021**, *21*, 2100147. [CrossRef]
168. Sun, S.; Cui, Y.; Yuan, B.; Dou, M.; Wang, G.; Xu, H.; Wang, J.; Yin, W.; Wu, D.; Peng, C. Drug delivery systems based on polyethylene glycol hydrogels for enhanced bone regeneration. *Front. Bioeng. Biotechnol.* **2023**, *11*, 1117647. [CrossRef]
169. Washington, M.A.; Balmert, S.C.; Fedorchak, M.V.; Little, S.R.; Watkins, S.C.; Meyer, T.Y. Monomer sequence in PLGA microparticles: Effects on acidic microclimates and in vivo inflammatory response. *Acta Biomater.* **2018**, *65*, 259–271. [CrossRef]
170. Wu, Z.; Yuan, K.; Zhang, Q.; Guo, J.J.; Yang, H.; Zhou, F. Antioxidant PDA-PEG nanoparticles alleviate early osteoarthritis by inhibiting osteoclastogenesis and angiogenesis in subchondral bone. *J. Nanobiotechnol.* **2022**, *20*, 479. [CrossRef]
171. Liu, Y.; Hong, H.; Xiao, Y.; Kwok, M.L.; Liu, H.; Tian, X.Y.; Choi, C.H.J. Dopamine Receptor-Mediated Binding and Cellular Uptake of Polydopamine-Coated Nanoparticles. *ACS Nano* **2021**, *15*, 13871–13890. [CrossRef] [PubMed]
172. Sun, L.; Zheng, C.; Webster, T.J. Self-assembled peptide nanomaterials for biomedical applications: Promises and pitfalls. *Int. J. Nanomed.* **2016**, *12*, 73–86. [CrossRef] [PubMed]
173. Qiang, W.; Li, W.; Li, X.; Chen, X.; Xu, D. Bioinspired polydopamine nanospheres: A superquencher for fluorescence sensing of biomolecules. *Chem. Sci.* **2014**, *5*, 3018–3024. [CrossRef]
174. Hing, K.A. Bone repair in the twenty–first century: Biology, chemistry or engineering? *Philos. Trans. R. Soc. A Math. Phys. Eng. Sci.* **2004**, *362*, 2821–2850. [CrossRef]
175. Raeburn, J.; Cardoso, A.Z.; Adams, D.J. The importance of the self-assembly process to control mechanical properties of low molecular weight hydrogels. *Chem. Soc. Rev.* **2013**, *42*, 5143–5156. [CrossRef]
176. Liyanage, W.; Ardoña, H.A.M.; Mao, H.-Q.; Tovar, J.D. Cross-Linking Approaches to Tuning the Mechanical Properties of Peptide π-Electron Hydrogels. *Bioconjug. Chem.* **2016**, *28*, 751–759. [CrossRef]
177. Maslovskis, A.; Guilbaud, J.-B.; Grillo, I.; Hodson, N.; Miller, A.F.; Saiani, A. Self-assembling peptide/thermoresponsive polymer composite hydrogels: Effect of peptide–polymer interactions on hydrogel properties. *Langmuir* **2014**, *30*, 10471–10480. [CrossRef]
178. Adhikari, B.; Nanda, J.; Banerjee, A. Pyrene-containing peptide-based fluorescent organogels: Inclusion of graphene into the organogel. *Chemistry* **2011**, *17*, 11488–11496. [CrossRef] [PubMed]
179. Cao, W.; Zhang, X.; Miao, X.; Yang, Z.; Xu, H. γ-Ray-responsive supramolecular hydrogel based on a diselenide-containing polymer and a peptide. *Angew. Chem. Int. Ed. Engl.* **2013**, *52*, 6233–6237. [CrossRef]
180. Fichman, G.; Schneider, J.P. Dopamine Self-Polymerization as a Simple and Powerful Tool to Modulate the Viscoelastic Mechanical Properties of Peptide-Based Gels. *Molecules* **2021**, *26*, 1363. [CrossRef]
181. Falcone, N.; Andoy, N.M.O.; Sullan, R.M.A.; Kraatz, H.-B. Peptide-Polydopamine Nanocomposite Hydrogel for a Laser-Controlled Hydrophobic Drug Delivery. *ACS Appl. Bio Mater.* **2021**, *4*, 6652–6657. [CrossRef] [PubMed]

gels

MDPI

Article

Gastric Acid-Protective and Intestinal Targeted Nanogels Enable Anti-Bacterial Activity of Cefquinome

Xianqiang Li [1,†], Tianhui Wang [2,†], Shuo Han [2,†], Jinhuan Liu [2,3], Xiuping Zhang [2], Zhiqiang Zhou [4], Ali Sobhy Dawood [5] and Wanhe Luo [2,*]

1 College of Biomedicine and Health, Anhui Science and Technology University, Chuzhou 233100, China; lixianqiang89@sina.com
2 Engineering Laboratory for Tarim Animal Diseases Diagnosis and Control, College of Animal Science and Technology, Tarim University, Alar 843300, China; w3505506223@163.com (T.W.); 15645977635@163.com (S.H.); liujinhuan0830@163.com (J.L.); zxpkdy@126.com (X.Z.)
3 College of Veterinary Medicine, Sichuan Agricultural University, Chengdu 611130, China
4 Instrumental Analysis Center, Tarim University, Alar 843300, China; zhou2011519@sina.com
5 Infectious Diseases, Faculty of Veterinary Medicine, University of Sadat City, Sadat City 32897, Egypt; ali.dawood@vet.usc.edu.eg
* Correspondence: luowanhe0728@163.com
† These authors contributed equally to this work.

Abstract: To enhance the antibacterial activity of cefquinome (CEF) against *Escherichia coli*, a Carboxymethylcellulose sodium (CMCNa)/D-Mannosamine hydrochloride (DMH)-based nanogels delivery system capable of protecting CEF from gastric acid degradation while enabling intestinal sustained release and targeted antibacterial enhancement was developed. Systematic research was conducted on the best formulation, physicochemical characteristics, stability, gastrointestinal fluid-responsiveness, and antibacterial activity of the optimal formulation. The results showed that the optimized CEF nanogels demonstrated an enhanced loading capacity (13.0% ± 1.7%) and encapsulation efficiency (52.2% ± 1.0%). CEF nanogels appeared as uniform transparent spheres with a smooth surface under transmission electron microscopy and exhibited a three-dimensional porous network via scanning electron microscopy. More importantly, stability studies revealed that the CEF nanogels hold satisfactory stability. In addition, the formed CEF nanogels could effectively avoid the destruction of CEF by gastric acid in simulated gastric juice. In addition, they had the effect of slow and targeted release in the simulated intestinal tract. Compared to the free CEF, CEF nanogels have stronger antibacterial activity against *Escherichia coli*. In short, the prepared CEF nanogels had stronger antibacterial activity than CEF through sustained and targeted release.

Keywords: cefquinome (CEF); *Escherichia coli*; sustained release and targeted release; carboxymethylcellulose sodium (CMCNa); D-mannosamine hydrochloride (DMH)

1. Introduction

Animal-derived diarrhea, predominantly caused by pathogenic *Escherichia coli* (*E. coli*), is one of the most prevalent diseases in the livestock industry. This disease induces growth retardation, reduced production performance, and results in high mortality rates, leading to substantial economic losses in animal husbandry [1–3]. Currently, antibiotic therapy remains the primary approach for treating *E. coli*-associated diarrhea [4]. Cefquinome sulfate (CEF), a fourth-generation cephalosporin, has a broad-spectrum antibacterial action, low toxicity, and good stability, which has led to its widespread use in veterinary clinics [5].

The bactericidal effect of CEF is achieved through the inhibition of bacterial cell wall synthesis, demonstrating remarkable efficacy against Gram-negative bacteria, such as *E. coli* [6]. However, significant limitations hinder its application in veterinary clinic: (1) oral administration of CEF is compromised by gastric acid degradation, drastically reducing its bioavailability; (2) conventional formulations lack sustained-release and targeted delivery capabilities, resulting in insufficient drug accumulation at infection sites, which not only diminishes therapeutic efficacy, but also increases the risk of bacterial resistance due to frequent administration [7,8]. Consequently, the development of a drug delivery system capable of protecting CEF from gastric acid degradation, while enabling sustained and targeted delivery, is urgently required to enhance its antimicrobial performance.

More and more nanocarrier systems are being used to enhance the antibacterial activity of CEF, such as CEF oily nanosuspension, CEF proliposomes, and CEF gelatin microspheres [5,7,8]. The larger particle size, the lower loading capacity (LC), and the reduced encapsulation efficiency (EE) of these nanocarrier systems are the main constraints that reduce and hinder the antibacterial activity of CEF. Recently, nanogels as a novel class of drug delivery systems have gained substantial attention in biomedicine due to their unique physicochemical properties [9–11]. Nanogels are three-dimensional crosslinked networks formed by hydrophilic or amphiphilic polymers through physical or chemical interactions. They are characterized by high LC and EE, excellent biocompatibility, and adjustable drug release profiles [12]. Compared to other nanoscale drug delivery systems such as liposomes, nanogels exhibit distinct advantages: (1) the porous structure enables efficient encapsulation of both hydrophobic and hydrophilic drugs; (2) controlled drug release can be achieved by modulating crosslinking density or environmental responsiveness (e.g., pH, temperature, or enzyme sensitivity); (3) surface functionalization facilitates targeted delivery. For instance, pH-sensitive nanogels maintain structural integrity in the acidic gastric environment (pH 1.5–3.5), shielding drugs from degradation, while undergoing swelling or dissociation in the neutral-to-alkaline intestinal environment (pH 6.5–7.5) to achieve site-specific release [13,14]. These characteristics make nanogels ideal carriers for oral antibiotic delivery systems. The nanogels are critical for constructing orally administered nanogel systems. Carboxymethylcellulose sodium (CMCNa), an anionic polysaccharide derivative, has been extensively utilized as a nanogels matrix due to its high-water solubility, biodegradability, and low toxicity. In gastric acidic conditions (pH < 3), the carboxyl groups (-COO^-) on CMCNa) chains undergo protonation (-COOH), reducing hydrophilicity and forming a dense hydrogel network that effectively separates encapsulated drugs from gastric acid. CMCNa-based nanocarriers significantly enhance the gastric stability of acid-labile drugs such as insulin or probiotics. Furthermore, the negative surface charge of CMCNa minimizes nonspecific adhesion to intestinal mucosa via electrostatic repulsion, prolonged and extended intestinal retention, and enhanced localized therapeutic effects [15]. On the other side, D-Mannosamine hydrochloride (DMH), a positively charged amino sugar derivative, exhibits targeting specificity attributed to the abundant Type 1 fimbriae on *E. coli* surfaces [16]. These fimbriae express mannose-specific adhesins (FimH) at their tips, which selectively recognize and bind to mannose derivatives. By conjugating DMH onto nanogel surfaces, active targeting of *E. coli* can be achieved through FimH-DMH ligand–receptor interactions [13]. This targeting strategy not only enhances drug enrichment at infection sites but also minimizes collateral damage to commensal microbiota, thereby reducing resistance risks.

Given this, a multifunctional nanogels delivery system with "gastric acid protection, intestinal sustained release, and bacterial targeting" was designed, in which the negatively charged CMCNa and positively charged DMH were used as the matrix, and CEF was encapsulated through electrostatic action. The CMCNa component leverages gastrointestinal fluid-responsive behavior to establish dual-phase regulation: a gastric acid-resistant barrier and controlled intestinal release. Simultaneously, DMH mediates active targeting to enhance antibacterial efficacy against *E. coli*. More importantly, the nanogel's sustained-release properties prolong drug action duration, and reduce dosing frequency (Figure 1). Thus, it is hypothesized that the multifunctional nanogel delivery system with "gastric acid protection, intestinal sustained release, and bacterial targeting" has obvious gastrointestinal fluid-responsiveness and excellent antibacterial activity through sustained and targeted release. The optimal formulation, physicochemical properties, gastrointestinal fluid-responsive performance, stability, and antibacterial activity have been studied systematically. This work aims to improve the antimicrobial activity of CEF against *E. coli* by protecting CEF from gastric acid degradation and achieving a sustained and targeted effect.

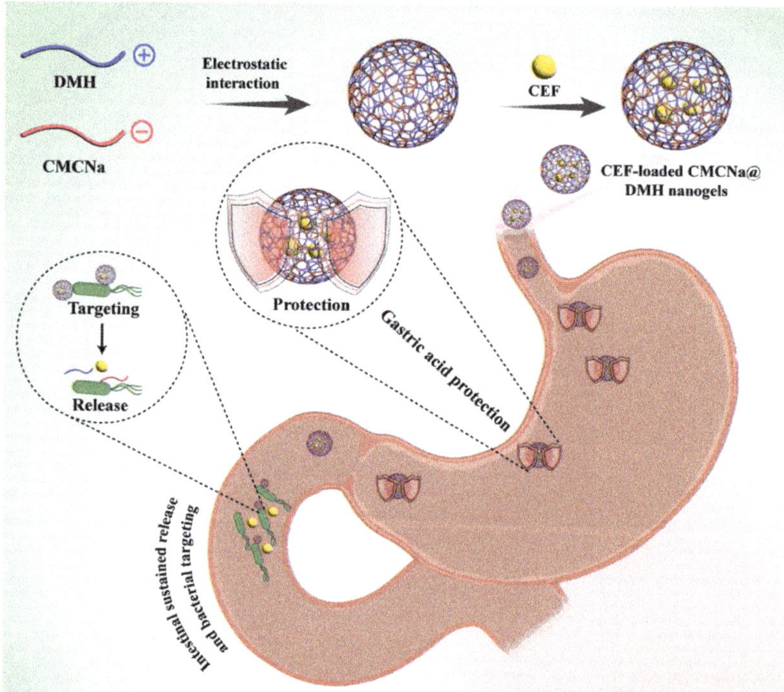

Figure 1. Schematic diagram of a multifunctional nanogel-based delivery system featuring "gastric acid protection, intestinal sustained release, and bacterial targeting", designed to enhance the antibacterial efficacy of CEF against *E. coli* through sustained release and targeted release.

2. Results and Discussion

2.1. Formulation Optimization

LC and EE are often used to screen for the optimal nanoformulation. The larger the LC and EE, the more drugs are encapsulated. The result was entirely the product of random errors, even though it was in the formulation. When LC is at its maximum, the optimal amount and proportion of the nanogels are obtained [17,18]. By determining the relationship between the generated response surfaces and the controllable input parameters, the response surface approach facilitates the investigation and modeling the formulation difficulties and process parameters. It does this by fusing mathematical and statistical methods [19]. To obtain a suitable estimate of the prediction variance across the whole model design space, thirteen experimental runs with three repeated center points were needed. Table 1 displays the trial design and outcomes produced by the Design-Expert tool. Using different concentrations of CMCNa (50, 100, and 200 mg/mL) and DMH (10, 20, and 40 mg/mL) as variables, and LC and EE as evaluation indices, the optimal formula was screened. The concentrations of auxiliary materials (CMCNa and DMH) were too high or too low; the LC and EE of the CEF nanogels will be affected. High concentration of auxiliary materials leads to high weight of the whole CEF nanogels; the calculated LC and EE of CEF nanogels were relatively low. The low concentrations of auxiliary materials make it difficult for CEF to be encapsulated, thus, the LC and EE of CEF nanogels were also relatively low. Therefore, the appropriate concentration of auxiliary materials will get the maximum LC and EE of CEF nanogels. Following the analysis, the quadratic polynomial regression equation linking the LC to three components and the thirteen groups' findings was shown in Tables S1 and S2 (A: CMCNa; B: DMH):

$$LC = 14.04 + 1.13 \times A + 0.4976 \times B - 0.4714 \times AB - 1.64A^2 - 0.8397 \times B^2 \quad (1)$$

Table 1. Single-factor experimental design and responses for CEF nanogels.

Run	CMCNa (mg/mL)	DMH (mg/mL)	LC (%)	EE (%)
1	50	10	9.4	46.4
2	200	10	12.7	48.6
3	50	40	11.5	47.4
4	200	40	12.8	50.5
5	50	20	10.8	50.3
6	200	20	13.3	51.5
7	100	10	12.0	50.3
8	100	40	13.1	51.3
9	100	20	13.2	52.8
10	100	20	13.2	52.8
11	100	20	13.2	52.8
12	100	20	13.2	52.8
13	100	20	13.2	52.8

The quadratic polynomial regression equation between the EE and three factors was (A: CMCNa; B: DMH):

$$EE = 54.1 + 1.12 \times A + 0.6828 \times B + 0.2951 \times AB - 2.9 \times A^2 - 2.85 \times B^2 \quad (2)$$

The residual lack of fit was not significant ($p > 0.05$), as evidenced by the highly substantial discrepancies between the different treatments of the LC and EE models ($p < 0.0001$). The regression equation coefficients R^2, adjusted R^2, and adjusted R^2 were 0.9841, 0.9727, and 0.8959 for EE, and 0.9951, 0.9916, and 0.9296 for LC, respectively, reflecting the range of response values. More importantly, $|\text{adjusted } R^2 - \text{pre } R^2| < 0.2$ (LC and EE), demonstrating that both prediction models were reliable. Three-dimensional response surface images were generated based on the above data (Figure 2A,B). The optimized CEF nanogels, according to Design-Expert software 8.0, were 193.2 mg/mL CMCNa and 27.5 mg/mL DMH. The LC and EE predicted by the software were 13.7% and 52.8%, respectively (Figure 2C). Subsequently, the optimal formulation was verified by producing CEF nanogels with 195 mg/mL CMCNa and 28 mg/mL DMH. The LC and EE of the prepared CEF nanogels were 13.0% ± 1.7% and 52.2% ± 1.0%, respectively. Thus, the optimal preparation method for the CEF nanogels designed by the Box–Behnken response surface technique was accurate and reliable.

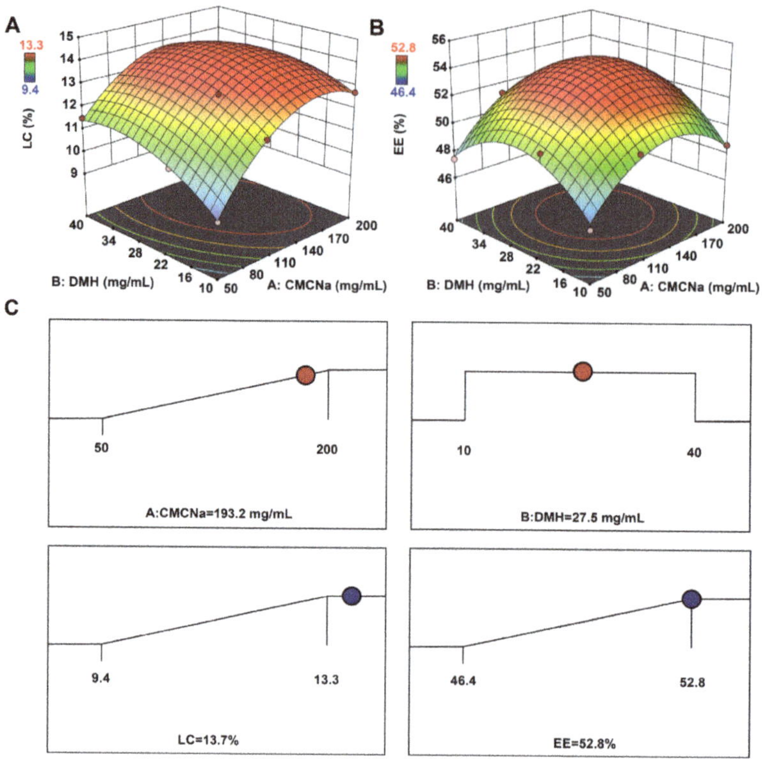

Figure 2. Optimization of CEF nanogels. Three-dimensional arrangement for response surface images of the different concentrations of CMCNa and DMH to LC (**A**) and EE (**B**). (**C**) The optimal formulation predicted by Design-Expert software.

2.2. Characterization

In recent years, an increasing number of CEF delivery platforms have been used to enhance the antibacterial activity of drugs. For example, to improve the strategy of CEF in the treatment of animal bacterial infection, a novel oily nanosuspension was designed to improve the stability and bioavailability of CEF, reduce muscle irritation, and the cost of production. However, the particle size (≈750 nm) and PDI (≈0.82) of the CEF oily nanosuspension were relatively large, which may reduce the therapeutic efficacy of the CEF. This may be attributed to the preparation method of the CEF oily nanosuspension [5]. The CEF proliposomes prepared by the solid-dispersion method combined with efferent vesicle hydration had an EE of only 63.21% and an LC of only 4.04%. The lower LC and EE greatly reduce the efficacy of the drug and increase the cost of the drug [8]. CEF gelatin microspheres were prepared as a sustained-release formulation using the emulsion chemical cross-linking technique. However, the mean diameter was 8.80 ± 0.78 μm. Large particle size is not conducive to sufficient interaction between the formulation and bacteria, thereby reducing the antibacterial activity of CEF [7]. In this study, a multifunctional nanogels delivery system with "gastric acid protection, intestinal sustained release, and bacterial targeting" was designed by the electrostatic action between CMCNa and DMH. The combination of gastric protection and *E. coli*-targeted delivery using DMH is an innovative strategy that was recently reported in veterinary drug delivery. Thus, the appearance, pH, TEM, mean size, ZP, PDI, SEM, and FTIR spectrum of optimal CEF nanogels were systematically evaluated in this study. The consistent, clear, transparent color of the CEF nanogels in the bottle provided preliminary confirmation of their good hydrogel stability (Figure 3A). The pH of CEF nanogels was 7.0. The CEF nanogels were found to be smooth and spherical by TEM investigation (Figure 3B). Additionally, CEF nanogels' EDS showed that C, N, O, and Na were evenly distributed throughout the nanogels, which provided ample evidence for the successful construction of nanogels delivery system through the electrostatic action between CMCNa and DMH (Figure 3C). In addition, the mean size, ZP, and PDI of CEF nanogels were 116.9 ± 1.2 nm (Figure 3D), −17.8 ± 0.4 mV (Figure 3E), and 0.14 ± 0.05, respectively, which demonstrated the homogeneous dispersion and nanoscale nature of the CEF nanogels. SEM of freeze-dried CEF nanogels showed a three-dimensional network structure (Figure 3F), and this high specific surface area characteristic may enhance its drug loading ability and drug release performance. The FTIR spectra of CEF, CMCNa, DMH, and CEF nanogels are shown in Figure 3G. Each component's physicochemical interactions were examined using FTIR spectroscopy. For example, the electrostatic interaction contacts between CMCNa and DMH can result in frequency shifts or absorption peak splitting. The distinctive peaks for DMH at 1518, 1628 and 2056 cm^{-1}, CMCNa at 1431 and 1628 cm^{-1}, and CEF at 1043 and 1663 cm^{-1} vanished from the spectrum of CEF nanogels, and new characteristic peaks (1028 and 1597 cm^{-1}) were visible instead, which may be attributed to the electrostatic action between CMCNa and DMH. Thus, CEF nanogels were successfully prepared by the electrostatic action between CMCNa and DMH.

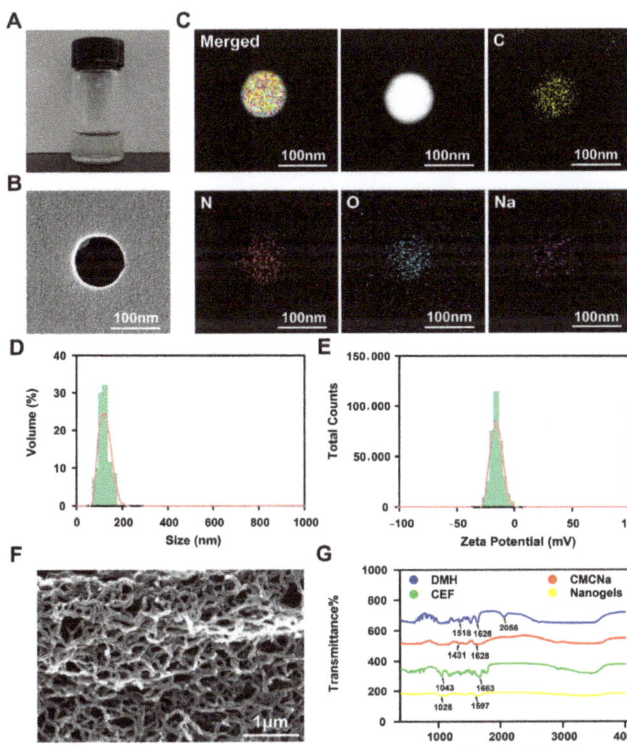

Figure 3. Characterization of CEF nanogels. Appearance (**A**), TEM (**B**); EDS (**C**); size distribution (**D**); Zeta potential (**E**); SEM (**F**); FTIR (**G**).

2.3. Stability

To investigate the stability of CEF nanogels, influencing-factor experiments, which included high temperature (40 °C), high humidity (90% ± 5%), and intense light (4500 ± 500 L×) in the drug stability tester (Figure 4G), were carried out by using their appearance, size, ZP, PDI, EE, and LC as an evaluation indicator. There were no significant differences in appearance (always clear transparent color in the bottle) (Figure 4A), size (about 120 nm) (Figure 4B), ZP (about −18.0 mV) (Figure 4C), PDI (about 0.2) (Figure 4D), EE (about 52%) (Figure 4E), and LC (about 13%) (Figure 4F) on the fifth and tenth days. It is suggested that the prepared CEF nanogels hold satisfactory stability. Thus, the results indicated that nanocarrier systems can effectively improve the stability of drugs.

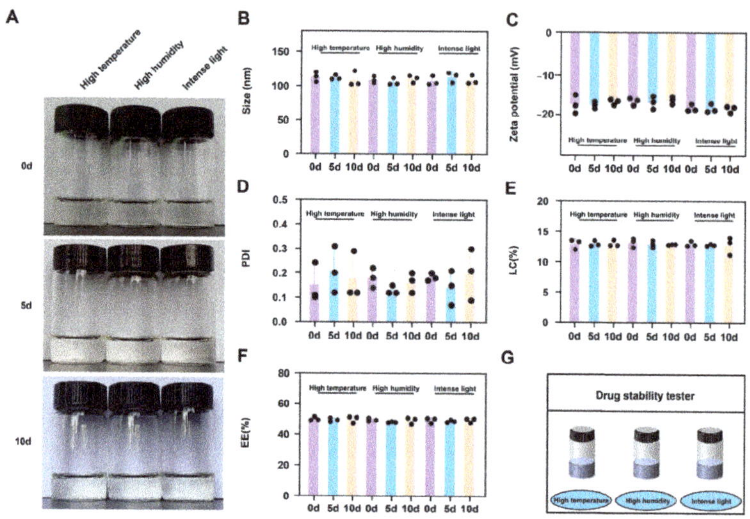

Figure 4. The influence factors test (high temperature, high humidity, and intense light) of CEF-loaded CMCNa@DMH nanogels. Appearance (**A**); size (**B**); ZP (**C**); PDI (**D**); LC (**E**); EE (**F**); schematic diagram of stability of CEF nanogels incubated at 40 °C, 90% ± 5% humidity, and 4500 ± 500 L× for illumination (**G**).

2.4. Gastrointestinal Fluid-Responsive Performances

This work comprehensively assessed the CMCNa@DMH nanogels loaded with CEF's gastrointestinal fluid-responsive performance in different microenvironments (SGJ, SIF, and gastrointestinal fluid; pH 7.4 and pH 5.5). The cefquinome-loaded nanogel exhibited distinct gastrointestinal fluid-responsive drug release profiles, demonstrating differential structural stability and release kinetics under various physiological and pathological environments. The CEF nanogels showed limited drug release in SGF, with only 30.2% ± 4.0% cumulative release over 24 h (Figure 5A,B), whereas, in SIF, a significantly higher release (95.5% ± 4.0%) was observed (Figure 5C,D), indicating inherent enteric solubility. To better mimic gastrointestinal transit, a dynamic release model (2 h in SGF followed by about 20 h in SIF) was employed. During the gastric phase, the CEF nanogels maintained structural integrity with only 18.5% ± 2.7% drug release, consistent with typical gastric emptying time (~2 h). Upon the intestinal phase, rapid structural disintegration occurred, triggering a burst release (93.5% ± 4.0% cumulative release), which confirmed efficient intestinal-targeted delivery (Figure 5E,F). Moreover, the CEF nanogels displayed pH-dependent release behavior in simulated physiological (pH 7.4) and infection microenvironments (pH 5.5). At neutral pH (7.4), 68.3% ± 4.6% of the CEF was released within 24 h (Figure 5G,H), whereas, under weakly acidic conditions (pH 5.5), the release was significantly suppressed (34.3% ± 4.4%) (Figure 5I,J). This pH-responsive characteristic maintains sustained drug release in acidic infection sites, which prolongs local therapeutic effects, and more importantly, accelerates clearance in neutral tissues to minimize systemic toxicity.

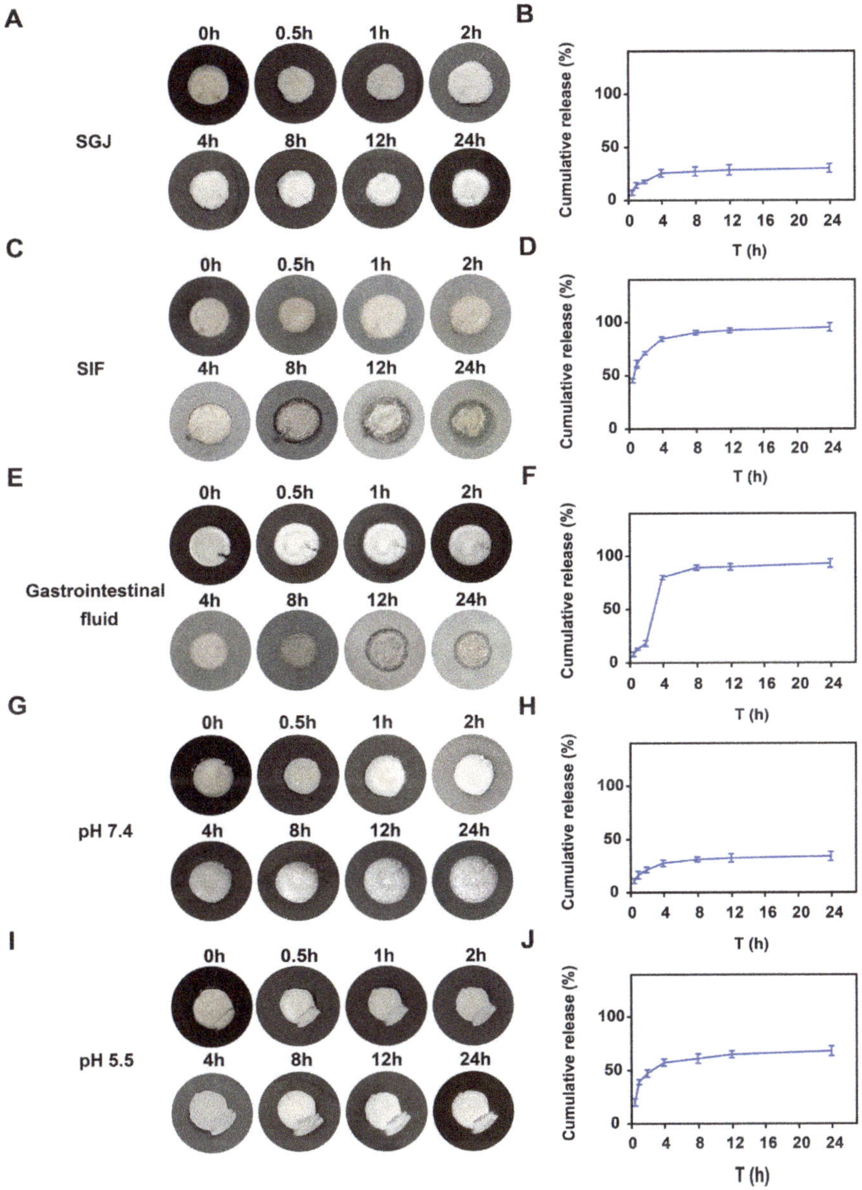

Figure 5. Morphology change and in vitro release of CEF-loaded CMCNa@DMH nanogels in SGJ (**A**,**B**), SIF (**C**,**D**), simulated gastrointestinal fluid (**E**,**F**), pH 7.4 (**G**,**H**), and pH 5.5 (**I**,**J**).

2.5. In Vitro Antibacterial Activity

The in vitro antibacterial activity of CEF and CEF-loaded CMCNa@DMH nanogels against isolates of *E. coli* was demonstrated in Figure 6. *E. coli* isolates had MICs of 1.0 and

0.5 μg/mL for CEF and CEF nanogels, respectively (Figure 6A). *E. coli* isolates showed inhibitory zones of 2.24 ± 0.07 cm for CEF and 2.75 ± 0.08 cm for CEF nanogels (Figure 6B,C). *E. coli* isolates were thus more susceptible to the antibacterial action of CEF nanogels than CEF. The delivery strategy of nanogels may enhance the antibacterial effectiveness of CEF through targeted and sustained release, according to this dose–response relationship. Additionally, the live/dead bacterial staining kit was used to treat the mixture of *E. coli* isolates with CEF or CEF nanogels. As demonstrated by the increase in dead bacteria (colored red) and decrease in living bacteria (colored green), the results showed that CEF nanogels had more bactericidal efficacy than CEF (Figure 6D). This synergistic effect may originate from the "drug storage effect" of the nanogels delivery system, that is, maintaining the local effective drug concentration through the sustained release characteristics, while the targeting effect of DMH enhances the drug-bacteria interaction. After the *E. coli* isolates were treated with CEF nanogels, SEM showed that the *E. coli* isolates had more holes and lysis. After treatment with CEF nanogels, the cell wall of *E. coli* isolates showed obvious holes and cytoplasm leakage, indicating that nanogels delivery system may synergistically enhance the bactericidal effect of CEF by destroying the integrity of bacterial membrane (Figure 6E). The synergistic mechanism of "structural damage drug penetration" is consistent with previous research reports on enhancing the antibacterial effect of Gram-negative bacteria by nanogels delivery system.

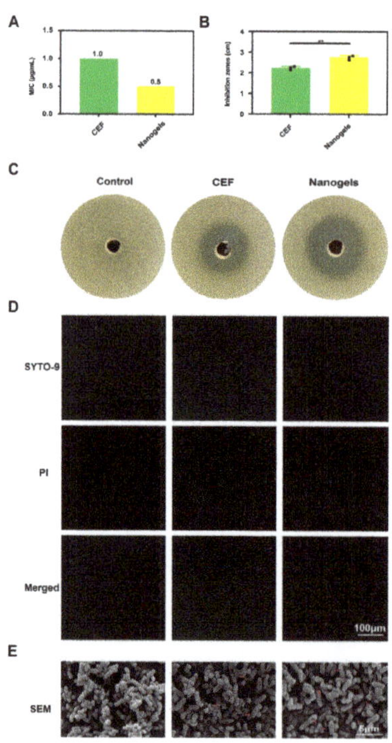

Figure 6. In vitro antibacterial activity of CEF nanogels against *E. coli* isolates. (**A**) MICs; (**B**,**C**) inhibition zones. (**D**) Live/dead bacterial staining images; (**E**) SEM images. (** $p < 0.01$).

3. Conclusions

In this study, a multifunctional nanogel delivery system with "gastric acid protection, intestinal sustained release, and bacterial targeting" was designed for animal-derived diarrhea caused by *E. coli*. Physicochemical characterization proved that the CEF nanogels were successfully prepared and had obvious gastrointestinal fluid-responsiveness and satisfactory stability. Moreover, the prepared CEF nanogels had stronger antibacterial activity against *E. coli* than CEF through sustained and targeted release. Therefore, the multifunctional nanogel delivery system (CEF nanogels) prepared in this study is expected to provide a new nano preparation for animal diarrhea caused by *E. coli*.

4. Materials and Methods

4.1. Materials

DMH, CEF (content: 97%), simulated gastric juice (SGJ), and simulated intestinal fluid (SIF) were purchased from Macklin (Shanghai, China). CMCNa was obtained from Suzhou Intelligent Manufacturing Research Institute (Suzhou, China). Phosphate-buffered saline (PBS) and tryptone soy broth (TSB) were provided by Dingyuan Biotechnology Co., Ltd. (Alar, China). Shanghai Bestbio Biotechnology Co., Ltd. provided a live/dead illuminated bacterial viability kit (Shanghai, China). The engineering laboratory for the diagnosis and control of animal diseases in Tarim, China, supplied the *E. coli* isolates (The *E. coli* isolates were isolated from piglet manure in a Henan farm; Henan, China).

4.2. Formulation of CEF-Loaded CMCNa@DMH Nanogels

The CEF-loaded CMCNa@DMH nanogels, composed of CEF, CMCNa, and DMH, were formulated by electrostatic action. Briefly, CMCNa (50, 100, or 200 mg), DMH (10, 20, or 40 mg), and CEF (1 mg) were added to 1 mL of ultrapure water with stirring to completely dissolve to obtain CMCNa solution, DMH solution, and CEF solution, respectively. Subsequently, the dissolved DMH solution was added dropwise to the CMCNa solution by using magnetic stirring at 800 RPM for one hour. To create CEF-loaded CMCNa@DMH nanogels, the CEF solution was then added dropwise (1 drop/10 s) to the CMCNa/DMH mixed solution while being magnetically stirred for one hour at 800 RPM. The freshly prepared CEF nanogels were kept at room temperature before further usage and tests. Meanwhile, the pH of CEF nanogels was measured. Briefly, 10 mL of ultrapure water was added to 0.1 mL of CEF nanogels, and shook it at 100 rpm for 24 h at room temperature until swelling equilibrium occurs. The pH of the hydrogel was then measured directly by the pH meter (PHG-2081, Shanghai Botuo Instrument Co., Ltd., Shanghai, China).

4.3. Box–Behnken Response Surface Analysis

The Design-Expert 8.0 program (State-Ease, Inc., Minneapolis, MN, USA) precisely identified the optimal values of DMH and CMCNa. LC and EE were applied as assessment indices. Table 1 displays factors and values of the Box–Behnken design [19].

4.4. Physicochemical Characterization

The surface morphology of CEF-loaded CMCNa@DMH nanogels was characterized using their appearance and TEM. Briefly, the freshly prepared CEF nanogels were observed in a bottle. Additionally, CEF nanogels were diluted 100 times and subjected to an ultrasonic cleaner (BL3-120A, Shanghai Jianglai Biotechnology Co., Ltd., Shanghai, China) for one hour each. Transmission electron microscopy (TEM, JEM-2100Plus, JEOL, Tokyo, Japan) was then used to investigate the CEF nanogels, and energy dispersive spectroscopy (EDS; X-Max N 150; Oxford, UK) was used to determine the elemental analysis. Following the lyophilization of the CEF nanogels using a lyophilizer (FDU-1200, Beijing Songyuan Huaxing Biotechnology Co., Ltd., Beijing, China), scanning electron microscopy (SEM, APREO, Thermo Scientific Inc., Waltham, MA, USA) was used to examine the morphology of the freeze-dried CEF nanogels. Additionally, the mean size, zeta potential (ZP), and polydispersity index (PDI) of CEF-loaded CMCNa@DMH nanogels were measured using the Zetasizer ZX3600 (Malvern Instruments, Malvern, UK). Finally, Fourier transform infrared (FTIR) spectra of CEF, CMCNa, DMH, and CEF-loaded CMCNa@DMH nanogels were analyzed using an FTIR spectrophotometer (Nicolet iS50, Thermo Scientific Inc., Waltham, MA, USA), respectively.

4.5. Gastrointestinal Fluid-Responsive Release

In this study, the gastrointestinal fluid-responsiveness of CEF-loaded CMCNa@DMH nanogels in different microenvironments (SGJ, SIF, and gastrointestinal fluid; pH 7.4 and pH 5.5) was evaluated. Briefly, the lyophilized CEF-loaded CMCNa@DMH nanogels were initially placed in SGJ (2 h) and subsequently in SIF (8 h) to assess the gastrointestinal fluid-responsive performance. Simultaneously, the lyophilized CEF-loaded CMCNa@DMH nanogels were initially placed in pH 7.4 and pH 5.5. At various time points, the morphological variations were observed in different microenvironments. Concurrently, the CEF-loaded CMCNa@DMH nanogels' cumulative curves in various microenvironments were shown [20].

4.6. Stability Evaluation

The stability of CEF-loaded CMCNa@DMH nanogels was evaluated using influence-factor studies, which comprised high temperature (40 °C), high humidity (90% ± 5%), and bright light (4500 ± 500 L×) at the Drug stability tester (WD-2A, Guangzhou Huruiming Instrument Co., Ltd., Guangzhou, China). The CEF nanogels were put in a container and incubated for 10 days at 40 °C, 90% ± 5% humidity, and 4500 ± 500 L× for illumination to perform the high temperature test. In order to evaluate the differences in their appearance, mean size, ZP, PDI, LC, and EE, samples were taken on the fifth and tenth days [14].

4.7. In Vitro Antibacterial Activity Studies

4.7.1. Broth Macrodilution Method

The minimum inhibitory concentrations (MICs) of CEF and CEF-loaded CMCNa@DMH nanogels against *E. coli* isolates were studied using the broth microdilution method [14]. Briefly, serial dilutions of CEF or CEF nanogels in TSB broth were prepared. A final bacterial concentration of 1×10^6 CFU/mL was then attained for each tube using *E. coli* isolates. As a negative control, PBS was employed. The lowest quantity that, after 24 h of incubation at 37 °C, inhibited the visible growth of bacteria was determined to be the MICs of CEF or CEF nanogels against *E. coli* isolates.

4.7.2. Bacterial Inhibition Zones

The inhibition zones of CEF and CEF nanogels against *E. coli* isolates were estimated [14]. Briefly, an aseptic plate was filled with 15 milliliters of agar medium. Following the solidification of the agar, 0.1 mL of bacterial fluid containing 1×10^6 CFU/mL of *E. coli* isolates was added, along with an additional 5 mL of agar medium. Once set, the appropriate straw was used to create holes in the solid agar. Then, either 50 μL of CEF or CEF nanogels were introduced. As a negative control, PBS was employed. The size of the inhibitory zones was measured and recorded after the *E. coli* isolates were cultured for 24 h at 37 °C in an incubator with 5% CO_2.

4.7.3. Analysis of Live/Dead Bacterial Staining

Furthermore, the live/dead bacterial staining method was used to systematically assess the antibacterial properties of CEF and CEF nanogels [15]. In short, *E. coli* isolates were mixed with CEF or CEF nanogels. After a two-hour incubation period, all samples were processed using the live/dead fluorescent bacterial viability kit. Eventually, 5 μL of the bacterial suspension that was placed onto the slide was examined using a laser confocal microscope (A1RHD25&-SIM, Nikon, Tokyo, Japan). In this investigation, physiological saline served as a negative control.

4.7.4. Morphological Analysis

SEM was used to observe the morphological changes in *E. coli* isolates treated with CEF and CEF nanogels [15]. In conclusion, *E. coli* isolates (1×10^6 CFU/mL) were cultivated in triplicate on a cover glass for 24 h at 37 °C using CEF or CEF nanogels (all 1 × MIC). Subsequently, 2.5% glutaraldehyde was used to fix the samples for two hours at 4 °C. The sample was dried using ethanol concentrations of 30%, 50%, 70%, 90%, 95%, and 100% for a total of 20 min after the surfaces had been cleaned twice for 15 min each. Subsequently, each sample was gold sputtered and coated by a fully automatic ion sputtering instrument (Cressington 108Auto, Beijing Zhongxing Bairui Technology Co., Ltd., Beijing, China) for 120 s with a working current of 25 mA. The final gold spray thickness of each sample was about 10 nm, then analysed using SEM. PBS was employed as a negative control.

4.8. Statistical Analysis

The experimental data are expressed as Mean ± S.D. and analyzed by one-way ANOVA using the SPSS 19.0 software, followed by Tukey's post-hoc test for multiple comparisons. The sample size (n = 3/group) was determined based on a power analysis ($\alpha = 0.05$, power = 0.80), ensuring adequate sensitivity to detect group differences. Statistical significance was set at * $p < 0.05$.

Supplementary Materials: The following supporting information can be downloaded at: https://www.mdpi.com/article/10.3390/gels11070503/s1, Table S1. ANOVA of the LC model. Table S2. ANOVA of the EE model.

Author Contributions: Conceptualization, X.L., S.H., J.L., X.Z. and W.L.; Methodology, X.L., T.W., S.H., Z.Z. and W.L.; Writing—original draft, A.S.D. and W.L.; Writing—review & editing, A.S.D. and W.L.; Funding acquisition, X.L. All authors have read and agreed to the published version of the manuscript.

Funding: This work was financially supported by the Natural Science Foundation of Anhui Provincial Education Department (2024AH040059), Innovation and Entrepreneurship Training Program for College Students (202510757069), National Natural Science Foundation of China (32460904), the second group of Tianshan Talent Training Program: Youth Support Talent Project (2023TSYCQNTJ0033) and Natural Science Support Program of Xinjiang Production and Construction Corps (2024DA029).

Institutional Review Board Statement: The authors confirm that they have adhered to international standards for the protection of animals used for scientific purposes. The use of mice and all the experimental protocols concerning the handling of mice were complied with either the ARRIVE guideline and carried out in accordance with the National Research Council's Guide for the Care and Use of Laboratory Animals, Animal Science Academy of Tarim University's Ethics Committee (approved number: 2023008, date of approval 10 March 2023).

Informed Consent Statement: Not applicable.

Data Availability Statement: The data used to support the findings of this study are available from the corresponding author upon request.

Acknowledgments: The authors extend their gratitude to Guo Xin from Scientific Compass (www.shiyanjia.com) for providing invaluable assistance with the XRD analysis.

Conflicts of Interest: The authors declare no conflicts of interest.

References

1. Wang, L.; Liu, N.; Gao, Y.; Liu, J.; Huang, X.; Zhang, Q.; Li, Y.; Zhao, J.; Wang, J.; Zhao, G. Surveillance and Reduction Control of *Escherichia coli* and Diarrheagenic *E. coli* During the Pig Slaughtering Process in China. *Front. Vet. Sci.* **2021**, *8*, 735076. [CrossRef]
2. Van Den Honert, M.S.; Gouws, P.A.; Hoffman, L.C. *Escherichia coli* Antibiotic Resistance Patterns from Co-Grazing and Non-Co-Grazing Livestock and Wildlife Species from Two Farms in the Western Cape, South Africa. *Antibiotics* **2021**, *10*, 618. [CrossRef]
3. Ribeiro, J.; Silva, V.; Monteiro, A.; Vieira-Pinto, M.; Igrejas, G.; Reis, F.S.; Barros, L.; Poeta, P. Antibiotic Resistance among Gastrointestinal Bacteria in Broilers: A Review Focused on *Enterococcus* spp. and *Escherichia coli*. *Antibiotics* **2023**, *13*, 1362. [CrossRef] [PubMed]
4. Thuthikkadu Indhuprakash, S.; Karthikeyan, M.; Gopal, G.; Ambi, S.V.; Sekaran, S.; Palaniappan, B.; Diraviyam, T. Antibody therapy against antibiotic-resistant diarrheagenic *Escherichia coli*: A systematic review. *Immunotherapy* **2021**, *13*, 1305–1320. [CrossRef] [PubMed]
5. Mao, Y.; Chen, Y.; Liu, C.; He, X.; Zheng, Y.; Chen, X.; Wang, Y.; Chen, W.; Wu, Y.; Shen, Y.; et al. Cefquinome Sulfate Oily Nanosuspension Designed for Improving its Bioavailability in the Treatment of Veterinary Infections. *Int. J. Nanomed.* **2022**, *17*, 2535–2553. [CrossRef] [PubMed]
6. Li, S.; Yu, N.; Tang, Y.; Liu, C.; Zhang, Y.; Chen, X.; Wu, H.; Li, X.; Liu, Y. Pharmacokinetics and relative bioavailability study of two cefquinome sulfate intramammary infusions in cow milk. *Front. Vet. Sci.* **2024**, *11*, 1384076. [CrossRef] [PubMed]
7. Zhang, S.; Dai, W.; Lu, Z.; Lei, Z.; Yang, B.; He, B.; Zhou, H.; Cao, J. Preparation and evaluation of cefquinome-loaded gelatin microspheres and the pharmacokinetics in pigs. *J. Vet. Pharmacol. Ther.* **2018**, *41*, 117–124. [CrossRef] [PubMed]
8. Li, D.; Chen, S.; Dou, H.; Wu, W.; Liu, Q.; Zhang, L.; Shen, Y.; Shu, G.; Yuan, Z.; Lin, J.; et al. Preparation of cefquinome sulfate cationic proliposome and evaluation of its efficacy on Staphylococcus aureus biofilm. *Colloids Surf. B Biointerfaces* **2019**, *182*, 110323. [CrossRef] [PubMed]
9. Wang, Z.; Zhang, P.; Yin, C.; Li, Y.; Liao, Z.; Yang, C.; Liu, H.; Wang, W.; Fan, C.; Sun, D.; et al. Antibiotic-Derived Carbon-Nanodot-Decorated Hydrogel for Reactive Oxygen Species-Enhanced Anti-Infection Through Biofilm Damage. *Adv. Funct. Mater.* **2023**, *33*, 2300341. [CrossRef]
10. Luo, Y.; Cui, L.; Zou, L.; Zhao, Y.; Chen, L.; Guan, Y.; Zhang, Y. Mechanically strong and on-demand dissoluble chitosan hydrogels for wound dressing applications. *Carbohydr. Polym.* **2022**, *294*, 119774. [CrossRef]
11. Wu, J.; Wang, W.; Shen, J.; Zhou, N.; Li, Y.; Tang, B.; Zhang, M. A Thermosensitive Hydrogel with Efficient NIR Photothermal Conversion as Injectable Wound Dressing for Accelerating Skin Wound Healing. *Adv. Funct. Mater.* **2024**, *34*, 2312374. [CrossRef]
12. López-Iglesias, C.; Markovina, A.; Nirmalananthan-Budau, N.; Resch-Genger, U.; Klinger, D. Optically monitoring the microenvironment of a hydrophobic cargo in amphiphilic nanogels: Influence of network composition on loading and release. *Nanoscale* **2024**, *16*, 9525–9535. [CrossRef]
13. Knipe, J.M.; Strong, L.E.; Peppas, N.A. Enzyme- and pH-Responsive Microencapsulated Nanogels for Oral Delivery of siRNA to Induce TNF-α Knockdown in the Intestine. *Biomacromolecules* **2016**, *17*, 788–797. [CrossRef]
14. Luo, W.; Zhang, M.; Jiang, Y.; Ma, G.; Liu, J.; Dawood, A.S.; Xie, S.; Algharib, S.A. Manipulated Slow Release of Florfenicol Hydrogels for Effective Treatment of Anti-Intestinal Bacterial Infections. *Int. J. Nanomed.* **2025**, *20*, 541–555. [CrossRef]
15. Luo, W.; Liu, J.; Zhang, M.; Jiang, Y.; Sun, B.; Xie, S.; Sobhy Dawood, A.; Attia Algharib, S.; Gao, X. Florfenicol core-shell composite nanogels as oral administration for efficient treatment of bacterial enteritis. *Int. J. Pharm.* **2024**, *662*, 124499. [CrossRef] [PubMed]
16. Ma, N.; Cai, K.; Zhao, J.; Liu, C.; Li, H.; Tan, P.; Li, Y.; Li, D.; Ma, X. Mannosylated MOF Encapsulated in Lactobacillus Biofilm for Dual-Targeting Intervention Against Mammalian Escherichia coli Infections. *Adv. Mater.* **2025**, 202503056. [CrossRef] [PubMed]
17. Asadi, K.; Azarpira, N.; Heidari, R.; Hamidi, M.; Yousefzadeh-Chabok, S.; Nemati, M.M.; Ommati, M.M.; Amini, A.; Gholami, A. Trinitroglycerin-loaded chitosan nanogels accelerate angiogenesis in wound healing process. *Int. J. Biol. Macromol.* **2024**, *278 Pt 3*, 134937. [CrossRef] [PubMed]
18. Zhang, Y.; Zuo, R.; Song, X.; Gong, J.; Wang, J.; Lin, M.; Yang, F.; Cheng, X.; Gao, X.; Peng, L.; et al. Optimization of Maduramicin Ammonium-Loaded Nanostructured Lipid Carriers Using Box-Behnken Design for Enhanced Anticoccidial Effect against Eimeria tenella in Broiler Chickens. *Pharmaceutics* **2022**, *14*, 1330. [CrossRef] [PubMed]
19. Asfour, M.H.; Kassem, A.A.; Salama, A. Topical nanostructured lipid carriers/inorganic sunscreen combination for alleviation of all-trans retinoic acid-induced photosensitivity: Box-Behnken design optimization, in vitro and in vivo evaluation. *Eur. J. Pharm. Sci.* **2019**, *134*, 219–232. [CrossRef] [PubMed]
20. Long, T.; Tan, W.; Tian, X.; Tang, Z.; Hu, K.; Ge, L.; Mu, C.; Li, X.; Xu, Y.; Zhao, L.; et al. Gelatin/alginate-based microspheres with sphere-in-capsule structure for spatiotemporal manipulative drug release in gastrointestinal tract. *Int. J. Biol. Macromol.* **2023**, *226*, 485–495. [CrossRef] [PubMed]

gels

MDPI

Article

Comparative Physicochemical and Pharmacotechnical Evaluation of Three Topical Gel-Cream Formulations

Ramona Pârvănescu [1,2], Cristina Trandafirescu [1,2], Adina Magdalena Musuc [3,*], Emma Adriana Ozon [4], Daniela C. Culita [3], Raul-Augustin Mitran [3], Cristina-Ionela Stănciulescu [5] and Codruța Șoica [2,6]

[1] Department of Pharmaceutical Chemistry, "Victor Babes" University of Medicine and Pharmacy, 300041 Timisoara, Romania; ramona.parvanescu@umft.ro (R.P.); trandafirescu.cristina@umft.ro (C.T.)
[2] Research Center for Experimental Pharmacology and Drug Design (X-Pharm Design), "Victor Babes" University of Medicine and Pharmacy, Eftimie Murgu Square, No. 2, 300041 Timisoara, Romania; codrutasoica@umft.ro
[3] Institute of Physical Chemistry—Ilie Murgulescu, Romanian Academy, 202 Spl. Independentei, 060021 Bucharest, Romania; dculita@icf.ro (D.C.C.); rmitran@icf.ro (R.-A.M.)
[4] Department of Pharmaceutical Technology and Biopharmacy, Faculty of Pharmacy, "Carol Davila" University of Medicine and Pharmacy, 6 Traian Vuia St., 020956 Bucharest, Romania; emma.budura@umfcd.ro
[5] Dermatology Department, Faculty of Medicine, University of Medicine and Pharmacy Craiova, 2 Petru Rares St., 200349 Craiova, Romania; medicine@umfcv.ro
[6] Department of Pharmacology—Pharmacotherapy, "Victor Babes" University of Medicine and Pharmacy, 300041 Timisoara, Romania
* Correspondence: amusuc@icf.ro

Abstract: In the context of modern dermocosmetic development, multifunctional topical gel-cream formulations must be efficient for both therapeutic efficacy and cosmetic applications. This study presents a comparative physicochemical and pharmacotechnical analysis of three topical gel-cream formulations developed by Brand Chanand®: Acne Control Cleanser (ACC), Acne Face Cream (AFC), and Gentle Cream Cleanser Serum Control, Regenerating, Hydrating, Calming (IRC). Each formulation is enriched with a specific blend of bioactive compounds, including botanical oils, vitamins, and proteins, designed to treat acne, to support skin regeneration, and to maintain the skin barrier. A multidisciplinary approach was used, including Fourier Transform Infrared Spectroscopy with Attenuated Total Reflectance (FTIR-ATR), differential scanning calorimetry (DSC), rheological evaluation, pH and density determination, spreadability analysis, and oxidative stability testing to evaluate the products. Antioxidant capacity was assessed through multiple in vitro assays. The results demonstrated that all three gel-cream formulations exhibit pseudoplastic rheological behaviour, suitable for topical application. AFC showed the highest oxidative stability and antioxidant activity, while IRC presented superior spreadability and cosmetic efficacy, likely due to its complex composition. ACC displayed faster absorption and was ideal for targeted use on oily or acne-prone skin. The differences observed in the stability and performance suggest that the ingredient synergy, base composition, and solubility profiles show notable variations in dermato-cosmetic formulations. These findings highlight the formulation–performance relationship in topical gel-cream formulations and support the development of new cosmetic products tailored for sensitive and acne-prone skin.

Keywords: gel-cream formulations; natural cosmetic formulations; oxidative stability; antioxidant capacity; skin barrier function

1. Introduction

The domain of cosmetic science has evolved significantly in recent years, integrating multidisciplinary research from dermatology, chemistry, materials science, and biotechnology [1–3]. Among the most dynamic segments of this field are dermato-cosmetic products, which not only satisfy aesthetic requirements but also offer therapeutic benefits, especially for sensitive and acne-prone skin. Acne vulgaris and its associated conditions are chronic dermatological disorders that affect a wide range of the population, often requiring long-term management through cleansers, moisturizers, and anti-inflammatory formulations [4]. In this context, modern cosmetic creams are expected to exhibit both efficacy and biocompatibility.

Topical formulations such as gel-cream products represent multifunctional compounds that combine active ingredients with carefully engineered bases. These gel-creams are promoted as suitable for sensitive skin and are formulated to perform specific tasks, ranging from cleansing and sebum regulation to skin barrier repair and hydration [5]. Their performance depends not only on the biological activity of the ingredients but also on their physicochemical properties, including pH, viscosity, spreadability, and resistance to oxidative degradation [6,7]. These formulations represent advanced dermato-cosmetic systems based on naturally derived active compounds and are optimized for therapeutic efficacy and skin tolerance [8].

In order to optimize formulation development, a comprehensive evaluation of these products is essential. Analytical techniques such as Fourier Transform Infrared Spectroscopy with Attenuated Total Reflectance (FTIR-ATR), and differential scanning calorimetry provide valuable insights into chemical interactions and thermal behaviour under controlled heating regimes, while rheological testing helps to assess the application and product viscosity behaviour. Additionally, oxidative stability is a crucial parameter for assessing the shelf life and safety of the products.

This study aims to conduct a comparative analysis of three topical gel-cream formulations developed by Brand Chanand® (The products formulations are established by Research & Developed Prop. 65 California Compliant USA and the products are produced in Bucharest, Romania, by Skincores LLC, Bucharest, Romania): Acne Control Cleanser (ACC), Acne Face Cream (AFC), and Gentle Cream Cleanser Serum Control, Regenerating, Hydrating, Calming (IRC) using a combination of physicochemical, pharmacotechnical, oxidative stability evaluations, antioxidant capacity and in vivo investigations of the cosmetic products behavior. By integrating results from multiple methodologies, the research aims to better understand how formulation characteristics influence the product performance and the stability related to their final scope. Such an integrated approach is essential for controlling future developments in the dermato-cosmetic formulations and ensuring advancement in the cream-based gel formulation design.

2. Results and Discussion

2.1. Organoleptic Properties

The organoleptic evaluation of the three gel-cream formulations—ACC, AFC, and IRC—was performed by direct observation and tactile assessment under standardized laboratory conditions [9,10]. The results are shown in Table 1.

Table 1. The organoleptic evaluation of gel-cream formulations.

Products	Color	Odor	Texture
ACC	white	odor characteristic of the components	Soft, greasy, and relatively easily absorbed into the skin
AFC	white	odor characteristic of the components	More compact, less greasy, and relatively easily absorbed into the skin
IRC	white-gray	odor characteristic of the components	Slightly oily, fluid

2.2. Density and pH Determination

The density and pH values of the studied creams (ACC, AFC, and IRC) were determined and are presented in Table 2. From Table 2, a difference in density was observed between AFC (0.99 g/cm^3) and ACC (0.62 g/cm^3) formulations. This is attributed to the distinct compositions. AFC, which is a semisolid cream, contains a higher proportion of lipid-based ingredients, whereas ACC, being a cleanser, includes more water and surfactants, resulting in a lower bulk density with a fluid gel-cream formulation.

Table 2. The density and pH values of gel-cream formulations.

Products	Density (g/cm^3) *	pH (22 °C) *
ACC	0.62 ± 0.02	6.02 ± 0.03
AFC	0.99 ± 0.03	5.81 ± 0.02
IRC	0.73 ± 0.01	5.05 ± 0.02

* Data are expressed as mean ± SD (n = 3).

All three gel-cream formulations exhibited a slightly acidic pH, which falls within the physiological pH range of human skin (4.5–6.5). This is favourable for maintaining the integrity of the skin barrier, supporting the microbiome, and minimizing the risk of irritation. The differences in density among the formulations reflect their varying compositions and textures, with AFC showing the highest density, consistent with its more compact consistency.

2.3. Spreadability Assessment

The spreadability of the three gel-cream formulations was evaluated using the extensometric method, with results recorded for five weights weighing 182.35 g, 232.35 g, 282.35 g, 382.35 g, and 682.35 g. The results are given in Figure 1.

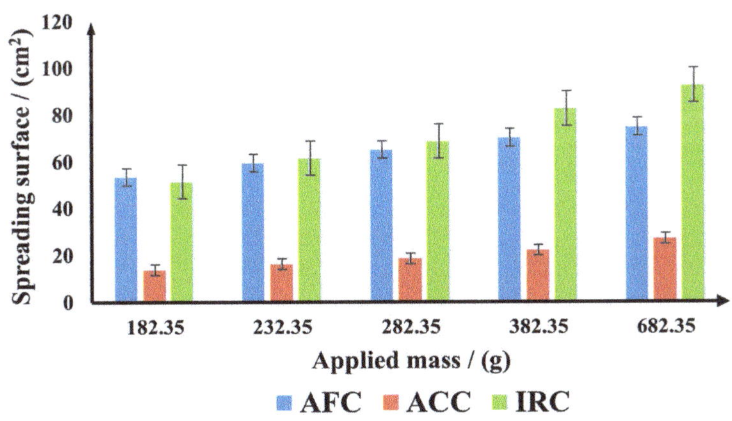

Figure 1. The spreading properties of the studied gel-cream formulations.

The data from Figure 1 revealed notable differences among the products:

(i) ACC showed the lowest spreadability values. This suggests a lower spreading performance compared to the other two gel-cream formulations. The ACC formulation was designed to have a higher viscosity, allowing for a prolonged contact time. Such a profile is advantageous for localized treatments, oily or acne-prone skin, where quick absorption is preferred, even though the spreadability is lower, as the gel-cream formulation was designed.

(ii) AFC is classified second in terms of spreadability, showing a consistent increase in spreading surface throughout the evaluation, although it remained below IRC. Its profile indicates a balanced formulation, offering both good spreadability and effective absorption. This makes it suitable for general daily use, especially for individuals with normal to combination skin types.

(iii) IRC exhibited the highest spreadability values throughout the entire applied mass, increasing progressively. This suggests that IRC has the greatest spreading capacity, potentially allowing it to cover a larger surface area with a smaller amount of product. Its high spreadability implies slower absorption, making it suitable for extended hydration and barrier function. As such, IRC is particularly appropriate for dry or very dry skin, and its use may be especially suitable as a night-time treatment.

These differences in spreadability align with the intended therapeutic goals and targeted skin types of each product, highlighting the importance of rheological and sensory characteristics in topical gel-cream formulations.

2.4. Oxidative Stability Assessment

The oxidative stability of the studied gel-cream formulations was assessed by monitoring the variation in oxygen pressure during accelerated oxidation. The obtained pressure curves reflect the consumption of oxygen as lipid oxidation progresses. A characteristic inflection point on the curve indicates the product's intrinsic resistance to oxidation, marking the onset of accelerated oxygen uptake that correlates with the initial formation of rancid odors and degradation products. The induction period (IP), determined by the intersection of tangent lines drawn before and after the inflection point, was used for the quantitative measure of the oxidative stability. A longer IP indicates a greater resistance to lipid peroxidation and a longer shelf life under oxidative stress. The results are presented in Table 3.

Table 3. Induction period values of the studied gel-cream formulations.

Products	Induction Period (min)
ACC	28.54
AFC	64.38
IRC	0.40

According to Table 3, among the tested gel-cream formulations, AFC demonstrated the highest IP, signifying superior oxidative stability. This is attributed to its composition of highly stable ingredients and a robust antioxidant profile, which effectively protects against oxidative degradation.

In contrast, ACC contains a higher proportion of vegetable oils rich in unsaturated fatty acids, such as *Abyssinian seed oil* and *Mango seed* butter, which, despite their nourishing properties, are more vulnerable to oxidation. The inclusion of vitamin E in ACC provides partial antioxidant protection; however, it is insufficient to fully mitigate the susceptibility of these oils to lipid peroxidation. This results in a moderately lower IP compared to the AFC.

The IRC formulation, while designed for enhanced cosmetic efficacy through a complex blend of active ingredients, lacks a comprehensive antioxidant system. Consequently, it exhibited the shortest induction period, indicating a higher tendency for oxidative degradation under the test conditions.

These findings highlight the essential role of each gel-cream formulation composition in oxidative stability, with implications for product shelf life, packaging choices, and recommended storage conditions. Formulations with longer IPs, such as AFC, are expected to maintain their efficacy and sensory qualities over extended periods, whereas those with lower IPs, like IRC, may require additional antioxidant fortification or protective packaging to ensure product integrity.

2.5. Fourier Transformed Infrared Spectroscopy—Attenuated Total Reflectance (FTIR-ATR) Analysis

The FTIR-ATR spectra of the three analysed samples are shown in Figure 2a ACC, (b) AFC, and (c) IRC, and were used to characterize the gel-cream formulations based on the mentioned active components presented in Table S1 in the Supplementary Materials.

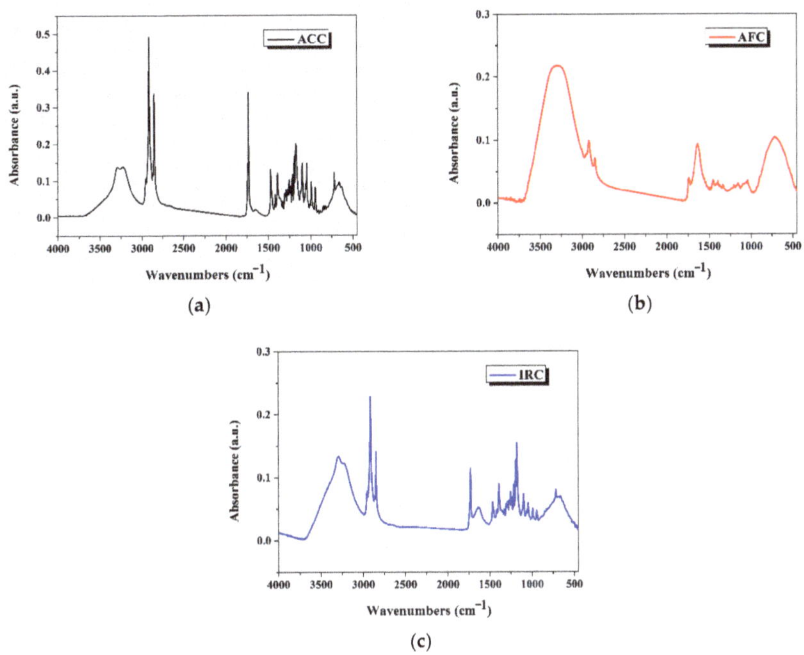

Figure 2. The FTIR-ATR spectra of (**a**) ACC, (**b**) AFC, and (**c**) IRC.

The main FTIR-ATR peaks of the ACC formulation (Figure 2a) are represented in Table S2 from the Supplementary Materials. The FTIR-ATR spectrum of the ACC nourishing formulation (Figure 2a) reveals the following bands: the broad band resulted from the overlapping of O-H and N-H bands of stretching vibration centered at 3291.9 cm^{-1} and 3226.3 cm^{-1}, which confirms the presence of alcohols, carboxylic acids, or amines, matching well with hydrating agents like *Abyssinian seed* oil, as it is mentioned in the ACC composition. Strong aliphatic symmetric and asymmetric C–H stretching vibration bands, which appear at 2914.9 cm^{-1} and 2849.3 cm^{-1}, support the presence of oils and fatty compounds (from *Abyssinian seed* oil) in the ACC composition. Carbonyl functional bands (C=O stretching vibration), which appear near 1729.8 and 1640 cm^{-1}, are indicative of esters (from butters/oils) and amides (from rice proteins). The amide I band at 1640 cm^{-1} supports the presence of protein-based ingredients such as rice protein. The two absorption bands at 1469.5 cm^{-1} and 1392.4 cm^{-1} are assigned to CH_2 and CH_3 bending vibrations of the ethyl and methyl groups. The C–O stretching vibrations of ester bonds and C–N stretching vibrations between 1300 and 1050 cm^{-1} suggest the presence of esters, alcohols, and possibly sugar derivatives from natural extracts [11,12].

The main FTIR-ATR peaks of the AFC anti-acne cream formulation (Figure 2b) are represented in Table S3 from the Supplementary Materials. The FTIR-ATR spectrum of the AFC anti-acne cream formulation (Figure 2b) reflects the presence and the synergy between hydrating active ingredients (betaine), lipid-replenishing agents (phytosterol esters), biological extracts (*Chlorella* extract), and antioxidants (vitamin E) [13–15].

The main FTIR-ATR peaks of the IRC intensive repair complex cream cleanser formulation (Figure 2c) are represented in Table S4 from the Supplementary Materials. The FTIR-ATR spectrum of IRC formulation confirms the strong moisturizing and barrier-repair properties (due to the presence of functional groups O–H, C–O, amide from the panthenol, niacinamide, and betaine compounds), the presence of lipids and antioxidants (based on the presence of C–H stretches, ester C=O, esters from mango seed butter, the anti-inflammatory and soothing actives (based on the presence of the bands which correspond to niacinamide and panthenol compounds) and the presence of the mild protein-based cleansing agents (from rice protein, algae extract) based on the presence of the amide I (1636.3 cm^{-1}) band [16,17]. The spectrum from Figure 2c is fully consistent with the stated main composition of the IRC formulation.

The FTIR-ATR spectral analyses of the ACC, AFC, and IRC formulations confirm the presence of the most important functional groups that correspond to most of the specified active ingredients.

2.6. *Differential Scanning Calorimetry (DSC)*

DSC analyses of the samples were carried out for all samples between −20 and 200 °C, at a temperature change rate of 10 °C min^{-1} (Figure 3).

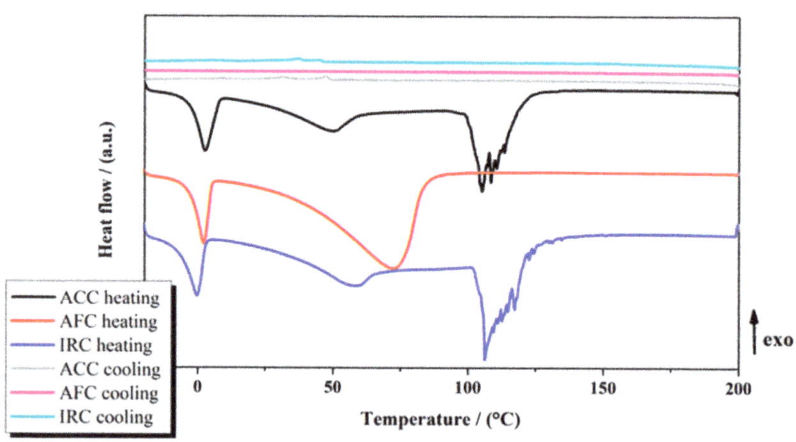

Figure 3. DSC analyses of the studied gel-cream formulations.

Water melting can be noticed for all samples during the heating cycle. An endothermic transition between 20 and 70 °C can also be noticed. This transition represents the melting of the organic components. Finally, water evaporation occurs after 100 °C for the ACC and IRC samples. Water evaporation seems to overlap with the organic melting for the AFC sample. The DSC events were confirmed by optical microscopy (Figure 4), exemplified for ACC formulation. The sample's melting and water evaporation can be noticed. In Figure 4, the melting process is indicated by the visible transition from a solid-like structure to a more fluid, less defined morphology, as observed under thermal microscopy during controlled heating. The water evaporation is suggested by the formation of microbubbles and gradual reduction in sample opacity, which occur concurrently with temperature increase.

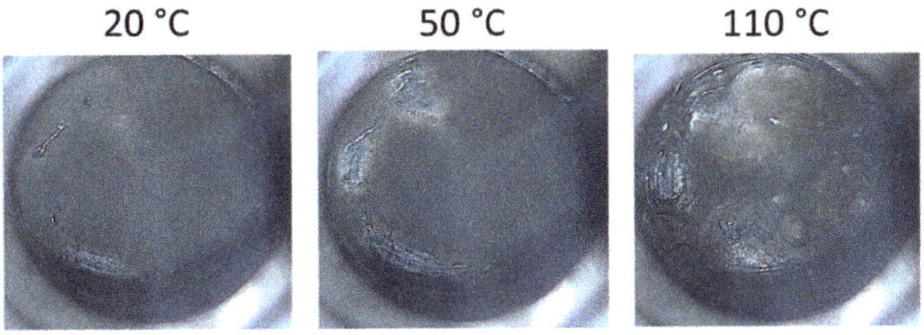

Figure 4. Representative optical microscopy images of the ACC sample at different temperatures (20 °C, 50 °C, and 110 °C).

The organic melting temperature varies between 29.8 °C and 40.4 °C. The water content was computed from the heat of fusion values, and it varies between 25.5 and 58.1%wt. (Table 4).

Table 4. Thermal data and water content are computed from the water heat of fusion values.

Products	H_2O Melting		Organic Melting		H_2O Evaporation		H_2O (%wt.)
	T (°C)	ΔH (Jg^{-1})	T (°C)	ΔH (Jg^{-1})	T (°C)	ΔH (Jg^{-1})	
ACC	−2.9	136.4	29.8	103.3	100.1	400.2	40.8
AFC	−2.8	194.1	39.1	1290.7			58.1
IRC	−6.3	85.0	40.4	60.2	103.1	316.0	25.5

2.7. Rheology Analysis

Rheology method represents an important step in evaluating the practical handling and performance of topical dermocosmetic creams during various stages of their usage, including application, mixing, storage, and administration [18]. The flow and deformation behaviour of these formulations directly influence their spreadability on the skin, their maintained homogeneity when mixed or blended, and their stability during storage to prevent phase separation. Additionally, rheological properties affect the efficiency and consistency of pumping or dosing mechanisms used in manufacturing and packaging. Understanding and optimizing the rheological characteristics is consequently essential to ensure user-friendly products that bring the intended scope while maintaining physical stability and aesthetic, cosmetically appealing throughout their use [19,20]. The obtained dynamic viscosity values were used to assess the flow behaviour of the formulations, with a focus on non-Newtonian characteristics and structural recovery after shear stress, which are important properties for the stability and performance of topical dermocosmetic products.

Figure 5a–c shows the graphical representation of data obtained from rheology measurements.

From Figure 5, it was observed that all three gel-cream formulations exhibit a pseudoplastic (shear-thinning) rheological behaviour, as the viscosity shows a decrease as shear rate increases throughout the entire examined shear rate range, which is highly required for topical applications. These formulations remain relatively viscous or semisolid at rest, ensuring the product's stability and the ease of handling, but become more fluid under shear stress, facilitating easy dispersion during application on the skin. ACC and IRC presented lower viscosity values and smoother flow profiles, revealing lighter textures. These properties contribute to easier application and rapid absorption during usage, and they represent essential characteristics that are particularly beneficial for cleansers and repair creams intended for daily or frequent use. Contrary to ACC and IRC formulations, AFC has a higher viscosity, suggesting a denser and more structured consistency. This increased resistance to flow may enhance the occlusive effects by creating a protective barrier on the skin surface to minimize and prevent water evaporation, providing a prolonged contact with the skin, and increasing the efficacy of its active anti-acne compounds. These rheological differences between the three formulations reflect not only the compositional differences between them but also their intended dermatological use.

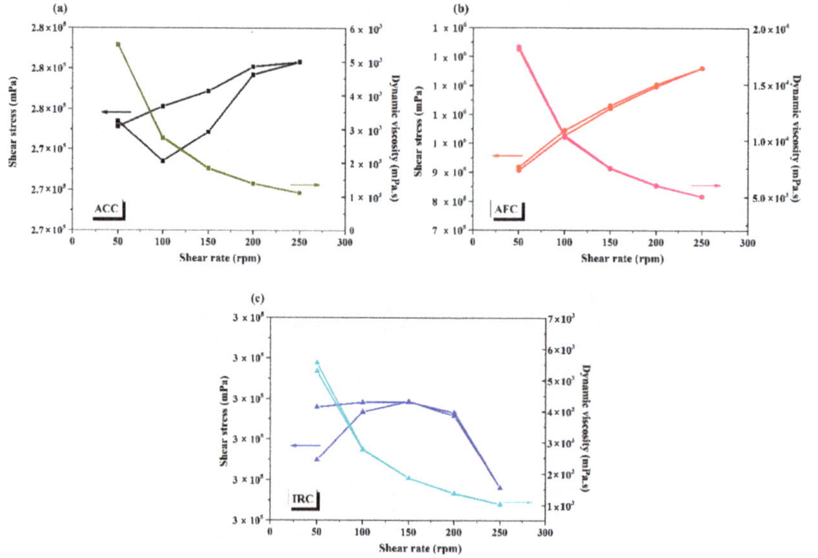

Figure 5. Variation in dynamic viscosity and shear stress as a function of shear rates in (**a**) ACC, (**b**) AFC, and (**c**) IRC.

2.8. Antioxidant Activity

2.8.1. DPPH Radical Scavenging Activity

Figure 6 presents the percentage of DPPH radical scavenging activities exhibited by the samples and the positive controls (vitamin C 0.175 mM, 0.35 mM, and 0.7 mM).

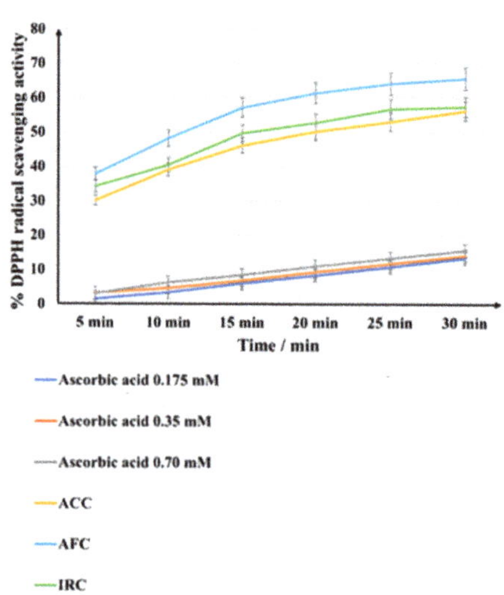

Figure 6. DPPH radical scavenging activities were exhibited by the samples and the positive controls.

All cosmetic products outperformed the reference ascorbic acid, which is considered to have strong antioxidant properties. The highest scavenging of DPPH radicals (up to 65.72% after 30 min) was observed for AFC cream. ACC and IRC showed quite similar performances, with the IRC formulation showing a slightly higher antioxidant effect (57.53% after 30 min). It should be noted that all three products exhibited a higher electron donor capacity after the first 5 min than any of the ascorbic acid samples used as a reference. The RSA percentage increases gradually over time in all samples, increasing more rapidly in the first 20 min, after which the rise is maintained, but the differences between 20 and 30 min are not marked.

2.8.2. ABTS Radical Scavenging Activity

The ABTS radical scavenging ability of the samples is presented in Figure 7.

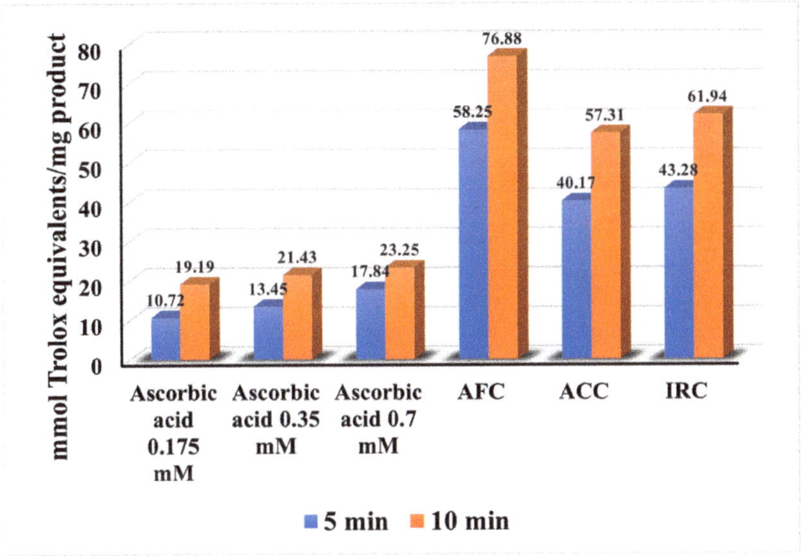

Figure 7. ABTS radical scavenging abilities of the samples and the positive controls.

In agreement with the data obtained for the DPPH scavenging effect, the samples showed a similar behavior. For ascorbic acid, the performance gradually increases with concentration, and for the cosmetic products, AFC still shows the highest antioxidant efficacy, both after 5 and 10 min, with an inhibition of 58.25% and 76.88%, respectively. However, the results show that all products, regardless of their physical system or composition, have a higher radical scavenging activity than ascorbic acid, as a control. As in the DPPH analysis, the lowest ABTS scavenging activity of the cosmetics was observed for ACC with 40.17% after 5 min and 57.31% after 10 min.

2.8.3. FRAP Assay

The FRAP values of the samples (μmol equivalent of Fe^{2+} ($FeSO_4$)/L) recorded at 5 and 30 min are shown in Figure 8.

The results of the FRAP assay are consistent with the findings of the other two in vitro antioxidant capacity studies, with the cosmetic products showing a much higher efficiency than the ascorbic acid reference solutions. As found in the previous analyses, the antioxidant ability of the tested products increases in the order IRC < ACC < AFC.

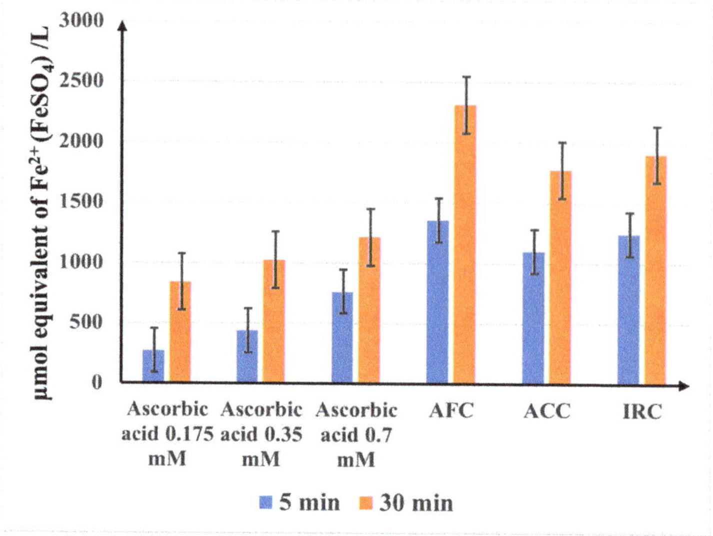

Figure 8. FRAP assay results.

According to the product's labels, several compounds with known antioxidant properties were included in the formulations. In particular, all three tested products contain vitamin E, which possesses a well-known high antioxidant function [21] mainly by protecting lipophilic compounds from oxidative damage [22]. However, the antioxidant mechanism of vitamin E is to scavenge free lipid peroxyl radicals, which are by-products of the chain reaction of lipid peroxidation. This mechanism is most effective in protecting the lipid membranes of the cell, and vitamin E is abundant [23].

The results of the in vitro analyses to prove the antioxidant capacity of the products have shown that the anti-acne cream (AFC) has the highest potential to inhibit reactive oxygen species (ROS) for all three methods. It can be assumed that the addition of *Chlorella vulgaris* extract and phytosterol esters from *Crambe abyssinica* may contribute to the antioxidant capacity of the cream, probably through a synergetic effect. Adhoni et al. [24] revealed that *Chlorella vulgaris* contains a large amount of flavonoids and phenols, two secondary metabolites with antioxidant qualities. Putri et al. [25] also found a high proportion of fatty acids in the phytochemical composition of the green microalgae, which can act as antioxidant molecules [26]. Flavonoids can prevent lipid oxidation and scavenge free radicals [27]. Phenolic compounds can donate hydrogen, and their antioxidant effect can be achieved either at the end of the radical chain reactions or during the neutralization reaction of the free radicals that start the oxidation process. The amount of hydroxyl groups in the chemical structure determines the antioxidant performance of phenolic and flavonoid components [26]. Wu et al. [28] discovered a significant content of β-carotene, ascorbic acid, and tocopherols, molecules with known antioxidant properties, in the chemical composition of *Chlorella vulgaris* in addition to the compounds mentioned above. On the other hand, Siti et al. [29] demonstrated that chlorophyll is the bioactive compound responsible for the antioxidant properties of *Chlorella vulgaris* extract. The authors carried out the analyses on different cosmetic products, varying various factors such as the amount of extract, the methods for its incorporation in the base, or the type of product. The results led to the conclusion that only by increasing the chlorophyll content can the antioxidant capacity be enhanced, regardless of the other technological factors. According to Chatzikonstantinou et al. [30] findings, of all Chlorella strains, C. vulgaris proved to exhibit the greatest antioxidant activity.

Regarding the phytosterol esters from *Crambe abyssinica*, Iwassa et al. [31] reported that their significant antioxidant efficiency is mainly due to the content of β-sitosterol. According to González-Larena et al. [32], the antioxidant ability of the crambe seeds' phytosterols increases with the β-sitosterol concentration.

The AFC product also contains betaine, whose antioxidant effect is the subject of intensive research, although the theories about its mechanism of action are controversial. While Alirezaei et al. [33,34] have conducted several studies suggesting that the antioxidant capacity of betaine is due to the increase in antioxidase activity, Balkan et al. [35] have proven that there is no correlation between these. The study conducted by Erman et al. [36] showed that betaine increases the activity of SOD (Superoxide Dismutase). Zhang et al. [37] conducted an important study and concluded that the three methyl groups of betaine are essential for its antioxidant activity and found that the mechanism is based on the enhancement in nonenzymatic antioxidant defenses by forming a protective membrane around the cells.

The results of the investigations on the antioxidant potency of AFC in the present study revealed its high performance, and it is assumed that this is due to the additional effect of the components, as they can rely on multiple studies that prove their individual efficiency.

It is interesting to note that both ACC and IRC have a lower antioxidant effect than AFC, although they contain crambe seed oil, which, in addition to phytosterol esters, also contains high amounts of tocopherols, especially γ-tocopherol, which is considered a stronger antioxidant than α-tocopherol [38]. There are several explanations for this: the oily phase, which acts more slowly, the inhibitory effect of other ingredients in the products, or the low concentration of oil in the formulations.

In addition, both products (ACC and IRC) contain rice proteins and mango butter, both of which have been shown to have an intense antioxidant effect. The results of the study by Chen et al. [39] suggest that rice proteins have strong ABTS radical scavenging activity and also antihyaluronidase and antityrosinase activity, which is beneficial for cosmetic applications. As found in several recent studies [40,41], the hydrogen donor activity of the aromatic amino acid hydroxyl groups contributes to their high capacity for scavenging radicals, and certain side-chain groups or the particular peptide structure can donate protons or electrons.

Various studies have attributed the antioxidant effect of mango butter to different ingredients. Nunez-Selles et al. [42] proved that it includes stable fats with a high proportion of saturated fatty acids, phospholipids, and various phenolic substances, and they assume a synergistic effect of these substances. Ahmed et al. [43] found that tocopherols and carotenoids may also be involved in the antioxidant activity of mango seed butter. According to the study of Y. Y. Soong and P. J. Barlow [44], mango butter possesses a high phenolic and tocopherols content, a high source of phytosterols such as stigmasterol, β-sitosterol, and campesterol, and has a strong antioxidant activity. Maldonado-Celis et al. [45] found that the antioxidant ability of mango butter is due to the high content of polyphenols, phytosterols, sesquiterpenoids, and microelements like selenium, copper, and zinc.

In addition to these ingredients, IRC also contains other effective antioxidant ingredients: niacinamide, cranberry oil, betaine, and panthenol.

Zhen et al. [46] demonstrated that niacinamide inhibits particulate matter 2.5 (PM2.5)-induced ROS generation and interrupts PM2.5-induced oxidation of various molecules, such as lipids, proteins, and DNA. Abdullah et al. [47] also found that niacinamide significantly suppresses oxidative stress in vivo and supports the repair of damaged DNA.

Cranberry oil has a high concentration of bioactive compounds, especially flavonoids, which are known to have antioxidant properties [48]. It also contains anthocyanins, which have anti-inflammatory and antioxidant qualities through their aglycones and anthocyanidins. Proanthocyanidins, flavonols, primarily quercetin and myricetin glycosides, and triterpenoids, of which ursolic acid is the predominant one, are also abundant in cranberries [49]. It has been shown to possess antioxidant qualities in cancer cell lines [50].

Betaine is a naturally occurring substance that has been extensively researched as an antioxidant in human health, but its antioxidant mechanism is still unknown. According to an interesting and extensive study developed by Zhang et al. [51], betaine exhibited minimal free radical scavenging action, according to radical scavenging assays. However, erythrocyte hemolysis and cellular antioxidant activity (CAA) tests ascertained betaine's antioxidant potential. The antioxidant activity of betaine was not caused by the gene expression and activity of antioxidases, according to the results of quantitative PCR and enzyme activity detection kits. By controlling the methionine–homocysteine cycle, betaine raised the amounts of nonenzymatic antioxidants, S-adenosylmethionine (SAM), and methionine, according to an analysis of its impact on the metabolism of sulfur-containing amino acids using high-pressure liquid chromatography. Furthermore, it was discovered that betaine's three methyl groups are crucial to its antioxidant properties. The potential explanation was that a strong protective membrane was created around cells to stop oxidative stressors from causing ROS production and cell damage due to the hydrophilicity of betaine's carboxyl and the hydrophobicity of its three methyl groups. The antioxidant mechanism of betaine was discovered to improve nonenzymatic antioxidant defenses through the formation of a protective layer around cells and the methionine–homocysteine cycle.

The body quickly oxidizes panthenol, a naturally occurring amine-containing diol, to pantothenic acid, or vitamin B5. Research showing that panthenol has moisturizing and anti-inflammatory qualities when applied to the skin supports its use in cosmetic formulations [52]. In an extensive study, Wang et al. [53] demonstrated that panthenol possesses proangiogenic, antibacterial, anti-inflammatory, and antioxidant qualities that can restore the mechanical and electrophysiological characteristics of skin and hasten wound closure.

The results show that IRC has better efficacy than ACC, which is probably due to the additional ingredients. However, IRC revealed a weaker antioxidant capacity than AFC in all three analyses, which cannot be explained by the number of compounds contained. The differences in the antioxidant performance of the three cosmetic products may be due to a synergistic effect between the ingredients, to the base used, or to the type of cosmeceutical form, or even to the different solubility of the ingredients in various solvents.

2.9. *In Vivo Investigations of the Cosmetic Products' Behavior*

2.9.1. pH on the Skin Surface

The human skin not only serves as a barrier against external infections, but also harbors a diverse microbiome that includes viruses, fungi, bacteria, and archaea. Disorders of the skin microbiome can impair immune function and lead to autoimmune and inflammatory diseases. The pH value is a key characteristic of the skin for the microbiome. Cosmetic skincare products are essential for maintaining the microbial balance as they interact with the skin's pH and microbiome. Products with unphysiological pH levels can disrupt the skin microbiome. A combination electrode, consisting of an H^+ ion-sensitive electrode and an additional reference electrode, is the basis for the Skin-pH-Meter PH 905 measurements. The results of the skin pH measurements are represented in Figure 9.

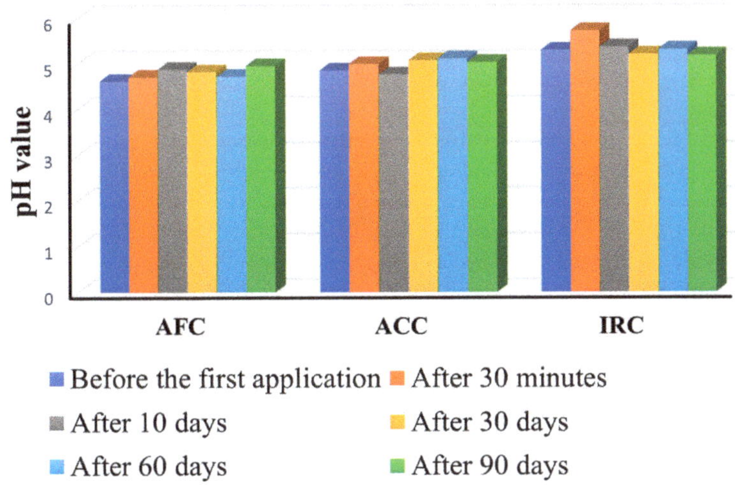

Figure 9. Skin pH measurements.

As an obvious conclusion, none of the products alter the pH of the skin, which means that they are well tolerated even with long-term use.

However, the behavior of the products is different for the three formulations. AFC gradually increases the skin pH to the highest recorded value after 3 months of daily use (4.95 ± 0.31 compared to 4.62 ± 0.53 before use). ACC also increases the skin pH, but the highest value (5.11 ± 0.54) was measured after 60 days of constant use, while it decreases slightly after 90 days (5.03 ± 0.60). IRC manifests differently, leading to a remarkable increase in pH 30 min after the first application (5.72 ± 0.67 compared to 5.29 ± 0.84 before the first application), but the value slowly decrease over time inducing, after 90 days of application, a final pH value lower (5.18 ± 0.71) than before application.

Although there were some differences in skin pH between volunteers, with subject no. 17 (age 29) having the lowest pH prior to application (4.4), and subject no. 3 (age 47), having the highest pH value at the beginning of the study (5.4), the trend was similar during the study period. Considering that IRC has the lowest pH (5.05) of all three products, its manifestation after application on the skin is not surprising. Nevertheless, the change in skin pH is not linear for any of the products. There are variations between different time intervals, but it is significant that there are no differences in responses between subjects.

In summary, an increased variety of the natural skin pH was observed during the course of the investigation. According to the Shannon diversity index [54], none of the test products significantly alter the diversity of the skin microbiome. Janssens-Böcker et al. [55] proved that using low-pH skincare products does not alter the diversity of the skin microbiota and may even improve skin microbiome diversity and health by lowering the numbers of some harmful bacteria. The acidic pH of the stratum corneum appears to play an important role both in the antimicrobial defense of the skin and in the formation of the permeability barrier [56]. The pH of the skin changes greatly throughout the stratum corneum, which presumably plays a role in regulating enzymatic activity and skin renewal [57]. Numerous endogenous factors, including skin moisture, perspiration, sebum, anatomic location, genetic predisposition, and age, influence the pH of the skin [58]. Variations in pH have been linked to the etiology of skin conditions such as irritant contact dermatitis, atopic dermatitis, ichthyosis, acne vulgaris, and Candida albicans infections [59]. According to Schmid-Wendtner et al. [60] findings, the prevention and treatment of certain skin conditions may benefit from the use of skin products with a pH of roughly 6.

2.9.2. Hydration Level

Improving skin hydration can lower sebum production, enhance the function of the skin barrier, and lower the risk of hyperkeratinization and colonization by microorganisms. Thus, topical anti-acne products with moisturizing properties may be more useful for the treatment of acne, particularly in individuals with dry, irritated skin. In addition, a more moisturizing formulation leads to better adherence to the treatment [61]. Corneometry is currently one of the most widely used methods in the field of dermocosmetics. The experts of the EEMCO (European group on efficacy measurement and evaluation of cosmetics and other products) expressly recommend the Corneometer® (Cologne, Germany) for testing the moisture content of the skin [62].

The stratum corneum, the uppermost layer of the skin, is used as a dielectric medium in the analysis based on capacitance measurements. Its dielectric properties change with increasing water content. Water has a higher dielectric constant (81) than most other substances (usually <7), being the basis for the measurement [63]. When Hua et al. compared Courage + Khazaka corneometry with other devices, they found that while the results for certain skin attributes were related to the measurements of other devices, the results for skin hydration and TEWL showed minimal variability [64]. According to Holm et al. [65], corneometry is a useful non-invasive tool for measuring the severity of atopic eczema in patients.

The results of the skin hydration levels are presented in Figure 10.

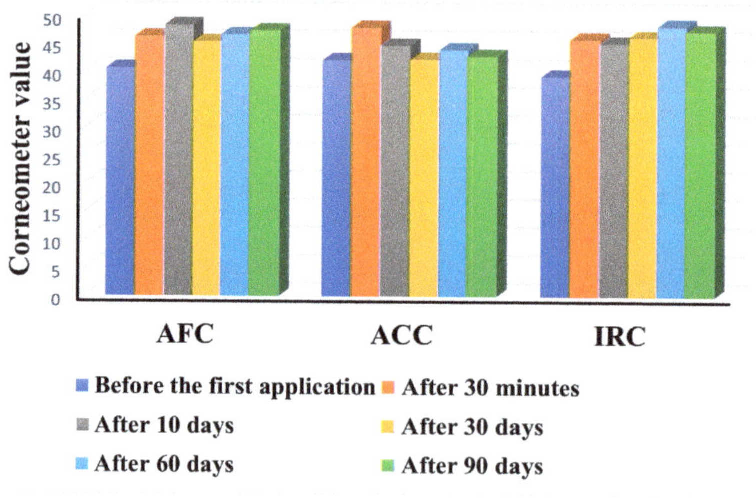

Figure 10. Skin hydration level.

All three products were found to notably increase the skin's moisture content after a single application. Even after three months of daily use, all three formulations were found to be moisturizing, but the performance of each product was different. The highest increase in skin hydration was achieved by IRC with a value of 47.22 ± 2.02 after 90 days, compared to 39.17 ± 4.18 before the first application. A similar behavior was also observed for AFC, with a final value of 47.28 ± 1.7 compared to 40.52 ± 2.47 at the beginning. ACC showed the weakest effect with a slight increase from 41.98 ± 3.25 to 42.74 ± 2.59 after 90 days. While AFC and IRC led to a constant increase in hydration over time, AFC showed a fluctuating behavior post-application.

In addition, the performance of the products in six of the subjects differed from the mean behavior registered in the other participants. For subject no. 5 (age 38), only AFC led to an increase in skin hydration, while IRC and ACC had no effect on the parameter. Subject no. 17 (age 29) showed a significant decrease in hydration level after 90 days of ACC application (from 48.06 to 42.13). Subject no. 20 (age 50) showed no change in hydration level at any time following ACC and IRC application. Subject no. 22 (age 27) and subject no. 34 (age 25) showed a significant increase in hydration after the application of ACC. The 90-day application of IRC in subject no. 36 (age 27) resulted in a slight decrease in skin hydration.

The moisturizing ability of the three products can be explained by their components. In AFC, the extract of *Chlorella vulgaris* and the phytosterol esters from *Crambe abyssinica* in particular help to retain moisture in the skin due to the content of amino acids, vitamins, and fatty acids, which leads to increased hydration [66]. IRC also contains *Crambe abyssinica* oil and betaine, which are known for their moisturizing effects [67]. Meanwhile, ACC also contains a large amount of *Crambe abyssinica* oil.

Skin damage caused by excessive dryness or oiliness can be prevented by moisturizing the skin, which also helps to prevent common skin conditions such as acne. In addition to protecting the skin barrier and reducing the formation of excess oil that can clog pores and lead to further acne breakouts, a moisturizing agent also helps maintain adequate moisture levels [68]. The use of moisturizers as supportive therapy has been shown to improve the treatment of some dermatological conditions [69].

2.9.3. Melanin Content

An important factor in the development of acne is inflammation, which causes capillary hyperplasia, prolonged vasodilation, and aberrant melanin synthesis, which in turn leads to postinflammatory erythema (PIE) and postinflammatory hyperpigmentation (PIH). While PIH is more common in people with darker complexions, PIE mainly affects people with lighter skin tones [70]. A significant percentage of acne patients experience PIH over an extended period of time, which emphasises the need for effective treatment methods. Therefore, anti-acne products should have effective properties to reduce pigmentation alterations. The results of the melanin content are presented in Figure 11.

The results indicate that all three tested products lead to a reduction in the melanin content of the skin after prolonged use. However, the behaviour of the products is different. While AFC and IRC show a slight increase in the melanin value 30 min after the first application, only ACC leads to a decrease in the parameter after the first application and maintains this decrease constant over time, from 63.44 to 52.96. Nevertheless, the greatest decrease in melanin was recorded after the application of AFC, with a decrease in the median value from 64.15 before the test to 50.42 after three months of daily application. The same pattern as with the AFC was observed with the IRC, but the decrease was much smaller in this case, from 69.8 to 61.39. However, in two subjects (no. 22—age 27 and no. 17—age 29), the melanin content was not affected by IRC, with final values similar to the initial values, but they responded with a reduction after the application of ACC and AFC. Also, one subject (no. 38—age 46) showed an increase in melanin content after the application of ACC (from 59.84 to 62.16), but a decrease after the application of AFC and IRC. It is important to note that in all subjects, the melanin content decreased after the continuous application of ACC and AFC, and only in 9 out of 40 (22.5%), the parameter also decreased after the first application of AFC. In the remaining 31 subjects (77.5%), the melanin content increased slightly but decreased again after long-term use.

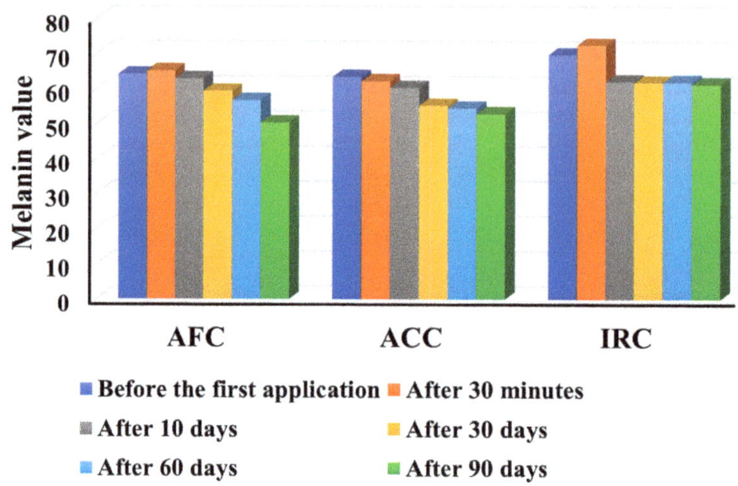

Figure 11. Melanin content.

The results demonstrate the positive effect of all three products on reducing hyperpigmentation of the skin, with AFC showing the highest efficacy, but ACC showing a constant behavior.

Chlorella vulgaris extracts have been found to suppress melanogenesis by inhibiting tyrosinase, a key enzyme in melanin synthesis [71]. In addition, Cho et al. demonstrated that betaine reduces the amount of melanin in the cells by directly inhibiting the activity of the tyrosinase enzyme and downregulating MITF at both the transcriptional and post-translational levels. Three signaling pathways seem to be involved simultaneously: activation of the ERK signaling pathway, AKT-GSK3β activation, and PKA-CREB repression [72]. Moreover, the study conducted by Kamei et al. [73] proved that vitamin E suppresses the activity of tyrosinase, a crucial cascade enzyme involved in melanin synthesis in melanoma cells, by 34%, apart from the 28% inhibition of melanin synthesis in B16 cells. According to the results of the present study, the combination of these ingredients in the AFC formulation appears to lead to increased efficacy in reducing the melanin content of the skin. According to the study by Kim H-K [74], melanin production in HRM-2 mice was significantly and strikingly reduced by the radish extract. Additionally, the radish extract cream showed superior skin-whitening and anti-wrinkle properties in humans, demonstrating its strong whitening effects. Its presence in the ACC formulation probably gave rise to its constant and pronounced anti-melanogenic activity. On the other hand, IRC contains niacinamide that can both enhance PIH and decrease melanosome transfer from melanocytes to adjacent keratinocytes [75].

2.9.4. Degree of Erythema

Skin erythema is one of the most common symptoms of acne, and following an inflammatory reaction, angiogenesis leads to acne-related erythema [76]. One of the aims of dermatocosmetic anti-acne products is to reduce erythema. The degree of erythema after application of a skin care product is also a measure of its tolerability and is recommended to be assessed for each new formulation developed. The results of the erythema index are presented in Figure 12.

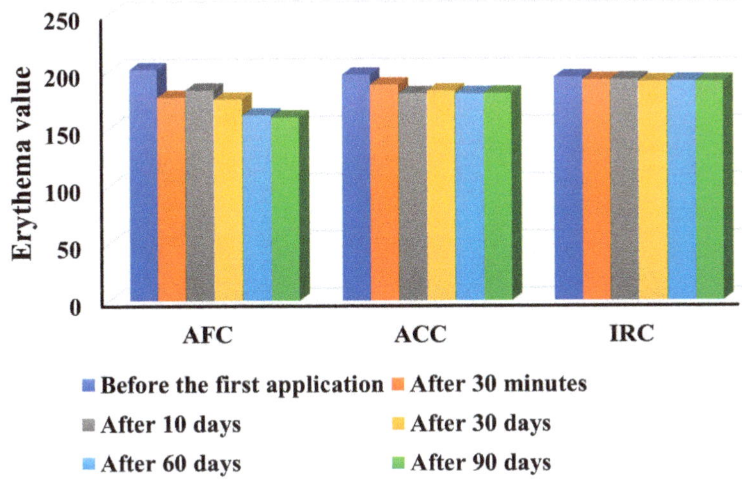

Figure 12. Erythema index.

It was found that all products diminished the degree of erythema in most subjects, resulting in a decreased mean haemoglobin index value. The most obvious decrease in erythema degree was reported for AFC, which reduced the index by 20.65% from 201.4 before any treatment to 159.8 after 90 days of use. Even 30 min after the first application of AFC, most subjects showed an abrupt decrease in the score. This means that the AFC cream has a good effect on the acne erythema and at the same time reduces the skin irritation caused by the anti-acne active ingredients, making it mild for the skin and easy to tolerate.

Various studies have proven the regenerative and soothing effect of each of its components: phytosterol esters from *Crambe abyssinica* [77], *Chlorella vulgaris* extract [78], betaine [79], and vitamin E [80]. It is interesting to note that the erythema value was not increased in any of the test subjects during the AFC application. The lowest decrease was registered after the application of IRC, but no increase in the index was recorded in any of the patients. Only one subject (no. 40—age 32) did not show a change in the erythema value on any of the test days. This proves that IRC is well tolerated even with prolonged use. This is not surprising as its composition is based on non-aggressive ingredients such as niacinamide, panthenol, *Crambe abyssinica* oil, betaine, and rice proteins. Regarding the behaviour of ACC, overall, it reduces the erythema index with the lowest value recorded after the first 10 days of application, a value that is maintained until the end of the study. Nevertheless, 11 (275.5%) of the subjects reported a slight increase in the parameter during the use of ACC, but no visible irritation occurred on the skin surface.

2.9.5. Transepidermal Water Loss (TEWL)

As a vital component of the body's metabolism, water is continuously evaporating from the skin. The unit of measurement for water content (Transepidermal Water Loss, or TEWL) is $g/m^2/h$. However, water loss will increase as soon as the skin's barrier function is compromised, even if the damage is minimal and imperceptible to the naked eye. Its measurement is a fundamental measurement in all types of topical product applications and an essential parameter for assessing the skin's water barrier performance. Skin's barrier capability and resistance are directly connected, and both are dependent on the stratum corneum's level of moisture [81]. The results of transepidermal water loss (TEWL) are presented in Figure 13.

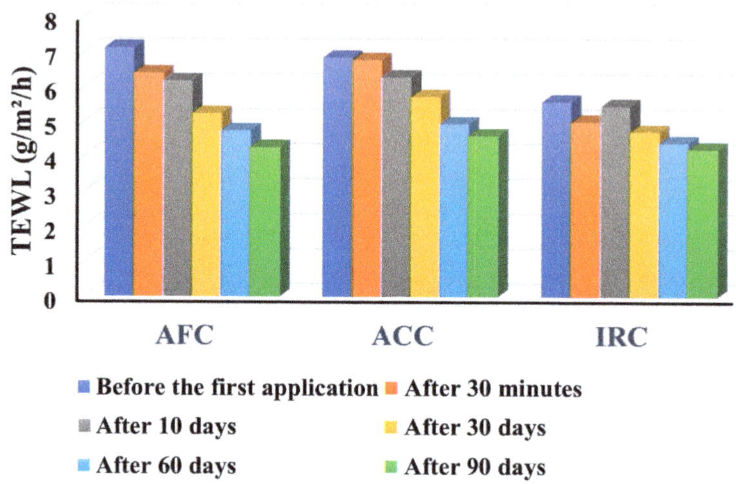

Figure 13. Transepidermal water loss (TEWL).

The three dermatocosmetic products reduced the TEWL from the initial value to a constant application over 90 days. For all three samples, TEWL decreased even immediately after the first application, and for ACC and AFC, this trend persists, gradually decreasing over time. In the case of IRC, the value recorded after 10 days is higher than the value recorded 30 min after the first application, but from this point onwards it decreases steadily over time. However, some different behaviors were observed. In the case of AFC, subjects no. 1 (age 38) and no. 15 (age 50) showed an increase in TEWL in the first 30 days, and the parameter only began to decrease after 60 days of use. In contrast, subject no. 31 (age 25) showed only a slight change in the indicator, from 4.43 at the beginning of use to 4.37 after 90 days. For ACC, seven of the subjects (175.5%) showed a consistent decrease in TEWL from the first application to the end of the study, while subject no. 37 (age 48) was the only subject to show an increase in the parameter after 90 days of use (from 6.55 to 7.06). For IRC, subjects no. 10 (age 33) and no. 29 (age 45) showed a significant decrease in TEWL from 5.78 and 5.42 at baseline to 3.05 and 3.20, respectively, after three months of daily use.

The results prove a drastic reduction in TEWL after the application of all tested products, which helps to retain hydration and a healthy skin state by forming a protective layer on top of the skin. The skin's capacity to retain moisture or the integrity of the skin barrier function can be determined by measuring TEWL [82]. Clinical data indicates a strong correlation between acne and skin barrier dysfunction. The skin's capacity to hold onto moisture is improved by a decrease in TEWL or an enhancement in skin barrier function [83]. Using moisturizers concurrently as an adjuvant acne treatment has therapeutic effects and improves skin condition by reducing inflammation and irritation [84]. As a result, acne and skin conditions can recover rather quickly. The study by Gala M. proved that regular application of moisturizers greatly enhanced skin hydration; repaired or strengthened the skin barrier; decreased skin oiliness; lessened the visibility of acne and prevented the emergence of new acne; decreased skin redness; lessened the visibility of blemishes or lightening them; and lowered the quantity, intensity and visibility of pores.

The registered results are in line with the results of the study by Morin et al., which proved that skin hydration is based on two processes and can thus be explained. The first hydration process takes place in the first few minutes after application of the product and follows first-order kinetics. Their results confirm that the process is primarily related to the filling of cavities and not to hydration-induced changes in the molecular components of the stratum corneum, which would require longer equilibration times. The second hydration process occurs at least one hour after application and has a slower rate with a linear progression. This process is thought to be caused by hydration-related changes in the stratum corneum, including changes in the kinetics and molecular structure of the proteins and lipids of the stratum corneum, the enlargement of corneocytes, and/or the development of water inclusions [85].

2.9.6. Skin Topography

The skin's surface topography is made up of scales, wrinkles, and lines. A network-like structure made up of primary and secondary lines can be recognized as a polygon. Measurements of skin surface roughness are often used in dermatological treatment and research [86]. The complex structure of human skin, its mechanical behavior, and its microscale topography all play a role in its ability to tolerate topical products. Some dermatological products can damage the skin and impair its functionality [87]. Skin topography analysis is an important test that provides important information about the behavior of the product on the skin during its continuous use.

SELS parameters, surface, texture, and ageing parameters were determined. The SELS parameters (Surface Evaluation of the Living Skin): SEr, SEsc, SEsm, and SEw represent the roughness, desquamation dryness, smoothness, and wrinkles of the skin. A higher SEr value indicates greater roughness, while a lower SEsc value signifies less desquamation/dryness. Conversely, a lower SEsm value indicates smoother skin, and a higher SEw value suggests more wrinkles. The surface parameters are represented by the surface area (if it is high, the skin quality is poor) and the volume (if it is high, the skin is hydrated). The texture parameters are represented by contrast (a low value indicates a good skin condition), entropy (a high value means a well hydrated skin), variance (a high value indicates a rough skin), energy (a high value reveals a young, hydrated, elastic skin) and homogeneity (a high value shows a hydrated skin). The ageing parameters are made up of the anisotropy index, which indicates the directionality of the lines (high values are characteristic of old skin), and the total number of cells—polygons between the lines (a high value is an indicator of young skin).

Black and white images of the skin show wrinkles and black lines, skin peeling represented by very large pixels, and light-coloured areas representing plateaus of the skin's microrelief. 3D color images show differences in the height and roughness of the skin surface. The results of skin topography parameters for AFC are presented in Table 5.

The results of the study show that AFC has a positive effect on the properties of the skin after the first application, which increases with long-term use, resulting in a significant reduction in roughness and dryness and a marked improvement in skin hydration, quality, and suppleness. In addition, it showed a significant anti-ageing effect, which is reflected in the reduction in the SEw value and the anisotropy index, as well as in the increase in the total number of polygons. Figure 14 registered for subject no. 2 (age 25) shows the images of skin topography registered for some subjects during the application of AFC.

Table 5. Skin topography indicators for AFC.

Parameter		Before the First Application	After 30 min	After 10 Days	After 30 Days	After 60 Days	After 90 Days
SELS	SEr	1.76 ± 0.91	2.38 ± 1.11	1.91 ± 0.71	1.94 ± 0.58	2.02 ± 0.49	2.53 ± 0.83
	SEsc	1.10 ± 0.04	0.06 ± 0.01	0.04 ± 0.03	0.02 ± 0.02	0.01 ± 0.01	0.01 ± 0.01
	SEsm	498.12 ± 21.25	495.21 ± 12.44	424.48 ± 27.19	439.42 ± 19.68	406.27 ± 15.61	385 ± 18.47
	SEw	159.71 ± 15.86	158.8 ± 4.75	121.45 ± 8.18	115.96 ± 10.85	104.55 ± 9.52	82.96 ± 8.81
Surface parameters	Surface area	655.74 ± 37.94	614.28 ± 28.44	620.07 ± 9.57	603.16 ± 21.18	583.66 ± 25.13	554.55 ± 17.40
	Volume	101.07 ± 22.46	111.47 ± 16.29	112.89 ± 0.14	117.48 ± 23.79	119.51 ± 18.75	122.01 ± 21.39
Texture parameters	Contrast	1.27 ± 0.22	1.08 ± 0.65	1.19 ± 0.71	1.11 ± 0.33	1.09 ± 0.28	1.05 ± 0.17
	Entropy	1.51 ± 0.57	1.64 ± 0.82	1.55 ± 0.77	1.54 ± 0.85	1.57 ± 0.82	1.61 ± 0.62
	Variance	4.65 ± 1.66	4.19 ± 1.21	4.38 ± 1.35	4.43 ± 1.29	4.55 ±1.85	4.50 ± 1.67
	Energy	0.02 ± 0.01	0.02 ± 0.01	0.02 ± 0.01	0.02 ± 0.01	0.02 ± 0.01	0.02 ± 0.01
	Homogeneity	1.4 ± 0.85	1.37 ± 0.99	1.38 ± 0.87	1.48 ± 0.54	1.47 ± 0.69	1.48 ± 0.71
Anisotropy	Anisotropy index	20.85 ± 8.69	19.42 ± 7.15	18.99 ± 8.48	17.89 ± 5.38	18.22 ± 8.04	17.51 ± 6.29
	The total number of cells (polygons)	59 ± 13	61 ± 18	70 ± 15	72 ± 16	75 ± 13	75 ± 9

The skin before the application of AFC registered for subject no. 2 (age 25) (Figure 14A) shows a moderate roughness, a slightly irregular relief, a slight peeling, a moderately hydrated and smooth skin, and a clear presence of fine wrinkles. It can be seen that skin roughness decreases in the long term, which is a clear sign of improved skin texture. The SEsc parameter gradually decreases and reaches its minimum after 90 days (Figure 14F), which indicates a clear smoothing of the skin. The SEw parameter decreases significantly up to 90 days, indicating a reduction in fine lines. The skin becomes smoother after application of the cream, especially between 30 and 90 days. The texture parameters improve significantly up to 30–90 days, indicating a smoother, more even, and younger texture. The relatively constant number of cells indicates stable epidermal activity, with no signs of inflammation or excessive regeneration.

The 50-year-old subject exhibited skin with mild roughness, indicating moderate skin relief and smoothness, with a moderate to high SEw score indicating the onset of structural changes in the skin (Figure S1 from the Supplementary Materials). The beginnings of photo-ageing are evident, but no significant peeling is observed. After application of the cream, a decrease in skin roughness is observed, and peeling is significantly reduced, indicating good skin hydration with surface smoothing and active cell regeneration. A homogenization of the skin texture and a reduction in the depth of fine lines are also observed, indicating improved hydration, probably also due to the stimulation of collagen synthesis, given the increase in volume.

At baseline, the facial skin of subject 18 (Figure S2 from the Supplementary Materials) has moderate SEr and SEw values, and the skin appears to be fairly smooth and slightly wrinkled. SEsc is very low, which is a good indicator that the skin is well hydrated (no visible scales). The texture appears quite even (moderate contrast and entropy). After applying the cream, the skin condition changes for the better. The surface parameters indicate a smoothing of the macrorelief of the skin and a stabilization of the skin. The texture becomes more homogeneous, smoother, and even, with active skin regeneration and subsequent stabilization. As a conclusion, the skin of all subjects notably improved its microrelief and mechanical properties after the continuous application of AFC during 90 days.

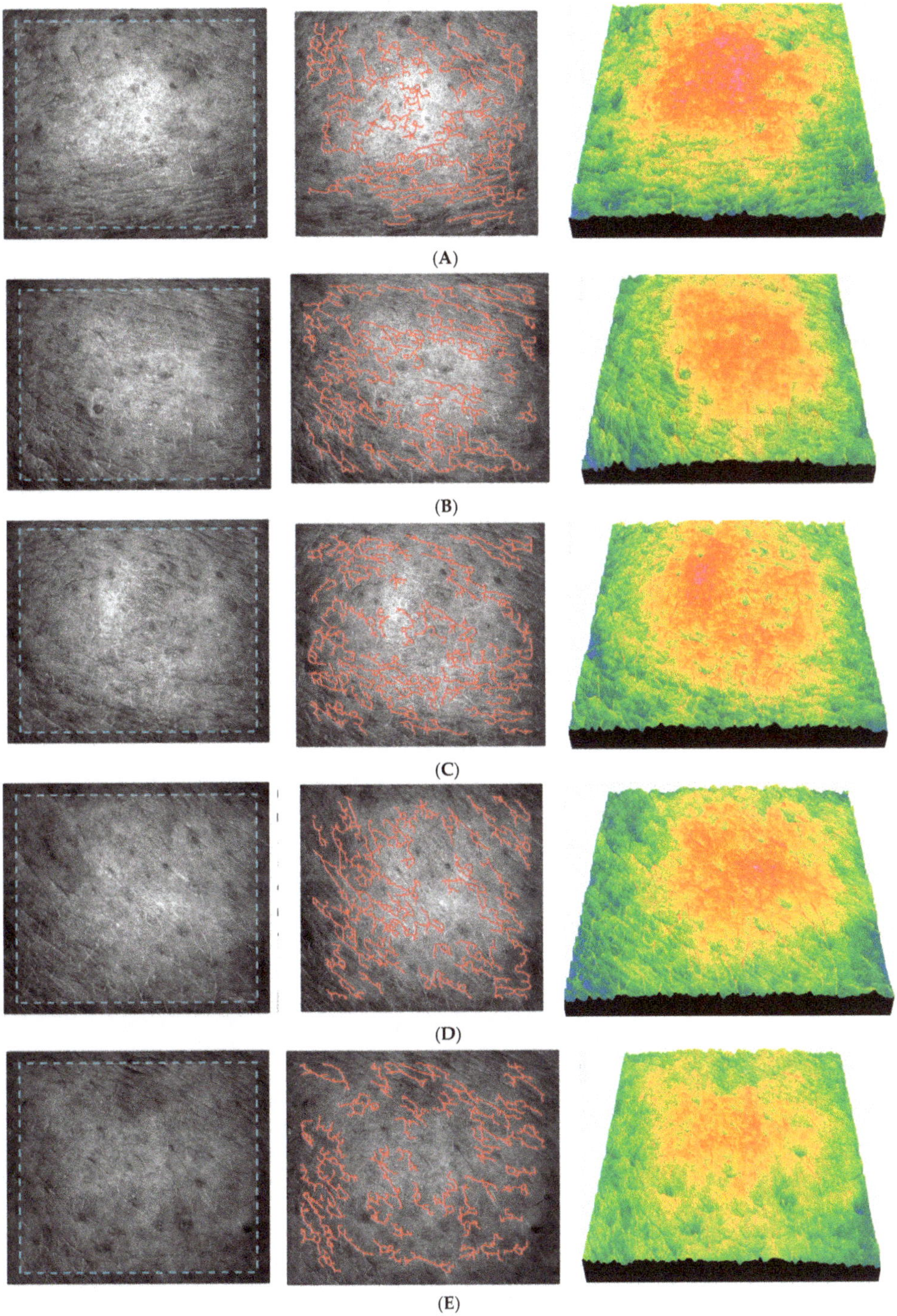

Figure 14. *Cont.*

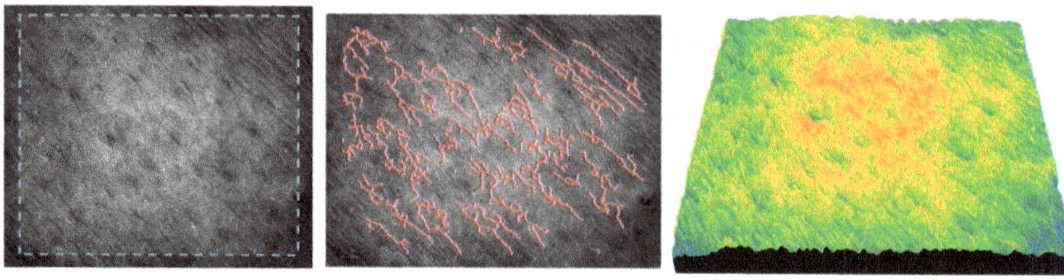

(F)

Figure 14. The images registered for subject no. 2 (age 25) when using AFC: (**A**) before the first application; (**B**) at 30 min after the first application; (**C**) after 10 days; (**D**) after 30 days; (**E**) after 60 days; (**F**) after 90 days.

The mechanical properties change in parallel with the biological changes that take place in the epidermis during cell development. The uppermost skin layer and the stratum corneum are commonly identified with different mechanical responses [88]. Compared to the initial physiological state [89], the apparent stiffness of the stratum corneum decreases by orders of magnitude when the corneocytes are hydrated and swell due to water uptake [90]. Due to the presence of essential amino acids (including proline, lysine, and glycine) and peptides in the composition of *Chlorella vulgaris* extract, it has been shown to enhance the production of collagen, increase skin suppleness, and reduce the visibility of wrinkles and fine lines [91]. *Chlorella vulgaris* extract also contains large amounts of polysaccharides that bind moisture, improve the skin barrier, and increase hydration [92]. The vitamin B complex (B1, B2, B3, B6, B12) it contains improves the overall tone and texture of the skin, stimulates cell metabolism, and promotes skin regeneration. Alpha-linolenic acid (ALA), an essential fatty acid, helps to maintain the lipid barrier of the skin, reducing irritation and dryness [93].

The results of skin topography parameters for ACC are presented in Table 6.

Table 6. Skin topography indicators for ACC.

Parameter		Before the First Application	After 30 min	After 10 Days	After 30 Days	After 60 Days	After 90 Days
SELS	SEr	1.92 ± 0.83	2.01 ± 1.05	2.05 ± 0.97	2.03 ± 0.67	2.12 ± 0.84	2.15 ± 0.92
	SEsc	0.93 ± 0.52	0.54 ± 0.44	0.53 ± 0.28	0.37 ± 0.20	0.31 ± 0.14	0.21 ± 0.07
	SEsm	514.75 ± 29.18	417.93 ± 34.02	482.96 ± 17.25	450.48 ± 26.94	447.15 ± 13.72	405.81 ± 19.14
	SEw	164.6 ± 10.23	159.14 ± 15.15	147.77 ± 12.45	139.99 ± 20.47	131.12 ± 17.61	128.97 ± 9.44
Surface parameters	Surface area	690.61 ± 41.13	601.14 ± 29.52	648.08 ± 27.11	639.79 ± 34.58	638.10 ± 28.36	626.02 ± 30.02
	Volume	101.16 ± 13.20	103.21 ± 12.78	103.88 ± 17.63	111.70 ± 14.22	112.74 ± 20.96	118.80 ± 18.19
Texture parameters	Contrast	1.35 ± 0.41	0.97 ± 0.68	1.24 ± 0.55	1.16 ± 0.70	1.14 ± 0.59	1.09 ± 0.65
	Entropy	1.44 ± 0.75	1.42 ± 0.49	1.41 ± 0.62	1.39 ± 0.57	1.40 ± 0.68	1.36 ± 0.66
	Variance	5.08 ± 2.01	5.11 ± 1.77	4.95 ± 1.53	4.74 ± 1.08	4.58 ± 1.24	4.45 ± 1.62
	Energy	0.01 ± 0.00	0.01 ± 0.00	0.01 ± 0.00	0.01 ± 0.00	0.01 ± 0.00	0.02 ± 0.01
	Homogeneity	1.39 ± 0.48	1.43 ± 0.27	1.39 ± 0.72	1.39 ± 0.83	1.40 ± 0.76	1.43 ± 0.44
Anisotropy	Anisotropy index	24.47 ± 3.09	21.68 ± 3.74	24.11 ± 5.13	21.94 ± 4.95	20.87 ± 3.86	20.8 ± 4.07
	The total number of cells (polygons)	57 ± 16	67 ± 18	60 ± 17	61 ± 12	64 ± 11	67 ± 17

Similar to AFC performance, ACC also improves the skin's microrelief and mechanical properties when applied over a longer period of time, but its efficiency is lower. However, evaluation of the skin by light scattering shows a significant decrease in roughness and an increase in smoothness, indicating a more uniform appearance in depth, and the fine lines become less pronounced. The reduction in surface area indicates that the skin becomes more uniform on the surface. The texture parameters indicate that the skin is more moisturized, and the homogeneity of the skin is improved. The change in the total cell count indicates stable cell activity, with a clear improvement, but no greater enhancement than for AFC. Some representative images were selected for the presentation (Figure 15).

With test subject no. 7, both roughness and dryness decrease, the skin becomes smoother, and wrinkles are reduced. The uniformity of the skin also improves, and the relief becomes less pronounced. The texture parameters indicate a natural, more even, and less rigid texture. The total number of cells has increased after a continuous 90-day application of ACC.

In subject no. 26 (Figure S3 from the Supplementary Materials), the behavior is different, and after the application of ACC, an increase in roughness, a strong deterioration of the superficial skin layer towards the end, a possible excessive peeling (dryness), and a decrease in skin smoothness were observed. This indicates a more uneven appearance in depth, and the fine lines become more pronounced, which is a sign of dehydration. The increase in surface area indicates that the skin is becoming more irregular on the surface, and the volume variations emphasize an increase in skin relief. In the texture parameters, it can be observed that the skin becomes more contrasted and "textured", which is a sign of irregularity, and that the uniformity of texture and homogeneity of the skin decrease. The fluctuations in the total cell count indicate unstable cell activity, with no clear improvement, but no clear regression either. ACC appears to cause irritation, dryness, or aggression of the skin in subject no. 26, aged 49 years. Compared to the other test subjects, however, this appears to be an isolated case, and the behavior could be triggered by a sensitivity to one of the product's ingredients.

For subject no. 37 (Figure S4 from the Supplementary Materials), the roughness decreases after the constant application of ACC, which means a regeneration of the epidermis and an improvement of the surface. The skin becomes smoother, finer, and the anti-wrinkle effect appears. A temporary inflammatory reaction or structural expansion is observed, but the increase in volume is a sign of hydration and replenishment of the skin. The skin texture parameters indicate a possible unevenness of the texture in certain phases, a temporary unevenness, and a slightly disorganized structure in the long term. The increase in the number of cells is a sign of increased cellular activity and regeneration of the epidermis. The high anisotropy at the end (90 days) could indicate an uneven reorganization of the dermal fibers. Overall, ACC seems to have more positive effects on young people than on older people.

The results of the study by Zhang et al. [94] indicate that rice protein hydrolysate is essential for skin protection due to its high antioxidant capacity, its effective protection of skin tissue, and its inhibition of water loss. Furthermore, the rice protein hydrolysate has been shown to diminish human face wrinkles by 11.8% [95], block the development of aging symptoms in mice [96], and lower the melanin content of human epidermal melanocyte cells [97].

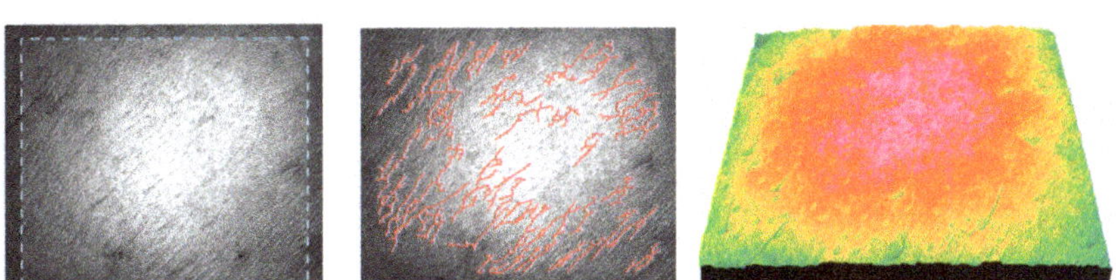

(A)

Figure 15. *Cont.*

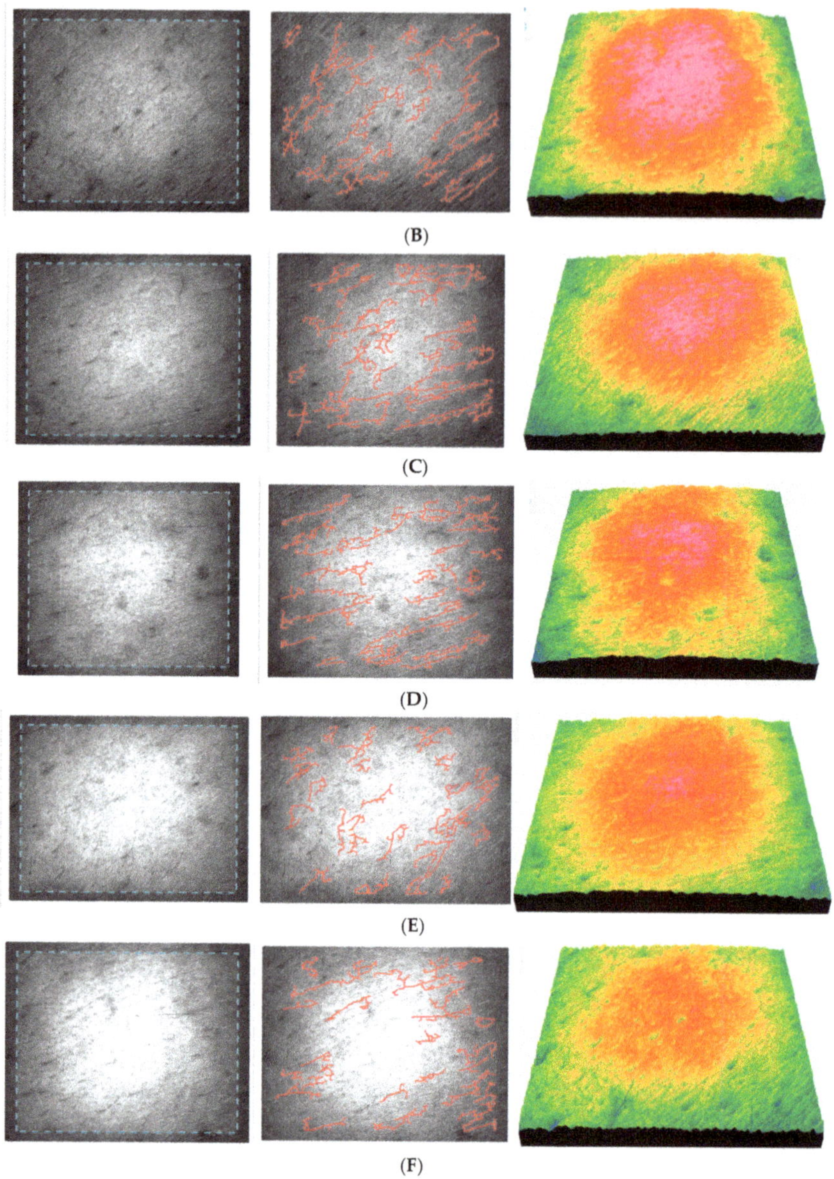

Figure 15. The images registered for subject no. 7 (age 26) when using ACC: (**A**) before the first application; (**B**) at 30 min after the first application; (**C**) after 10 days; (**D**) after 30 days; (**E**) after 60 days; (**F**) after 90 days. Image size: approximately 10 mm × 8 mm.

The results of skin topography parameters for IRC are presented in Table 7.

It can be seen that IRC produces the greatest improvement in skin topography of all three products analyzed. The positive effect was observed from the first application and significantly improved the biophysical properties of the skin during continuous application, with the highest point being reached after 90 days of use. It appears to be suitable for all skin types, both young and mature, with a marked improvement in the overall quality of the skin, especially texture, internal organization, and cellular activity. Roughness slowly diminished and smoothness improved significantly, with fine lines softened in the long term. The internal organization of the skin has improved according to the anisotropy index, and cell activity has considerably improved. The images registered for subject 9 (Figure 16) highlight a positive course with an important reduction in skin roughness. The smoothness of the skin is improved in the long-term application, accompanied by a clear reduction in fine lines and wrinkles. The surface parameters signal a clear improvement in skin uniformity in the long term, and a significant cellular recovery was detected.

Table 7. Skin topography indicators for IRC.

Parameter		Before the First Application	After 30 min	After 10 Days	After 30 Days	After 60 Days	After 90 Days
SELS	SEr	1.81 ± 0.25	2.10 ± 0.36	2.73 ± 0.54	2.98 ± 0.28	2.85 ± 0.60	4.06 ± 0.52
	SEsc	0.88 ± 0.19	0.64 ± 0.11	0.56 ± 0.20	0.50 ± 0.16	0.44 ± 0.09	0.43 ± 0.11
	SEsm	428.12 ± 27.18	404.95 ± 17.26	378.29 ± 20.15	366.40 ± 14.74	290.48 ± 12.03	251.01 ± 23.55
	SEw	137.97 ± 33.14	107.94 ± 25.32	100.12 ± 19.78	97.94 ± 12.96	96.55 ± 16.75	60.14 ± 21.44
Surface parameters	Surface area	796.17 ± 43.23	755.32 ± 27.42	759.08 ± 37.55	735.15 ± 29.14	684.56 ± 22.68	672.5 ± 20.91
	Volume	112.75 ± 14.48	126.32 ± 16.51	116.61 ± 12.16	116.06 ± 25.39	116.76 ± 23.08	128.21 ± 18.77
Texture parameters	Contrast	2.01 ± 0.30	1.51 ± 0.24	1.99 ± 0.11	1.87 ± 0.33	1.67 ± 0.28	1.10 ± 0.27
	Entropy	1.41 ± 0.17	1.35 ± 0.08	1.39 ± 0.15	1.36 ± 0.04	1.36 ± 0.12	1.37 ± 0.23
	Variance	6.98 ± 0.75	6.69 ± 0.35	6.02 ± 0.61	5.76 ± 0.46	5.61 ± 0.50	4.75 ± 0.27
	Energy	0.01 ± 0.00	0.01 ± 0.00	0.01 ± 0.00	0.02 ± 0.01	0.02 ± 0.01	0.02 ± 0.01
	Homogeneity	1.33 ± 0.18	1.39 ± 0.26	1.39 ± 0.45	1.46 ± 0.38	1.47 ± 0.49	1.52 ± 0.35
Anisotropy	Anisotropy index	26.3 ± 5.04	24.06 ± 3.78	23.12 ± 5.01	22.91 ± 3.98	21.47 ± 3.26	21.28 ± 4.15
	The total number of cells (polygons)	73 ± 13	76 ± 10	82 ± 14	81 ± 15	88 ± 11	90 ± 16

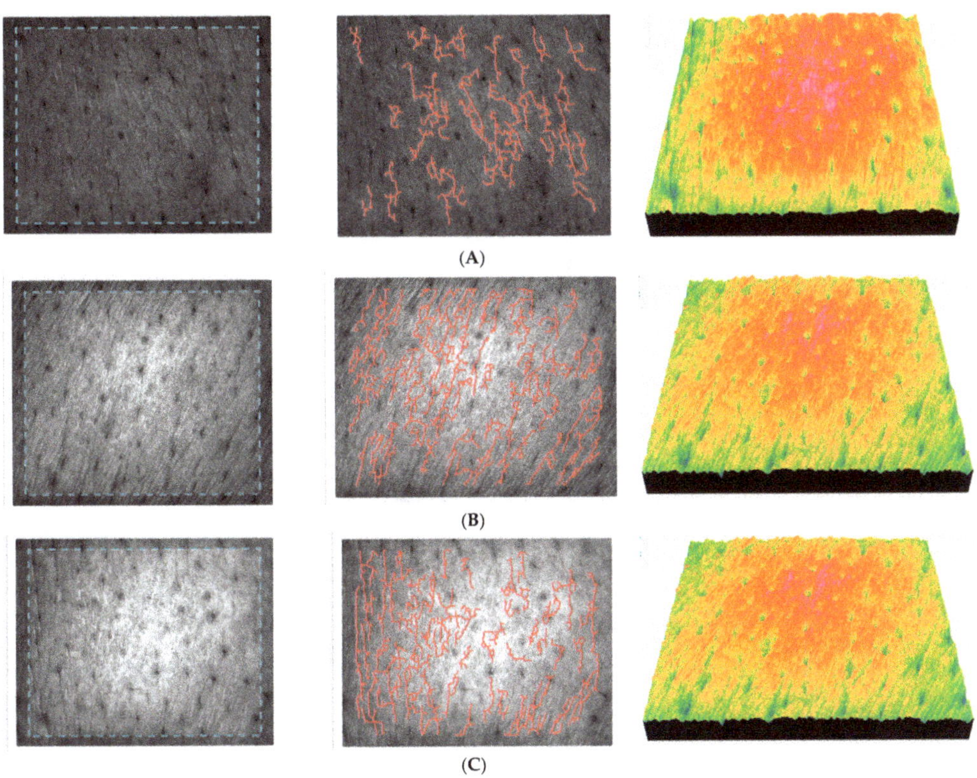

Figure 16. *Cont.*

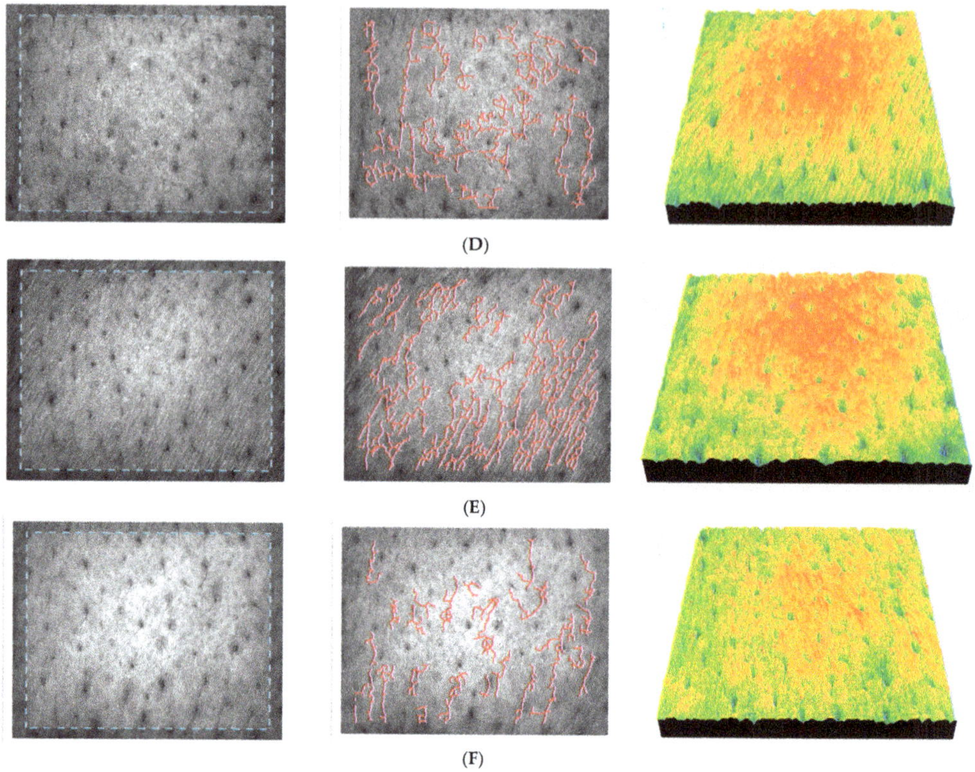

Figure 16. The images registered for subject no. 9 (age 24) when using IRC: (**A**) before the first application; (**B**) at 30 min after the first application; (**C**) after 10 days; (**D**) after 30 days; (**E**) after 60 days; (**F**) after 90 days. Image size: approximately 10 mm × 8 mm.

The data for subject no. 14 (age 47) (Figure S5 from the Supplementary Materials) indicate that the roughness of the skin has decreased, accompanied by strong hydration, followed by excellent soothing and restoration of smoothness. The fine lines were initially accentuated (signs of dehydration/contracture), but after daily use, they are significantly reduced. Texture is more uniform, balanced, and normalized compared to baseline. The anisotropy index indicates that the internal organization of the skin is largely restored, and the cellular regeneration is active.

The results recorded for subject no. 15 (Figure S6 from the Supplementary Materials) shows a constant improvement in skin quality. The skin is less rough and becomes smoother, while the fine wrinkles are significantly improved. The uniformity of the skin is partially restored, as is hydration, which is also confirmed by the texture parameters. The change in the total cell count attests to clearly activated cell regeneration, a sign of a positive adaptive reaction of the skin.

To summarize, IRC proved to be the most effective of the three products in terms of improving the skin's microrelief. It was followed by the AFC and then the ACC. The IRC behavior can be explained by the high content of rice protein hydrolysate and vitamin E. Mango butter has also been proven to reduce wrinkles and roughness due to its bioactive components such as phytosterols, tocopherols, and triterpenes [98]. The study conducted by Mandawgade et al. [99] showed that mango butter results in exceptional softness, actively restoring moisture for improved skin protection and rebuilding a naturally occlusive, protective skin barrier, leaving skin feeling smooth, moisturized, and silky. However, Camargo et al. [100] demonstrated that panthenol in skin care formulations has an enhanced protective impact in maintaining skin integrity after 30 days of treatment and leads to a remarkable reduction in TEWL. Also, niacinamide, included in the IRC formulation, was revealed to considerably lower pigmentation, inflammation, and oxidative stress in the skin [101]. Marques et al. stated that niacinamide may be able to partially prevent and/or reverse a number of biophysical alterations linked to skin aging through a variety of multimodal methods [102]. In conclusion, IRC has a very balanced formulation that contributes to strong skin activity by restoring skin functionality and preventing premature ageing.

3. Conclusions

The present study shows a comprehensive analysis of three commercially available dermocosmetic gel-cream formulations designed for sensitive and acne-prone skin: ACC (Acne Control Cleanser), AFC (Acne Face Cream), and IRC (gentle cream cleanser serum control, regenerating, hydrating, calming). Through a combined physicochemical assessment, such as spectroscopic analysis (FTIR-ATR), differential scanning calorimetry (DSC), rheological evaluation, spreadability testing, oxidative stability measurements, and antioxidant capacity, the key performance parameters and formulation characteristics that influence their efficacy were evaluated.

The results highlighted that all three gel-cream formulations exhibit pseudoplastic, shear-thinning behaviour, which is advantageous for topical application and ensures ease of spreading. Notably, AFC demonstrated superior oxidative stability, as evidenced by its extended induction period, and maintained a robust antioxidant capacity. In contrast, although IRC provided excellent spreadability and cosmetic efficacy, it was ideal for extensive skin coverage and prolonged hydration. ACC, with its formulation rich in vegetable oils and active constituents such as rice proteins and vitamin E, offers rapid absorption.

These results emphasise the importance and synergy of formulation composition and used ingredients, by influencing the overall performance of topical cosmetic products. The differences observed among ACC, AFC, and IRC highlight that not only the presence but also the compatibility and solubility of active ingredients within the formulation matrix are essential for achieving the desired use and sensory properties. In conclusion, the present study contributes to the optimization of dermocosmetic formulations. The in vivo investigations of the cosmetic products' behaviour demonstrate a good efficiency on the skin as they were designed.

4. Materials and Methods

4.1. Materials

Three dermatologically tested topical gel-cream formulations developed by Brand Chanand®: Acne Control Cleanser (ACC), Acne Face Cream (AFC), and Gentle Cream Cleanser Serum Control, Regenerating, Hydrating, Calming (IRC), were used in the present study. All products are recommended for sensitive skin and are formulated with synergistic blends of bioactive compounds designed for cleansing, moisturizing, and therapeutic purposes [103].

4.2. Methods

4.2.1. Physico-Chemical Determinations

Organoleptic Characteristics

Physico-chemical testing of the gel-cream formulations was performed to evaluate their physical properties such as color, odor, and texture [10].

Determination of Density and pH

The pH was measured using a calibrated ExStik pH meter (model PH110) (Extech, Taiwan, Taiwan), under controlled laboratory conditions. Density was determined by applying the classical formula, defined as the ratio of mass to volume, using precisely weighed and volumetrically measured cream samples. Each determination was made for three experiments, and the results are expressed as mean ± standard deviation.

Spreadability Study

Spreadability was assessed using the extensometric method with the Ojeda Arbussa apparatus, which quantifies the spreading area under standardized mechanical pressure, at five points. On a glass plate, 1 g of each hydrogel was placed in the middle of a circle with a diameter of 2 cm. After a second glass plate with a 182.35 g weight was applied to the surface, the diameter of the circle filled by the gel was measured. After a 2-min rest period, weights weighing 50 g, 100 g, 150 g, 200 g, and 500 g were placed successively on the upper glass plate, and measurements were taken after each individual weight was added. The diameter of the circle occupied by the gel was then measured [104]. The following formula (Equation (1)) was used to determine the spreading area occupied by the hydrogel:

$$S = \pi r^2 \quad (1)$$

where S is the spreading area (mm^2) and r is the radius (mm).

Oxidative Stability Test

Lipid auto-oxidation is an important factor that can significantly reduce the shelf life and efficacy of cosmetic products, especially formulations rich in unsaturated oils or active ingredients sensitive to oxygen. To evaluate the oxidative stability, expressed as induction period, of the studied gel-cream formulations, the Velp OXITEST reactor (Velp Scientifica, Usmate, Italy), which accelerates the oxidation process under controlled and reproducible conditions, was used. The test involves subjecting the cream samples to elevated oxidative stress by exposing them to a temperature of 90 °C and a pressure of 6 atm in the presence of pure oxygen. Small amounts of product (5–10 g) were placed in the oxidation chamber, where oxygen consumption is continuously monitored. As the oxidation reaction progresses, oxygen is consumed, leading to a decrease in internal pressure. The sharp drop in oxygen pressure indicating the onset of significant oxidation was determined using the OXISoft™ 3.0.0 software, which is integrated with the Velp OXITEST system.

The induction period (IP) is determined as the time (in hours and minutes) until a sharp drop in oxygen pressure is detected, signalling the onset of significant oxidation. This point correlates with the formation of primary oxidation products, such as hydroperoxides, and is commonly associated with early signs of rancidity or changes in sensory and functional properties. Two calculation methods were considered for determining the IP (i), the least squares method, which fits a curve to the oxygen consumption data, and (ii) the graphical method used as a supplementary recalculation approach if needed.

A longer induction period indicates a higher resistance of the gel-cream to oxidative degradation, and thus, greater shelf-life stability under real storage conditions. This parameter is particularly relevant for formulations containing plant oils, unsaturated fatty acids, or antioxidants, and is essential for determining packaging, storage, and formulation optimization.

Fourier Transform Infrared Spectroscopy (FTIR-ATR) Analysis

Fourier-transform infrared (FTIR) spectra were recorded using a JASCO FT/IR 4700 spectrophotometer (Tokyo, Japan) equipped with a monolithic diamond attenuated total reflectance (ATR) accessory (Tokyo, Japan). Spectra were collected over the wavenumber range of 4000–400 cm^{-1} at a 45° incident angle, with 64 scans accumulated at a resolution of 4 cm^{-1}.

Differential Scanning Calorimetry (DSC) Analysis

Differential scanning calorimetry (DSC) analyses were carried out using a Mettler Toledo DSC 3 calorimeter (Greifensee, Switzerland), under 100 mL min^{-1} nitrogen flow, at a heating rate of 10 °C min^{-1}. Optical microscopy images were acquired in situ, during the DSC analysis, using an Olympus SC50 digital microscope (Tokyo, Japan), at a frame rate of 1 image min^{-1}.

Rheology

Rheological measurements were performed using a B-One Plus rotational viscometer (Lamy Rheology Instruments, Champagne du Mont d'Or, France) equipped with a TE 95 spindle. The specified amount of cream was introduced into the measurement vessel, and the spindle was immersed up to the marked level to ensure reproducibility and accurate contact. Tests were conducted at various rotational speeds: 50, 100, 150, 200, and 250 rpm, with each speed maintained for 20 s. The temperature was kept constant at 22 °C throughout the experiment to eliminate viscosity variations due to thermal fluctuations. The hysteresis curves, represented as the variation in shear stress as a function of shear rate during ascending and descending shear cycles, were evaluated to determine the rheological properties of the analysed samples.

4.2.2. Antioxidant Activity

Three methods (ABTS, DPPH, and FRAP) were used to evaluate the antioxidant activity of the cosmetic products, and the results were compared with ascorbic acid used as a positive control. DPPH, ABTS, and TPTZ were purchased from Sigma-Aldrich Chemie GmbH, Schnelldorf, Bayern, Germany.

Preparation of the Samples

1 g of each product was mixed with 10 mL of ethanol and sonicated for 15 min, then centrifuged at 7500 rpm for 15 min. Finally, the mixtures were filtered through a 0.45 µm cellulose acetate filter.

DPPH Radical Scavenging Activity

It was determined according to the method established by Brand-Williams et al. [105]. The sample solutions were mixed with DPPH solution and sonicated for 10 min. At 517 nm, the absorbance values were measured every five minutes for 30 min, and the results are expressed as the percentage decrease in optical density from the starting value.

The DPPH scavenging efficiency (radical scavenging activity (RSA%) was calculated according to Equation (2):

$$RSA\% = \frac{(Abs_0 - Abs_p)}{Abs_0} \times 100 \quad (2)$$

where Abs_0 is the absorbance of DPPH solution (reference) at t_0 (initial optical density); Abs_p is the absorbance of the samples measured at different periods of time t (sample optical density).

ABTS Radical Scavenging Activity

A previously described method was used to evaluate the total antioxidant capacity [106]. ABTS and potassium persulfate reacted for 12 h at room temperature in the dark to form the cationic radical $ABTS^{\bullet+}$. At 734 nm, the absorbance of the working reagent was 0.70 ± 0.02. After the addition of the samples, the decrease in absorbance at 734 nm was measured after 5 and 10 min, and the results were calculated in relation to a Trolox calibration curve. The final data were displayed as mmol Trolox equivalents/mg product.

FRAP Assay

The FRAP assay was evaluated according to the method described by Benzie IFF and Strain JJ [107]. 5 and 30 min after preparation, the absorbances at 593 nm were measured for the samples combined with FRAP solution. Fe^{2+} calibration curves in methanol were used to calculate the FRAP values (μmol equivalent of Fe^{2+} ($FeSO_4$)/L).

All analyses were performed in triplicate. The results are presented as mean values with corresponding error bars representing standard deviations.

4.2.3. In Vivo Investigations of the Cosmetic Products' Behavior

Various biophysical properties of the skin were determined with the appropriate Multi Probe Adapter MPA 6 device (manufactured by Courage + Khazaka electronic GmbH, Cologne, Germany) probes: pH (with Skin-pH-Meter PH 905 (Cologne, Germany)), hydration level (with Corneometer® CM 825), melanin content and degree of erythema (with Mexameter® MX 18, Courage + Khazaka electronic GmbH, Cologne, Germany) and transepidermal water loss (with Tewameter® TM Hex, Courage + Khazaka electronic GmbH, Cologne, Germany). Skin topography was determined by image analysis with the Visioscan® VC 20plus, also manufactured by Courage + Khazaka electronic GmbH, Cologne, Germany.

Study Design

The experiments were carried out on the facial skin of 40 healthy volunteers. The test subjects, who identified themselves as women, were between 18 and 50 years old, with a mean age of 35.25 ± 17.25. They were informed about the products to be applied to the skin and gave their informed verbal and written consent. Each volunteer was given a code number (1–40) according to their enrollment order. The subjects declared that they did not suffer from any skin disease or sensitivity. Eight of the volunteers were smokers, and two of them were vegetarians.

The analyses were performed at the same time (9 am), under the same temperature (22 ± 0.5 °C) and humidity conditions (45%), on the forehand, right and left cheeks, at a distance of at least 5 cm from the eyes. The subjects applied the products every evening before going to bed and left them on the skin surface all night (around 7 h). During this time, they were asked not to use any other skin products. The following test areas were considered: AFC was applied on the right cheek, AFC on the left cheek, and IRC on the forehand. The application area was 4×4 cm^2, which ensured sufficient clearance for the measurement probe inside each site (the probes are approximately 12 cm in diameter). The measurements were realized at six different times: before the first application, after 30 min, 10 days, 30 days, 60 days, and 90 days after the first application. The results are given as mean ± SD.

The study was conducted in accordance with the Declaration of Helsinki and approved by the Commission for University and Scientific Ethics and Deontology of the University of Medicine and Pharmacy of Craiova (no. 72/11 May 2021).

Supplementary Materials: The following supporting information can be downloaded at: https://www.mdpi.com/article/10.3390/gels11070532/s1, Figure S1: The images registered for subject no. 15 (age 50) when using AFC: (**A**) before the first application; (**B**) at 30 min after the first application; (**C**) after 10 days; (**D**) after 30 days; (**E**) after 60 days; (**F**) after 90 days; Figure S2: The images registered for subject no. 18 (age 35) when using AFC: (**A**) before the first application; (**B**) at 30 min after the first application; (**C**) after 10 days; (**D**) after 30 days; (**E**) after 60 days; (**F**) after 90 days; Figure S3: The images registered for subject no.26 (age 49) when using ACC: (**A**) before the first application; (**B**) at 30 min after the first application; (**C**) after 10 days; (**D**) after 30 days; (**E**) after 60 days; (**F**) after 90 days; Figure S4: The images registered for subject no. 37 (age 48) when using ACC: (A) before the first application; (**B**) at 30 min after the first application; (**C**) after 10 days; (**D**) after 30 days; (**E**) after 60 days; (**F**) after 90 days; Figure S5: The images registered for subject no. 15 (age 50) when using IRC: (**A**) before the first application; (**B**) at 30 min after the first application; (**C**) after 10 days; (**D**) after 30 days; (**E**) after 60 days; (**F**) after 90 days; Figure S6: The images registered for subject no. 15 (age 50) when using IRC: (**A**) before the first application; (**B**) at 30 min after the first application; (**C**) after 10 days; (**D**) after 30 days; (**E**) after 60 days; (**F**) after 90 days. Table S1: Composition of gel-cream formulations according to Chanand; Table S2: The functional groups for the ACC nourishing formulation, their peak position, and the identified possible source ingredients; Table S3: The functional groups for the AFC anti-acne cream formulation, the peak position, and possible source ingredients; Table S4: The functional groups for the IRC formulation, their peak position, and the identified possible ingredients.

Author Contributions: Conceptualization, A.M.M. and E.A.O.; methodology, E.A.O. and A.M.M.; software, C.-I.S.; validation, R.P., E.A.O. and A.M.M.; formal analysis, R.P., C.T., D.C.C., R.-A.M., C.-I.S. and C.Ș.; investigation, R.P., C.T., D.C.C., R.-A.M., C.-I.S. and C.Ș.; resources, R.P.; data curation, R.P.; writing—original draft preparation, A.M.M. and E.A.O.; writing—review and editing, A.M.M. and E.A.O.; supervision, A.M.M. and E.A.O.; funding acquisition, R.P. All authors have read and agreed to the published version of the manuscript.

Funding: We would like to acknowledge Victor Babes University of Medicine and Pharmacy, Timișoara, for their support in covering the costs of publication for this research paper.

Institutional Review Board Statement: The study was conducted according to the Declaration of Helsinki and approved by the Institutional Ethics Committee of the University of Medicine and Pharmacy Craiova, code 72/11 May 2021 for studies involving humans.

Informed Consent Statement: Informed consent was obtained from all subjects involved in the study.

Data Availability Statement: Data are contained within the manuscript.

Conflicts of Interest: The authors declare no conflicts of interest.

References

1. Aonsri, C.; Kuljarusnont, S.; Tungmunnithum, D. Discovering Skin Anti-Aging Potentials of the Most Abundant Flavone Phytochemical Compound Reported in Siam Violet Pearl, a Medicinal Plant from Thailand by In Silico and In Vitro Assessments. *Antioxidants* **2025**, *14*, 272. [CrossRef] [PubMed]
2. Grech, V.S.; Kefala, V.; Rallis, E. Cosmetology in the Era of Artificial Intelligence. *Cosmetics* **2024**, *11*, 135. [CrossRef]
3. Tafuro, G.; Costantini, A.; Piatto, M.; Lucchetti, S.; Francescato, S.; Busata, L.; Baratto, G.; Semenzato, A. Eco-Designing Cosmetic Products while Preserving the Sensorial-Application Properties: An Instrumental Approach toward Sustainable Formulations. *Cosmetics* **2024**, *11*, 60.
4. Kim, H.J.; Kim, Y.H. Exploring Acne Treatments: From Pathophysiological Mechanisms to Emerging Therapies. *Int. J. Mol. Sci.* **2024**, *25*, 5302. [CrossRef]

5. Marie-Carole Kouassi, Michel Grisel, Ecaterina Gore, Multifunctional active ingredient-based delivery systems for skincare formulations: A review. *Colloids Surf. B Biointerfaces* **2022**, *217*, 112676. [CrossRef]
6. Neacșu, S.M.; Hîncu, L.; Vlaia, L.L.; Lupuliasa, D.; Scafa-Udriște, A.; Mihai, S.; Olteanu, G.; Grumezescu, A.M.; Ene, R.; Marin, R.C.; et al. Eco-Friendly Extraction and Formulation of Black Sea Shark Liver Oil-Based Emulgel for Anti-Inflammatory and Healing Dermatocosmetic Applications. *Gels* **2025**, *11*, 222. [CrossRef]
7. Ferdaus, M.J.; Mahmud, N.; Talukder, S.; Silva, R.C.D. Characteristics and Functional Properties of Bioactive Oleogels: A Current Review. *Gels* **2025**, *11*, 69. [CrossRef]
8. Karwal, K.; Mukovozov, I. Topical AHA in Dermatology: Formulations, Mechanisms of Action, Efficacy, and Future Perspectives. *Cosmetics* **2023**, *10*, 131. [CrossRef]
9. Chelu, M.; Popa, M.; Ozon, E.A.; Pandele Cusu, J.; Anastasescu, M.; Surdu, V.A.; Calderon Moreno, J.; Musuc, A.M. High-Content *Aloe vera* Based Hydrogels: Physicochemical and Pharmaceutical Properties. *Polymers* **2023**, *15*, 1312. [CrossRef]
10. Galdorfini, B.; De Almeida, M.G.J.; Antonio, M.; Isaac, V.L.B. Cosmetics' Quality Control. In *Latest Research into Quality Control*; Akyar, I., Ed.; InTech: London, UK, 2012.
11. Szmatoła, M.; Chrobak, J.; Grabowski, R.; Iłowska, J.; Woch, J.; Szwach, I.; Semeniuk, I.; Drabik, J.; Wrona, M.; Kozdrach, R.; et al. Spectroscopic Methods in the Evaluation of Modified Vegetable Base Oils from *Crambe abyssinica*. *Molecules* **2018**, *23*, 3243. [CrossRef]
12. Miedzianka, J.; Walkowiak, K.; Zielińska-Dawidziak, M.; Zambrowicz, A.; Wolny, S.; Kita, A. The Functional and Physicochemical Properties of Rice Protein Concentrate Subjected to Acetylation. *Molecules* **2023**, *28*, 770. [CrossRef]
13. Kitamura, Y.; Iwasaki, T.; Saito, M.; Mifune, M.; Saito, Y.; Sato, K.; Yomota, C.; Tanamoto, K. Standard infrared absorption spectrum of betaine and optimal conditions for its measurement. *Shokuhin Eiseigaku Zasshi* **2006**, *47*, 232–236. [CrossRef] [PubMed]
14. Ganeson, Y.; Paramasivam, P.; Palanisamy, K.M.; Govindan, N.; Maniam, G.P. LCMS and FTIR profiling of microalga *Chlorella* sp. for cosmetics and skin care applications. *Clean. Water* **2024**, *2*, 100028. [CrossRef]
15. Rungchang, S.; Kittiwachana, S.; Funsueb, S.; Rachtanapun, C.; Tantala, J.; Sookwong, P.; Yort, L.; Sringarm, C.; Jiamyangyuen, S. Nondestructive Determination of Tocopherol and Tocotrienol in Vitamin E Powder Using Near- and Mid-Infrared Spectroscopy. *Foods* **2024**, *13*, 4079. [CrossRef]
16. Wawrzyńczak, A.; Nowak, I.; Feliczak-Guzik, A. SBA-15- and SBA-16-Functionalized Silicas as New Carriers of Niacinamide. *Int. J. Mol. Sci.* **2023**, *24*, 17567. [CrossRef]
17. Kaur, G.; Kaur, D.; Kansal, S.K.; Garg, M.; Krishania, M. Potential cocoa butter substitute derived from mango seed kernel. *Food Chem.* **2022**, *372*, 131244. [CrossRef] [PubMed]
18. Wang, S.; Kislalioglu, M.S.; Breuer, M. The effect of rheological properties of experimental moisturizing creams/lotions on their efficacy and perceptual attributes. *Int. J. Cosmet. Sci.* **1999**, *21*, 167–188. [CrossRef]
19. Lee, I.A.; Maibach, H.I. Pharmionics in dermatology: A review of topical medication adherence. *Am. J. Clin. Dermatol.* **2006**, *7*, 231–236. [CrossRef] [PubMed]
20. Huynh, A.; Garcia, A.G.; Young, L.K.; Szoboszlai, M.; Liberatore, M.W.; Baki, G. Measurements meet perceptions: Rheology–texture–sensory relations when using green, bio-derived emollients in cosmetic emulsions. *Int. J. Cosmet. Sci.* **2021**, *43*, 11–19. [CrossRef]
21. Wolf, G. The discovery of the antioxidant function of vitamin E: The contribution of Henry A. *Mattill. J. Nutr.* **2005**, *135*, 363–366. [CrossRef]
22. Didier, A.J.; Stiene, J.; Fang, L.; Watkins, D.; Dworkin, L.D.; Creeden, J.F. Antioxidant and Anti-Tumor Effects of Dietary Vitamins A, C, and E. *Antioxidants* **2023**, *12*, 632. [CrossRef]
23. Shahidi, F.; Pinaffi-Langley, A.C.C.; Fuentes, J.; Speisky, H.; de Camargo, A.C. Vitamin E as an essential micronutrient for human health: Common, novel, and unexplored dietary sources. *Free Radic. Biol. Med.* **2021**, *176*, 312–321. [PubMed]
24. Adhoni, S.A.; Thimmappa, S.C.; Kaliwal, B.B. Phytochemical Analysis and Antimicrobial Activity of *Chlorella vulgaris* Isolated from Unkal Lake. *J. Coast. Life Med.* **2016**, *4*, 368–373.
25. Putri, T.W.; Raya, I.; Natsir, H.; Mayasari, E. *Chlorella* sp.: Extraction of fatty acid by using avocado oil as solvent and its application as an anti-aging cream. *J. Phys.* **2018**, *979*, 012009.
26. Putri, T.W.; Nursida, N.F.; Raya, I. Antioxidant Activity of *Chlorella vulgaris* Used As an Antioxidant Cream. *J. Phys. Conf. Ser.* **2021**, *1899*, 012030.
27. Treml, J.; Smejkal, K. Flavonoids as potent scavengers of hydroxyl radicals. *Food Sci. Food Saf.* **2016**, *15*, 720–738. [CrossRef]
28. Wu, L.C.; Ho, J.A.A.; Shieh, M.C.; Lu, I.W. Antioxidant and antiproliferative activities of Spirulina and Chlorella water extracts. *J. Agric. Food Chem.* **2005**, *53*, 4207–4212.
29. Agustina, S.; Aidha, N.N.; Oktarin, E. The extraction of antioxidants from *Chlorella vulgaris* for cosmetics. *IOP Conf. Ser. Mater. Sci. Eng.* **2021**, *1011*, 012057.
30. Chatzikonstantinou, M.; Kalliampakou, A.; Gatzogia, M. Comparative analyses and evaluation of the cosmeceutical potential of selected *Chlorella* strains. *J. Appl. Phycol.* **2016**, *29*, 179–188. [CrossRef]

31. Iwassa, I.J.; Saldaña, M.D.A.; Cardozo-Filho, L.; da Silva, C. Yield and quality parameters of pretreated crambe seed oil extracted using C_3H_8, CO_2 and C_3H_8 + CO_2 mixtures under pressurized conditions. *J. Supercrit. Fluids* **2021**, *175*, 105277. [CrossRef]
32. González-Larena, M.; Garcia-Llatas, G.; Clemente, G.; Barberá, R.; Lagarda, M.J. Plant sterol oxides in functional beverages: Influence of matrix and storage. *Food Chem.* **2015**, *173*, 881–889. [CrossRef]
33. Alirezaei, M.; Jelodar, G.; Ghayemi, Z.; Mehr, M.K. Antioxidant and methyl donor effects of betaine versus ethanol-induced oxidative stress in the rat liver. *Comp. Clin. Pathol.* **2014**, *23*, 161–168. [CrossRef]
34. Alirezaei, M.; Khoshdel, Z.; Dezfoulian, O.; Rashidipour, M.; Taghadosi, V. Beneficial antioxidant properties of betaine against oxidative stress mediated by levodopa/benserazide in the brain of rats. *J. Physiol. Sci.* **2015**, *65*, 243–252. [CrossRef] [PubMed]
35. Balkan, J.; Öztezcan, S.; Küçük, M.; Çevikbaş, U.; Koçak-Toker, N.; Uysal, M. The effect of betaine treatment on triglyceride levels and oxidative stress in the liver of ethanol-treated guinea pigs. *Exp. Toxicol. Pathol.* **2004**, *55*, 505–509. [CrossRef]
36. Erman, F.; Balkan, J.; Cevikbaş, U.; Kocak-Toker, N.; Uysal, M. Betaine or taurine administration prevents fibrosis and lipid peroxidation induced by rat liver by ethanol plus carbon tetrachloride intoxication. *Amino Acids* **2004**, *27*, 199–205. [CrossRef] [PubMed]
37. Zhang, M.; Zhang, H.; Li, H.; Lai, F.; Li, X.; Tang, Y.; Min, T.; Wu, H. Antioxidant Mechanism of Betaine without Free Radical Scavenging Ability. *J. Agric. Food Chem.* **2016**, *64*, 7921–7930. [CrossRef]
38. Santos, K.A.; Bariccatti, R.A.; Cardozo-Filho, L.; Schneider, R.; Palú, F.; da Silva, C.; da Silva, E.A. Extraction of crambe seed oil using subcritical propane: Kinetics, characterization and modeling. *J. Supercrit. Fluids* **2015**, *104*, 54–61. [CrossRef]
39. Chen, H.-J.; Dai, F.-J.; Chen, C.-Y.; Fan, S.-L.; Zheng, J.-H.; Huang, Y.-C.; Chau, C.-F.; Lin, Y.-S.; Chen, C.-S. Evaluating the Antioxidants, Whitening and Antiaging Properties of Rice Protein Hydrolysates. *Molecules* **2021**, *26*, 3605. [CrossRef]
40. Gomes, M.H.G.; Kurozawa, L.E. Improvement of the functional and antioxidant properties of rice protein by enzymatic hydrolysis for the microencapsulation of linseed oil. *J. Food Eng.* **2020**, *267*, 109761. [CrossRef]
41. Phongthai, S.; Amico, S.D.; Schoenlechner, R.; Homthawornchoo, W.; Rawdkuen, S. Fractionation and antioxidant properties of rice bran protein hydrolysates stimulated by in vitro gastrointestinal digestion. *Food Chem.* **2018**, *240*, 156–164. [CrossRef]
42. Núñez Sellés, A.J.; Durruthy Rodríguez, M.D.; Rodríguez Balseiro, E.; Nieto González, L.; Nicolais, V.; Rastrelli, L. Comparison of Major and Trace Element Concentrations in 16 Varieties of Cuban Mango Stem Bark (*Mangifera indica* L.). *J. Agric. Food Chem.* **2007**, *55*, 2176–2181.
43. Abdalla, A.E.M.; Darwish, S.M.; Ayad, E.H.E.; El-Hamahmy, R.M. Egyptian mango by-product 2: Antioxidant and antimicrobial activities of extract and oil from mango seed kernel. *Food Chem.* **2007**, *103*, 1141–1152. [CrossRef]
44. Soong, Y.Y.; Barlow, P.J. Antioxidant Activity and Phenolic Content of Selected Fruit Seeds. *Food Chem.* **2004**, *88*, 411–417. [CrossRef]
45. Maldonado-Celis, M.E.; Yahia, E.M.; Bedoya, R.; Landázuri, P.; Loango, N.; Aguillón, J.; Restrepo, B.; Guerrero Ospina, J.C. Chemical Composition of Mango (*Mangifera indica* L.) Fruit: Nutritional and Phytochemical Compounds. *Front. Plant Sci.* **2019**, *10*, 1073. [CrossRef] [PubMed]
46. Zhen, A.X.; Piao, M.J.; Kang, K.A.; Fernando, P.D.S.M.; Kang, H.K.; Koh, Y.S.; Yi, J.M.; Hyun, J.W. Niacinamide Protects Skin Cells from Oxidative Stress Induced by Particulate. Matter. *Biomol. Ther.* **2019**, *27*, 562–569. [CrossRef]
47. Abdullah, K.M.; Alam, M.M.; Iqbal, Z.; Naseem, I. Therapeutic effect of vitamin B3 on hyperglycemia, oxidative stress and DNA damage in alloxan induced diabetic rat model. *Biomed. Pharmacother.* **2018**, *105*, 1223–1231. [CrossRef]
48. Boira, C.; Jolibois, J.; Durduret, A.; Tiguemounine, J.; Szewezyk, C.; De Tollenaere, M.; Scandolera, A.; Reynaud, R. Cranberry Oil: A Potent Natural Intimate Care Ingredient Displaying Antioxidant and Anti-Inflammatory Effects and Promoting Beneficial Vaginal *Lactobacillus*. *Int. J. Mol. Sci.* **2025**, *26*, 2176. [CrossRef]
49. Sedbare, R.; Raudone, L.; Zvikas, V.; Viskelis, J.; Liaudanskas, M.; Janulis, V. Development and Validation of the UPLC-DAD Methodology for the Detection of Triterpenoids and Phytosterols in Fruit Samples of *Vaccinium macrocarpon* Aiton and *Vaccinium oxycoccos* L. *Molecules* **2022**, *27*, 4403. [CrossRef]
50. Šedbarė, R.; Janulis, V.; Pavilonis, A.; Petrikaite, V. Comparative In Vitro Study: Assessing Phytochemical, Antioxidant, Antimicrobial, and Anticancer Properties of *Vaccinium Macrocarpon* Aiton and *Vaccinium oxycoccos* L. Fruit Extracts. *Pharmaceutics* **2024**, *16*, 735. [CrossRef]
51. Zhang, M.; Wu, X.; Lai, F.; Zhang, X.; Wu, H.; Min, T. Betaine Inhibits Hepatitis B Virus with an Advantage of Decreasing Resistance to Lamivudine and Interferon α. *J. Agric. Food Chem.* **2016**, *64*, 4068–4077. [CrossRef]
52. Gehring, W.; Gloor, M. Effect of topically applied dexpanthenol on epidermal barrier function and stratum corneum hydration. Results of a human in vivo study. *Arzneimittelforschung* **2000**, *50*, 659–663. [CrossRef]
53. Wang, H.; Duan, C.; Keate, R.L.; Ameer, G.A. Panthenol Citrate Biomaterials Accelerate Wound Healing and Restore Tissue Integrity. *Adv. Healthc. Mater.* **2023**, *12*, 2301683. [CrossRef] [PubMed]
54. Shannon, C.E. A mathematical theory of communication. *Bell Syst. Tech. J.* **1948**, *27*, 379–423.
55. Janssens-Böcker, C.; Doberenz, C.; Monteiro, M.; de Oliveira Ferreira, M. Influence of Cosmetic Skincare Products with pH < 5 on the Skin Microbiome: A Randomized Clinical Evaluation. *Dermatol. Ther.* **2025**, *15*, 141–159. [CrossRef]

56. Lukić, M.; Pantelić, I.; Savić, S.D. Towards Optimal pH of the Skin and Topical Formulations: From the Current State of the Art to Tailored Products. *Cosmetics* **2021**, *8*, 69. [CrossRef]
57. Eyerich, S.; Eyerich, K.; Traidl-Hoffmann, C.; Biedermann, T. Cutaneous Barriers and Skin Immunity: Differentiating A Connected Network. *Trends Immunol.* **2018**, *39*, 315–327.
58. Van Smeden, J.; Janssens, M.; Gooris, G.; Bouwstra, J. The important role of stratum corneum lipids for the cutaneous barrier function. *BBA Mol. Cell Biol. Lipids* **2014**, *1841*, 295–313.
59. Elias, P.M. The how, why and clinical importance of stratum corneum acidification. *Exp. Dermatol.* **2017**, *26*, 999–1003.
60. Schmid-Wendtner, M.H.; Korting, H.C. The pH of the skin surface and its impact on the barrier function. *Skin Pharmacol. Physiol.* **2006**, *19*, 296–302. [CrossRef]
61. Dréno, B.; Pécastaings, S.; Corvec, S. Cutibacterium acnes (*Propionibacterium acnes*) and acne vulgaris: A brief look at the latest updates. *J. Eur. Acad. Dermatol. Venereol.* **2018**, *32*, 2–14.
62. Berardesca, E.; Loden, M.; Serup, J.; Masson, P.; Rodrigues, L.M. The revised EEMCO guidance for the in vivo measurement of water in the skin. *Skin Res. Technol.* **2018**, *24*, 351–358. [CrossRef]
63. Courage + Khazaka Electronic GmbH. Brochure Corneometer® CM 825. Available online: https://www.courage-khazaka.com/en/scientific-products/corneometer-cm-825 (accessed on 19 December 2024).
64. Hua, W.; Fan, L.M.; Dai, R.; Luan, M.; Xie, H.; Li, A.Q.; Li, L. Comparison of two series of non-invasive instruments used for the skin physiological properties measurements: The DermaLab® from Cortex Technology vs. the series of detectors from Courage & Khazaka. *Skin Res. Technol.* **2017**, *23*, 70–78. [PubMed]
65. Holm, E.A.; Wulf, H.C.; Thomassen, L.; Jemec, G.B. Instrumental assessment of atopic eczema: Validation of transepidermal water loss, stratum corneum hydration, erythema, scaling, and edema. *J. Am. Acad. Dermatol.* **2006**, *55*, 772–780. [PubMed]
66. Putri, T.W.; Nursida, N.F.; Raya, I. The effectiveness of *Chlorella vulgaris* cream applied to male and female rats. *Natl. J. Physiol. Pharm. Pharmacol.* **2020**, *10*, 1118–1121.
67. Nicander, I.; Aberg, P.; Ollmar, S. The use of different concentrations of betaine as a reducing irritation agent in soaps monitored visually and non-invasively. *Skin Res. Technol.* **2003**, *9*, 43–49. [CrossRef]
68. Gala, M.Y.N.; Snehal, S.M.; Sujeet, N.C.; Rahul, R.R.; Mane, A.; Pandit, S.; Alok Ranjan, S.; Avijit, C.A. Effect of plant-based paraben free Venusia max cream on skin hydration in healthy individuals with dry skin. *J. Clin. Investig. Dermatol.* **2021**, *9*, 4.
69. Lynde, C. Moisturizers for the treatment of inflammatory skin conditions. *J. Drugs Dermatol.* **2008**, *7*, 1038–1043.
70. Shucheng, H.; Zhou, X.; Du, D.; Li, J.; Yu, C.; Jiang, X. Effects of 15% Azelaic Acid Gel in the Management of Post-Inflammatory Erythema and Post-Inflammatory Hyperpigmentation in Acne Vulgaris. *Dermatol. Ther.* **2024**, *14*, 1293–1314. [CrossRef]
71. Mirajkar, R.; Ingale, A.; Vanne, M.; Mane, S.; Shinde, J.; Gade, P.; Sakhare, P. Prebiotic *Chlorella vulgaris*: A novel ingredient for skincare products targeting hyperpigmentation and acne. *Int. J. Res. Publ. Rev.* **2025**, *6*, 17031–17034.
72. Cho, B.R.; Jun, H.J.; Thach, T.T.; Wu, C.; Lee, S.J. Betaine reduces cellular melanin content via suppression of microphthalmia-associated transcription factor in B16-F1 murine melanocytes. *Food Sci. Biotechnol.* **2017**, *26*, 1391–1397. [CrossRef]
73. Kamei, Y.; Otsuka, Y.; Abe, K. Comparison of the inhibitory effects of vitamin E analogues on melanogenesis in mouse B16 melanoma cells. *Cytotechnology* **2009**, *59*, 183–190. [CrossRef] [PubMed]
74. Kim, H.-K. The Processed Radish Extract Melanogenesis in Humans and Induces Anti- Photoaging Effects in Ultraviolet B-Induced Hairless Mouse Model. *Int. J. Adv. Cult. Technol.* **2019**, *7*, 125–136. [CrossRef]
75. Hakozaki, T.; Minwalla, L.; Zhuang, J.; Chhoa, M.; Matsubara, A.; Miyamoto, K.; Greatens, A.; Hillebrand, G.G.; Bissett, D.L.; Boissy, R.E. The effect of niacinamide on reducing cutaneous pigmentation and suppression of melanosome transfer. *Br. J. Dermatol.* **2002**, *147*, 20–31. [CrossRef]
76. Abdlaty, R.; Hayward, J.; Farrell, T.; Fang, Q. Skin erythema and pigmentation: A review of optical assessment techniques. *Photodiagnosis Photodyn. Ther.* **2021**, *33*, 102127. [CrossRef] [PubMed]
77. Burnett, C.L.; Fiume, M.M.; Bergfeld, W.F.; Belsito, D.V.; Hill, R.A.; Klaassen, C.D.; Liebrel, D.; Marks, J.G., Jr.; Shank, R.S.; Slaga, T.J.; et al. Safety Assessment of Plant-Derived Fatty Acid Oils. *Int. J. Toxicol.* **2017**, *36* (Suppl. S3), 51S–129S. [CrossRef]
78. Machmud, E.; Ruslin, M.; Waris, R.; Asse, R.A.; Qadafi, A.M.; Achmad, H. Effect of the application of *Chlorella vulgaris* ointment to the number of fibroblast cells as an indicator of wound healing in the soft tissue of pigears. *Pesqui. Bras. Odontopediatria Clín. Integr.* **2020**, *20*, e5012. [CrossRef]
79. Chen, A.; An, Y.; Huang, W.; Xuan, T.; Zhang, Q.; Ye, M.; Luo, S.; Xuan, X.; He, H.; Zheng, J.; et al. Highly Water-Preserving Zwitterionic Betaine-Incorporated Collagen Sponges with Anti-oxidation and Anti-inflammation for Wound Regeneration. *Front. Cell Dev. Biol.* **2020**, *8*, 491. [CrossRef]
80. Keen, M.A.; Hassan, I. Vitamin E in dermatology. *Indian Dermatol. Online J.* **2016**, *7*, 311–315. [CrossRef]
81. Björklund, S.; Engblom, J.; Thuresson, K.; Sparr, E. A water gradient can be used to regulate drug transport across skin. *J. Controll. Release* **2010**, *143*, 191–200.

82. Kulthanan, K.; Trakanwittayarak, S.; Tuchinda, P.; Chularojanamontri, L.; Limphoka, P.; Varothai, S. A double-blinded, randomized, vehicle-controlled study of the efficacy of moisturizer containing licochalcone A, decanediol, L-carnitine, and salicylic acid for prevention of acne relapse in Asian population. *Biomed. Res. Int.* **2020**, *2020*, 2857812.
83. Gala, M.; Aich, B.; Bhureddy, S.; Muchhala, S.; Veligandla, K.C.; Rathod, R.; Samal, A.R.; Choudhury, A.A.; Kotak, B.; Sethi, S.; et al. Skin moisturizing and anti-acne effect of acne moisturizer in healthy adult subjects with mild-to-moderate acne-an open label, single arm clinical study. *CosmoDerma* **2023**, *3*, 85. [CrossRef]
84. Chularojanamontri, L.; Tuchinda, P.; Kulthanan, K.; Pongparit, K. Moisturizers for acne: What are their constituents? *J. Clin. Aesthet. Dermatol.* **2014**, *7*, 36–44. [PubMed]
85. Morin, M.; Ruzgas, T.; Svedenhag, P.; Anderson, C.D.; Ollmar, S.; Engblom, J.; Björklund, S. Skin hydration dynamics investigated by electrical impedance techniques in vivo and in vitro. *Sci. Rep.* **2020**, *10*, 17218. [CrossRef]
86. Trojahn, C.; Dobos, G.; Schario, M.; Ludriksone, L.; Blume-Peytavi, U.; Kottner, J. Relation between skin micro-topography, roughness, and skin age. *Skin Res. Technol.* **2015**, *21*, 69–75. [CrossRef]
87. Diosa, J.G.; Moreno, R.; Chica, E.L.; Villarraga, J.A.; Tepole, A.B. Changes in the three-dimensional microscale topography of human skin with aging impact its mechanical and tribological behavior. *PLoS ONE* **2021**, *16*, e0241533. [CrossRef]
88. Wu, K.S.; van Osdol, W.W.; Dauskardt, R.H. Mechanical properties of human stratum corneum: Effects of temperature, hydration, and chemical treatment. *Biomaterials* **2006**, *27*, 785–795. [PubMed]
89. Persson, B.N.J.; Kovalev, A.; Gorb, S.N. Contact mechanics and friction on dry and wet human skin. *Tribol. Lett.* **2013**, *50*, 17–30.
90. Gerhardt, L.C.; Strässle, V.; Lenz, A.; Spencer, N.D.; Derler, S. Influence of epidermal hydration on the friction of human skin against textiles. *J. R. Soc. Interface* **2008**, *5*, 1317–1328. [PubMed]
91. de Melo, R.G.; de Andrade, A.F.; Bezerra, R.P. Viana Marques, D.A.; da Silva, V.A., Jr.; Paz, S.T.; de Lima Filho, J.L.; Figueiredo Porto, A.L. Hydrogel-based *Chlorella vulgaris* extracts: A new topical formulation for wound healing treatment. *J. Appl. Phycol.* **2019**, *31*, 3653–3663.
92. Lu, B.; Hu, H.; Yang, G.; Pan, M.; Wang, Y.; Zhang, J.; Zhang, J.; Zhang, J. Ultrasound-assisted green and efficient extraction of polysaccharides from *Chlorella vulgaris* using deep eutectic solvents and improving their performance. *New J. Chem.* **2024**, *48*, 4426–4436.
93. Bertoloni dos Santos, B.; Morocho-Jácome, A.L.; Prieto, Z.A.; Morowvat, M.H.; Lima, F.V.; Velasco, M.V.R.; de Carvalho, J.C.M.; Baby, A.R. Algae materials for cosmetics and cosmeceuticals. In *Developments in Applied Microbiology and Biotechnology: Algae Materials*; Arunkumar, K., Arun, A., Raja, R., Palaniappan, R., Eds.; Academic Press: Cambridge, MA, USA, 2023; pp. 285–312.
94. Zhang, R.; Wei, Y.; Zhang, J.; Cai, M.; Lu, L.; Fang, L.; Qin, X.; Gu, R. Protection effects of rice protein hydrolysate on UVB-irradiated photodamage in Hartley guinea pigs skin and human skin fibroblasts. *J. Funct. Foods* **2021**, *82*, 104504. [CrossRef]
95. Li, H.; Wan, Y.; Zeng, X.; Wu, Z.; Gong, S. Study on the anti-aging effects of rice-protein polypeptides. *Flavour Fragr. Cosmet.* **2015**, *6*, 37–40.
96. Dai, L.; Chen, Y.; Hu, T.; Liu, P.; Li, B.; Wang, F. Study on antioxidant effect of rice peptide on D-galactose-induced aging mice. *Sci. Technol. Food Ind.* **2013**, *34*, 330–332.
97. Zhang, R.; Wei, Y.; Li, M.; Cai, M.; Gu, R.; Ma, Y.; Wang, J. Melanogenesis effects of rice protein hydrolysate and its characteristic peptides Leu-Leu-Lys, Leu-Pro-Lys, and pyroGlu-Lys on UVB-induced human epidermal melanocyte cells. *Food Funct.* **2020**, *11*, 8757–8767. [PubMed]
98. Bhattacharya, K.; Shukla, V.K. Mango butter in cosmetic formulations. *Cosmet. Toil.* **2002**, *117*, 65–70.
99. Mandawgade, S.D.; Patravale, V.B. Formulation and evaluation of exotic fat based cosmeceuticals for skin repair. *Indian J. Pharm. Sci.* **2008**, *70*, 539–542. [CrossRef]
100. Camargo, F.B., Jr.; Gaspar, L.R.; Maia Campos, P.M. Skin moisturizing effects of panthenol-based formulations. *J. Cosmet. Sci.* **2011**, *62*, 361–370.
101. Boo, Y.C. Mechanistic Basis and Clinical Evidence for the Applications of Nicotinamide (Niacinamide) to Control Skin Aging and Pigmentation. *Antioxidants* **2021**, *10*, 1315. [CrossRef]
102. Marques, C.; Hadjab, F.; Porcello, A.; Lourenço, K.; Scaletta, C.; Abdel-Sayed, P.; Hirt-Burri, N.; Applegate, L.A.; Laurent, A. Mechanistic Insights into the Multiple Functions of Niacinamide: Therapeutic Implications and Cosmeceutical Applications in Functional Skincare Products. *Antioxidants* **2024**, *13*, 425. [CrossRef]
103. Available online: https://chanand.com/ (accessed on 2 April 2025).
104. Burloiu, A.M.; Ozon, E.A.; Musuc, A.M.; Anastasescu, M.; Socoteanu, R.P.; Atkinson, I.; Culita, D.C.; Anuta, V.; Popescu, I.A.; Lupuliasa, D.; et al. Porphyrin Photosensitizers into Polysaccharide-Based Biopolymer Hydrogels for Topical Photodynamic Therapy: Physicochemical and Pharmacotechnical Assessments. *Gels* **2024**, *10*, 499. [CrossRef]
105. Brand-Williams, W.; Cuvelier, M.E.; Berset, C. Use of a free radical method to evaluate antioxidant activity. *LWT—Food Sci. Technol.* **1995**, *28*, 25–30. [CrossRef]
106. Re, R.; Pellegrini, N.; Proteggente, A.; Pannala, A.; Yang, M.; Rice-Evans, C. Antioxidant activity applying an improved ABTS radical cation decolorization assay. *Free Radic. Biol. Med.* **1999**, *26*, 1231–1237. [CrossRef] [PubMed]

107. Benzie, I.F.F.; Strain, J.J. The ferric reducing ability of plasma (FRAP) as a measure of 'antioxidant power': The FRAP assay. *Anal. Biochem.* **1996**, *239*, 70–76. [CrossRef] [PubMed]

MDPI AG
Grosspeteranlage 5
4052 Basel
Switzerland
Tel.: +41 61 683 77 34

Gels Editorial Office
E-mail: gels@mdpi.com
www.mdpi.com/journal/gels

www.ingramcontent.com/pod-product-compliance
Lightning Source LLC
Chambersburg PA
CBHW061819210926
51850CB00006B/753
* 9 7 8 3 7 2 5 8 7 6 0 7 5 *